MW01165092

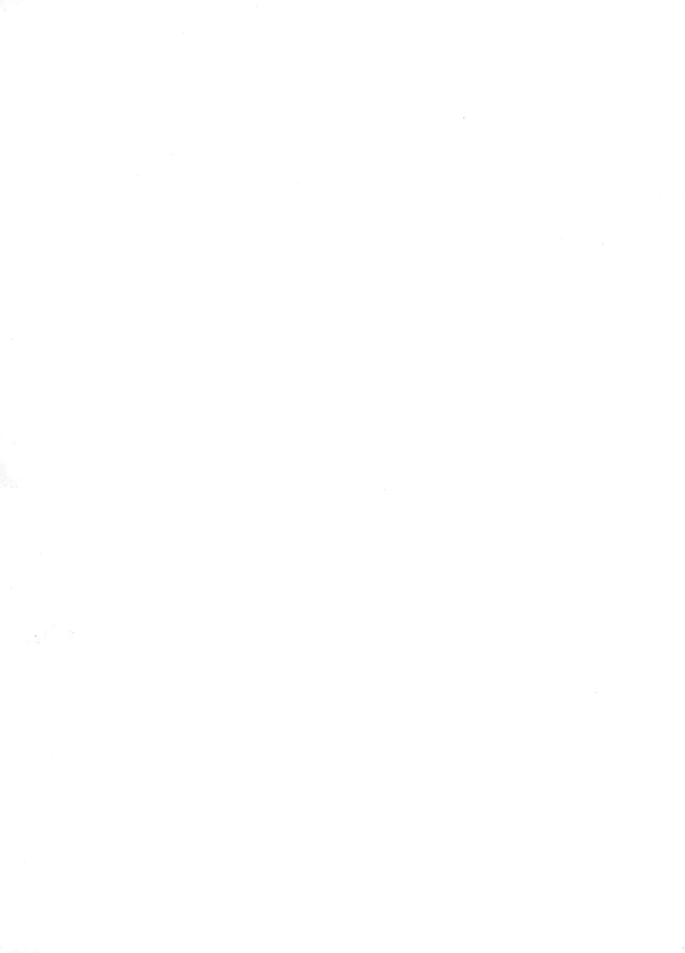

Clinical Allergy

Current Clinical Practice

Neil S. Skolnik, *Series Editor*

For other titles published in this series, go to
www.springer.com
select the subdiscipline
search for your title

Gerald W. Volcheck

Clinical Allergy

Diagnosis and Management

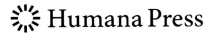 Humana Press

Gerald W. Volcheck
Consultant, Division of Allergic Diseases, Mayo Clinic
Rochester, MN
Assistant Professor of Medicine, College of Medicine,
Mayo Clinic

Series Editor
Neil S. Skolnik
Abington Memorial Hospital
Abington, PA 19001
USA

ISBN 978-1-58829-616-0   e-ISBN 978-1-59745-315-8
DOI: 10.1007/978-1-59745-315-8

Library of Congress Control Number: 2008936256

© 2009 Mayo Foundation for Medical Education and Research. All rights reserved. This book is protected by copyright. No part of it may be reproduced, stored in a retrieval system, or transmitted in any form by any means, electronic, mechanical, recording, or otherwise, without written permission from Mayo Foundation, Section of Scientific Publications, Plummer-10, 200 First Street SW, Rochester, MN 55905.

Care has been taken to confirm the accuracy of the information presented and to describe generally accepted practices. However, the authors, editors, and publisher are not responsible for errors or omissions or for any consequences from application of the information in this book and make no warranty, express or implied, with respect to the contents of the publication.
The authors, editors, and publisher have exerted efforts to ensure that drug selection and dosage set forth in this text are in accordance with current recommendations and practice at the time of publication. However, in view of ongoing research, changes in government regulations, and the constant flow of information relating to drug therapy and drug reactions, the reader is urged to check the package insert for each drug for any change in indications and dosage and for added warnings and precautions. This is particularly important when the recommended agent is a new or infrequently employed drug.
Some drugs and medical devices presented in this publication have Food and Drug Administration (FDA) clearance for limited use in restricted research settings. It is the responsibility of health care providers to ascertain the FDA status of each drug or device planned for use in their clinical practice.

Cover illustration: Figure 6, Chapter 2, "Environmental Allergens"

Printed on acid-free paper

9 8 7 6 5 4 3 2 1
springer.com

To my wife Mary Margaret and children Joseph and Allison for their love, encouragement, and support.

Series Editor's Introduction

Diseases exacerbated by allergy, as well as primary allergic disorders, are among the most common disorders seen by primary care physicians. Seldom does an office session occur where there are not two or three patients with some manifestation of allergic disease ranging from asthma, to allergic rhinitis, to urticaria. The science of allergy and immunology has exploded over the last two decades, making it important for physicians to have an effective reference to help update their knowledge of the field. In a recent survey conducted by the Academy of Family Physicians, 50–60% of family doctors responded that they had a moderate to high need for further allergy education.[1]

Clinical Allergy: Diagnosis and Management by Dr. Volcheck is an excellent, detailed overview of the field of allergy, with an eye toward relevance and the right level of detail for busy primary care physicians. Dr. Volcheck presents the evidence clearly and gives clear opinions and recommendations when the evidence still falls short. Starting with an overview of the immune response, then discussing environmental allergens, the book then addresses details of allergy testing and immunotherapy. This chapter is particularly well done and answers relevant, ongoing, natural questions that come up in all primary care offices, which I have not seen well answered in general articles on the topic.

Dr. Volcheck then discusses the specific allergic-influenced diseases including allergic rhinitis, ophthalmic allergies, asthma, urticaria and angioedema, atopic dermatitis, drug allergies, food allergies, anaphylaxis, and stinging insect allergies. As I read through this book, I was amazed at how many topics were covered in which I had clinical questions while seeing patients, and which the chapters of the book readily answered.

In summary, *Clinical Allergy: Diagnosis and Management* by Dr. Volcheck from Mayo Clinic is a valuable addition to the literature and is effective at answering the many questions that come up in the day-to-day care of patients with allergic diseases. It deserves a place on our shelves as a book of study, understanding, and reference.

Abington, Pennsylvania, USA   Neil Skolnik

---

[1] American Academy of Family Physicians, Continuing Medical Education Topics Surveys, April 2006, accessed at http://www.aafp.org/online/en/home/aboutus/specialty/facts/30.html, Feb 2008

Preface

The purpose of this book is to provide a practical clinical overview for the common disorders encountered in the specialty of allergy. Allergic diseases affect nearly one-fourth of the population and cause or contribute to significant chronic illness. Because allergic diseases are so common, they are seen by a wide variety of health care providers. With this in mind, *Clinical Allergy: Diagnosis and Management* has been designed to be easily readable and to provide clinically applicable information for both the nonallergist and the allergist. The text is not encyclopedic. Instead, the intent is to unravel the mystery of allergy and to provide a logical framework for the evaluation and management of allergic disorders. The introductory chapters focus on the human immune response, environmental allergens, and the different types of allergy testing. The subsequent chapters focus on the common allergic conditions seen in the office or clinic, including rhinitis and rhinosinusitis, allergic eye disease, asthma, urticaria and angioedema, atopic and contact dermatitis, drug allergy, food allergy, anaphylaxis, and stinging insect allergy. "Cross-talk" between chapters helps show the interrelationships among the various allergic disorders. The chapters begin with a review of pathophysiologic mechanisms and then consider a clinically structured approach to diagnosis and management of the disorders. In addition to pharmacologic treatment, the importance of nonpharmacologic management and patient education is emphasized. The primary clinical pearls of daily clinical management of the allergic patient are highlighted by the clinical vignettes at the end of each chapter.

The book is designed for primary care providers, medical students, residents, and junior allergy fellows. Senior allergy fellows and seasoned allergists will also likely find practical, clinically useful information in this book.

I am indebted to Susan R. Miller, John P. Hedlund, Roberta Schwartz, and Dr. O.E. Millhouse for their superb editorial assistance, to Drs. Mark D.P. Davis and Keith H. Baratz for providing excellent photographs of allergic skin and eye disorders, and to the medical students, residents, fellows, colleagues, and most importantly the patients who bring these pages to life.

Rochester, Minnesota, USA   Gerald W. Volcheck

Contents

Chapter 1
Overview of the Human Immune Response

Abbreviations APC: antigen-presenting cell; BCR: B-cell receptor; COX: cyclooxygenase; CpG: cytosine-phosphate-guanine; FcR: Fc receptor; FcεRI: Fcε receptor I; GM-CSF: granulocyte-macrophage colony-stimulating factor; H: histamine; HLA: human leukocyte antigen; ICAM: intercellular adhesion molecule; IL: interleukin; IL-1Ra: interleukin-1 receptor antagonist; IL-2R: interleukin-2 receptor; IFN: interferon; LFA: leukocyte function-associated antigen; LPB: LPS-binding protein; LPS: lipopolysaccharide; LT: leukotriene; MBL: mannose-binding lectin; MBP: major basic protein; MHC: major histocompatibility complex; NK: natural killer; PAMP: pathogen-associated molecular pattern; PG: prostaglandin; PLA: phospholipase A; SCF: stem cell factor; TCR: T-cell receptor; TGF: transforming growth factor; TLR: toll-like receptor; TNF: tumor necrosis factor; TXA: thromboxane A; VCAM: vascular cell adhesion molecule.

1.1 Introduction

The immune system is a vast network that involves many interacting constituents. This chapter provides an overview of the immune system to establish a sense of the communication and checks and balances between the cells and mediators that provide immune protection and the process that occurs in allergic or hypersensitivity responses.

The immune response does not occur in a strictly linear pattern. Although allergen exposure activates the allergic immune response, the subsequent immune cell and mediator cascade includes numerous intersecting positive and negative feedback loops. Initially, it is difficult to visualize all the interconnecting pieces of the immune response. The chapter presents the response chronologically, acknowledging that multiple processes occur simultaneously. The chapter begins with the innate immune response because this is the body's first response to a foreign protein. This is followed by the acquired immune response, which is activated just after the innate immune response. Both of these processes subsequently work together interdependently. Next, the key components of the acquired immune response are reviewed, with the focus on antigen presentation, the major histocompatibility

G.W. Volcheck, *Clinical Allergy: Diagnosis and Management*
DOI: 10.1007/978-1-59745-315-8_1, © 2009 Mayo Foundation for Medical
Education and Research

complex (MHC), and T- and B-cell interaction and activation. As knowledge of the immune system has evolved, a major focus has been on cytokines, the secretory proteins that function as mediators of immune and inflammatory reactions. The cytokines, as presented, are grouped by their physiologic activity, which further underscores the intricate communication between the various cell types of the immune system. This emphasizes how the predominance of certain cytokine subsets determines the type of immune response that occurs (cytotoxic, humoral, cell-mediated, or allergic). The chapter ends with an overview of the allergic response, with a focus on how current and experimental immunomodulatory medications may be used to attenuate the allergic response.

1.2 Innate Immune System

The innate immune system represents the host's first line of defense against pathogens from the environment. Unlike the acquired immune system in which gene elements are rearranged somatically to produce specific antigen-binding molecules, the innate immune system contains responses that are encoded by the genes in the host's germline. These elements are present from the outset and do not require previous exposure: they are inborn. This system recognizes foreign matter, such as that contained by microbes, that is not present in the host. The innate and acquired immune systems work in concert to fight pathogens. The differences between these two systems are outlined in Table 1.1.

The innate immune system contains many components. The first line of the body's defense against invaders includes physical barriers such as skin (epithelial barriers) and mucous membranes. The three major interfaces between the body and

Table 1.1 Differences Between Innate and Acquired Immunity

Feature	Innate	Acquired
Specificity	Microbe molecular patterns	Microbial antigens
		Nonmicrobial antigens
		Distinct antibody molecule production
Receptors	Encoded in germline	Encoded by genes
	Limited diversity	Produced by somatic recombination of gene segments
		Great diversity
Distribution of receptors	Nonclonal	Clonal
Discrimination of self vs. nonself	Yes, only recognize foreign molecular patterns	Yes, however, based on selection against self-reactive lymphocytes
Primary cells involved	Epithelial cell, monocyte/macrophage, neutrophil, natural killer cell	T-cell, B-cell

the external environment are the skin, the gastrointestinal tract, and the respiratory tract. The organs of the integumentary, gastrointestinal, and respiratory systems have multiple specialized features that help repel foreign invaders; for example, the lactic acid in sweat maintains an acidic pH that prevents bacterial colonization, and the epithelia lining the respiratory tract contain a flowing layer of mucus that sweeps away foreign substances. In addition, these areas are lined by epithelia that can produce peptide antibiotics to kill bacteria and intraepithelial lymphocytes that likely signal the presence of a pathogen. To cause infection, bacteria, viruses, and parasites must first penetrate these physical barriers. In addition to preventing infection, these physical barriers decrease allergen exposure. Disruption of the epithelial lining and mucous membranes increases allergen exposure, thus resulting in a greater chance of sensitization and a greater allergic response in persons genetically predisposed to the development of allergy.

After the pathogen penetrates the physical barriers, it encounters the second line of defense, namely, the immune cells and proteins of the innate immune system. The innate immune system is manned primarily by macrophages, neutrophils, natural killer (NK) cells, complement, and soluble, bioactive proteins and molecules. The primary function of these cells and proteins is to destroy any invading pathogen. These components and their function in relation to the innate immune response are discussed briefly below.

Macrophages are the primary first-line cells of the innate immune response. They are able to migrate to areas of invasion and phagocytose the pathogen. Macrophages are derived from monocytes. Monocytes are produced in the bone marrow and circulate for approximately 24 hours before settling in the tissue where they become tissue macrophages. Monocytes contain lysosomes and organelles needed to synthesize secretory and membrane proteins. Monocytes, like neutrophils, can be attracted to an area of inflammation through the three-phase endothelial attachment process (described below). The specific chemoattractants differ somewhat for neutrophils and monocytes because these cells have different chemokine and cytokine receptors. Therefore, the chemokines, cytokines, and other mediators released by the immune cells determine whether monocytes, neutrophils, or other leukocytes are attracted to the area of inflammation. This pattern of released mediators attracting different cell types holds throughout the various types of immune reactions. Basically, the body signals for what it needs to fight the pathogen.

A tissue macrophage survives for approximately 3 months. When the macrophage encounters inflammatory mediators, it is activated. Interferon (IFN)-γ released by the surrounding cells and lipopolysaccharide (LPS) and mannose, microbial markers, are potent macrophage activators. Macrophages have receptors for IFN-γ, LPS, and mannose which when occupied activate the macrophage. Upon activation, many new proteins are synthesized by the macrophage, and the macrophages become avid phagocytes that engulf foreign particles and cellular debris. Before activation, macrophages are relatively dormant and serve as "scavenger" cells in the tissues. Activated macrophages also secrete a large variety of biologically active substances into the surrounding tissues. These include enzymes, cytokines, nitric oxide, complement components, coagulation factors, and reactive oxygen species.

Their functions include antimicrobial activity, remodeling of the extracellular matrix, leukocyte chemotaxis, and facilitation of the healing process. In addition to their work in the innate immune response, macrophages are one of the most important types of antigen-presenting cells (APCs). In this capacity, macrophages process foreign substances and then present them to T-lymphocytes, thereby initiating the acquired immune response. (The acquired immune response is discussed in detail below.)

The neutrophil is the most potent phagocyte. Neutrophils contain granules that store bactericidal agents and enzymes that kill and digest an ingested microorganism. After neutrophils mature in the bone marrow, they are released into the circulation, where they form approximately one-half to two-thirds of all circulating leukocytes. Neutrophils are programmed to die by apoptosis only 12 hours after entering the circulation. This requires the bone marrow to devote nearly 60% of hematopoietic activity to the production of neutrophils. Once in the circulation, neutrophils migrate to an area of inflammation. They leave the circulation and enter the tissue through a process in which they adhere to the activated endothelium, migrate through the vessel walls, and invade the affected tissues, where their phagocytic or cytotoxic activity occurs. This process of margination occurs in three phases (Fig. 1.1):

1. Selectin-mediated phase – In this phase, the circulatory neutrophils come into contact with the vessel wall, allowing P-selectin and E-selectin molecules on the activated endothelium to bind mucins on the neutrophils, which slows down the neutrophils and causes them to "roll" along the endothelium. The expression of P-selectin and E-selectin on the endothelium comes from interleukin (IL)-1 and tumor necrosis factor (TNF) released by macrophages in response to a pathogen.

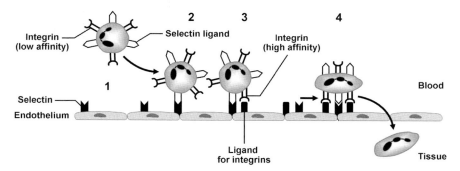

Fig. 1.1 Migration of blood leukocytes to area of infection. (1) Macrophages that have been activated by microbes produce cytokines (tumor necrosis factor, interleukin-1) that activate endothelial cells to produce selectins, ligands for integrins, and chemoattractants. (2) Selectins "slow down" blood neutrophils. (3) Chemoattractants draw neutrophils to the area and stimulate integrin to a high-affinity state. (4) Integrins mediate firm attachment of the neutrophil to the endothelium, with subsequent migration into the tissue

2. Activation phase – In this phase, chemokines, cytokines, complement components, and other chemicals secreted by endothelial cells and other cell types in
   inflamed tissue attract leukocytes. This attraction occurs through leukocyte
   surface receptors strengthening the attachment of the leukocyte to the
   endothelium.
3. Firm attachment – In this phase, integrins from the neutrophils, Mac-1 and
   leukocyte function-associated antigen (LFA)-1, bind to intercellular adhesion
   molecule (ICAM)-1 on the activated endothelial cells, leading to a stable,
   molecular contact; that is, the selectins start applying the brakes to the neutrophils, and the integrin-ICAM binding brings the neutrophils to a stop. Once
   attached, the neutrophils emigrate into the tissue, where they begin the process of
   engulfing bacteria.

The NK cells comprise about 10% of the lymphocytes in the blood and peripheral
lymphoid organs. They are able to kill infected cells and produce IFN-γ. As part of
the innate immune system, NK cells do not express immunoglobulins or T-cell
receptors but are able to recognize host cells that have been infected. NK cells are
activated by IL-12, which is usually supplied by macrophages. Once activated, NK
cells release cytoplasmic granule proteins into the infected cell and induce apoptotic
cell death. The release of IFN-γ by NK cells stimulates macrophages to kill phago-
cytosed microbes and also to secrete IL-12, which further activates NK cells, creating a positive feedback loop. The perpetuation of the process is necessary to kill
microorganisms.

Recently, research has focused on how the innate immune system recognizes
microorganisms. In addition to molecules such as LPS and mannose that are
detected by immune cell receptors, a large area of study involves toll-like receptors
(TLRs). TLRs are transmembrane receptors that signal the presence of microbes by
recognizing the presence of pathogen-associated molecular patterns (PAMPs).
TLRs are found principally on macrophages and dendritic cells but also on neutrophils, eosinophils, epithelial cells, and keratinocytes. Ten human TLRs have
been defined. Activation of most TLRs induces a cellular response that initiates cell
activation and cytokine release and results in acute and chronic inflammation. The
activation of most TLRs elicits mediators that, in addition to fighting a pathogen
through the innate immune response, skew CD4+ helper T-cells toward a Th1
response. Of note, cytosine-phosphate-guanine (CpG) DNA activation of TLR9 can
divert an established Th2 response to a Th1 response. This type of diversion may
help dampen an allergic response to an allergen. The Th1 and Th2 types of T-cell
response are reviewed in detail in the section on T-cells, and the role of CpG DNA
as an immunomodulatory agent in atopic disease is reviewed in the section on
current and experimental immunomodulatory treatment.

The complement pathway consists of several interacting serum proteins that
have a key role in innate immunity. The complement system is composed of more
than 25 proteins that work together to destroy pathogens. These proteins are derived
primarily from the liver and macrophages. Complement can be activated in three
ways. In the innate immune system, it can be activated, independently of antibody,
by the alternative pathway and the lectin pathway. In the acquired immune response,

complement is activated by the classic pathway (discussed below). The most abundant complement protein is C3, which is continuously broken down in the body into smaller reactive proteins. These proteins either attach to invaders or are neutralized. In the alternative pathway, microbial-bound C3 interacts with other serum complement components (factors B and D) to form a highly reactive compound capable of activating the rest of the complement system. In the lectin pathway, mannose-binding lectin (MBL), a protein synthesized in the liver and present in blood and tissues, binds to a pathogen through a mannose–MBL bond. After being bound, proteases are released that clip C3, which then activates the entire complement system. Once activated, the complement cascade proteins provide protection in three ways: (1) by creating a disruption in the microbial surface membrane through membrane attack complexes that kill the cell, (2) by opsonizing the cell membrane, which enhances killing by host cells, and (3) by serving as chemoattractants for leukocytes. The complement cascade is shown in Fig. 1.2.

Soluble proteins and bioactive molecules such as lysozyme, MBL, LPS-binding protein (LPB), soluble CD14, complement, and defensins provide innate defense against pathogens. Lysozyme is found in human saliva, mucus, and other secretions. MBL, derived from the liver, has little direct effect on the pathogen but through opsonization allows for host recognition and destruction of the pathogen.

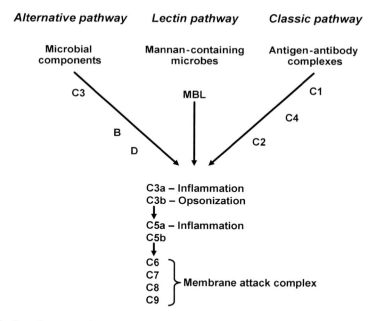

Fig. 1.2 Complement pathway. The complement system may be activated by three different pathways. They all form C3b, an opsonin, which also initiates the late steps of complement activation, resulting in the formation of the membrane attack complex. C3a and C5a bind to receptors on neutrophils and stimulate inflammatory reactions. *MBL* mannose-binding lectin

LPB and soluble CD14 are humoral proteins that are able to bind LPS. Defensins are small peptides that are produced and stored within human granulocytes and specialized epithelial cells. They can be found in the mucus lining of various epithelial tracts. These effector proteins of the innate immune system target microbial surfaces such as peptidoglycan of cell walls, glycoproteins, glycolipids, LPS, and microbial membranes. These interactions help the host destroy the invading pathogen by digestion of the cell wall, opsonization, complement activation, and membrane lysis.

Although the innate and acquired immune systems are often described as separate arms of the immune response, they act together, with the innate response initiating the host defense and the acquired response becoming prominent later. The innate immune system provides signals that allow antigen-specific T- and B-cells to undergo rearrangement and clonal expansion, as discussed below. The acquired immune system is also able to release signals that either propogate or limit the innate immune response. Clearly, synergy between these two systems is essential for an effective immune response. The acquired immune system has the primary role in specific IgE-mediated allergic disease through the production of IgE; however, the innate immune system also has an important role by allowing or not allowing allergen exposure through epithelial barriers and by providing the initial signals to the type of acquired immune response that will occur.

1.3 Acquired Immune System

The acquired immune system differs significantly from the innate immune system in the way it recognizes and processes pathogens. The innate immune system mainly recognizes substances such as distinctive carbohydrates, lipids, and N-formylated peptides that are not found in the host, but the acquired immune system most commonly targets proteins that may or may not be foreign to the host. The protein focus reflects the antigen specificity of T-lymphocytes, whose antigen receptors only recognize the complexes formed by peptides bound to MHC proteins on the surface of APCs. These proteins are targeted with extreme specificity, with the acquired immune system being able to discriminate between proteins on the basis of a single amino acid or conformational change. Through somatic rearrangment of gene elements, T-cells synthesize antigen-binding molecules specific to the protein. This provides immune memory; consequently, subsequent contacts with the protein initiate a rapid and vigorous response. Similarly, through their diverse receptors, B-cells can recognize nearly any organic molecule. B-cells, however, are not MHC restricted and can recognize proteins, polysaccharides, lipids, nucleic acids, and small chemicals in their soluble (immunoglobulin) or cell surface–associated form. Through somatic hypermutation, B-cells are also able to increase their affinity for their specific antigen. B- and T-cells work closely together to optimize the acquired immune response. The process of the acquired immune system is quite complex and is discussed below in detail.

1.3.1   Immunogens and Allergens

An immunogen is a molecule or collection of molecules that is able to induce an immune response in a host. The vast range of immunogens includes microorganisms, foreign tissue grafts, and proteins in pollens and food. Antigens and allergens are subsets of immunogens. An antigen triggers an immune response through an immunoglobulin or T-cell receptor. Allergens elicit an immune response ultimately through an IgE-mediated mechanism. Proteins are the most potent immunogens. Other classes of molecules such as lipids and carbohydrates are also able to elicit immune responses, primarily when they are linked to a protein such as a lipoprotein or glycoprotein. Allergens are discussed in detail in Chap. 2.

1.3.2   Antigen-Presenting Cells

The acquired immune response is triggered when an antigen encounters a specialized class of cells called antigen-presenting cells (APCs). APCs have the ability to capture the antigen and present it so that it can be recognized by T-lymphocytes. Without the aid of APCs, T-lymphocytes are not able to respond to the antigen because they do not have the necessary specificity and they are not present in significant numbers where the antigens are found in the body. In addition to antigen recognition, a second costimulatory signal is required for T-cell activation. APCs are able to provide both class I and class II MHC–peptide display and provide the necessary costimulatory signals to activate naïve T-cells. The primary APCs are dendritic cells, macrophages, and B-lymphocytes. Their relationship with the T-cell through antigen presentation and costimulation helps determine the type and extent of the immune response.

Dendritic cells are present in nearly all tissues, including surface epithelia and lymphoid organs, allowing them to encounter foreign pathogens in the skin, respiratory and gastrointestinal tracts, and blood and lymph organs. Dendritic cells have a large surface area for contacting immunogens and also have numerous surface receptors that can recognize and bind pathogens. Dendritic cells are activated when their surface receptors recognize a microbial pathogen or when activated by cytokines such as TNF. The pathogens are captured by phagocytosis, receptor-mediated endocytosis, or pinocytosis. Once the immunogens are engulfed by an APC, they undergo a series of alterations called antigen processing. This process involves the cleavage of the immunogen into short peptides. These peptides associate with MHC proteins within the APC and are transported to the APC surface. The presented peptide–MHC complex can then be detected by specific T-cells. Without antigen processing, the T-cell is not able to recognize the pathogen. A T-lymphocyte that comes into direct contact with an APC with the MHC–peptide complex becomes activated under two conditions: (1) if it expresses a T-cell receptor that is able to recognize and bind the specific

MHC–peptide complex and (2) a costimulatory signal is applied. Dendritic cells can be seen at various stages of maturity. The immature dendritic cells only express surface receptors that capture microbial antigens. In addition to expressing surface receptors that capture antigens, mature dendritic cells also express high levels of MHC molecules and costimulators that enable them to interact with and stimulate T-cells.

Macrophages are found throughout body tissues. They are activated by stimulatory cytokines such as IFN-γ. After being activated, they are able to engulf antigen, complex it with MHC peptides, and present it to T-cells. They tend to be less mobile than dendritic cells. They stay in their initial tissue and restimulate T-cells. In cell-mediated immune reactions, macrophages phagocytose microbes and display the antigens of these microbes to effector T-cells. The T-cells in turn release signals that activate the macrophages to kill the microbes.

An activated B-cell is able to act as an APC for T-cells. Although B-cells are able to independently induce effector function on antigen recognized by their membrane-bound B-cell receptor (BCR) and by immunoglobulin, their role in antigen presentation is also important. The B-cell recognizes the antigen on its BCR, internalizes the antigen, and complexes it with MHC II molecules for presentation to T-cells. This occurs primarily in memory or activated B-cells, because naïve B-cells express small amounts of MHC II and costimulatory molecule B7. Because BCRs have a high affinity for antigen, they serve as highly efficient APCs. B-lymphocytes ingest protein antigens and display them to helper T-cells, the process of which is important for the development of amplified, clonal humoral immune responses.

1.3.3 *Major Histocompatibility Complex*

The MHC proteins are also referred to as human leukocyte antigens (HLAs). They are membrane proteins on cells that display peptide antigens for recognition by T-lymphocytes. MHC proteins are separated into two primary classes, each of which is recognized by one of the two major subsets of T-lymphocytes. Class I MHC proteins, which occur on nearly all somatic cell types, present antigens to CD8 T-cells (cytotoxic cells); class II MHC proteins, which are found primarily on dendritic cells, macrophages, and B-lymphocytes, present antigens to CD4 T-cells (helper cells). Therefore, almost any cell can present antigens to cytotoxic T-cells, but only macrophages, dendritic cells, and B-lymphocytes usually present antigen to helper T-cells. Three separate genes, *HLA-A*, *HLA-B*, and *HLA-C*, code for classic MHC class I proteins. These are located on chromosome 6. Many different forms of genes encode the three class I HLA proteins. Each class I MHC protein pairs with a monomorphic β_2-microglobulin to make up the complete class I MHC molecule. β_2-Microglobulin is encoded on chromosome 15. Class II MHC molecules are formed by polypeptides called α and β; there is no class II MHC β_2-microglobulin.

There are three classic MHC class II gene loci, *HLA-DP*, *HLA-DQ*, and *HLA-DR*, on chromosome 6, which includes genes for one α-polypeptide and at least one β-polypeptide. Multiple different alleles exist for each locus; thus, there are many alternative versions of each MHC gene, resulting in proteins with different sequences. This MHC polymorphism benefits the host by increasing the likelihood of being able to present antigens from new pathogens. MHC genes are codominantly expressed, and each person inherits one set of these genes from each parent; therefore, any cell can express six different class I molecules. Because the α- and β-chains of the class II molecules are polymorphic, up to 10–20 different class II molecules can be synthesized.

The HLA class I molecules bind peptide antigens by the α-chain folding into two α-helices and forming a physical groove that binds the peptide. Generally, peptides bound in the grooves of HLA class I molecules are derived from proteins synthesized within the cell; these include ordinary cellular proteins as well as proteins encoded by viruses and other pathogens that have infected the cell. Because almost every cell in the human body has HLA class I molecules on its surface, CD8 T-cells are able to check all these cells to determine whether they have been infected by a pathogen and whether they should be destroyed. Unlike peptides presented by HLA class I molecules, the peptides that are presented by HLA class II molecules are not endogenously synthesized but rather are derived from exogenous proteins that were taken up by the APC by phagocytosis and degraded enzymatically into peptides. HLA class II molecules occur exclusively on cells of the immune system, primarily APCs (dendritic cells, macrophages, and B-cells). They combine with proteins that were outside the cell but then brought in and readied for presentation to the CD4 helper T-cell.

MHC molecules ensure that T-cells only recognize cell-associated protein antigens and that the correct type of T-cell (CD4+ helper T-cell or CD8+ cytotoxic T-cell) responds to the antigen. Characteristics of MHC antigen processing are summarized in Table 1.2.

Table 1.2 MHC Antigen Processing

Feature	Class I MHC	Class II MHC
Peptide–MHC complex	Polymorphic α chain	Polymorphic α chain
	β_2-Microglobulin	Polymorphic β chain
	Peptide; only α chain binds with peptide	Peptide; both chains interact with peptide
Antigen-presenting cells	All nucleated cells	Dendritic cells
		Mononuclear phagocytes/ macrophages
		B-lymphocytes
Responsive T-cells	CD8+ T-cells	CD4+ T-cells
Source of antigens	Proteins synthesized in the cell	Proteins internalized from extracellular environment

MHC major histocompatibility complex

1.4 T- and B-Cells in the Acquired Immune Response

Specific antigen recognition is performed by the membrane-bound antibodies on B-cells (BCR) and the T-cell receptor (TCR) complex on T-cells. These receptors detect their specific antigen, which initiates the cell response. B- and T-cell antigen receptors are clonal; each clone of lymphocytes has a unique receptor. Antibodies may be membrane-bound antigen receptors of B-cells or secreted proteins, immunoglobulins; however, TCRs exist only on membrane receptors of T-cells. Both cell antigen receptors are attached to internal molecules whose function is to deliver or relay the activation signals that are triggered by antigen recognition. The specific characteristics of the T- and B-lymphocytes are discussed below.

1.4.1 T-Lymphocytes

The T-lymphocyte is the director of the acquired immune response. The interaction of the APC and the MHC–peptide complex with the T-cell determines the type of immune response that will occur. T-cells cannot interact themselves with antigen; they recognize antigen bound to the specialized molecules on the APC. T-cells interact with these through the TCR. The two types of TCR are a heterodimer composed of α- and β-chains and one composed of δ- and γ-chains. The α-chain and the β-chain each contain one variable (V) region and one constant (C) region. The α–β TCR accounts for nearly all T-cell helper and cytotoxic activity. The physiologic role of the γ–δ TCR is less clear. This chapter focuses on the α–β TCR.

The α- and β-chains are polymorphic, so a large number of different TCR α–β dimers occur, each capable of recognizing a particular combination of peptide and MHC. The number of complexes that can be recognized by the TCR is a function of the recombination of the variable, diversity, and joining gene segments of the β-chain and the variable and joining segments of the α-chain. Diversity is enhanced further by imprecise joining of these segments and the insertion of nongermline-encoded nucleotides (N regions) between segments by the enzyme terminal deoxynucleotidyltransferase during the rearrangement process. This allows for exponential diversity of the TCR and the ability to adapt to the presentation of the peptide–MHC complex. The TCR is thought to be as diverse as the BCRs. Of interest, each TCR recognizes as few as one to three residues of the MHC–peptide complex. Therefore, T-cells can distinguish between complex microbes on the basis of small amino acid differences.

The recognition of appropriately presented antigen activates T-cells to proliferate, differentiate, and perform their effector functions. For activation, the TCR is associated with a complex of four proteins designated CD3. The CD3 chains serve as transduction signals allowing the TCR to convert the recognition of the peptide–MHC complex into intracellular signals for activation. Several molecules contribute to T-cell signaling and subsequent activation. This process consists of the intracellular production of biochemical intermediate products, enzyme activation, and gene transcription whose products mediate the responses of T-cells. The primary activating factors are protein tyrosine kinases, phospholipases, and tyrosine phosphatases.

In addition to the signals triggered by the TCR and CD3, a second set of signals is required for full activation. TCR activation alone, without the second signal, induces the T-cell to enter an anergic state, where it remains viable but refractory to stimulation by antigen. The most important second signal is CD28, a homodimer on the surface of nearly all CD4 T-cells and approximately one-half of CD8 T-cells. CD28 binds B7-1 (CD80) and B7-2 (CD86) cell surface molecules found on the APCs (i.e., dendritic cells, macrophages, and activated B-cells). The requirement for costimulation ensures that naïve T-cells are activated fully by microbial antigens, because microbes stimulate the expression of B7 costimulators on APCs. The combination of TCR stimulation and the interaction of CD28 with the B7 ligands fully activates T-cells. The affinity of TCRs is low compared with that of BCRs; therefore, the binding of T-cells to APCs is strengthened by accessory molecules. Because of this, the contact between T-cells and the APC is stable long enough for signaling to occur. These include the CD4 or CD8 coreceptor and integrins on the T-cell. The major T-cell integrin involved in binding to the APCs is LFA-1, which binds to ICAM-1 on APCs. LFA-1 is in a low-affinity state on resting naïve T-cells; however, with chemokine exposure from cells of the innate immune system, it is activated into a high-affinity state. Other molecules that contribute to increase costimulatory signals for T-cells are CD40 ligand on T-cells and CD40 on APCs. This interaction activates the APCs to express more B7 costimulators and to secrete IL-12 and other cytokines that enhance T-cell differentiation. The APC–T-cell interaction in T-cell activation is summarized in Fig. 1.3. The outcomes of T-cell activation depend on the type of T-cell and how and when it is triggered. Two primary groups of T-cells with very different functions are CD4 helper T-cells and CD8 killer T-cells.

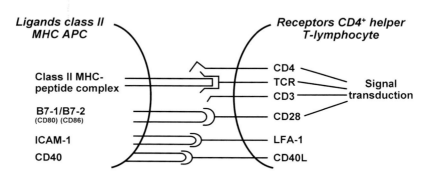

Fig. 1.3 T-cell activation. The initiation of the T-cell response requires multiple ligand–receptor interactions between the antigen-presenting cell (APC) and T-cell. The two primary interactions are T-cell receptor (TCR) binding to the presented major histocompatibility complex (MHC) class II–peptide complex and the costimulatory signal B7-1/B7-2 with CD28. CD8+ T-cells use most of the same molecules except that the TCR, coupled with CD8 instead of CD4, recognizes MHC class I–peptide complexes. *ICAM* intercellular adhesion molecule; *LFA* leukocyte function-associated antigen

1.4.1.1 Helper T-Cell (CD4⁺)

CD4 on the surface of helper T-cells stabilizes the interaction between the T-cell and APC by interacting with the domain of the antigen-presenting class II MHC molecule. CD4 also amplifies the TCR activation signal.

When the helper T-cell is activated by the peptide/MHC complex–TCR and the B7–CD28 interactions, another important event occurs. CD40L is upregulated on the surface of the T-cell. The interaction of CD40L with CD40 on the APC results in the production of cytokines by both the T-cell and APC. These cytokines have an important role in helper T-cell function. When the naïve T-cells are first activated, the major cytokine released is IL-2, a T-cell growth factor. Activation also enhances the ability of T-cells to bind and respond to IL-2 by upregulating the expression of the IL-2 receptor. This allows for T-cell proliferation and an increase in the number of antigen-specific T-cells. When activated with subsequent exposure, the effector T-cells can differentiate into functionally distinct effector subsets depending on the cytokines and costimulatory signals they receive during the activation process. The result is the production of several different patterns of cytokine release from helper T-cells, which defines their function. Activated helper T-cells produce cytokines that further regulate the activities of T-cells, B-cells, monocyte-macrophages, and other effector cells of the immune system. Helper T-cells provide signals that stimulate cell-mediated immune responses and B-cell differentiation into antibody-producing cells. Cytokine release also has a critical role in whether the response to an antigen is atopic or nonatopic.

Th1-Th2 Cells

Helper T-cells differentiate into subsets of effector cells that produce distinct sets of cytokines that perform different functions. The two general subsets are the Th1 subset and Th2 subset. Th1 and Th2 cells are from common CD4 helper T-cells that have the capability to differentiate into either subset. The cytokine milieu surrounding the T-cell appears to have the major role in determining whether the T-cell will become a Th1 or Th2 cell. IL-12, produced by activated macrophages usually in response to infection, causes antigen-primed naïve T-cells to differentiate into Th1 cells. The Th1 cells then produce IFN-γ to kill the microbes. In contrast, the presence of IL-4 during an immune response promotes the differentiation of naïve T-cells into Th2 cells. The original source of the IL-4 responsible for Th2 differentiation is not clear, but it may be the naïve T-lymphocytes themselves. The activation and products of Th1 and Th2 cells are summarized in Fig. 1.4.

Th1 cells produce IL-2, IFN-γ, and TNF-β. These cytokines promote macrophage and other phagocytic cell activity that results in the intracellular killing of pathogens. IL-2 is a growth factor that stimulates cytotoxic lymphocytes and NK cells to proliferate. IFN-γ, likely the most important cytokine produced by Th1 cells, acts on activated B-cells to promote the production of antibody isotypes such as IgG1 that stimulate phagocytosis of microbes. These antibodies bind microbes and

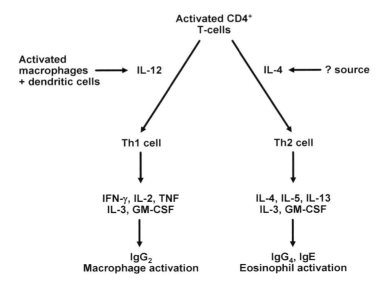

Fig. 1.4 Th1 and Th2 CD4⁺ helper T-lymphocytes. Activated CD4⁺ T-cells differentiate into Th1 and Th2 phenotypes depending on the cytokine milieu. Th1 cells produce cytokines that activate phagocytes to kill ingested microbes and stimulate the production of antibodies that promote the ingestion of microbes by phagocytes. Th2 cells produce cytokines that stimulate IgE production and eosinophil activation. *GM-CSF* granulocyte-macrophage colony-stimulating factor; *IFN* interferon; *IL* interleukin, *TNF* tumor necrosis factor

phagocyte receptors, facilitating activation of complement. IFN-γ is also an important activator of macrophages. TNF activates primed macrophages and NK cells. The overall effect of Th1 cells is to potentiate both engulfment and killing of pathogens by phagocytes. This pathway is essential in protecting the host; however, if dysregulated, it can be associated with autoimmune disorders associated with the destruction of host tissues, as in diabetes mellitus, multiple sclerosis, and inflammatory bowel disease.

In contrast to Th1 cells, Th2 cells do not make IL-2, IFN-γ, or TNF-β but instead secrete a different set of cytokines, primarily IL-3, IL-4, IL-5, IL-9, IL-10, IL-13, and IL-25. These Th2 cytokines act together to chemoattract B-cells, mast cells, basophils, and eosinophils and promote B-cell immunoglobulin class switching to IgE, the immunoglobulin bound uniquely by Fcε receptors on mast cells and basophils. IgE is the critical immunoglobulin in causing the allergic response. This type of reaction is effective protection against large parasites that can be killed by eosinophils but are too large to be engulfed by macrophages. This response is also helpful against mucosal infection. Specifically, IL-4 stimulates the production of IgE antibody and IL-5 activates eosinophils. In addition, cytokines produced by Th2 cells inhibit the activation of macrophages. Therefore, Th2 cells may also serve to limit the tissue injury that accompanies Th1 cell-mediated protective immunity.

Generally, Th1 cells support cell-mediated immune responses against viruses and bacteria, and Th2 cells support mucosal, antiparasitic, and allergic responses.

In most immune responses, helper T-cells show a combination of Th1 and Th2 features. After prolonged immunization, however, the response can become predominantly Th1- or Th2-like. Understanding the factors that govern whether a T-helper response adopts a Th1- or Th2-type response is important for modulating the allergic response. Normally, a T-cell would not be expected to have a Th2 response to a harmless protein antigen such as food or pollen, but this appears to occur in patients with allergic disease. Research has focused on using various methods to "reprogram" the immune response from an allergic Th2 response in atopic patients toward a nonallergic Th1 response with antigen exposure. Recent evidence suggests that the dysregulated immune system involved in allergy and asthma cannot be explained fully by the Th1–Th2 dichotomy. Another mechanism contributing to the allergic response likely involves T-regulatory cells.

Treg, Th3, and TR1: Regulatory T-Cells

In addition to Th1 and Th2 subsets of T-cells, regulatory T-cell subsets have been studied recently, primarily in mouse models. These serve to dampen the immune response. The regulatory T-cell subsets include IL-10-producing cells called T-repressive 1 (TR1) cells, CD25$^+$ regulatory T-cells called Treg cells, and Th3 lymphocytes that produce the immunosuppressive cytokines TGF-β and IL-10. These are important in actively suppressing or terminating immune responses. Thymus-derived Treg cells constitutively express CD25, the IL-2 receptor, and the transcription factor foxp3. They are important for the prevention of autoimmunity by responding to thymic expression of self-antigens. Th3 lymphocytes function to provide mucosal tolerance and, through the production of transforming growth factor (TGF)-β help provide antigen-specific IgA production. They are not thought to be important in allergen protection but rather to provide self-tolerance and mucosal immunity. TR1 cells, however, through the production of IL-10, are thought to have a key role in reducing allergen-specific T-cell responses in healthy subjects and in those treated with immunotherapy. It has been proposed that immune suppression of the regulatory T-cells may be involved in a Th2-skewed immune response among atopic individuals.

1.4.1.2   Cytotoxic T-Cell (CD8$^+$)

Cytotoxic T-cells function to eliminate cells that express foreign antigens on their surface, such as virus-infected cells. When a cell is infected by a virus, immunogenic viral proteins are processed and the resulting peptides appear as surface complexes with the MHC class I molecule. In addition to serving as a marker for cytotoxic T-cells, the CD8$^+$ molecule stabilizes the interaction between the T-cell and APC by binding to the peptide-loaded class I MHC molecules on the target cell. This interaction between the TCR, CD8, and peptide–MHC complex is the first signal for T-cell activation and serves to induce high-affinity IL-2 receptors on the T-cell. The second signal required for activation is IL-2, which is secreted by nearby activated Th1 lymphocytes. Therefore, both CD8$^+$ and CD4$^+$ (Th1) cells specific for viral antigens are activated near one another. These two signals enable the cytotoxic T-cell to acquire cytotoxic activity, enabling it to eliminate the cell to which it is bound as well as other cells bearing the same peptide–MHC class I complex. The elimination can occur through the release of cytotoxic toxins into the target cell or the induction of apoptosis of the target cell. Cytotoxic T-cells deliver perforin and granzyme B onto the surface of target cells. After being taken inside the cell, they induce cell apoptosis. Cytotoxic lymphocytes also bind to the Fas molecule on the surface of the target cell with their own Fas ligand. This interaction triggers apoptosis of the target cell. Importantly, the cytotoxic T-cell also proliferates, giving rise to additional cytotoxic T-cells with the same antigen specificity, thus enhancing the host response.

1.4.2 B-Lymphocytes and Immunoglobulins

B-cells represent approximately 15% of peripheral blood leukocytes and are defined by the production of immunoglobulins. Immunoglobulins are able to bind antigens and, unlike TCR which recognizes only short linear peptides bound in the groove of MHC class I and class II molecules, are able to recognize complex, three-dimensional antigens.

B-cells differentiate from hematopoietic stem cells in the bone marrow by the production of IL-7 by bone marrow stromal cells. Their surface immunoglobulins are assembled in a process similar to that used for the production of the TCR. The immunoglobulin molecules are composed of two identical heavy chains and two identical light chains encoded by genes that are assembled from gene segments. Both heavy and light chains have a variable component. The variable regions of the heavy and light chains are brought together to form the antigen-binding domain of the molecule (Fab). The heavy chain constant regions form the Fc domain of the molecule that is responsible for most of the effector functions of the immunoglobulin, such as binding to Fc receptors and activating complement. A diagram of immunoglobulin is shown in Fig. 1.5.

Assembly of the immunoglobulin begins with the joining of the Dh and Jh segments in the heavy chain genes. The cell then joins a Vh segment. Because of errors in V/D/J joining, approximately 50% of pro-B-cells die in the marrow. Successful V/D/J rearrangement results in synthesis of heavy chain proteins. The heavy chain proteins complex with surrogate light chains, which can be transiently displayed on the surface membranes of the immature B-cells. There, they receive a signal halting any further heavy chain rearrangement and gain the ability to rearrange the light chain genes. Once a light chain protein appears, it associates with the existing heavy chains and the resulting four chain units are transported to the cell surface as membrane IgM. All the immunoglobulin molecules produced by a given B-lymphocyte have identical antigen specificity and light chain type. Because of the mixing that occurs to make the final heavy chain and light chain genes, the receptors on B-cells are so diverse that collectively they can likely recognize any

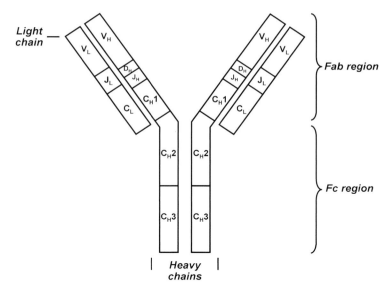

Fig. 1.5 An antibody molecule is composed of two identical heavy (H) chains and two identical light (L) chains, with each chain containing one variable (V) region and one constant (C) region. The Fab region binds the antigen. The Fc region mediates effector functions by binding to the cell surface receptors of phagocytes, natural killer cells, or the C1 complement protein. *D* diversity segment; *J* joining segment

organic molecule that exists. As B-lymphocytes mature, they acquire additional surface molecules: IgD, complement receptors CR1 and CR2, the lectin-like oligosaccharide-binding protein CD23, and adhesion proteins LFA-1, ICAM-1, and CD22. The cells also acquire class II MHC proteins, which enable them to present antigen to T-cells. They also begin surface expression of CD40, a protein critical for T-cell interaction. All these molecules can have a role in the activation of B-cells.

B-cell signaling requires the activation of Igα and Igβ chains that associate with the heavy chain protein enabling signaling to take place. For this to occur, BCRs need to be clustered together to bring enough Igα and Igβ molecules together to send a strong signal to the inside of the cell. This can occur when the BCR binds to an epitope that is repeated many times on a single antigen, when the BCR binds to epitopes on individual antigens that are close together on the surface of an invader, or when the BCR binds to epitopes on antigens that are clumped together. A second signal is required with this. In T-cell independent activation, the second signal is usually supplied by cytokines of the innate immune system. Activation can also be enhanced by the binding of complement to the complement receptor on the B-cell. This greatly amplifies signaling.

In response to certain antigens such as those with repeated epitopes, naïve B-cells can be activated with little or no T-cell help, but this typically is not the case. The naïve B-cell usually requires two signals: the clustering of BCRs with their associated signaling molecules and a second T-cell-dependent costimulatory signal. The best characterized costimulatory signal comes from the helper T-cell. In this interaction, CD40L from the helper T-cell combines with CD40 from the B-cell, sending the costimulatory signal and allowing B-cell activation. After a B-cell has been activated, it develops a memory for the antigen, so that with subsequent exposure the requirements for reactivation are less stringent. Thus, they are more efficient in clearing a later attack. One of the new proteins expressed on an activated B-cell is the receptor for IL-2. IL-2 is a growth factor that stimulates B-cell proliferation. This forms a clone of B-cells that have identical BCRs. Once the B-cells have been activated and have proliferated, they can further mature in three main ways: class switching, affinity maturation in which mutations and selection can increase affinity for the antigen, and further development into a plasma cell (Fig. 1.6).

Once a B-cell has been activated, it is ready to produce IgM antibodies, the default antibody class. Class switching results from a specialized DNA rearrangement in the expressed heavy chain gene that places a new Ch sequence adjacent to the V/D/J exon. As switching occurs, it does not change the structure of the V/D/J exon and, thus, does not affect antigen specificity. The choice of the new Ch isotype is influenced by cytokines and other factors acting on the B-cell. TGF-β in the microenvironment results in the production of IgA. Exposure of the activated B-cell to IL-4 promotes switching to IgE. IFN-γ promotes switching to IgG1. If an isotype switch occurs and the cell continues to divide, its products, both memory and plasma cells, express the new heavy chain isotype. Memory cells in subepithelial regions most commonly express IgA, whereas IgM and IgG memory cells are predominant peripherally.

1.4.2.1   IgG

IgG constitutes approximately 75% of the total serum immunoglobulins. There are four subclasses based on differences in the Fc region. The relative concentrations are IgG1 60–70%, IgG2 15–20%, IgG3 5–10%, and IgG4 2–5%. IgG is the only

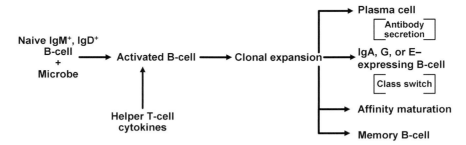

Fig. 1.6 B-cell and antibody immune response. Naïve B-cells recognize antigen and, with the aid of helper T-cells, become activated. B-cells proliferate and expand clonally. The B-cell can develop into a plasma cell, switch classes, or develop greater antigen affinity and become a memory B-cell

class of immunoglobulin that can cross the placenta. IgG is capable of fixing complement in the following order: IgG3 > IgG1 > IgG2 > IgG4. Although IgG4 is not able to fix complement by the classic pathway, it activates complement through the alternative pathway. Macrophages bear surface receptors that bind IgG1 and IgG3 by their Fc fragments. The binding of IgG to the Fc receptor (FcR) activates the macrophage, which then can function in a cytotoxic fashion. In addition, antibody that binds bacteria through the process of opsonization can facilitate phagocytosis by macrophages through Fc–FcR interaction. NK cells can bind to the Fc region of IgG3 antibodies; therefore, IgG3 can bind both antigen with its Fab region and the NK cell with its Fc region. This process is called antibody-dependent cellular toxicity. IgG antibodies have the longest half-life, approximately 3 weeks, whereas IgM antibodies have a half-life of only 1 day.

1.4.2.2   IgA

IgA is the predominant immunoglobulin class in the mucosal immune system. Secretory IgA provides the primary defense mechanism against local infections though its presence in saliva, tears, bronchial secretions, and nasal mucosa and secretions of the small intestines. The unique tail of the IgA makes it resistant to acids and enzymes found in the digestive tract. IgA exists in the serum, constituting approximately 15% of the total serum immunoglobulins. IgA, however, is not able to fix complement because C1 does not bind to its Fc region.

1.4.2.3   IgM

IgM constitutes approximately 10% of normal immunoglobulins and is prominent in the early immune response to most antigens. It is the major immunoglobulin expressed on the surface of B-cells and is the most efficient complement-fixing immunoglobulin. In addition to binding the invader, the IgM antibody is able to bind, because of its pentameric structure, two or more molecules of C1 together in the Fc region, thereby triggering the complement cascade on the invader's surface. IgM antibodies are also effective at binding viruses and preventing them from infecting cells.

1.4.2.4   IgE

IgE is the primary allergy antibody. It binds with high affinity to Fcε receptor type I found on mast cells and basophils. IgE does not activate complement and is not able to transfer through the placenta. IgE synthesis is initiated when allergen is taken up by the APC, processed, and presented to a T-cell. The propensity toward Th2 development and IgE production has a strong genetic basis. The complex is recognized by the TCR, resulting in the activation of the T-cell and the production of IL-4, IL-13, and CD40L

(CD154). IL-4 and IL-13 activate transcription, and the CD40L–CD40 interaction activates the DNA switch recombination, resulting in the isotype class switch to IgE.

The sequence of events in the development of immediate hypersensitivity reactions consists of the production of IgE antibodies in response to an antigen, binding of IgE to FcεRI of mast cells, cross-linking of the bound IgE by reintroduced antigen, and release of mast cell mediators. Immediate hypersensitivity reactions have diverse clinical and pathologic features, all of which are secondary to mediators produced by mast cells in different amounts in different tissues. The primary products of mast cell activation are vasoactive amines, proteases, prostaglandins, leukotrienes, and cytokines.

1.4.2.5 B-Cell Maturation

Somatic hypermutation is a late event in the maturation of B-cells. It typically occurs after class switching has taken place. Somatic hypermutation involves changing the rearranged antibody gene that encodes the antigen-binding region of the antibody. This process results in a fine tuning of antigen specificity by the BCR. The changes that have resulted in an increased ability to bind the antigen are propagated by a greater proliferation of those cells because their higher affinity results in a greater stimulation when exposed to the antigen. The net result is B-cells that are better adapted to defend against the pathogens. These changes are controlled primarily by helper T-cell cytokines; therefore, B-cells that are activated without T-cell help usually do not undergo somatic hypermutation.

The final step in the maturation of B-cells produces either a plasma cell or memory cell. Plasma cells are able to secrete large amounts of immunoglobulin. The primary shift in plasma cells is the ability to secrete immunoglobulin rather than producing only membrane-bound immunoglobulin. Plasma cells can produce 2,000 antibodies per second and most survive only a few days. If a proliferating B-cell does not differentiate into a plasma cell, it reverts to the resting state to become a memory B-cell. Memory B-cells typically have already undergone class switching and somatic hypermutation, so they are well prepared to defend against reexposure to a pathogen.

1.5 Lymphoid Tissues

Cellular interactions are necessary for a protective immune response. To produce memory against most protein antigens, T-cell help is needed to generate high-affinity antibody. To accomplish this, the immune system of a naïve subject needs to bring antigen-specific B-cells together with antigen-specific T-cells and antigen-containing APCs. The major role of the secondary lymphoid tissues is to aid these interactions. The secondary lymphoid organs typically contain zones enriched for B-cells, called follicles, and other zones enriched for T-cells. The B-cell zones contain clusters of follicular dendritic cells that bind antigen-antibody complexes and provide sites adapted for B-cell maturation, somatic mutation, and selection of high-affinity

B-cells. The T-cell zones contain a large number of potent APCs for T-cell activation. Endothelial venules in lymph nodes, Peyer patches, and mucosal-associated lymphoid tissues contain specialized vascular structures for recruitment of naïve B- and T-cells into the tissue. Afferent lymphatic vessels provide entry of antigen-containing APCs from peripheral tissues into lymph nodes, and efferent lymphatics export antigen-experienced cells back into the circulation. These secondary lymphoid tissues are essential for the induction of an efficient, protective immune response.

1.6   Tolerance: Distinguishing Self from Nonself

A remarkable characteristic of the immune system is the ability to react to an inordinate number of antigens without reacting against itself. The unresponsiveness to self-antigens is termed immunologic tolerance. This occurs despite continuous self-antigen exposure to the immune system. A breakdown in immunologic tolerance results in autoimmunity. Several mechanisms contribute to immunologic tolerance; they can be divided into central tolerance and peripheral tolerance. Central tolerance occurs when self-tolerance is assessed by the thymus for T-cells and by the bone marrow for B-cells. Peripheral tolerance occurs when mature lymphocytes encounter self-antigens in the peripheral tissues.

When T-cells enter the thymus from the bone marrow, they do not express CD4, CD8, or TCR. As they migrate through the thymus, they start to rearrange the gene segments for the TCR and, subsequently, CD3, CD4, and CD8. They undergo a process of negative selection, in which the T-cells are exposed to dendritic cells that have migrated to the thymus, where they present self-peptides displayed by the MHC molecules on their surface. The T-cells that recognize the self-peptides and MHC complex are killed. In addition, there is a positive selection process, whereby the T-cell needs to recognize self-MHC. This will be required later for antigen recognition. As the T-cells finish this process, they retain the TCR and either the CD4 or CD8 coreceptor, but not both. Of all the T-lymphocytes that progress through the thymus selection process, approximately 3% survive.

Peripherally, T-cell tolerance can be induced by anergy, activation-induced cell death, or immune suppression. Anergy is the functional inactivation of T-lymphocytes that occurs when these cells recognize self-antigens but lack the necessary second signal that is needed for full T-cell activation. These inactive cells eventually die; thus, peripheral tolerance induction can result in either anergy or death. Activation-induced cell death occurs when an activated T-cell is repeatedly stimulated, sensitizing the cell to its Fas proteins. The Fas–Fas ligand interaction between the T-cell and target triggers an internal death program that prevents the T-cell from continuing to respond. Therefore, self-antigens may delete specific T-cells because these antigens are continuously present and capable of repeatedly stimulating the lymphocytes. Immune suppression may develop under the control of regulatory T-cells. It is thought that these T-cells which produce IL-10 and TGF-β are able to block the activation of lymphocytes and macrophages. The mechanism of their development is not clear.

Self-polysaccharides, self-lipids, and self-nucleic acids are not recognized by T-cells. These antigens induce tolerance in B-lymphocytes to prevent autoantibody production. Central and peripheral tolerance in B-lymphocytes is similar to that of T-cell tolerance. In the bone marrow, negative selection of B-cells eliminates lymphocytes with high-affinity receptors for self-antigens. Peripherally, mature B-lymphocytes that encounter self-antigens become anergic and cannot respond to the self-antigen because they do not receive T-cell help. The peripheral tolerance of T-cell-independent self-antigens is not clear.

1.7 Cytokines

The multidirectional communication among the cells of the immune system is controlled by soluble mediators called cytokines. As mentioned above, cytokines have a critical role in determining host defense, tissue repair, and inflammation (e.g., whether a naïve helper T-cell develops into a Th1 type or Th2 type T-cell) in response to a pathogen. Multiple cytokines have been identified. To gain a better understanding of their various roles, cytokines are grouped below on the basis of the cells that produce them and the function they serve instead of being described in numerical order.

1.7.1 Cytokines Produced by Antigen-Presenting Cells

Cytokines derived from APCs are effective in vigorously mounting the host immune response to a pathogen and, thus, help produce the cellular infiltrate of the host tissue characteristic of inflammation. The primary cytokines involved include TNF, IL-1, and IL-6 but also IL-8, IL-12, IL-15, IL-18, IL-23, and IL-27. These cytokines are produced by mononuclear phagocytic cells during the processing of antigen and presentation to T-cells and also through the innate immune system after nonhost pathogens have been recognized.

TNF includes TNF-α and TNF-β. TNF-α is derived from mononuclear phagocytes, neutrophils, activated lymphocytes, NK cells, endothelial cells, and mast cells. TNF-β is derived primarily from lymphocytes. The most potent inducer of TNF by monocytes is LPS, acting through TLR-2 and TLR-4. The TNFs have numerous functions. TNF-α is an important inducer of the acute phase response. TNF induces fever, fibrosis of arthritic joints, and cachexia and is the primary endogenous mediator of toxic shock and sepsis. It interacts with endothelial cells to induce adhesion molecules such as ICAM-1, vascular cell adhesion molecule (VCAM)-1, and E-selectin. TNF costimulates T-cell activation, induces IL-2 and IFN-γ receptors, and induces T-cell cytokine production. TNF also promotes B-cell proliferation and enhances immunoglobulin expression. TNF is a potent activator of neutrophils, mediating adherence, chemotaxis, degranulation, and respiratory burst. It induces antitumor immunity through direct cytotoxic effects on tumors and by stimulating antitumor immune responses. TNF was investigated initially as a therapeutic agent because of its immunostimulating and antineoplastic effects; however, its extensive side effect profile precluded its use. Currently, however, anti-TNF is used in the treatment of rheumatoid arthritis and is being studied for possible treatment of moderate to severe asthma.

IL-1 is produced primarily by monocytes but also by endothelial cells, keratinocytes, synovial cells, osteoblasts, neutrophils, glial cells, and numerous other cells. The production of IL-1 is stimulated by endotoxin, microorganisms, antigens, and other cytokines. TNF and IL-1 share numerous biologic activities. IL-1 produces fever, lethargy, sleep, and anorexia, and contributes to the hypotension of septic shock. It also stimulates the production of acute phase response proteins and inhibits the production of albumin. IL-1 activates T-lymphocytes by enhancing the production of IL-2 and the expression of IL-2 receptors. IL-1 also augments B-cell proliferation and increases immunoglobulin synthesis. IL-1 receptor antagonist (IL-1Ra) binds to the IL-1 receptor without transducing biologic activities, thereby serving as a cytokine antagonist. IL-1Ra is secreted naturally in inflammatory processes and is thought to modulate the potentially deleterious effects of IL-1 in the natural course of inflammation.

IL-6 is produced primarily by mononuclear phagocytic cells but also by T- and B-lymphocytes, fibroblasts, endothelial cells, keratinocytes, hepatocytes, and bone marrow cells. Like TNF and IL-1, IL-6 induces fever and the production of acute phase proteins. IL-6 augments B-cell differentiation into mature plasma cells and immunoglobulin secretion. It also mediates T-cell activation, growth, and differentiation and some anti-inflammatory effects. IL-6 inhibits IL-1 and TNF synthesis and stimulates the synthesis of IL-1Ra. This activity is unique to IL-6 because IL-1 and TNF upregulate each other.

IL-12 is derived from monocytes, macrophages, B-cells, dendritic cells, Langerhans cells, polymorphonuclear cells, and mast cells. It activates and induces proliferation, cytotoxicity, and cytokine production of NK cells. IL-12 also augments the proliferation of T-helper and cytotoxic lymphocytes. Of note, IL-18 is not derived from lymphocytes or NK cells but from the liver, lung tissue, pancreas, kidney, and skeletal muscle. The biologic activity of IL-18 is similar to that of IL-12. It is part of the final common pathway used by IL-1 and TNF for ICAM-1 expression. IL-23 is secreted by activated dendritic cells and is a potent inducer of IFN-γ. It is thought to contribute to the differentiation of Th1 lymphocytes. IL-15 is produced by mononuclear phagocytic cells, epithelium, and fibroblasts. Its activity is similar to that of IL-2; it is a T-cell growth factor, it participates in the differentiation of NK cells, and it stimulates B-cell growth and differentiation.

1.7.2   Cytokines in the Humoral Immune Response

In the bone marrow, B-lymphocyte maturation occurs through the stimulation of lymphoid stem cell factors IL-7 and IL-11. IL-7 is produced by stromal tissue of the bone marrow and thymus and then interacts with the lymphoid precursors, guiding them toward maturation. After the B-cells leave the bone marrow, T-cells and their cytokines have the major roles in isotype switching and the activation of mature B-cells into immunoglobulin-secreting cells and their final differentiation into plasma cells. IgE isotype switching is triggered by IL-4 and IL-13. IgA is triggered by TGF-β, and IgG4 is triggered by IL-10. Other cells that contribute to B-cell maturation include IFN-γ, IL-1, IL-2, IL-5, IL-6, IL-12, IL-15, and IL-21.

1.7.3 Cytokines in the Cellular and Cytotoxic Immune Response

Cellular immunity refers to an adaptive immune response to a specific antigen through T-cells, resulting in the clonal selection and expansion of the antigen-specific lymphocytes to eliminate pathogens and to generate memory cells. Many cytokines are involved in cell-mediated immunity, including IL-2, IL-15, IL-16, IL-17, IL-21, TNF-β, and IFN-γ. IL-2 is the most important cytokine in this regard. It is secreted by activated T-lymphocytes stimulated by antigen and the interaction of the B7 molecules with CD28. At the time IL-2 is secreted, the high-affinity IL-2 receptor (IL-2R) is also expressed. The binding of secreted IL-2 to IL-2R-positive T-cells induces clonal proliferation that ensures only those T-cells specific for the antigen inciting the immune response become activated. Because IL-2 has a very short half-life in the circulation, it acts primarily as an autocrine or paracrine mediator. In addition to its role as a T-cell growth factor, IL-2 is also involved in the activation of NK cells, B-cells, cytotoxic T-cells, and macrophages.

Cytotoxic responses are directed primarily against virus-infected and neoplastic cells by CD8 lymphocytes and NK cells. Cytokines that activate cytotoxic immunity include IL-2, IL-4, IL-5, IL-6, IL-7, IL-10, IL-11, IL-12, IL-15, TNF, and the IFNs. The three members of the IFN family are α, β, and γ. IFN-α and IFN-β are derived primarily from monocytes, macrophages, B-lymphocytes, and NK cells. They inhibit viral replication within virus-infected cells, protect uninfected cells from infection, and stimulate antiviral immunity by cytotoxic lymphocytes and NK cells. IFN-γ, however, is produced by T-cells and NK cells and has only mild antiviral activity. Its primary role is in cell-mediated immunity. IFN-γ increases MHC class I and II molecule expression and increases mononuclear cell activity, including adherence, phagocytosis, the respiratory burst, and nitric oxide production. These activities contribute to the accumulation of macrophages at the site of cellular immune responses. IFN-γ also stimulates killing by NK cells and neutrophils. Like IL-1 and TNF, IFN-γ induces ICAM-1, stimulating the adherence of granulocytes to endothelial cells.

1.7.4 Cytokines in the Allergic Immune Response

1.7.4.1 IgE

The regulation of IgE is primarily through IL-4, IL-13, and IFN-γ. IL-4 is derived from helper T-cells, eosinophils, basophils, and mast cells. It induces the immunoglobulin isotype switch from IgM to IgE. In eosinophils and mast cells, IL-4 is preformed and can be released rapidly in allergic inflammatory responses. In addition, IL-4 stimulates MHC class II molecules, B7, CD40, surface IgM, and low-affinity IgE receptor (CD23) expression by B-cells. IL-4 also influences T-lymphocyte growth, differentiation, and survival. It favors the initial differentiation of naïve helper T-cells toward a Th2 phenotype. IL-4 also prevents the apoptosis of T-lymphocytes and helps create steroid resistance. In addition, IL-4 has anti-inflammatory effects by downregulating nitric oxide, IL-1, IL-6, and TNF while stimulating IL-1Ra. IL-4 induces the expression of VCAM-1 on endothelial cells, increasing the adhesiveness of T-cells, eosinophils, basophils, and monocytes, but not neutrophils, to the endothelium. IL-4 also stimulates mucus production, which contributes to dysfunction in the asthmatic airway.

IL-13 shares biologic activities with IL-4, rendering the same effect on mononuclear phagocytic cells, endothelial cells, epithelial cells, and B-cells. Unlike IL-4, however, IL-13 does not have an effect on T-lymphocyte growth, differentiation, and survival. IFN-γ inhibits IL-4-mediated expression of low-affinity IgE receptors and the isotype switch to IgE.

1.7.4.2   Eosinophilia

The primary eosinophil-activating cytokines are IL-5, IL-3, and granulocyte-macrophage colony-stimulating factor (GM-CSF). IL-5 is the most important eosinophil activator; it is derived from helper T-cells, mast cells, and probably eosinophils themselves. IL-5 stimulates eosinophil production, chemotaxis, activation, secretion, and cytotoxicity. It increases eosinophil survival by blocking apoptosis. IL-3 and GM-CSF prolong eosinophil survival and activate eosinophils by increasing their degranulation, cytotoxicity, and response to chemoattractants. Both IL-3 and GM-CSF also support the growth of dendritic cells, neutrophils, and macrophages.

1.7.4.3   Mast Cell Proliferation and Activation

The most important cytokine for mast cell growth and proliferation is stem cell factor (SCF or c-kit ligand). Mast cell precursors circulate in the blood and home to tissues, where they mature under the influence of SCF, which is derived from bone marrow stromal cells, endothelial cells, and fibroblasts. Several cytokines may also contribute to mast cell proliferation, including IL-3, IL-5, IL-6, IL-9, and IL-11. IL-4 upregulates the expression of FcεRI on mast cells. IFN-γ decreases mast cell numbers.

1.7.5   Anti-Inflammatory Cytokines

The cytokines with primarily anti-inflammatory effects are TGF-β and IL-10. TGF-β is produced primarily by chondrocytes, osteocytes, fibroblasts, platelets, activated macrophages, and some T-cells. It is a stimulant of fibrosis, promoting wound healing and scar formation. TGF-β inhibits T-cell proliferation and cytokine production, B-cell proliferation and antibody production, and NK activity. Although TGF-β acts as a negative feedback regulator that dampens immunologically mediated reactions, it does have some proinflammatory activity. It is a chemoattractant for neutrophils and monocytes, and it increases expression of adhesion proteins on monocytes.

IL-10 is produced by Th1 and Th2 lymphocytes, cytotoxic T-cells, B-lymphocytes, mast cells, and mononuclear phagocytic cells. IL-10 has widespread anti-inflammatory effects, by inhibiting the production of IFN-γ and IL-2 by Th1 lymphocytes, of IL-4 and IL-5 by Th2 lymphocytes, of IL-1, IL-6, and TNF by monocytes, of IgE synthesis by IL-4 and IFN-γ, and of TNF by NK cells. Constitutive expression of IL-10 by cells in the respiratory tract is critical in the induction and maintenance of tolerance to allergens. IL-10 enhances isotype switching to IgG4 and functions as a growth factor for cytotoxic T-cells. Overall, IL-10 inhibits cytokines associated with cellular immunity and allergic inflammation, while stimulating humoral and cytotoxic immune responses.

1.8   Chemokines

Chemokines are a group of small molecules able to induce chemotaxis in various cells, including neutrophils, monocytes, lymphocytes, eosinophils, fibroblasts, and keratinocytes. Although their function was described originally as inflammatory, being produced at the site of infection or inflammation, and for the recruitment of leukocytes, new functions are being recognized. They also are involved in lymphocyte trafficking, hematopoiesis, and immune surveillance. Homeostatic chemokines typically are found in specific tissues or organs, whereas inflammatory chemokines can be produced by many different cell types in multiple locations. Nearly 50 chemokines and 20 chemokine receptors have been described.

The chemokines share considerable homology and are categorized on the basis of the positioning of the N-terminal cysteine residues. The C–X–C subfamily is characterized by the presence of an amino acid between the first two cysteines; the C–C family has the first two cysteine residues adjacent to each other. These groups can be distinguished by their target cells. The C–X–C group targets primarily neutrophils and the C–C group targets primarily monocytes and T-cells. Various cells can express multiple chemokine receptors, and there is significant overlap in function.

C–X–CL8 (IL-8) is the most important chemoattractant for polymorphonuclear cells. It is derived from numerous cells, including mononuclear phagocytes, endothelial cells, epithelial cells, T-cells, eosinophils, neutrophils, fibroblasts, keratinocytes, and hepatocytes. It appears relatively late in the inflammatory response. In addition to being chemotactic, C–X–CL8 also stimulates neutrophil degranulation, the respiratory burst, and adherence to endothelial cells. CCL3 also activates polymorphonuclear cells.

Chemokines can have a direct effect on T-cell differentiation. CCL3, CCL4, and CCL5 promote a Th1-cell response by directly augmenting IFN-γ-producing Th1-lymphocytes and by increasing IL-12 production from APCs. A Th2 response is mediated by CCL2, CCL7, CCL8, and CCL13, all of which inhibit IL-12 production from APCs and increase IL-4 production from activated T-cells.

Eosinophilia results from the selective recruitment of eosinophils by CCL3, CCL5, and CCL11 (eotaxin). CCL11 is produced by eosinophils, macrophages, mast cells, T-cells, airway smooth muscle cells, and fibroblasts.

Cytokines and chemokines important in allergy and asthma are summarized in Table 1.3.

Table 1.3 Important Cytokines and Chemokines in Allergy and Asthma

Cytokine/chemokine	Produced principally by	Activity
Interleukin-4	Th2 cells	IgE isotype switch
	Mast cells	Cofactor for mast cell growth
		Induction of VCAM-1
		Generation of interleukin-4 -producing (Th2) lymphocytes
Interleukin-13	Th2 cells	IgE isotype switch
		Induction of VCAM-1
Interleukin-5	Th2 cells, mast cells	↑ Eosinophil survival, chemotaxis, degranulation and activation
CCL2 (MCP-1)	Monocytes/macrophages, neutrophils, dendritic cells, eosinophils	Recruitment Th2-type cells
		Basophil chemotaxis and histamine release
Interleukin-10	T-cells, B-cells, mast cells, monocytes/macrophages	Suppression of Th2 response
Transforming growth factor-β	T-cells, macrophages, platelets, chondrocytes, fibroblasts	Inhibition of interleukins 4 and 13
		IgA isotype switch
Interferon-γ	Th1 cells, natural killer cells	Inhibition of interleukins 4 and 13
Interleukin-1, tumor necrosis factor-α	Macrophages	Induction of VCAM-1, ICAM-1 and E-selectin
Stem cell factor	Stromal cells, fibroblasts, epithelial cells	Mast cell growth and differentiation
CCL3 (MIP-1α), CCL4 (MIP-1β), CCL5 (RANTES)	Monocytes/macrophages, T-cells, neutrophils	Promote development of interferon-γ-producing Th1 lymphocytes
CCL7 (MCP-3), CCL8 (MCP-2), CCL13 (MCP-4)	Monocytes/macrophages, fibroblasts	↑ Interleukin-4 production from T-cells leading to Th2 phenotype

ICAM intercellular adhesion molecule; *VCAM* vascular cell adhesion molecule

1.9   Complement

The complement system can be activated by the innate system through the alternative and lectin pathways, as mentioned above. It also can be activated by antigen–antibody complexes through the classic pathway. The antigen–antibody complex provides the activating signal for the complement cascade by the activation of C1, C4, and C2. This activation produces C3 convertase, which cleaves and activates C3. The primary products include the C3a fragment, which is a potent anaphylatoxin, and C3b, which binds to the activating antigen, leading to the destruction of the antigen either through serving as a target for the complement membrane attack complex or as an opsonin by binding to the complement receptors on the surfaces of the neutrophils and macrophages (Fig. 1.2).

1.10   Inflammatory Cells

1.10.1   Eosinophils

Eosinophils develop and mature in the bone marrow from CD34$^+$ progenitor cells and are released into the peripheral blood as mature cells. After release from the bone marrow, eosinophils circulate in the blood and can be attracted into tissue. The blood half-life is 8–18 hours. Most eosinophils are located in the gut and lungs. They are brought from the blood to the tissue by IL-4 and IL-13, which upregulate CCL11 expression by bronchial epithelial cells and fibroblasts and by increasing endothelial cell VCAM-1 expression. Platelet-activating factor and leukotriene B$_4$ (LTB$_4$) are also potent eosinophil chemotactic factors. The major signaling mechanism for eosinophil activation is not clear. There does not appear to be functional Fcε receptor I (FcεRI) on eosinophils. In vitro eosinophils can be activated by agarose beads coated with IgG, IgA, or secretory IgA. Eosinophils can be primed by several mediators, including IL-3, IL-5, GM-CSF, CC chemokines, and platelet-activating factor.

Eosinophils release granule-stored cationic proteins, newly synthesized eicosanoids, and cytokines. Major basic protein (MBP) accounts for more than 50% of the protein mass of eosinophil granules. In patients with asthma, the levels of MBP in the serum and bronchoalveolar lavage fluid correlates with bronchial hyperresponsiveness. Additional eosinophil granule proteins include eosinophil-derived neurotoxin and eosinophil cationic protein. They also are thought to contribute to the pathogenesis of asthma. Eosinophils are a major source of cysteinyl leukotrienes, particularly leukotriene C$_4$ (LTC$_4$) and are the principal LTC$_4$ synthase-producing cells in asthmatic bronchial mucosa. Although eosinophils produce smaller amounts of cytokines than other inflammatory cells, they have been shown to produce IL-1, TGF-β, IL-3, IL-4, IL-5, IL-8, and TNF-α.

Peripheral blood and tissue eosinophilia are seen in allergic disease, asthma, and helminth infections. In allergic disease and asthma, eosinophils have a proinflammatory role, in which eosinophil mediators contribute to mucosal inflammation and bronchial hyperresponsiveness.

1.10.2 Mast Cells

The mast cell is a tissue-based inflammatory cell of bone marrow origin that upon activation responds with immediate and delayed release of inflammatory mediators. Mast cells are the main cells implicated in the pathogenesis of allergic diseases on the basis of their activation through FcεRI-bound antigen-specific IgE and the large number of active mediators released by the cell. In the lungs, mast cells occur in bronchial airway connective tissues and in peripheral intra-alveolar spaces. In the skin, they are near blood vessels, hair follicles, sebaceous glands, and sweat glands.

Human mast cells arise from CD34$^+$ pluripotent stem cells. Mast cell precursors circulate in the blood and migrate into tissues, where they differentiate under the influence of SCF. Cytokines affect mast cell development. IL-4 upregulates the expression of FcεRI, IL-5 promotes the proliferation in the presence of SCF, and IFN-γ decreases the number of mast cells. In addition to activation by FcεRI, mast cells are also activated by C3a, C5a, nerve growth factor, and IgG.

Mast cell mediators typically are grouped into preformed mediators, newly synthesized mediators, and cytokines. Preformed mediators are contained within secretory granules that are released within minutes after activation. The principal granule products are histamine, serine proteases, tryptase, carboxypeptidase A, and proteoglycans (heparin and chondroitin sulfate E). Histamine is the most important mediator and has wide-ranging effects, depending on the site of release.

The newly formed mediators include prostaglandins and leukotrienes. The major prostaglandin produced is prostaglandin D$_2$ and the major leukotrienes are LTC$_4$, LTD$_4$, and LTE$_4$. Numerous cytokines are released from mast cells, including TNF-α, IL-4, IL-3, GM-CSF, IL-5, IL-6, IL-8, and IL-16. Human mast cells also produce chemokines, including CCL3 (macrophage inflammatory protein 1α).

The immediate reaction induced by mast cell activation includes the following: in the skin, erythema, edema, and pruritus; in the upper airway, sneezing, rhinorrhea, and mucous secretion; in the lungs, cough, wheezing, and mucous secretion; in the gastrointestinal tract, nausea, vomiting, diarrhea, and cramping; and in the cardiovascular system, tachycardia and hypotension. Reactions may be followed 6–24 hours later by a late phase reaction. This may manifest as another episode of anaphylaxis or contribute to persistent asthma. Mast cell activation is summarized in Fig. 1.7.

1.10.3 Basophils

Basophils are granulocytes that share features with mast cells, such as FcεRI expression, Th2 cytokine expression, and histamine release. Basophils develop from CD34$^+$ pluripotent stem cells, differentiate in the bone marrow under the influence

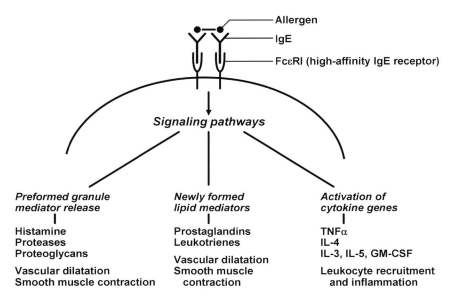

Fig. 1.7 Mast cell activation. *GM-CSF* granulocyte-macrophage colony-stimulating factor; *IL* interleukin; *TNF* tumor necrosis factor

of IL-3, and circulate in the periphery. They comprise less than 1% of peripheral blood leukocytes. Basophils are activated by FcεRI. The result is granule exocytosis and mediator release. Basophils produce histamine, leukotrienes, IL-4, and IL-13. Unlike mast cells, they do not produce prostaglandin (PG) D$_2$ or IL-5. The physiologic role of basophils has not been clearly defined. Because they express FcεRI, it is reasonable to assume that they participate in allergic reactions. Studies have identified basophils in lung tissue from patients who died of asthma. They also have been seen in tissues and airway fluids after experimental allergen challenge.

1.11 Primary Mediators of Inflammation

1.11.1 Histamine

Histamine is a major biogenic amine in human mast cells and basophils. It is formed by decarboxylation of the amino acid histidine by histidine decarboxylase in the Golgi apparatus of mast cells and basophils. Histamine is stored in secretory granules (2–5 pg per cell), where it is ionically bound to heparin or proteoglycan. It is secreted spontaneously at low levels by mast cells. Normal urine histamine concentrations range from 5–15 µg per 24 hours; normal plasma levels are 0.5–2 nM. An increased rate of secretion and higher levels are found with mast cell activation.

When activation occurs, the granules swell and histamine, along with proteases and proteoglycans, is expelled into the local extracellular environment by compound exocytosis. Histamine exerts many effects on various tissues pertinent to the immediate phase of the allergic response. It induces vasodilatation, increases vasopermeability, stimulates contraction of bronchial and intestinal smooth muscle, and increases mucus production. Histamine has a significant role in the majority of signs and symptoms associated with an allergic or anaphylactic reaction, including pruritus, urticaria, rhinorrhea, sneezing, wheeze, abdominal cramping, diarrhea, and hypotension. It is rapidly metabolized, within 1 or 2 minutes, making it difficult to measure during an allergic reaction. The major enzymatic pathways of histamine breakdown are methylation (70%) by histamine N-methyltransferase or oxidation (30%) by diamine oxidase. The initial methylation product is N-methylhistamine, which is excreted by the kidney and may be quantified in the urine as a measure of histamine release. N-methylhistamine can be oxidized further to methylimidazole acetic acid. Oxidation of histamine by diamine oxidase results in imidazole acetic acid. This intermediate product is further metabolized to riboside-N-3-imidazole acetic acid.

Histamine receptor antagonists have been helpful in identifying the role of histamine in different organ systems. Histamine (H_1) receptor antagonists have been found to be helpful in the treatment of allergic rhinoconjunctivitis, local and systemic anaphylactic reactions, and urticaria. They are able to inhibit approximately 75% of the skin wheal and flare responses induced by allergen. In experimental studies, H_1 antagonists inhibit nearly 50% of allergen-invoked bronchoconstriction, although they have not been shown to be helpful in the treatment of asthma. The lack of efficacy of H_1 antagonists in asthma suggests that cellular events other than mast cell mediator release are important in the pathophysiologic mechanism of asthma.

Histamine stimulation of H_2 receptors on gastric parietal cells promote the secretion of gastric acid. Selective H_2 receptor antagonists have shown to be effective for gastroesophageal reflux disease but have little to do with allergic disease. When combined with H_1 receptor antagonists, H_2 receptor antagonists may help in the treatment of urticaria and systemic mastocytosis, but they do not add to H_1 antagonists in the treatment of allergic rhinoconjunctivitis.

1.11.2   Arachidonic Acid Metabolism

Eicosanoids are made up of prostaglandins, leukotrienes, lipoxins, and thromboxanes. Prostaglandins and leukotrienes are important mediators of inflammation in asthma and allergic reactions. These molecules are synthesized de novo from membrane phospholipids in response to cell stimulation by allergen, infection, inflammation, or trauma. All eicosanoids are synthesized from arachidonic acid, which occurs in the cell membrane phospholipids of numerous cells (mast cells, neutrophils, eosinophils, and macrophages). The first and rate-limiting step in eicosanoid production is the release of arachidonic acid from the phospholipids by phospholipase A_2 (PLA_2) enzymes. PLA_2 is activated by the receptor-mediated influx of calcium

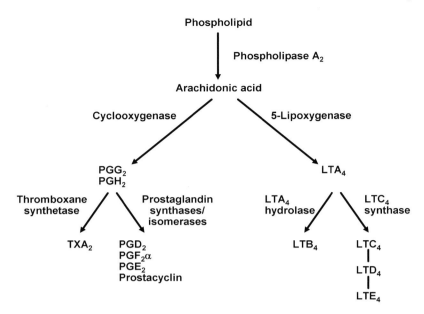

Fig. 1.8 Primary lipid mediator synthetic pathways. *LTA–LTE* leukotrienes A, B, C, D, and E; *PGD–PGH* prostaglandins D, E, F, G, and H; *TXA* thromboxane A

ions into the cell. Activation of this enzyme results in free arachidonic acid that can enter the arachidonic acid cascade, where it is transformed primarily by cyclooxygenases (COXs) or lipoxygenases. The products of COXs are thromboxanes and prostaglandins, and the products of lipoxygenases are lipoxins and leukotrienes. The final products of arachidonic acid metabolism depend on the type of cell, type of stimulus, and regulatory processes. The synthetic pathways for the primary lipid mediators are shown in Fig. 1.8.

1.11.3 Cyclooxygenase Products: Prostaglandins

Free arachidonic acid is metabolized to prostaglandins by COX enzymes. COX is found in two forms: COX-1 is the constitutive form found in almost all cell types, and COX-2 is the inducible form, activated by proinflammatory cytokines, growth factors, and endotoxin. The generation of prostaglandins by COX-2 in macrophages, mast cells, and infiltrating polymorphonuclear leukocytes is associated with pain, inflammation, and pyrexia. COX activity produces the unstable intermediate prostaglandin H_2, which is converted into prostaglandins (PGD_2, $PGF_2\alpha$, PGE_2, PGI_2), or thromboxane A_2 (TXA_2) by individual synthases.

PGD_2, $PGF_2\alpha$, $9\alpha11\beta$-PGF_2, and TXA_2 are powerful constrictors of airway smooth muscle. Although they are less potent bronchoconstrictors than cysteinyl leukotrienes, they are released in large molar amounts. In the lung, macrophages produce TXA_2 and $PGF_2\alpha$. TXA_2 is also synthesized by platelets. The most abundant COX product generated by human lung mast cells is PGD_2. Although histamine is produced by mast cells and basophils, only mast cells release PGD_2. PGD_2 is metabolized to $9\alpha11\beta$-PGF_2, another potent bronchoconstrictor. Although TXA_2 has not itself been evaluated in humans for bronchoconstrictor activity because of its instability, thromboxane receptor antagonists have reduced baseline bronchial responsiveness to cholinergic agonists in subjects with asthma. Conversely, prostacyclin and PGE_2 have bronchoprotective action. Prostacyclin is made by vascular endothelial cells and vascular and nonvascular smooth muscle cells. PGE_2 is generated by airway epithelial cells and alveolar macrophages. The protective activity of PGE_2 seems to be exerted by a reduction in the release of leukotrienes and other mediators by eosinophils, neutrophils, and macrophages rather than its limited bronchodilator effect. Nonselective COX inhibitors such as aspirin appear to have little effect on airway tone or inflammation in most situations. This is likely because they block the production of both the bronchoconstrictor and bronchodilator prostaglandins, thereby having a neutral effect. The exception to this occurs in patients who have aspirin-exacerbated respiratory disease, in which significant worsening of their underlying asthma occurs with aspirin use. Although the exact mechanism is not understood completely, it does appear that significant leukotriene production has a major role.

1.11.4   Lipooxygenase Products: Leukotrienes

During stimulus-specific cell activation, arachidonic acid is translocated to the 5-lipoxygenase activating protein and converted to 5-hydroperoxyeicosatetraenoic acid and then to unstable leukotriene A_4 (LTA_4) by 5-lipoxygenase. LTA_4 serves as the precursor for both LTB_4 and cysteinyl leukotrienes. LTA_4 is converted to LTB_4 by LTA_4 hydrolase or to the cysteinyl leukotriene LTC_4 by LTC_4 synthase. LTC_4, the first of the cysteinyl leukotrienes, can be cleaved further into the cysteinyl leukotrienes LTD_4 and LTE_4.

The type and amount of leukotrienes produced depend on the cell and the local inflammatory, especially cytokine, environment. LTB_4 is produced primarily by alveolar macrophages, monocytes, and neutrophils, whereas the cysteinyl leukotrienes are produced primarily by eosinophils, mast cells, and basophils. LTB_4 is a proinflammatory lipid mediator. It is a potent chemotactic agent for neutrophils and eosinophils, and it promotes neutrophil adherence to vascular endothelial cells, facilitating the accumulation of granulocytes at the site of inflammation. LTB_4 also stimulates neutrophil degranulation and superoxide generation and IL-6 production from human monocytes. The cysteinyl leukotrienes were formerly known as the slow-reacting substances of anaphylaxis. They are able to induce airway, gastrointestinal, and mesangial smooth muscle contraction. LTC_4 and LTD_4 are potent bronchoconstrictors. The cysteinyl leukotrienes also serve as chemotactic agents for leukocytes, particularly eosinophils, increase the permeability of the vascular endothelium, and stimulate bronchial mucus secretion. They are released during allergen-mediated asthma and allergic rhinoconjunctivitis.

1.12   Allergic Response to an Allergen: Summary

The following is a step-wise summary of a type I IgE-mediated hypersensitivity reaction to an allergen (keep in mind the various interacting components of the immune system reviewed in this chapter).

1. Allergen exposure: the initial step of an allergic reaction is allergen exposure. It can occur through contact with the skin, the mucosal epithelium of the eyes, respiratory system (nose, upper airway, lungs), and the digestive system (mouth, esophagus, gastrointestinal tract), and even through the vascular system in the context of intravenous administration of medication.
2. At each of these contact areas, APCs are able to come into contact with the allergen, take in the allergen, process the allergen, and combine the allergen product, typically a peptide, with MHC II.
3. The peptide–MHC II complex is brought to the surface of the APC and presented to a $CD4^+$ helper T-cell.
4. In persons genetically predisposed and in the presence of IL-4, the $CD4^+$ T-cells differentiate into Th2 lymphocytes. T- and B-cell interaction induces the clonal expansion of allergen-specific T- and B-cells.
5. Th2 lymphocytes release cytokines, particularly IL-4 and IL-13, which induce isotype switching in newly generated IgM-bearing B-cells from mu to epsilon, resulting in the subsequent production of IgE.
6. IgE antibody via the Fc portion binds to high-affinity receptors specific for the IgE heavy chain on mast cells (FcεRI), "coating" the mast cells with IgE.
7. Upon further allergen exposure, cross-linking of the mast cell-bound IgE by allergen triggers the activation of mast cells.
8. Mast cell degranulation results in the release of the preformed mediators, namely histamine, heparin, tryptase, protease, and chemotactic cytokines, and the newly formed lipid mediators, namely, leukotrienes (LTB_4, LTC_4, and LTD_4), prostaglandins (PGD_2), and platelet-activating factor. These are the main components of the acute allergic reaction.
9. The late phase reaction is caused by leukocytes recruited by the release of cytokines from mast cells. The primary leukocytes of the late phase reaction are eosinophils, neutrophils, and Th2 cells.

1.13   Immune-Modulating Medications in Allergic Disease

On the basis of our knowledge of the immune system and the allergic response, numerous medications are used to inhibit the allergic response. The following is a list of experimental and currently used immunomodulatory medications for treating atopic disease. The focus is on their action on modulating the immune response.

1.13.1 CpG-DNA

CpG oligooxynucleotides mimic bacterial DNA and, thus, stimulate Th1-type cytokine responses. These nucleic acids activate the innate immune receptor TLR9, a receptor present on dendritic cells, leukocytes, and other cells that inhibit Th2 cells. CpG has been given alone or in combination with a protein allergen. The latter is performed to enhance immunogenicity to elicit a Th1 response to the allergen. Th1 responses lead to the production of IFN-γ, IL-12, IL-18, and IL-23, inhibiting Th2 responses. These agents have shown promise in animal models and have entered human clinical trials. An initial randomized, double-blind, placebo-controlled phase 2 trial of Amb a 1 (ragweed pollen allergen) conjugated to an immunostimulatory sequence of DNA given over a 6-week period before ragweed season showed clinical efficacy and safety. Additional clinical trials will determine whether the CpG DNA therapies are safe and effective in humans who have allergic rhinitis and asthma.

1.13.2 Omalizumab

Omalizumab is a humanized anti-IgE monoclonal antibody. It binds to the Fc portion of IgE, disrupting the ability of the IgE antibody to bind with its receptors (FcϵRI-high affinity and FcϵRII-low affinity). This prevents the IgE-mediated activation of mast cells and basophils. Omalizumab has also been shown to decrease the number of inflammatory cells that express CD4, IL-4, and FcϵRI by inhibiting the positive feedback loop. Clinically, omalizumab has been studied primarily in moderate to severe asthma, for which it has been shown to decrease the amount of corticosteroid required for disease management and to decrease the number of asthma exacerbations and hospitalizations. Currently, omalizumab therapy does not appear to result in a significant improvement in overall airflow obstruction.

1.13.3 Anti-TNF

TNF-α is an important proinflammatory cytokine that is important in the pathogenesis of chronic inflammatory disorders of the airways. It enhances the release of proinflammatory/chemotactic mediators and upregulation of adhesion molecules that facilitate the migration of eosinophils and neutrophils. TNF-α mRNA is expressed more frequently in the airways of people with asthma than in controls and increased levels are found with bronchoalveolar lavage in patients with asthma, including those provoked with allergen challenge. TNF-α has been shown to induce and potentiate airway hyperresponsiveness. TNF-α blockers have been found to be effective and well-tolerated in the treatment of rheumatoid arthritis refractory to conventional therapy. The commercially available TNF-α blockers include infliximab (a chimeric mouse/human monoclonal anti-TNF-α antibody), adalimumab (a fully human monoclonal anti-TNF-α antibody), and etanercept (a fusion protein combining two TNF receptors with a Fc fragment of human IgG1). Currently, there is little information on the use of TNF-α blocking agents in asthma. Retrospective analysis of patients receiving infliximab for rheumatoid arthritis showed significant improvement in FEV_1 and exercise tolerance. An open-labeled, uncontrolled trial of etanercept administered to patients with severe asthma showed improved lung function and improvement in asthma symptom scores. In small, randomized, placebo-controlled studies, etanercept and infliximab decreased asthma exacerbations and improved symptom scores in those with moderate to severe asthma, with less improvement in those with mild asthma. Although these preliminary results are encouraging, particularly for severe asthma, additional studies are needed to evaluate the role of TNF-α blocker in treating asthma.

1.13.4   Immunotherapy

Immunotherapy consists of the administration of allergen extracts to achieve clinical tolerance to the symptom-producing allergens. Immunotherapy has shown to be successful in the treatment of allergic rhinitis, allergic asthma, and venom hypersensitivity. Several mechanisms have been proposed to identify the immunologic response resulting in the clinical benefits of immunotherapy. Possible mechanisms of immunotherapy include induction of IgG4 blocking antibodies, long-term decrease in specific IgE, reduced recruitment of effector cells, altered T-cell cytokine release, T-cell anergy, and induction of regulatory T-cells. The main theme appears to be the effect of immunotherapy on allergen-specific T-cells, resulting in more of a Th1 cytokine pattern release (IFN-γ, TNF-α, IL-2, IL-12, and IL-18) as opposed to a Th2 cytokine release pattern (IL-4, IL-5, IL-9, and IL-13), and the induction of regulatory T-cells producing IL-10 when subsequently exposed to allergen. These modulatory T-cell changes likely also have a role in the clinical observations of the reduction of the development of new allergic sensitizations and inhibition of the development of asthma in patients with allergic rhinitis.

1.13.5   Corticosteroids

Corticosteroid molecules interact with an intracytoplasmic corticosteroid receptor that migrates into the nucleus, where it binds to DNA sequences known as glucocorticoid response elements. These elements affect target gene transcription.

The anti-inflammatory effects of corticosteroids result from the inhibition of transcription by direct gene element binding or by the production of proteins that have inhibitory effects on inflammatory target gene transcription. Corticosteroids affect the various arms of the immune system. Cytokines IL-1, IL-2, IL-6, IL-8, IFN-γ, and TNF-α are inhibited. Leukotriene synthesis is decreased by the production of lipocortin, which inhibits PLA$_2$. Nitric oxide synthetase is inhibited, thus decreasing the production of nitric oxide, an inflammatory mediator. Neutrophils, although increased in the circulation, are reduced at the site of inflammation by downregulation of endothelial and intercellular adhesion molecules. IL-8 inhibition also results in decreased activation of neutrophils. Eosinophil adherence and degranulation are inhibited. With the use of systemic corticosteroids, serum eosinophil levels are often undetectable. Monocyte-mediated effects are inhibited by the interference with recruitment, antigen processing, and MHC class II and IL-1 production. Immature lymphocytes and thymocytes are susceptible to corticosteroid-induced apoptosis, and T-cell proliferation in response to antigen is limited. Generally, immunoglobulin synthesis is not inhibited, but serum IgG levels may be decreased, possibly because of the increased metabolism of immunoglobulin.

1.13.6   Immunophilins

The immunophilins include cyclosporine, tacrolimus, and sirolimus. They inhibit T-cell activation through a series of calcium-dependent signal events involved in cytokine gene transcription. Cyclosporine and tacrolimus block the signal transduction pathway initiated by the TCR. By binding to calcineurin, they prevent the nuclear translocation of the nuclear factor of activated T-cells. Therefore, they inhibit the production of IL-2, IL-3, IL-4, IFN-γ, GM-CSF, and TNF-α. In atopic diseases, they are used most commonly to treat atopic dermatitis and severe chronic urticaria. They are used primarily to treat graft-versus-host disease after bone marrow transplantation and graft rejection of solid-organ transplants. In addition, cyclosporine has been effective in the treatment of autoimmune disorders, including psoriasis, Behçet syndrome, uveitis, rheumatoid arthritis, Crohn disease, polymyositis/dermatitis, aplastic anemia, and nephritic syndrome. Adverse effects include hypertension, susceptibility to infection, development of malignancies, and posttransplant lymphoproliferative disorder.

1.14   Summary

This overview of the immune response, with the focus on the allergic response, provides a glimpse of the complexity of the interactions between the cells and mediators of the immune system. Modulation of the immune system, particularly in

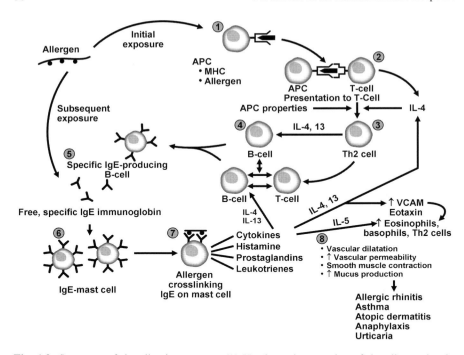

Fig. 1.9 Summary of the allergic response. (1) Uptake and processing of the allergen by the antigen-presenting cell (APC). The processed allergen with major histocompatibility complex (MHC) II is presented on the surface of the APC. (2) T-cell recognizes the allergen–MHC complex. (3) In the setting of interleukin (IL)-4 exposure and through properties of the APC, the T-cell becomes a Th2 cell. (4) Th2 cell release of cytokines and T- and B-cell interaction lead to the class switch of the B-cell to an allergen-specific IgE-producing B-cell. (5) IgE-producing B-cell produces free IgE immunoglobulin. (6) Fc portion of IgE binds to mast cells and basophils via the FcεRI receptor. (7) Subsequent allergen exposure results in crosslinking of mast cell-bound IgE and mast cell activation. (8) Mast cell releases multiple mediators, including histamine, prostaglandins, and leukotrienes, resulting in the immediate hypersensitivity response, and also cytokines and other mediators that recruit leukocytes and create the late phase allergic inflammation. *Barriers to the allergic response at the various steps include the following*: (1) Intact epithelial barriers. (2) Probable genetic predisposition; corticosteroids (decrease reactivity of CD4+–APC interaction). (3) Probable genetic predisposition; allergen-specific immunotherapy (decreases Th2 phenotype, increases interleukin [IL]-10); cytosine-phosphate-guanine (CpG)-DNA (decreases Th2 phenotype). (4) Allergen-specific immunotherapy (decreases Th2 phenotype, increases IL-10); CpG-DNA (decreases Th2 phenotype); immunophilins, including cyclosporine and tacrolimus (reduces activation state of T-cells); antimetabolites, including azathioprine, methotrexate, and cyclophosphamide (reduce effector function of activated B-cells). (5) IgE antibody, omalizumab (binds IgE). (7) Chromones, including cromolyn and nedocromil (attenuate mast cell mediator release). (8) H_1 antagonists (prevent histamine binding to target receptors); leukotriene (LT) receptor antagonists (prevent LTC_4, LTD_4, LTE_4 binding to target receptors). *VCAM* vascular cell adhesion molecule

attenuation of the allergic response, will likely become the cornerstone of treatment of allergic disease in the near future. The allergic immune response and the area in which current and experimental immunomodulators act are summarized in Fig. 1.9.

Suggested Reading

Abbas, A. K. and Lichtman, A. H. (2006) Basic immunology: functions and disorders of the immune system, 2nd ed, updated edition 2006–2007. Philadelphia: Elsevier Saunders.

Bochner, B. S. and Schleimer, R. P. (2001) Mast cells, basophils, and eosinophils: distinct but overlapping pathways for recruitment. Immunol. Rev. 179, 5–15.

Broide, D. H. (2005) DNA vaccines: an evolving approach to the treatment of allergic disorders. Allergy Asthma Proc. 26, 195–198.

Cazzola, M. and Polosa, R. (2006) Anti-TNF-α and Th1 cytokine-directed therapies for the treatment of asthma. Curr. Opin. Allergy Clin. Immunol. 6, 43–50.

Chaplin, D. D. (2006) Overview of the human immune response. J Allergy Clin. Immunol. 117, S430–S435.

Corry, D. B. and Kheradmand, F. (2006) Control of allergic airway inflammation through immunomodulation. J. Allergy Clin. Immunol. 117, S461–S464.

Creticos, P. S., Schroeder, J. T., Hamilton, R. G., et al. (2006) Immunotherapy with a ragweed-toll-like receptor 9 agonist vaccine for allergic rhinitis. N. Engl. J. Med. 355, 1445–1455.

Djukanovic, R., Wilson, S. J., Kraft, M., et al. (2004) Effects of treatment with anti-immunoglobulin E antibody omalizumab on airway inflammation in allergic asthma. Am. J. Respir. Crit. Care Med. 170, 583–593.

Erin, E. M., Leaker, B. R., Nicholson, G. C., et al. (2006) The effects of a monoclonal antibody directed against tumor necrosis factor-α in asthma. Am. J. Respir. Crit. Care Med. 174, 753–762.

Francis, J. N., Till, S. J., and Durham, S. R. (2003) Induction of IL-10+ CD4+ CD25+ T cells by grass pollen immunotherapy. J. Allergy Clin. Immunol. 111, 1255–1261.

Hayashi, T., Gong, X., Rossetto, C., et al. (2005) Induction and inhibition of the Th2 phenotype spread: implications for childhood asthma. J. Immunol. 174, 5864–5873.

Ngoc, P. L., Gold, D. R., Tzianabos, A. O., Weiss, S. T., and Celedon, J. C. (2005) Cytokines, allergy, and asthma. Curr. Opin. Allergy Clin. Immunol. 5, 161–166.

Prussin, C. and Metcalfe, D. D. (2006) IgE, mast cells, basophils, and eosinophils. J. Allergy Clin. Immunol. 117, S450–S456.

Sompayrac, L. (2003) How the immune system works. Malden, MA: Blackwell Publishing.

Steinke, J. W. and Borish, L. (2006) Cytokines and chemokines. J. Allergy Clin. Immunol. 117, S441–S445.

Tosi, M. F. (2005) Innate immune responses to infection. J. Allergy Clin. Immunol. 116, 241–249.

Yokoyama, W. M. (2005) Natural killer cell immune responses. Immunol. Res. 32, 317–325.

Chapter 2
Environmental Allergens

2.1 Overview of Allergens

An allergen is an antigen that is characterized by its ability to induce a specific IgE-mediated immune response with an associated clinical allergic reaction. Allergens come from a great variety of sources such as pollens, molds or fungal spores, mites, animals, venoms, drugs, food, and latex. Seasonal tree, grass, and weed pollens and fungal spores account for most outdoor airborne allergens. Dust mite, animals, cockroach, and fungal spores are the primary indoor airborne allergens. This chapter focuses on these airborne environmental allergens; venom, drug, food, and latex allergens are discussed in separate chapters. Most allergens are proteins or glycoproteins that are 5–60 kDa in size. However, some allergens include polysaccharides and low-molecular-weight substances. The allergenicity of an antigen is determined by several variables, primarily the genetic predisposition of the host and the solubility, size, stability, and conformational fold of the allergen. The complete complementary (cDNA) sequences have been determined for many allergenic proteins, but the composition of many other allergens is unknown. Multiple research techniques, including chemical, immunological, and biological techniques, are being used to purify and characterize the specific chemistry of allergens.

For an aeroallergen to be clinically significant, it must be buoyant, be present in significant numbers, and be able to induce an IgE-mediated response. Particle size is an important physical component of an allergen. Small size allows the particle to be carried by the wind and to be deposited within the respiratory mucosa and conjunctiva. Large particles, in comparison, settle more quickly except in high winds. Most airborne tree, grass, and weed pollens are 20–60 μm in diameter, fungal spores 3–30 μm in diameter, and mite particles 1–10 μm in diameter. The upper airway filters the larger allergens, with particles smaller than 7 μm depositing in the airways and those smaller than 3 μm making it to the distal alveoli. The conjunctivae and upper airways receive the largest amount of airborne allergens. Once an allergen has been inspired, allergenicity is also determined by the breakdown of pollen grains, the rapidity that various allergens are released from the pollen grain, the biochemical function of the allergens, and the intrinsic allergenicity of the protein.

G.W. Volcheck, *Clinical Allergy: Diagnosis and Management*
DOI: 10.1007/978-1-59745-315-8_2, © 2009 Mayo Foundation for Medical
Education and Research

For example, even if a pollen grain elutes a large amount of allergen, if it has low intrinsic allergenicity, such as pine pollen, there will only be a minimal allergic response. In addition, enzymatic properties of allergens, such as dust mite proteases, may facilitate an allergic response. The allergenic molecules generally are water soluble and can be leached from airborne particles. In some instances, immunochemical methods have shown that atmospheric allergens exist in ambient air in the absence of pollen grains. This elution of allergen from the pollen grain likely explains why allergens from large pollen grains are able to instigate an allergic reaction in the lower airways.

Each aeroallergen may contain one or more allergenic proteins that can initiate an allergic response. Proteins that bind to a majority of the IgE-enriched sera from sensitized patients are called major allergens. The proteins that bind to only a small percentage are termed minor allergens. The specific allergens are designated by the first three letters of the genus name and the first letter of the species name, followed by an Arabic numeral uniquely identifying the allergen. For example, a major allergen from *Alternaria alternata* is designated Alt a 1.

Currently, more than 200 tree, weed, and grass allergen extracts are available for testing through the major commercial vendors of allergen extracts. Choosing a clinically relevant panel for testing can be difficult. To make the most prudent choices, knowledge of plant taxonomy, allergenic cross-reactivity, and geographic distribution of the plant species is required. Allergenic cross-reactivity occurs when different proteins have a certain degree of homology and contain identical or similar specific IgE-binding epitopes. The following review of pollens focuses on the major allergens for the various geographic locations, with emphasis on cross-reactivity between the various allergens.

2.2 Pollens

The primary allergenic pollens come from anemophilous, or wind-pollinated, plants. These plants tend to have odorless, inconspicuous flowers. During pollination, the male genetic material is transferred from one plant to another. At this time, the local concentration of a pollen type can reach thousands of grains per cubic meter of air. In comparison, insect- or animal-pollinated, or entomophilous, plants, typically have colorful, fragrant flowers and tend to have sticky, heavy pollen, which possibly is allergenic in nature but does not come into contact with the respiratory mucosa in significant amounts to elicit an allergic response.

2.2.1 Pollen Counts

Airborne pollens can be measured and reported as a "pollen count." There are numerous methods for sampling the air. The two basic methods are passive and active sampling. Passive sampling simply collects particles from the air onto slides, plates, or traps by the force of gravity. This method is heavily biased toward the large particles and is not commonly used. In active sampling, particles are actively removed from the air by a mechanical or electrical device. The most commonly used active air-sampling devices are impaction devices that work by accelerating an airstream onto a sampling surface. This enables the particles to break free of the airstream and "impact" onto the collecting device. It is more difficult for smaller particles to break free of the airstream; therefore, measuring smaller particles, particularly fungal spores, is more difficult.

Two commonly used impaction devices are the Rotorod sampler and the Burkard spore trap. The Rotorod sampler consists of two plastic rods that are coated with silicone grease and rotated rapidly around a fixed circumference by an electric motor. The collector rods are then removed, stained, and analyzed under light microscopy. Pollen grains are identified by light microscopy at 400× magnification. The number of particles per cubic meter of air ($p\,m^{-3}$) is calculated from the volume of the atmosphere sampled. It has been shown to be more than 90% efficient at capturing pollen particles approximately 20 μm in diameter. The Burkhard spore trap consists of plastic tape or a standard microscope slide coated with silicone adhesive that is moved past an air intake orifice at a fixed speed. The tape or slide is stained and analyzed under light microscopy. The total particle recovery per day ($p\,m^{-3}$) can then be calculated. The Rotorod is the more widely used device in the United States and is less expensive than the Burkhard spore trap. The Burkhard spore trap has a greater acceleration velocity and is more efficient at collecting particles smaller than 10 μm (primarily fungal spores).

The pollen grains collected on the slides can be categorized by their surface characteristics. The outermost layer of the pollen grain, the exine, is prominently sculptured and may show apertures as circular pores, elongate furrows, or both. The pollen grains with pores alone are classified as porate and those with furrows alone as colpate; those with both are termed colporate. Depending on the number of apertures, pollens are labeled as monoporate, tricolpate, and so forth. When numerous apertures are present, the prefix "peri-" is used. "Stephano-" is used to refer to equatorial pores or furrows (Fig. 2.1). This nomenclature is used to help identify particular pollens.

Approximately 30 grains of pollen per cubic meter of air is required to cause an allergic reaction. Because of priming, the amount of pollen grains required to initiate symptoms at the beginning of the season is greater than at the end. An average person inhales about 10 m^3 of air per day, which would result in approximately 300–500 pollen grains per day to sustain an allergic reaction. The amount of allergen per pollen grain is variable and difficult to quantify. For ragweed pollen, it has been estimated there is 5 ng of Amb a 1 per pollen grain. This would result in the inhalation of approximately 2.2 μg of Amb a 1 on a daily basis during the ragweed season.

Various sampling devices can be used for indoor air sampling. Indoor sampling has been difficult, particularly for fungal allergens. Fungal spores can be collected on a greased microscope slide or a spore trap. Viable fungal spores can be collected through a vacuum pump and then grown on a culture plate. All houses have fungal

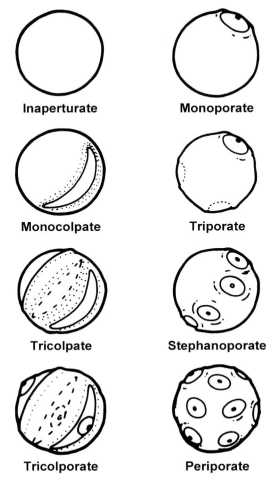

Fig. 2.1 Pollen apertural types

growth, but currently the amount of fungal growth or number of fungal spores associated with allergic symptoms is not known. When sampling for indoor particles, outside air should also be sampled. Most fungal spores originate outdoors, and if the findings are similar for outdoor and indoor sampling, the home is less likely to be the problem. Indoor dust samples can be collected with a vacuum cleaner. The material can be analyzed for specific allergens such as Der p 1 (dust mite) or Fel d 1 (cat) with immunoassay and the results expressed as micrograms of allergen per gram of dust collected. Unlike fungal allergens, quantitated exposure has been associated with increased risk of allergy sensitization or exacerbation. For dust mite allergen, more than 10 μg allergen per gram of dust has been associated with allergen sensitization and exacerbation. This type of analysis is most commonly performed in a research setting.

Although microscopy is still the standard analytical mode for aerobiology monitoring, culture analysis and immunoassay measurements have been used. Culture analysis applies to fungal spores only, not pollens, because only the fungi have the potential for culture media growth. This is helpful because many fungal spores are not sufficiently distinct morphologically for microscopic identification. Cultures are particularly useful in the speciation of *Aspergillus* and *Penicillium*. Disadvantages of the culture method are underestimation of the spore count and inability of all fungal spores to grow on ordinary culture media. Although immunoassays identify allergens directly, without dependence on the morphologic features of the materials sampled, their practical use is currently limited primarily to research centers where immunoassays of specific IgE, IgG, or monoclonal antibodies are available.

The air-sampling devices have increased our awareness and understanding of the airborne allergens. However, resultant pollen counts should be interpreted with caution because of the variability inherent in making these measurements. Collection factors that affect pollen counts include timing of the sample, location, and weather conditions.

Pollen and spore concentrations vary from year to year, day to day, and even hour to hour. The peak times noted at a sampling station are altered by the distance from the pollen source. For example, a sampler located next to a maple tree forest will accurately note when pollination is occurring. However, if the sample station is miles from the source, the peak time will be hours later because of the time needed for the pollen to travel. In addition, it is known that ragweed pollen is released between 6:30 and 8:30 am. At this time, however, the pollen is wet and does not become airborne. Later in the morning, as the pollen dries, it becomes airborne. Thus, ragweed pollen may not be measured at an elevated air sampler (on top of a tall building) until late in the afternoon because of the time required for mixing and transport. Most importantly in regard to time, it must be noted that published or broadcast pollen counts reflect the readings of the previous day.

The location of the air sampler has a direct effect on the air-sampling results. The air sampler should be placed on an elevated surface 16–20 ft above ground. The collecting device should be clear of any obstruction and placed away from trees that may affect the results. Legitimate concern has been raised about whether the sampling obtained from a community rooftop air sampler accurately reflects the eye- and nose-level pollen and spore exposure of a person. Compared with community rooftop samplers, personal samplers have shown differences in both the type and amount of pollen recovered. It should be emphasized that although a pollen count provides general information, it may be difficult to apply this information specifically to an individual. This emphasizes the importance of inquiring about the home and work landscape of the patient.

Weather conditions can affect the pollen count. For example, the wind front preceding a rainstorm usually causes a transient increase in pollen release, followed by a decrease in the pollen count for a few hours after the rain.

Another important variable is the skill of the pollen counter. Identification of the various tree, grass, and weed pollens and particularly fungal spores is difficult, and interobserver variability occurs even among experienced counters.

Even with these difficulties, allergic symptoms correlate positively with the atmospheric pollen counts. The main benefit derived from pollen and spore counts is the identification of the overall pattern to aid in predicting levels in the future.

In simplest terms, trees pollinate in the spring, grasses in the summer, and weeds in the late summer through the autumn. Mold spores do not have a definite seasonal pattern; they are present primarily throughout the warmer months when temperature and moisture conditions are suitable. The seasonal ranges are typical for these groups, but there are year-to-year differences in the onset, the peak pollen concentration, and the length of season for each pollen.

2.2.2   *Tree Pollens*

Tree pollen grains are 20–60 µm in diameter. Despite some cross-reactivity among tree pollen allergens, cross-reactivity is relatively uncommon. Several taxonomic classification systems have been used for trees. Trees are divided into the standard taxonomic categories of division, class, order, family, genus, and species. The closer two trees are related, for example, two trees in the same family as opposed to two trees in the same class, the greater the likelihood for cross-reactivity. Tree pollens are released during the spring season and are often considered the harbinger of the "allergy season." In the U.S. Midwest and Northeast, tree pollination typically occurs from late March to early June, but in Florida and California the season can span 6 months, January–June. The onset of the tree season is determined by seasonal development, primarily the number of warm days preceding pollination in the spring. The amount of pollen produced is affected by the soil moisture levels earlier in the season because this influences the number of buds that develop. In some tree species, the initiation of bud formation occurs during the previous spring; thus, the weather conditions of the previous spring can influence the following year's pollen load. This is unique to tree pollens because the grass and weed pollens depend primarily on the current growing season and weather pattern.

2.2.2.1   Tree Pollens: Division Magnoliophyta, Class Magnoliopsida

Ulmaceae Family (Elm, Hackberry)

Elm and hackberry species are included in the Ulmaceae family. These trees are distributed from the eastern United States through the central plains. Cross-reactivity has not been shown between these species. Although elm trees have been decimated by Dutch elm disease, they are not at risk for extinction because younger trees are relatively resistant to the disease. Elm pollination is intense for a short time, and individual trees may release their pollen load over 2–3 days. Not all elms pollinate in the spring: Chinese elm, red elm, September elm, and cedar elm pollinate in late summer or early autumn. Elm pollens are 25–35 μm in diameter, with a ring of pores around the equatorial circumference of the grain. The surface has rugulate sculpturing, which produces an almost peanut shell-like appearance. Selection of elm and hackberry species should be based on patterns of skin-test reactivity in patients and local tree populations.

Moraceae Family (Mulberry)

The Moraceae family includes the mulberry species, which are widely distributed across the United States from the eastern seaboard to Arizona. Mulberry trees, compared with elm trees, pollinate late in the tree season. No cross-reactivity is known between the Moraceae and Ulmaceae families. Certain members, primarily the mulberries and hops, are highly allergenic.

Plantanaceae species (sycamore) are important sources of pollinating tree allergens in North America and Western Europe. This includes the American sycamore, which is one of the largest broadleaf trees in eastern North America. It is common throughout the eastern United States and the Midwest and extends into southern Ontario. Pollen release occurs in March–May in the south-central and southeastern states and in May–June in the northern portions of the range. Despite shedding abundant pollen, most sycamores are of only moderate importance in allergic rhinitis; however, in California, they are a prominent cause of early spring allergic rhinitis. The pollen grains are typically 18–20 μm in diameter but can vary widely in size and shape. Grains are tricolpate, with a finely reticulate surface. Because there are no definitive studies of allergen cross-reactivity, testing should be determined by the type found in the region.

The family Juglandaceae includes the walnut, pecan, and hickory species distributed from the East Coast to the Rocky Mountains. The black walnut is distributed throughout the Northeast, across the Mississippi into the eastern Great Plains, and south into Texas. Its distribution is limited in the southeastern coastal plains and Florida. Pollination occurs in April–May in the southern regions and in May–June in the northern regions. Walnut pollen is shed in high quantities in the Northeast, but allergic rhinitis is better documented in the western states. Pecan, *Carya*, is shed in enormous amounts in April–June, but because of the large size of the pollen grains, long-range dispersal is not seen. Allergic rhinitis from pecan has been well documented, especially in areas where it is cultivated, the southeastern United States. Hickories account for 10–15% of the pollen load in May–June in the Northeast. Pollen grains of the *Juglans* are approximately 40 μm in diameter, with a granular surface texture and 6–15 pores distributed equatorially and over the dorsal hemisphere. Skin tests show positive correlations between hickory and pecan and a moderate correlation between these and black walnut. Testing should be dictated by regional aerobiological data.

Two closely studied orders of trees are the Fagales and Betulales, which include the oaks (Fagales), beeches (Fagales), and birches and alder (Betulales). They are scattered widely across the United States. There appears to be extensive cross-reactivity between these orders. Recombinant protein studies have shown a strong homology among the major alder allergen Aln g1 and the primary allergens of birch (Bet v 1), hornbeam (Car b 1), and oak (Que a 1).

Oaks of the genus *Quercus* are hardy trees of temperate climate, frequently found with pines. Oaks are identified by their fruit, the acorn, which is edible. Temperate oaks are wind pollinated and often are major inciters of pollinosis during late winter and early spring. In the southeastern and south-central states, live oaks and white oaks pollinate from February–April, with red oaks pollinating in March–May. In northern states, pollen release is usually in May–June. Oak pollen grains are 20–36 μm in diameter and are tricolpate or tricolporate, depending on the species (Fig. 2.2). Beech pollen release is mid-April–May. Although the pollen is buoyant and carried long distances from the source, it is much less abundant than oak and is of less allergenic importance. Birch is a member of Betulales, which also includes alder, hazel, hornbeam, and hop hornbeam. Birches shed enormous amounts of pollen, with a single catkin producing 6 million grains. Pollen release is from April–June. Birches are responsible for significant spring allergic rhinitis in the eastern United States and Canada and in northern Europe. IgE immunoblot cross-inhibition between birch and alder is almost complete. Birch pollen grains are 20–27 μm in diameter and triporate, with a smooth to slightly granular surface texture. Although birch, alder, beech, and oak have strong cross-allergenicity because of the high production of pollen and clear allergy potential, the trees used for testing should be selected on the basis of local prevalence and timing of allergy symptoms. In areas where oaks predominate, the use of a single oak should provide coverage for other oaks. The major birch pollen allergen Bet v 1 has been isolated. This allergen cross-reacts with a low-molecular-weight apple allergen, which helps explain the association between birch tree allergy and the oral allergy sensitivity with apple. This cross-reactivity appears to extend also to pear, celery, carrot, and potato allergens.

The order Salicales includes the willows (*Salix*), poplars, and cottonwoods (*Populus*). Willows are found throughout North America. They release white

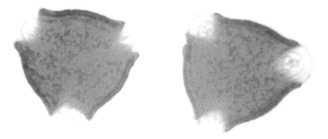

Fig. 2.2 Pollen grains of oak in polar position, with three furrow ends converging

tufted seeds in June. Willow pollen grains have a convex triangular shape and are approximately 25 μm in diameter. They are tricolporate with a reticulate surface. The poplars and cottonwoods are entirely wind pollinated, with separate male and female trees. Cottonwood pollen release is from April–May. Cottonwood seeds have buoyant cottonlike tufts that permeate the air, resembling a snowstorm. Patients may attribute their allergic symptoms to these seeds, but grass pollens are often the true cause. *Populus* pollen grains are 30 μm in diameter and spheroidal, without pores or furrows. The surface is finely granular. On the basis of skin-test correlation, the cross-reactivity among the willows, poplars, and cottonwoods is strong. There is also moderate cross-reactivity between the willows and members of Fagales.

Sapindales and Oleales are two orders within the subclass Rosidae. The Sapindale includes the Aceraceae family, which contains the maples and box elders. Maples are primarily prevalent east of the Great Plains, but they also are distributed in the Pacific Northwest and Rocky Mountains. Among the *Acer*, box elder is the most prolific airborne pollen producer; it accounts for the greatest percentage of *Acer*-induced allergic rhinitis. There does not appear to be significant cross-reactivity among members of the Aceraceae family, as indicated by the poor skin-test correlation between box elder and red maple. Also, no cross-reactivity has been noted with hazel, birch, or alder. Maple pollen grains are tricolpate, 23–36 μm in size, with a rugulate surface texture. The order Oleales includes olive and ash trees. Olive trees are particularly common in the southwest United States, and various species of ash trees are found throughout the United States and Canada. The oleales show significant cross-reactivity among themselves, and, of note, olive trees have also shown significant cross-reactivity with other tree species such as birch, pine, and cypress. Even though olive and ash cross-react, local tree populations should determine whether olive, ash, or both should be included in the clinical evaluation and therapy.

2.2.2.2   Tree Pollens: Division Pinophyta, Subdivision Pinicae

The order Coniferales includes three important tree families: Cupressaceae, Taxodiaceae, and Pinaceae. The Cupressaceae family includes the mountain cedar, Rocky Mountain cedar, white cedar, western red cedar, and eastern red cedar. The mountain cedar is a highly allergenic tree found in Texas and the Ozarks. In south and central Texas, the trees pollinate in mid-December–January and are the primary significant aeroallergen at that time of year. Further north, Rocky Mountain cedar pollinates in late February or March and continues as late as June. The white cedar is found in the Northeast, red cedar in the South and in central states, and the western cedar in the Northwest. The pollen grains of the cedars are 20–35 μm in diameter and have small verrucae scattered irregularly over the surface. The grains do not have pores. There is strong cross-reactivity among members of the Cupressaceae family, which allows a single species to be selected for skin testing and formulation of immunotherapy.

Other conifers, including pines, firs, spruces, and hemlock are not considered to be as important clinically. Even though pines produce copious amounts of buoyant pollen, sensitization is relatively low. This is thought to be due to possible evolutionary tolerance to pine protein or hindered elution of pine allergens because of the waxy resin on the pollen surface. Pine pollen grains have two prominent bladders, which give the grains a distinctive "Mickey Mouse hat" appearance (Fig. 2.3). The size of the grains, including the bladders, varies, 60–100 μm.

2.2.2.3 Tree Pollens: Summary

Because tree pollens have many unique allergens, the species used for testing often needs to be chosen at the level of the genus or family. This is determined by the regional distribution of the plant population and pollen aerobiology. Patterns of cross-reactivity are helpful, particularly in the family Fagaceae, in which only one oak tree may need to be selected, and the family Cupressaceae, in which only one cedar may need to be selected. However, although the elder and maple are in the same family, they do not appear to be cross-reactive. The use of these principles and an understanding of the native plant population provide the most effective means to measure tree pollen allergy. Examples of the most common allergens by geographic region (North America) are listed in Table 2.1. This is not an exhaustive list, and for specific skin testing, the local aerobiological tree pollen counts and the patient's home and work environment should be reviewed.

2.2.3   Grass Pollens

In contrast to tree pollens, grass pollens show remarkable cross-reactivity, but it is not complete. Grass pollens are plentiful in the months of May–July in the Northeast and Midwest, and the seasons are as long as 10–11 months in Florida and

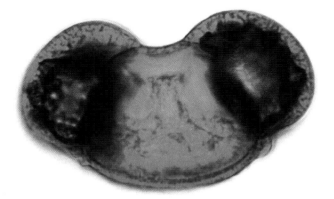

Fig. 2.3 Pine pollen grain. Two air bladders give the pollen grain a distinctive appearance

Table 2.1 Key pollen allergens in North America

Area	Trees (genus)	Grasses (subfamily)	Weeds (genus)
Northeast Connecticut, New York, Delaware, New Jersey, Massachusetts, Rhode Island, Maine, New Hampshire, Vermont, Pennsylvania, Maryland, District of Columbia, West Virginia	Mar–May Oak, white, red (*Quercus*) Elm, white (*Ulmus*) Cottonwood (*Populus*) Beech (*Fagus*) Ash, white (*Fraxinus*) Birch, yellow, paper (*Betula*) Maple, sugar (*Acer*) Aspen, cottonwood, poplar (*Populus*)	May–July June/Kentucky blue (Festucoideae) Orchard (Festucoideae) Timothy (Festucoideae) Sweet vernal (Festucoideae)	July–Sept Ragweed, short (*Ambrosia*) Plantain[a] (*Plantago*) Russian thistle (*Salsola*)
Southeast Kentucky, Tennessee, Georgia, South Carolina, North Carolina, Alabama, Mississippi, Virginia, Arkansas, Louisiana, Florida	Jan–May Elm (*Ulmus*) Ash, white, green (*Fraxinus*) Poplar (*Populus*) Oak, red, white (*Quercus*) Cottonwood (*Populus*) Hickory, pecan (*Carya*) Maple, red (*Acer*) Hackberry (*Celtis*) Cedar, red (*Juniperus*) Mulberry, red, white (*Morus*)	Apr–Nov June/Kentucky blue (Festucoideae) Timothy (Festucoideae) Orchard (Festucoideae) Bermuda (Eragrostoideae) Johnson (Panicoideae)	Aug–Oct Ragweed, short, giant (*Ambrosia*) Marsh elder, rough, burweed (*Iva*) Western water hemp (*Acnida*) Plantain[a] (*Plantago*) Pigweed (*Amaranthus*)
Midwest Ohio, Michigan, Indiana, Illinois, Minnesota, Wisconsin, Iowa, Missouri	Mar–May Elm, white (*Ulmus*) Box elder (*Acer*) Ash, white, green (*Fraxinus*) Oak, red, white (*Quercus*) Hickory, pecan (*Carya*) Mulberry, red (*Morus*) Juniper, red cedar (*Juniperus*) Maple, red, sugar, black, box elder (*Acer*) Birch, yellow, paper (*Betula*)	May–July June/Kentucky blue (Festucoideae) Orchard (Festucoideae) Timothy (Festucoideae) Bermuda (Eragrostoideae) Rye (Festucoideae)	July–Oct Ragweed, short, giant (*Ambrosia*) Burweed, marsh elder (*Iva*) Burning bush (*Kochia*) Russian thistle (*Salsola*)

(continued)

Table 2.1 (continued)

Area	Trees (genus)	Grasses (subfamily)	Weeds (genus)
Great Plains North Dakota, South Dakota, Kansas, Nebraska, Oklahoma, Texas, Colorado, Wyoming, Montana	Feb–May Cottonwood, aspen (*Populus*) Elm, white, cedar[b] (*Ulmus*) Ash, white, green (*Fraxinus*) Box elder (*Acer*) Oak, bur, white (*Quercus*) Mulberry, red (*Morus*) Red cedar, juniper (*Juniperus*) Mountain cedar, juniper[a] (*Juniperus*) Hackberry (*Celtis*) Willow, black (*Salix*)	May–July June/Kentucky blue (Festucoideae) Timothy (Festucoideae) Bermuda (Eragrostoideae)	July–Oct Ragweed, short, giant (*Ambrosia*) Burning bush (*Kochia*) Russian thistle (*Salsola*) Western water hemp (*Acnida*) Marsh elder, burweed (*Iva*) Plaintain[a] (*Plantago*)
Southwest Arizona, New Mexico, Nevada, Utah, California	Dec–May Mountain cedar (*Juniperus*) Ash, velvet (*Fraxinus*) Juniper, cedar (*Juniperus*) Elm (*Ulmus*) Mulberry, white (*Morus*) Olive (*Olea*) Oak (*Quercus*)	Apr–Sept Bermuda (Eragrostoideae) Johnson (Panicoideae)	June–Oct Ragweed, canyon, rabbit bush, burroweed[c] (*Ambrosia*) Russian thistle (*Salsola*) Sage (*Artemisia*) Scales (*Atriplex*)
Northwest Idaho, Oregon, Washington	Jan–May Alder, red, white (*Alnus*) Cedar, juniper (*Juniperus*) Cottonwood, black, aspen (*Populus*) Birch, paper (*Betula*) Box elder (*Acer*) Walnut, English (*Juglans*)	May–Aug June/Kentucky blue (Festucoideae) Sweet vernal (Festucoideae)	June–Sept Sorrel, dock (*Rumex*) Sage (*Artemisia*)

[a] Okla and Tex Dec–Mar
[b] Okla and Tex Aug–Oct
[c] Mar–May
[d] June–Aug

southern California. Grass pollens typically are 30–40 μm in diameter, and they usually are released in the afternoon. Most temperate grasses grow from seed each year, so the time of onset and the amount of pollen released depend on the moisture, sun exposure, and daily weather patterns of the season.

2.2.3.1 Grass Pollens: Division Magnoliophyta, Class Liliopsida

Most grass allergens are found in the family Poaceae, which includes the subfamilies Festucoideae, Eragrostoideae, and Panicoideae. These subfamilies are divided further into tribes. Members within a tribe would be expected to have more similarity than members of different tribes or subfamilies.

The subfamily Festucoideae contains the most important grass pollen allergens in North America. This subfamily consists of five tribes that account for the major northern pasture grasses. These tribes are Poeae (Kentucky bluegrass, orchard, fescue, brome, and ryegrass), Avenae (oat and velvet grass), Phalarideae (sweet vernal), Agrostideae (timothy, redtop, and foxtail), and Triticeae (western wheatgrass and the cereal grains). Kentucky bluegrass is one of the most important commercial perennial grasses in the United States. It produces abundant seed that is highly viable; it also is a strong sod builder and is used extensively for lawns. This grass is abundant throughout the northern states and mountainous regions but less common in southern states, where hot, dry summers cause it to wilt and "brown out." In the central states, pollen release begins in mid-May and peaks in June. It is estimated that Kentucky bluegrass, together with orchard grass, accounts for more grass pollinosis in the eastern United States than all other grasses combined. Commercially, timothy is the most important perennial grass in the United States. It is widely cultivated for hay. Timothy is grown in the Northeast, west to the Missouri River, and south to Missouri. Depending on the region, pollen release is between May–October. All members of the Festucoideae are strongly cross-reactive; timothy grass and sweet vernal may possess unique antigens.

The subfamily Eragrostoideae includes Bermuda grass, which is found primarily across the central and southern United States. It is resistant to drought and alkali and found in irrigated portions of the Southwest. In the warmer areas of its distribution, pollination occurs from February–December, but in the northern part of its range, pollination may only occur from July–October. Other tribe members include windmill, buffalo, and grama grasses of the western prairie. Bermuda grass also appears to contain unique allergens, with little cross-reactivity with temperate grasses.

The subfamily Panicoideae contains Bahia grass and Johnson grass, which are found primarily in southern North America. Despite being considered a southern grass, Johnson grass can be found through Iowa and Kansas and the western states. Pollination overlaps closely with the Bermuda grasses. Johnson grass shows moderate cross-reactivity with both northern pasture grasses and southern grasses. Bahia grass contains some unique allergens.

Fig. 2.4 Pollen grain of timothy grass. All grasses are monoporate, and various grasses usually are not distinguished on the basis of pollen count identification

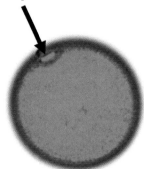

Because all grass pollen grains generally have a similar appearance, an effort is not usually made to describe individual species on pollen sampling. Grass pollen grains are all monoporate, spherical, and 22–122 μm in size (Fig. 2.4).

2.2.3.2 Grass Pollens: Summary

Because of extensive cross-reactivity among grasses, testing with timothy grass in combination with a single northern grass provides coverage in the Northeast and most of the Midwest. Species with less cross-reactivity and unique allergens, such as Bermuda, Bahia, and Johnson grasses, deserve individual consideration, particularly in the southern regions, where they are prominent.

Examination of grass pollen extracts with immunochemical methods has shown approximately 40 different antigens with variable ability to bind IgE. Grass pollen allergens have been categorized into eight groups on the basis of chemical and immunologic characteristics. Group I allergens are of major importance because with skin testing 90–95% of patients allergic to grass pollen have a reaction. High cross-reactivity has been observed between group I allergens from different grass species. Examples of grass group I allergens include Poa p 1 (Kentucky bluegrass), Phl p 1 (timothy), Cyn d 1 (Bermuda), Dac g 1 (orchard), and Sor h 1 (Johnson). Groups II–VIII show significant but lesser degrees of reaction among those with IgE sensitization.

The most commonly found grasses in different geographic regions are listed in Table 2.1.

2.2.4 Weed Pollens

Weed pollens are typically the "third wave" of the seasonal pollens; in the midwest and northeast United States, they are released in late July and are prevalent until the first hard frost. Ragweed is the most important cause of allergic rhinitis and pollen asthma in North America. The seasonal onset of weed pollen release depends on seasonal sunlight exposure, with flowering initiated by lengthening nights. Typically, the pollen is released during the early morning hours. Once released, dispersion is affected by wind and moisture. High temperature, wind, and dry air favor dispersal. Ragweed pollen travels a long distance and has been detected 400 miles out to sea. Because of the amount of spread, weed eradication is futile.

2.2.4.1 Weed Pollens: Subfamily Asteroideae

The subfamily Asteroideae contains four major allergenic tribes: Heliantheae (sunflower), Ambrosieae (short ragweed, giant ragweed, southern ragweed, western ragweed, false ragweed, slender ragweed, silver ragweed, and cocklebur), Anthemideae (mugwort, wormwood, prairie sage, and daisy), and Astereae (goldenrod). Ambrosieae and Anthemideae are significant allergens for essentially all of North America. The four ragweeds of major importance are giant, short, western, and false. Ragweeds are prolific pollen producers and are the predominant cause of late summer allergic rhinitis in the central and eastern states. In portions of the Northeast and south-central states, ragweed accounts for 75–90% of all pollen captured between August–October. Giant ragweed generally begins pollination 2–3 weeks before short ragweed. Cross-reactivity of crude extracts of the four major ragweeds is strong, based on RAST inhibition. There appears to be significant cross-reactivity within the Ambrosieae and Anthemideae tribes and between them. Typical ragweed pollen grains are triporate, with a mean diameter of approximately 20 μm. They are covered with broad-based conical spines that resemble spikes (Fig. 2.5). Mugwort is found mainly on the east coast and in the midwestern United States. The pollen grains are spheroidal and 15–30 μm in diameter. They have a thick exine and essentially no spines.

2.2.4.2 Weed Pollens: Order Chenopodiales (Chenopod-Amaranths)

The order Chenopodiales contains the family Chenopodiaceae, which includes lamb's-quarter, Russian thistle, burning bush (the Great Plains tumbleweeds), and the family Amaranthaceae, which includes pigweed. The Chenopod-Amaranth weeds are generally prolific producers of pollen and are major inducers of pollinosis throughout the Great Plains and western states. Pollination occurs from June–November, with peaks in August. Cross-reactivity varies among the Chenopod-Amaranth weeds. Russian thistle seems to be the most allergenically potent weed. Chenopod-Amaranth pollen grains are spheroid, 10–40 μm in size, and periporate. Pores are scattered evenly over the surface of the grain, which resembles a golf ball. Because of their similarities, Chenopod-Amaranth weeds are typically identified on the family level.

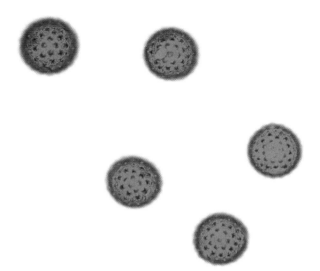

Fig. 2.5 Ragweed pollen grains. The grains are characterized by multiple broad-based conical spines, giving the grain a "spiked" appearance

2.2.4.3   Weed Pollens: Order Polygonales

The order Polygonales includes the family Polygonaceae, which contains sheep sorrel, swamp dock, and water dock. These are found throughout North America, especially in western North America. Sheep sorrel pollinates in late spring to early summer, and at the height of pollination, its pollen counts approach those of grasses. The allergenic importance of Sheep sorrel is probably underestimated because of the overlap with grass pollination. The pollen grains are spheroid, 22–30 μm in diameter, and tetracolporate, with globular, densely packed cytoplasmic starch granules. The cross-reactivity among these weeds is not well defined.

2.2.4.4   Weed Pollens: Order Scrophulariales

This order includes the family Plantaginaceae, which contains English and black-seed plantain. Unlike other weeds, this one sheds pollen primarily in May–June and, thus, can be confused with late tree or grass pollinosis. It is found throughout North America.

2.2.4.5   Weed Pollens: Summary

There does not seem to be significant cross-reactivity among the different orders of weed pollens, and representative pollens from the various orders are required for testing. Within the subfamily Asteroidieae, however, a ragweed may also cover for mugwort. Numerous ragweed tests do not need to be performed because, on the basis of cross-reactivity, one appears to be representative. In view of the limited information on cross-reactivity, individual species of Chenopod-Amaranth weeds are likely required.

Ragweed pollen extract contains more than 50 antigens, but only about one-half of them are allergens, as shown by their binding of specific IgE from ragweed-sensitive patients. Not all these allergens have been fully characterized. Two major ragweed allergens, Amb a 1 and Amb a 2, have been isolated, as have minor allergens Amb a 3, 5, 6, and 7. Techniques are available that allow direct quantitation of Amb a 1 in allergenic extracts to help assess the potency of the extract. In addition to the short ragweed allergens, other allergens have been characterized from other weeds, including Russian thistle (Sal p 1), mugwort (Art v 1-4), and lamb's-quarter (Che a 1).

The most common weeds are listed by geographic region in Table 2.1.

2.2.5   Environmental Control: Outdoor Pollens

Because pollen grains are ubiquitous during the season of release, complete avoidance is impossible. It is worthwhile informing patients that pollen is not found just in the vicinity of various trees, grasses, and weeds but occurs throughout the outdoor environment because of air mixing and travel. The overall strategy is to decrease large exposures to pollen. Although the following measures have not been studied rigorously, they help decrease exposure to pollen:

1. Avoid lawn mowing, gardening, or other activities involving hands-on exposure to tree, grass, and weed pollens
2. Keep house windows closed during pollen season
3. Perform outdoor activities in the early morning before pollens typically are dispersed
4. Place clothes in the wash or in a laundry bag and shower when entering the house after prolonged exposure outdoors

These recommendations may help decrease exposure to a large amount of pollen and, thus, decrease allergic symptoms. With the difficulty inherent in avoiding the outdoor atmospheric environment, these recommendations are not expected to render the patient symptom free.

2.3   Fungal Allergens

Fungi are eukaryotic, unicellular or multicellular, plantlike organisms that do not contain chlorophyll. They are mostly spore-bearing organisms that exist as saprophytes or parasites of animals and plants. Molds have been defined as a furry growth of microscopic fungi or fungi that produce microscopic reproductive structures. Thus, fungi and molds are not entirely synonymous, but the terms are often used interchangeably. The role of fungi in producing allergic and respiratory symptoms is well established and has been described since the early 1700s. More recently, fungal sensitivity has been shown with skin-test reactivity and inhalation challenge studies. Spore concentrations required to provoke symptoms depend on the species, for example, 50–100 m^{-3} for *Alternaria* and 3,000 m^{-3} for *Cladosporium*. Although fungal spores are thought to be causative agents of allergic reactions, other particles that become airborne, including mycelial fragments, may trigger an allergic reaction. Fungal spores are structurally different from pollens because the inhaled particles consist of entire living cells capable of growing and secreting allergens in vivo. In the natural environment, people are exposed to more than 100 species of airborne fungi. Colonies of the fungi *Aspergillus fumigatus*, *Alternaria alternata*, *Cladosporium herbarum*, *Penicillium*, and *Fusarium* are universally present in our environment; hence, there is no fungi-free environment.

2.3.1   Classification

The fungi constitute a very large and diverse set of organisms, and the taxonomy is complicated. Classification schemes have undergone numerous revisions to develop a system easier to follow. Most fungi produce sexual and asexual spores, and the taxonomy is based on spore characteristics such as size, shape, color, and surface ornamentation. The major taxonomic groups of fungi that are currently recognized are the ascomycetes, basidiomycetes, and zygomycetes. Some texts also refer to a separate group, the deuteromycetes, or Fungi Imperfecti. The deuteromycetes are an artificial grouping of asexual fungal stages and are primarily forms of ascomycetes that produce asexual spores called conidia. Deuteromycetes (Fungi Imperfecti) contains a large number of allergenic fungi that reproduce asexually by the differentiation of specialized hyphae called conidiophores. The species are characterized by the morphology of the conidia. The asexual ascomycetes (Deuteromycetes) include *Aspergillus*, *Penicillium*, *Alternaria*, *Cladosporium*, *Fusarium*, *Epicoccum*, *Drechslera*, and *Curvularia*.

Perhaps more useful to allergy is the ecological groupings of fungi (Table 2.2). These groupings pair fungi that sporulate in response to similar environmental conditions. This results in high spore counts of these types, with a similar exposure. The three general ecological types of fungi are the phyllophane fungi, basidiomycetes, and the soil and litter fungi.

Phyllophane fungi live on the surface of leaves, and most of them are deuteromycetes. Known allergens in this group are *Cladosporium*, *Alternaria*, *Epicoccum*, and *Curvularia*. Because phyllophane fungi live on the leaf surface, they have adapted to continual wetting and drying cycles, sunlight exposure, and exudates from the leaves. This hardiness also allows for survival in the indoor environment. The shower wall can mimic a leaf surface, with a wet-dry cycle and skin scales-soap residues that serve as a nutrient source. Although these fungi are

Table 2.2 Ecological classification of common allergenic fungi

Phyllophane
Alternaria
Cladosporium
Epicoccum
Curvularia
Basidiomycetes
Pleurotus
Ganoderma
Calvatia
Coprinus
Rusts
Smuts
Soil and litter
Penicillium
Aspergillus
Fusarium

detected indoors, they are primarily outdoor fungal allergens. The spores in this group are passively liberated. They must be positioned so that air currents can pick them up. Blowing wind is often sufficient to release them. These spores are like dust; thus, they are held by wet surfaces and become airborne in greater quantities during dry conditions. Dry, windy days during the growing season tend to have high spore concentrations of these fungi. Patients with a strong allergy to *Alternaria*, for example, may want to avoid walking in or near the woods on these days. Peak levels are typically found in the early afternoon, after the organisms have dried from the morning dew.

Basidiomycetes includes mushrooms, puffballs, and conks. Several basidiomycetes are known to produce allergens. Basidiomycetes typically live on plants or as decomposers of wood and are found primarily in shade trees, lawns, parks, or wherever wood becomes sufficiently wet to decay. Basidiomycetes also includes rust and smut fungi. They are the primary pathogens for plants and produce spores recognized as allergens. The prevalence of reactivity to basidiomycetes appears comparable to that of deuteromycetes, but very few commercial extracts are available. Unlike phyllophane fungi, the spores of the basidiomycetes are actively discharged. This propels the spores into the air currents; thus, they are not dependent on dry, windy conditions. The discharge can sometimes be seen as a puff or cloud of spores. The near-ground concentrations of basidiospores are frequently highest between midnight and 6 am.

The soil and litter fungi are primarily deuteromycetes. Well-known members of this group are *Penicillium*, *Aspergillus*, and *Fusarium*. *Penicillium* and *Aspergillus* are considered the most common indoor allergens, but they also are measured outdoors. These fungi can be found in moist soil, wet leaves, or other decaying organic matter. They are found indoors in indoor dust, particularly in high humidity. When cellulose building materials, for example, wallpaper, paper coating on wallboard, and acoustic ceiling tiles, are wet, they provide an environment for the fungi to flourish. Most soil and litter fungi passively release their spores. Disturbing mulch or decaying organic matter releases plumes of spores from soil and litter fungi. Patients allergic to *Aspergillus* or *Penicillium* should avoid old wet piles of leaves and avoid handling wet yard wastes and composting activities.

The rest of this section focuses on the characteristics of commonly encountered fungi allergens.

2.3.2   *Alternaria alternata*

Alternaria alternata, an ascomycete and deuteromycete, is one of the most important of the allergenic fungi. It is known to be an important cause of rhinoconjunctivitis and bronchospasm in patients with asthma. There is an association between *Alternaria* sensitization and life-threatening asthma. *Alternaria* is found in the air year round, with peak levels from late summer to autumn. *Alternaria* thrives best on plants in the field and decaying plant parts in the soil. Satisfactory substrates are found in the soil, on foods, and on textiles. Rotting wood, wood pulp, and compost are common sites. *Alternaria* is one of the most common mold spores found in house dust in homes in North America and Europe. Counts of *Alternaria* are highest on dry, windy days.

Recent advances have been made in characterizing the *A. alternata* allergens. The major allergenic fraction Alt a 1 has been cloned, but its biological function is unclear. About 90% of *Alternaria*-sensitive patients react positively to skin testing with this fraction. Minor allergens of *A. alternata* have also been isolated and characterized, including Alt a 2, Alt a 3, Alt a 4, Alt a 6, Alt a 7, Alt a 10, Alt a 11, and Alt a 12. Response rates to these allergens are in the range of 10–60%. Cross-reactivity among molds is difficult to assess because it is unclear how much protein similarity there is between life stages. Varying degrees of cross-reactivity have been shown between *Alternaria*, *Stemphylium*, and *Curvularia*. Alt a 1 is abundant in *Stemphylium*. The *Alternaria* spores are 20–60 µm long and club shaped. They are segmented, with both transverse and longitudinal septa, and easily recognizable on slides taken from air samplers.

2.3.3   *Aspergillus*

Aspergillus, a deuteromycete, is sometimes referred to as a "storage fungus" because it is found in stored grain, fruits, and vegetables. In a subset of patients with asthma, *Aspergillus* is a major factor in causing allergic bronchopulmonary aspergillosis (ABPA) (discussed in depth in chapter on asthma). ABPA is a unique entity – a marked hypersensitivity response characterized by an IgE and IgG response to *Aspergillus* that is associated with markedly elevated total IgE, eosinophilia, and bronchiectasis – that is separate from typical IgE-mediated allergic sensitivity. Besides *Aspergillus fumigatus*, which has the major role in ABPA, other species of *Aspergillus* have also been reported to cause more typical IgE-mediated allergic disease in humans. *Aspergillus*, unlike *Alternaria*, thrives on a substrate with a low moisture content. It is cultured from homes, particularly from basements, crawl spaces, and bedding. *Aspergillus* is of the dry spore type and is released by the wind during dry periods.

Numerous *Aspergillus* antigens have been identified. *Aspergillus fumigatus* extracts are generally prepared from culture filtrate material instead of spores. The allergen Asp f 1 has been cloned and found to be secreted from the fungus only during growth. In combination with Asp f 3 and Asp f 5, Asp f 1 has a sensitivity of 97% for diagnosing *Aspergillus* sensitivity.

Recombinant *Aspergillus* antigens may show promise in diagnosis of ABPA, for example, allergens Asp f 4 and Asp f 6 are only recognized by patients with ABPA, and Asp f 3 and Asp f 5 are recognized by patients with *Aspergillus* sensitivity who do or do not have ABPA.

2.3.4 *Cladosporium herbarum*

Cladosporium herbarum, a deuteromycete, is widely distributed in the environment and is a major source of fungal inhalant allergens (Fig. 2.6). Whereas *Alternaria alternata* is found more prominently in warm, humid climates, *Cladosporium* is the leading fungus in cooler climates, particularly Scandinavia. *Cladosporium* is considered a "field fungus" and requires a substrate with a relatively high moisture content. It is prevalent from spring through the autumn, and levels decrease sharply with the first hard frost.

Three major *Cladosporium herbarum* allergens have been purified and characterized: Cla h 1, Cla h 2, and Cla h 4. *Cladosporium* contains enolase, a highly

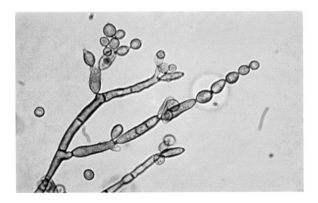

Fig. 2.6 Cladosporium

conserved major allergen in most fungi. Approximately 25–50% of patients allergic to *Alternaria* and *Cladosporium* show IgE binding to enolase.

2.3.5   Penicillium

Penicillium, a deuteromycete, is a prevalent indoor fungal allergen. *Penicillium* is referred to as a "storage fungus" because it is found in stored grain, fruits, and vegetables. In the presence of moisture, different species grow in particleboard and wallboard and behind paint. *Penicillium* is the green mildew often found on articles stored in basements. It is the third most common airborne allergen. Inhalation of *Penicillium* by sensitive persons can induce both immediate and late asthma responses in addition to rhinitis.

Many antigens from various species of *Penicillium* have been identified as allergens and characterized. The allergen Pen c 3 shows homology with Asp f 3 (*Aspergillus*), and Pen c 22 is similar to Asp f 22. IgE antibodies against *Penicillium* antigens have been found in 16–26% of asthmatic patients. *Penicillium* spores are 2–4 μm long and resemble a paint brush. *Penicillium* spores cannot be identified by microscopic observation alone because its features are similar to those of other spores such as *Aspergillus*. Culture is needed for identification.

2.3.6   Basidiomycetes

Basidiomycetes comprises the physically largest and most complex fungi. These include mushrooms, puffballs, rusts, and smuts. Despite being implicated as allergenic fungi, their allergens are not well characterized. *Ganoderma* has been widely studied as wood-decaying allergenic fungi. These fungi produce large shelflike fruiting bodies called rackets or conks. IgE-binding bands are mostly 18–82 kDa, but no purified antigens have been obtained.

2.3.7   Other Fungi

Although several fungi have been implicated in allergic disorders, they have not been characterized further to define reliable antigens. Other deuteromycetes that have commonly been implicated include *Helminthosporium*, *Fusarium*, *Aureobasidium* (Pullaria), *Curvularia*, and *Stemphylium*.

Helminthosporium and *Fusarium* are field fungi that propogate in the field and release their spores when the soil is disturbed. *Aureobasidium* (Pullaria) is a non-fermentative yeast that requires a sugary fluid for its substrate, primarily leaves. This is one of the wet-weather spores with counts that increase with the rain. Other wet-weather spores include *Trichoderma* and *Phoma*. Dry and wet fungal spore dispersion is summarized in Table 2.3.

Table 2.3 Fungal spore dispersion

Disperse in dry conditions
Alternaria
Cladosporium
Epicoccum
Curvularia
Helminthosporium

Disperse in wet conditions
Aureobasidium (Pullaria)
Trichoderma
Phoma

2.3.8   Avoidance of Fungal Allergens

Avoidance of fungal allergens can be divided into avoidance of indoor fungal exposure and avoidance of outdoor fungal exposure.

Fungal spore counts are highest in the living room, followed by the kitchen, bathroom, and bedroom. The principle for reducing indoor fungal exposure is to control indoor moisture. The relative humidity indoors should be kept below 50%. Leaks should be sealed to prevent the accumulation of water. Bathroom and kitchen ventilation should be increased with the use of exhaust fans. Air conditioning should be used during the summer months and at times of high levels of humidity. A dehumidifier should be used in the basement or other areas of dampness. Carpets, wallpaper, paneling, and heating and air conditioning systems should be observed carefully because they can harbor fungal spores. If marked contamination is noted, replacement may be necessary. Washable wallpaper and paneling can be treated with bleach and detergent solutions; however, care must be taken when applying these solutions. Replacement of carpeting with hardwood, tile, or other types of firm flooring is advantageous, particularly if dampness is a problem in the house.

Avoidance of outdoor fungal spores is similar to avoidance measures for tree, grass, and weed pollens. It is especially important to avoid cool damp areas such as composts or grain silos and farming activities such as cutting and bailing hay. Also, construction areas or other places where soil is being turned over should be avoided.

2.4   Indoor Allergens

2.4.1   Mite Allergens

House dust has been recognized as a source of respiratory allergy for many centuries. Mites are now accepted as the major source of allergens in house dust. These microarthropods have a worldwide distribution. Domestic mite is the term used for all mite species that can be found in an indoor environment. House dust mites live in carpets, soft furnishings, and mattresses. In addition to domestic mites, storage mites are found in stored grain, barns, hay, and straw. Some species of storage mites can be found in the house under specific conditions. Domestic mites contain many allergens; thus far, 19 groups of mite allergens have been characterized. The common house dust mites are *Dermatophagoides farinae* and *D. pteronyssinus*. The term *Dermatophagoides* means "skin eating." The two species names *pteronyssinus* and *farinae* mean "feather loving" and "flour," respectively. *D. farinae* but not *D. pteronyssinus*, can be found in baking mixes. *D. farinae* and *D. pteronyssinus* are found in most homes in humid climates in the United States. Studies have shown that houses in areas such as New Mexico and Arizona once believed to be too dry to support mite populations can contain significant levels of dust mite allergen.

Mites have an exoskeleton, jointed appendages, and a hemocoel. The life cycle of house dust mites consists of five stages: the egg, larva, protonymph, tritonymph, and adult. House dust mites have a well-developed digestive tract, including mouth parts, salivary glands, and gut. The digestive system produces spherical fecal pellets approximately 20 µm in diameter. The respiration of mites is cutaneous, and dehydration of the body regulates colonization and population growth. For successful completion of the life cycle, mites require a relative humidity of 70–90%. A temperature of 25°C is required for successful reproduction. The development of *D. farinae* and *D. pteronyssinus* from egg to adult takes 19–33 days.

Mite allergens can be detected in many areas of the house, including beds, carpets, upholstered furniture, and clothing. Mites are also present, but in fewer numbers, on leather-covered couches, wood furniture, and bare floors. Because beds provide the ideal temperature, food, and moisture, they are the ideal habitat for mites. Mite allergens are present in mite bodies, secreta, and excreta. Fecal particles contain the greatest proportion of mite allergen. Mite allergens have been characterized and labeled Der p 1-7 and Der f 1-7. A single dust mite contains approximately 0.02 µg of mite allergen. The mite allergens include cysteine proteases, serine proteases, amylase, glutathione transferases, and tropomyosins.

A seasonal variation has been observed in the number of house dust mites in house dust. In North America, mite growth is maximal during the summer months when indoor relative humidity conditions are most favorable for mite survival and breeding. The major factors governing mite propagation are temperature and humidity. When the relative humidity is less than 50%, and the temperature is above 25°C, mites are not able to survive more than 11 days because of dehydration. Mite allergens are consistently higher in the air during room disturbance (cleaning) than in undisturbed conditions. Mite allergens remain airborne for only a short time.

Mite allergen levels are usually greatest in humid locations and least in dry, high altitudes. The main domestic mite species in the United States are *D. pteronyssinus*, *D. farinae*, *Euroglyphus maynei*, and *Blomia tropicalis*. In temperate climates worldwide, *D. pteronyssinus* and *D. farinae* are the predominate house dust mites. In tropical and subtropical areas, *B. tropicalis* occurs with high frequency.

Cross-reactivity is a common feature among mite allergens, particularly those from closely related taxonomic species. In addition, mites contain species-specific allergens. The clinical relevance of cross-reacting allergens is not well understood.

Mite and allergen surveys in the United States indicate that in most geographic areas both *D. pteronyssinus* and *D. farinae* should be considered when diagnosing or treating patients with mite allergies. Although a house could only contain one species of mite, most houses are coinhabited by *D. pteronyssinus* and *D. farinae*. *E. maynei* and *B. tropicalis* are found in houses in humid climates, such as Florida and the Gulf Coast, but testing is limited by lack of diagnostic test reagents.

2.4.2 Mite Allergen Avoidance

The first line of treatment in allergy is to avoid the allergen if possible. With knowledge of the survival requirements of dust mites, environmental measures have been implemented to decrease exposure (Table 2.4). Several studies have used various environmental modifications, but the results have been mixed. The main conclusion of these studies has been that studies of environmental modification are difficult to conduct because of confounding allergen exposure, and a comprehensive program needs to be implemented for significant reduction of allergen exposure and subsequent clinical improvement. Single control measures are not effective in mite avoidance, and multiple methods are needed to affect the multiple factors that contribute to high levels of mites.

Environmental control can be helpful in several stages of the sensitization and disease processes. It can be used to prevent or delay sensitization or to control symptoms after an individual has been sensitized. There is a significant dose–response relation between exposure to mite allergens and subsequent sensitization. Institution

Table 2.4 Measures for avoiding indoor allergens

Dust mite
  Encase mattress, pillow in impermeable covers
  Wash bedding in hot cycle (55–60°C) weekly
  Replace carpets with wood or linoleum flooring
  Minimize upholstered furniture
  Limit dust-accumulating objects

Pet allergen
  Remove pet from home

If pet not removed:
  Keep pet out of main living area and bedroom
  Install HEPA filters in main living areas and bedroom

Fungi
  Reduce humidity in home to <50%
  Install HEPA filters in main living areas and bedroom
  Check home for signs of water damage, visible mold growth

Cockroach
  Remove food and water sources
  Use pesticide in bait form

HEPA high-efficiency particulate air

of allergen avoidance measures early in life has helped decrease the frequency of allergic symptoms caused by mites. Mite-sensitive patients studied in a setting with a low level of mites have also shown improved symptoms. Therefore, effective avoidance of mites, through a combination of methods, is clinically useful for preventing and treating dust mite allergy. Each indoor environment is unique and allergen levels vary from room to room; therefore, environmental control measures need to be tailored to each component of the house.

Interventions in the house have two interrelated objectives: (1) to decrease mite allergen levels and (2) to reduce human exposure. In selecting the methods used to accomplish this, the following need to be considered: the cost of the intervention, the ease with which it can be implemented, the safety of the intervention, and the expected benefit. A comprehensive plan requires several methods. The main intervention methods currently used include encasements, humidity reduction, washing and drying of bedding materials, vacuuming carpets, freezing soft toys and small items, and replacement of carpets, draperies, and upholstery.

Encasement of the mattress and pillows in mite-impermeable coverings is effective in reducing exposure to house dust mite allergens. To be effective, the pore size of the encasement should be 20 µm or less. This prevents entry of dust mite larvae, which can be as large as 50 µm. To be comfortable, these encasements should be vapor permeable and made from breathable fabrics. Various types of encasements are available, including plastic, finely woven cotton or satin, or nonwoven synthetics. After a mattress or pillow has been encased, little maintenance is required. Some manufacturers recommend wiping the encasements with a damp cloth at the time the bedding is being washed. Encasements are effective in trapping mites present in the mattress, and air-sampling studies have not shown a significant difference in mite allergen in rooms with an encased old mattress or an encased new mattress. Unexpectedly, new synthetic and non-feather pillows have been shown to contain more dust mite allergen than feather pillows. This may be explained by the more tightly woven fabric covers on feather pillows. Therefore, the covering is important, and apparently a feather pillow can be used if it is properly encased.

Moisture is critical for mite survival, and adjustment of the humidity in the house affects exposure to dust mite allergen. Maintaining the relative humidity below 50% is recommended for persons with dust mite allergy. Adult dust mites die in 5–11 days at temperatures of 25–34°C when exposed to a relative humidity of 40–50%. Seasonal fluctuations in levels of mite allergen parallel fluctuations in indoor relative humidity. The use of high-efficiency dehumidifiers and air conditioners in houses has been helpful in decreasing the relative humidity. In a humid temperate climate, the relative humidity can be maintained below 50%. Also, even when the relative humidity increases above 50% for less than 8 hours, the mite population is still restricted as long as the relative humidity is less than 50% the rest of the time. Higher humidity levels generally are recorded in basements; therefore, if possible, the basement should not be used for bedrooms.

The washing of sheets, pillow cases, blankets, and mattress pads at least weekly in hot (55°C) water kills mites and removes allergens. This is extremely important to do in conjunction with encasements, because the washing rids the environment of the current mite population. Washing in warm or cold water does not kill most mites, but does help reduce mite allergen because allergens are water soluble. Tumble drying blankets can kill mites if a temperature higher than 55°C is maintained for 10 minutes. Dry cleaning of fabrics can kill mites but does not remove all allergens.

Carpets, draperies, and upholstery fabrics provide an ideal environment for mites by holding moisture and nutrients. In humid climates, it is recommended where possible that carpets be replaced with hard surfaces. Also, draperies can be replaced with blinds or shades. In the most used areas of the house, fabric upholstery can be replaced with vinyl or leather coverings. Wooden furniture is also recommended.

In houses with carpeting, weekly vacuuming and frequent replacement of vacuum bags are recommended. Vacuum bags with two layers or a high-efficiency particulate air filter are recommended to help prevent aerosolization of allergens during vacuuming. After vacuuming is completed, the patient should stay out of the room for 30 min to allow aerosolized mite allergen to settle. Hot steam cleaning can remove mites and allergens from surfaces but does not eliminate deep populations of mites. Any residual water will increase the humidity and promote growth of the mite population.

Freezing soft toys, such as stuffed animals, and other small items at −17°C to −20°C for at least 24 hours is effective for killing the mite population on these objects. After the items have been frozen, they can be washed to remove the dead mites. In a cold climate, leaving mattresses and pillows outside for at least 24 hours can kill mites.

Other measures with questionable results have been reported for mite control. An air-cleaning or filtration system in undisturbed spaces does not help to decrease the mite population because the mites and their allergen have already settled out, which means that essentially mite-free air is being filtered. The cleaning of ducts has not been shown to be particularly helpful in reducing mite populations, likely because mites normally do not reside in heating, ventilating, and air conditioning systems. Additional studies are needed to determine whether duct cleaning helps reduce mite allergen in the air from heating vents. The use of chemicals and acaricides on carpets and upholstery has produced mixed results in the control of dust mites and their allergens. Although these agents possibly are useful in specific situations, their general use is not highly recommended.

2.5 Animal Allergens

Animal allergens, primarily mammals, are common causes of both acute and chronic allergic disease. People come into contact with animals at home and through occupational exposure and recreational activities. In the household environment, cat and dog allergy predominate, but other household pets such as mice, hamsters, guinea pigs, and gerbils are also sources of allergens. Exposure to pet allergens is not limited to direct contact. Dog and cat allergens become airborne and disperse and can stick to clothing. They are consistently found in houses and public buildings such as schools that do not contain pets. These concentrations are typically low, but they may be high enough to cause symptoms in sensitized persons. Occupations bring people into contact with animals, and allergy to laboratory animals is a worldwide occupational problem. Exposure occurs through the respiratory tract, conjunctiva, and skin. Common laboratory animals such as the mouse, rat, guinea pig, hamster, rabbit, and dog are effective as sensitizers. The highest concentrations of allergens are encountered during the emptying and cleaning of cages. In most cases, symptoms of laboratory animal allergy appear within 2–3 years of exposure; in contrast, cattle sensitivity in farmers can take more than 20 years to develop. Recreationally, horseback riding can produce sensitization and subsequent allergic symptoms with exposure to horses. Dander is the term used to describe desquamated epithelium. The dander contains many proteins that are highly allergenic. Hair itself is not an important allergen, but it harbors water-soluble proteins of epidermal or salivary origin that are important allergens. These proteins are important in pet allergy. Rodents, however, excrete significant amounts of allergenic protein in their urine. All these substances become part of the particulate matter of the air, where they are encountered to trigger respiratory allergy.

Over the past 20 years, the molecular structure, immunogenicity, and environmental distribution of major animal allergens have been defined and characterized. One intriguing finding is that almost all important mammalian respiratory allergens belong to the lipocalin family of proteins, with the exception of Fel d 1 of cat. Lipocalins are a large protein group found in vertebrate and invertebrate animals, plants, and bacteria, including milk allergen (Bos d 5) and cockroach allergen (Bla g 4). The overall amino acid identity between lipocalins is usually less than 20%. Lipocalins are typically small, extracellular proteins that are able to bind small, principally hydrophobic molecules, to attach to specific cell surface receptors, and to form covalent and noncovalent complexes with soluble macromolecules in hydrophilic environments. Lipocalins function as transport molecules and enzymes and show immunomodulatory activity. In animals, the majority of lipocalins are produced in the liver or secretory glands.

2.5.1 Cat Allergen

Cat allergens are the most studied of mammalian allergens. The major cat allergen, Fel d 1, is potent and elicits IgE responses in 90–95% of patients with cat allergy and accounts for 60–90% of the total allergenic activity of cat extracts. This allergen is found in the hair roots and sebaceous glands, in dander and saliva, and in high concentration in the anal glands. Its production is thought to be under hormonal control because castration decreases the production of Fel d 1. This allergen is secreted in copious amounts and accumulates in house dust at levels of up to 3,000 µg g^{-1} of dust. Fel d 2, cat serum albumin, is a minor allergen, causing IgE reactivity in about 20% of people allergic to cats.

Unlike dust mite allergen, cat allergens are very buoyant and sticky and can be found in high levels on walls and other surfaces in houses. Cat allergen has been shown to be carried on particles less than 1 µm to more than 20 µm in size. These smaller particles stay airborne for prolonged periods, which explains why people with cat allergy often experience symptoms on entering homes that have cats. Allergen levels less than 100 ng m^{-3} are capable of inducing upper and lower respiratory tract symptoms. These levels can be found in homes with or without cats, which suggests that even people without known cat exposure may have significant exposure. A relation has been shown between the number of cat owners in a classroom and the settled cat allergen level in that room. More important, levels of cat allergen in school classrooms are high enough to induce symptoms in children sensitized to cats. Once a cat has been removed from the house, the clinical benefit may not be seen for 4–6 months because of the persistence of the allergen. The allergen levels may decrease more quickly if extensive environmental control measures are undertaken.

2.5.2 Dog Allergen

Dogs can be a source of up to 20 allergens. The major allergen from dogs, Can f 1, accounts for about 50% of the IgE-binding capacity of dog hair and dander extract and for 60–70% of the IgE-binding capacity of the dog saliva preparation. Although Can f 1 is found mainly in dog saliva, it is also present in dog dander. It is absent or in very low concentration in the serum, urine, and feces. Can f 2 is a minor allergen, sensitizing 25% of people allergic to dogs. It is found in dog dander and saliva, and, like Can f 1, very little is found in the urine or feces.

Dog allergen shares several physical characteristics with cat allergen. Similar to cat allergen, it is buoyant and sticky. Dog allergens are carried on particles smaller than 5 µm. Dog allergen can be detected in houses and schools in the absence of a dog. Although the number and amount of antigens differ among dog breeds, there does not appear to be a "nonallergic" or even significantly "less allergic" breed.

2.5.3 Horse Allergen

The major horse allergen is Equ c 1, which is bound by specific IgE in 76% of people allergic to horses. It is found in high concentration in horse dander and saliva, but urine contains little of the allergen. Like cat allergen, horse allergen can cause marked symptoms on exposure to dander, and some people exhibit exquisite sensitivity. This tends to be easier to manage because of the absence of horse dander in the home.

2.5.4   Cow Allergen

The major respiratory allergen in cow dander is Bos d 2. About 90% of dairy farmers with cow sensitivity react to Bos d 2, which is found in the skin, specifically in the secretory cells of apocrine sweat glands and the basement membranes of the epithelium and hair follicles.

2.5.5   Mouse Allergen

Mouse allergens induce allergic symptoms in up to one-fourth of laboratory animal workers. The major mouse allergen, Mus m 1, is a major mouse urinary protein. In addition to being found in mouse urine, it is found in the serum, pelt, and liver. Mouse allergen has been shown to travel on particles 0.05–10 μm in size.

2.5.6   Rat Allergen

The major rat allergen, Rat n 1, is found primarily in the urine but also in the pelt and saliva. It is closely related to the mouse major urinary protein. About 60% of laboratory animal workers symptomatic to rat are sensitized to rat urinary proteins. The majority of rat allergens are found on particles smaller than 7 μm. Exposure is highly dependent on the type of activity being performed, with cleaning and feeding of the rats being associated with the highest levels of exposure.

2.5.7   Guinea Pig Allergen

The prevalence of sensitization to guinea pigs among personnel in laboratory animal facilities is approximately 30%. Of note, guinea pigs as pets have been associated with an increased risk for atopic eczema that has not been found with other pets, such as cats, dogs, or hamsters. Guinea pig allergens have been characterized only partially. The major allergen is Cav p 1, which has been purified from a hair extract.

2.5.8   Rabbit Allergen

Rabbits induce allergic symptoms in approximately 30% of laboratory animal workers. Allergy against rabbits develops rapidly and is more prevalent during 1 year of exposure than for other laboratory animals. The major allergen that has been identified is Ag r 1, which is found primarily in the saliva and, to lesser extent, in the fur.

2.5.9 Animal Allergen Environmental Control

For household pets that cause allergic symptoms in patients, the overall recommendation is simple, but not easy. The most appropriate recommendation is to remove the pet from the home. Health care providers should strongly recommend this approach. A high proportion of patients are unwilling to remove a household pet; therefore, alternative measures should be implemented. Most information about environmental controls relates to cat allergen. However, because of the similarities in the physical characteristics of allergens, the same measures can likely be adopted for households with a dog or other pet.

Reductions in airborne Fel d 1 allergens have been noted with a combination of air filtration, cat removal or washing, vacuum cleaning, and removal of furnishings. Air filtration may be more effective in decreasing cat allergen than dust mite allergen because of the buoyancy of the allergen. The high-efficiency particulate air (HEPA) filters conform to a strict standard of being able to filter out 99.97% of all particles larger than 3 μm. Airflow standards for this removal exist, so HEPA filters can be placed in a house according to the size of the area that the filter covers. Studies of cat washing have produced conflicting results. Cat washing generally results in a transient decrease in airborne cat allergens, but allergen levels return to baseline within a week. Studies that used a combination of a HEPA filter in the bedroom, encasements for mattresses and pillows, and keeping the cat out of the bedroom have reported improvement in clinical symptoms.

Overall, the recommendations for families who insist on keeping pets include (1) restricting the animal to one area of the house and keeping it out of the patient's bedroom and off heavy upholstery and other reservoirs for allergen collection, (2) use of a HEPA cleaner, especially in the patient's bedroom, and (3) use of mattress and pillow encasements. The use of tannic acid and other chemicals that purportedly render a pet "nonallergenic" may result in a transient, modest decrease in measurable allergen, but because the change is so small, this method is not recommended. Similarly, washing the cat or dog provides only a transient benefit and probably does not add significant improvement, especially considering the difficulty sometimes encountered with washing the pet.

A comprehensive plan should be implemented to decrease exposure to laboratory animal allergens by laboratory workers. Individually ventilated cage systems have been shown to decrease ambient rodent allergen levels. Automated cage-handling machines have been developed to reduce the exposure of persons emptying and cleaning soiled cages. The most effective personal protection against airborne allergens is with the use of ventilated, motorized helmets in which inhaled air is pumped through filters.

2.6 Cockroach Allergen

Cockroach allergen has been implicated as a major cause of asthma morbidity throughout the world. Approximately 40–60% of patients who have asthma and are from large cities, including New York, Chicago, Boston, Detroit, Washington D.C., and New Orleans, are sensitized to cockroach allergen. Cockroach allergy is strongly linked to socioeconomic factors and occurs wherever living conditions favor cockroach infestation. However, cockroach sensitization is not confined only to inner cities. Studies in Charlottesville, Virginia, and Wilmington, Delaware, have shown that cockroach sensitization can occur wherever substandard housing or apartment buildings sustain cockroach infestation.

The two major domestic cockroaches in North America are *Blatella germanica*, the German cockroach, and *Periplaneta americana*, the American cockroach. The German cockroach is most prevalent in the United States. It is brown and 16 mm long. They aggregate in dark, warm, humid spaces around water and food sources and rarely leave these areas except to feed at night. They seldom move across open spaces, and if they are seen during the day, it is an indication that large populations are present. The American cockroach is 38mm long and aggregates in dark humid spaces. They eat any organic food but are attracted to sweets and alcohol products.

Cockroach allergens are derived from saliva, fecal material, secretions, skin casts, debris, and dead bodies. Cockroach aeroallergen particles have physical properties similar to those of dust mite allergens. They are detectable in the air primarily after a disturbance and fall to the ground and settle rapidly. Unlike animal allergens, cockroach allergens are associated with larger particles and, thus, do not remain airborne long. Patients often are not aware of being allergic to cockroaches and do not immediately notice symptoms upon entering a house or building that has cockroaches.

Several allergens from cockroaches have been characterized. Allergens from the German cockroach include Bla g 1, Bla g 2, Bla g 4, Bla g 5, and Bla g 6, and those from the American cockroach are Per a 1, Per a 3, and Per a 7. Although most of the cloned allergens from these two cockroaches are species-specific, some cross-reactivity has been established. Testing should include all cockroaches endemic to the area.

2.6.1 Cockroach Environmental Control

To eliminate cockroaches from an infested house or building is difficult and often requires professional extermination. The first step in extermination is inspection. The inspection should help determine the hiding places and travel routes of the cockroaches. Insecticides are most effective and least toxic to the human residents if the hiding areas of the cockroaches are targeted. The inspection should also target the food and water sources that harbor the cockroaches. Integrated pest management uses selected placement of gels or baits to help minimize human exposure. In this system, gel spots are applied to cracks and crevices of cupboards or counters, without making the gels accessible to children or pets. The gels contain sugars and other attractants so the cockroaches carry the pesticides back to their primary living space.

Successful allergen removal also requires household cleaning. Before insecticides are applied, the house should be cleaned thoroughly to remove additional food sources, so the baits will be effective. After the insecticides have been applied, cleaning should be delayed for a week so the insecticides will not be disturbed. The cleaning should include thorough vacuuming and scrubbing of hard surfaces to remove allergen in sticky secretions. Because allergen is likely to be left on the walls, floors, appliances, countertops, and woodwork, these areas should be scrubbed with water and detergent.

Extermination is easier than allergen removal. The best one can expect is to decrease settled dust allergen concentrations by 95% with repeated cleaning for 6 months after extermination. The combination of thorough cleaning practices, proven extermination techniques, and consistent maintenance helps to decrease exposure and prevent infestation. The major clinically relevant aeroallergens are listed in Table 2.5.

Table 2.5 The major clinically relevant aeroallergens of North America[a]

Tree pollen
  Chinese elm (*Ulmus parvifolia*)[b,c]; Siberian elm (*Ulmus pumila*)[b,c]; elm (*Ulmus americana*)[b,c]
  Red oak (*Quercus rubra*)[b]; white oak (*Quercus alba*)[b]
  Paper birch (*Betula papyrifera*)
  Alder (*Alnus rubrum*)
  Box elder (*Acer negundo*)[b]; red maple (*Acer rubrum*)[b]
  Eastern cottonwood (*Populus deltoides*)
  Sycamore (*Platanus occidentalis*)
  White ash (*Fraxinus americana*)[b]; olive (*Olea europaea*)[b,c]
  Black walnut (*Juglans nigra*)
  Mulberry (*Morus rubra*)
  Mountain cedar (*Juniperus ashei*)
  Pecan (*Carya illinoinenis*)

Grass pollen
  Rye (*Lolium perenne*)[d,e]
  Timothy (*Phleum pratense*)[d,e]
  Meadow fescue (*Festuca elatior*)[d,e]
  Bermuda (*Cynodon dactylon*)[e]
  Johnson (*Sorghum halepense*)
  Bahia (*Paspalum notatum*)

Weed pollen
  Short ragweed (*Ambrosia artemisiifolia*)[e,f]
  English (narrow leaf) plantain (*Plantago lanceolata*)
  Mugwort (*Artemisia vulgaris*)
  Russian thistle (*Salsola kali*)

(continued)

Table 2.5 (continued)

Burning bush (*Bassia scoparia*)
Sheep (red) sorrel (*Rumex acetosella*)
Red root pigweed (*Amaranthus retroflexus*)
Indoor aeroallergens
Cat epithelium (*Felis domesticus*)[e]
Dog epithelium (*Canis familiaris*)
Arthropods (domestic mites: *Dermatophagoides farinae*[e]; *Dermatophagoides pteronyssinus*)[e]
Insects (German cockroach: *Blattella germanica*)

Fungi
Alternaria alternata[g]
Cladosporium (*C. cladosporioides*, *C. herbarum*)[g]
Penicillium (*P. chrysogenum*, *P. expansum*)[g]
Aspergillus fumigatus[g]
Epicoccum nigrum
Drechslera or *Bipolaris* type (e.g., *Helminthosporium solani*)[g]

From Li, J. T., Lockey, R. F., Bernstein, I. L., et al., Joint Task Force on Practice Parameters, American Academy of Allergy, Asthma and Immunology; American College of Allergy, Asthma and Immunology; Joint Council of Allergy, Asthma and Immunology (2003). Allergen immunotherapy: a practice parameter. Ann. Allergy Asthma Immunol. 90:12. Used with permission
[a]Compiled and selected in collaboration with the American Academy of Allergy, Asthma, and Immunology Immunotherapy committee and Allergen subcommittee for the identification of 35 key allergens in North America
[b]Extensive cross-reaction of species within the genus
[c]Apart from regional prevalences, are limited to local sites with substantial stands of these trees
[d]Extensively cross-react with one another and bluegrass, orchard, red top, and sweet vernal
[e]Allergens for which standardized extracts are commercially available
[f]Like all ragweeds, extensively cross-react with other species within their genus
[g]Species that are widely distributed and clinically important

2.7 Clinical Vignettes

2.7.1 Vignette 1

A 24-year-old woman reported symptoms of watery and itchy eyes, nasal congestion, itchy nose, and sneezing approximately 15 min after entering the furnished basement of her home. She does not notice any severe symptoms when she is in other areas of the house, but she does have some nasal congestion on a year-round basis. She also notes that her symptoms increase during the warmer months, particularly on days when she is outside for a long period. She does not have a history of asthma.

Comment: The symptoms described are compatible with an IgE-mediated reaction suggestive of airborne allergen sensitivity. In particular, the basement seems to cause problems, as do the warmer months. An environmental history with detailed information about the home often provides clues about the identity of the offending allergen.

Additional history disclosed that the house is 30 years old. There are no pets or a history of pets in the house. There is no smoking in the house, which has central heating and air-conditioning. Five years ago, during a flood, water seeped into the basement, which had standing water for a few days. No subsequent flooding has occurred, but the basement is typically damp. The basement flooring consists of carpet over a cement base. The carpet was placed after the flood. A dehumidifier is run intermittently.

Comment: The home has had water damage, and the basement continues to be damp. High moisture levels are conducive to both dust mite and mold growth. There are no pets, so cat and dog allergens are essentially ruled out. Additional information about the contents of the basement may be helpful.

The basement is divided into two sections: a carpeted area with a television, couch, and two soft chairs, and a back storage area, which contains old papers and books. A green mildew has been noted on the edges of the books and papers. The walls have some old water marks from the previous flood.

Comment: The green mildew found in the storage area is suggestive of *Penicillium* mold. Other mold growth is likely. The most common indoor molds are *Aspergillus* and *Penicillium*. The conditions are also optimal for dust mite growth. The symptoms that occur during the warmer months may be caused by outdoor molds and/or tree, grass, or weed pollens. Skin testing to these can help clearly identify the allergens.

Allergen skin testing was performed, and the patient had positive responses to *D. farinae, D. pteronyssinus, Penicillium, Aspergillus, Alternaria, Cladosporium,* and timothy grass.

Comment: Avoidance measures were reviewed in detail. By decreasing exposure to all the allergens throughout her living space, her allergic symptoms should improve. For the basement, all materials with evidence of mold contamination should be removed. A dehumidifier should be placed to keep the humidity less than 50%. Dust mite precautions should be implemented for both the basement and bedroom. Complete avoidance of outdoor grass pollen is essentially impossible. Historical review of the timothy grass pollen counts helps outline the months that would cause the most symptoms. It was recommended that during these months, the windows of the house, especially the bedroom window, be kept closed. It also was recommended that the patient shower and change clothes after significant outdoor exposure. The rest of the management plan reviewed the role of medications and immunotherapy.

2.7.2   Vignette 2

A 30-year-old man has a 10-month history of chronic rhinitis and itchiness of the eyes. He does not recall any similar symptoms before the last 10 months. There has been no seasonal variation in his symptoms. Environmental history discloses that he has lived in the same townhouse for the last 4 years. The townhouse is 7 years old. There has not been any problem with water contamination. The house is not damp. The patient does not have any pets.

Comment: Although allergic rhinitis can occur at any age, the onset is typically before age 30 years. In some instances, patients can have a history of childhood allergic rhinitis, which was seemingly dormant for many years and then recurred. The history of this patient did not confirm any childhood allergic rhinitis. His current home environment has not had any recent change. When evaluating a patient who has rhinitis, an occupational history should be obtained.

The patient reported that he has worked as a laboratory technician for the past 5 years, and approximately 1 year ago, he began working extensively on a project involving mice. He had not had any previous exposure to mice. At work, he uses nonlatex gloves. He did not identify any other change in his work environment.

Comment: This vignette emphasizes the importance of obtaining an occupational history when evaluating a patient who has rhinitis and eye symptoms. In this case, further evaluation was performed with skin testing to mouse, and the result was markedly positive. On the basis of this information, a plan was implemented to decrease exposure to mouse allergen. This included the use of protective clothing, glove exchange after mouse handling, and a high-efficiency filtration mask.

2.7.3   Vignette 3

A 10-year-old boy presented with a 2-year history of marked eye itching, sneezing, nasal congestion, and clear, watery rhinorrhea during April and May and also in August, September, and October. During the rest of the year he is essentially free of symptoms. With the eye and nose symptoms, he occasionally wheezes.

Comment: The symptoms described are classic for seasonal allergic rhinitis. The predominance of symptoms in the spring and autumn is usually from tree and weed pollens, respectively. Additional information about the child's activities and home landscape is usually helpful.

The mother reported that the boy loves sports and spends many hours outdoors playing baseball in the spring and football in the autumn. They recently moved to a newly built two-story house just outside town in a wooded area. The boy's bedroom is on the upper floor and has large windows. Although the home has air-conditioning, the family rarely uses it, preferring to keep the windows open. Birch and oak trees surround the house. Currently, the yard consists of wild grass and weeds.

Comment: The child's environment is conducive to seasonal pollen exposure. Living in a wooded area increases the exposure to tree pollen; however, significant exposure can occur with any outdoor exposure, whether in a wooded area or in the center of a city. Keeping the windows open increases exposure to pollen within the house.

Further evaluation was performed with skin prick testing to the tree, grass, and weed pollens and mold spores indigenous to the area. Positive results were found to maple, birch, oak, and alder trees and short ragweed. The tests to mold spores were nonreactive.

Comment: The family was counseled about avoidance measures for seasonal pollens. On the basis of pollen counts recorded over the years, the expected times of pollen release for the trees and short ragweed were reviewed. During these times, it was recommended that the windows of the house, especially the boy's bedroom, be kept closed. It also was recommended that the boy shower and change clothes after playing outdoors for an extended time. The rest of the management plan reviewed the role of medications and immunotherapy.

Suggested Reading

Bush, R. K. and Portnoy, J. M. (2001) The role and abatement of fungal allergens in allergic diseases. J. Allergy Clin. Immunol. Suppl. 107:S430–S440.

Chapman, M. D. and Wood, R. A. (2001) The role and remediation of animal allergens in allergic diseases. J. Allergy Clin. Immunol. Suppl. 107:S414–S421.

Custovic, A., Murray, C. S., Gore, R. B., and Woodcock, A. (2002) Controlling indoor allergens. Ann. Allergy Asthma Immunol. 88:432–441.

Eggleston, P. A. and Arruda, L. K. (2001) Ecology and elimination of cockroaches and allergens in the home. J. Allergy Clin. Immunol. Suppl. 107:S422–S429.

Frenz, D. A. (1999) Comparing pollen and spore counts collected with the Rotorod Sampler and Burkard spore trap. Ann Allergy Asthma Immunol. 83:341–347.

Horner, W. E., Levetin, E., and Lehrer, S. B. (2004) Aerobiology. Clin. Allergy Immunol. 18:125–149.

Solomon, W. R. (2002) Airborne pollen prevalence in the United States. In: L. C. Grammer, P. A. Greenberger (Eds.), Patterson's Allergic Diseases, 6th ed. Philadelphia: Lippincott Williams & Wilkins. pp. 131–144.

Vijay, H. M. and Kurup, V. P. (2004) Fungal allergens. Clin. Allergy Immunol. 18:223–249.

Weber, R. W. (2003) Patterns of pollen cross-allergenicity. J. Allergy Clin. Immunol. 112:229–239.

White, J. F. and Bernstein, D. I. (2003) Key pollen allergens in North America. Ann. Allergy Asthma Immunol. 91:425–435.

Chapter 3
Allergen Testing and Allergen Immunotherapy

Abbreviations AIC: Amb a 1-immunostimulatory DNA sequence conjugate; APC: antigen-presenting cell; HSA: human serum albumin; IFN: interferon; IL: interleukin; PNU: protein nitrogen units; RAST: radioallergosorbent test; SIT: allergen-specific immunotherapy (specific allergen immunotherapy); SLIT: sublingual immunotherapy.

3.1 Allergen Testing

The diagnosis and management of allergic disorders begins with a detailed symptom and environmental exposure history and physical examination. Once signs and symptoms compatible with an allergic disorder have been identified, allergy testing can be considered. The signs and symptoms that suggest an allergic disease are discussed in detail in the subsequent clinical chapters. Briefly, they include the following:

- Allergic rhinoconjunctivitis: watery and itchy eyes, nasal congestion, rhinorrhea, sneezing, nasal itch
- Allergic asthma: cough, wheeze, shortness of breath
- Medication allergy: pruritus, urticaria, angioedema, anaphylaxis
- Food allergy: pruritus, urticaria, angioedema, vomiting, diarrhea, anaphylaxis
- Stinging insect allergy: pruritus, urticaria, angioedema, wheezing, vomiting, diarrhea, anaphylaxis

Allergy testing helps the physician to determine if a patient's problem is indeed caused by allergy and to identify the specific problem allergens. After the culprit allergens have been identified, several therapeutic interventions may be instituted, including environmental modifications, pharmacotherapy, and immunotherapy. The major indications for allergy testing include rhinitis, asthma, suspected food allergy, suspected drug allergy, and suspected insect sting allergy. Other indications are atopic dermatitis, latex allergy, and occupational asthma. The results of allergy tests should not be viewed in isolation but always within the context of the patient's clinical history and physical examination results. Random allergy testing without a clear clinical reason for the testing is not recommended.

G.W. Volcheck, *Clinical Allergy: Diagnosis and Management*
DOI: 10.1007/978-1-59745-315-8_3, © 2009 Mayo Foundation for Medical Education and Research

The two major types of tests for IgE-mediated type I hypersensitivity reactions are skin tests and in vitro serum IgE specific antibody testing. These tests are used to assess for sensitivity to airborne allergens, foods, insect stings, and medications. The focus of this chapter is primarily on these two types of tests, with special emphasis on the advantages and disadvantages in various clinical scenarios (e.g., allergic rhinitis vs. drug allergy).

Specific organ challenge tests may facilitate or confirm the clinical diagnosis when the diagnosis is very suggestive but skin or in vitro tests (or both) are negative. However, testing should only be pursued with the realization that a severe anaphylactic reaction may occur. Specific conjunctival, nasal, and bronchial challenges can be performed. However, they should be performed in a testing center where there is experience in managing severe reactions and in quantitating the outcome with these types of procedures.

3.1.1   Skin Prick Testing

The two primary types of skin testing are skin prick and intradermal tests. Intradermal tests are also referred to as intracutaneous tests. The term *intradermal* is used in this chapter. They are reliable, cost-effective tests for diagnosing IgE-mediated diseases. Skin testing dates to the late 1800s, when initial testing consisted of placing pollen on abraded skin. Various forms of skin testing have been used over the years, mainly derivatives of the scratch test. Today, skin testing is performed most commonly by the skin prick route, in which diluted allergen is pricked into the skin surface. Several sharp objects may be used for skin prick tests, including a hypodermic or solid bore needle, lancet with or without a bifurcated tip, and multihead lancet devices. No single or multitest device appears to have a clear advantage. Optimal results are obtained by having a working familiarity with the device and using proper technique. In performing the skin prick test, a drop of allergen extract is placed on the skin, then pierced through by the instrument at a 45–60° angle to the skin, creating a small break in the epidermis, which allows the allergen solution to penetrate. This technique should not cause bleeding. The excess extract is removed with gauze or tissue paper. A variation of this is the puncture method, in which the device is held at a 90° angle to the skin and pushed through the extract into the epidermis. In the allergic patient, the allergen in the solution binds and cross-links specific IgE, triggering mast cell release of histamine and preformed and newly synthesized mediators. The mediators (primarily histamine) released at the site cause the formation of localized erythema, edema, and widespread flare, which peak at 15–20 minutes. The size of the wheal and the surrounding erythema are then recorded.

Currently, there is no standardized way for recording the results of skin prick tests. Qualitative scoring (0–4+) has been used, but the interpretation is quite variable from physician to physician. In this system, 1+ represents a wheal one quarter the size of the histamine control and 4+ represents a wheal twice as large as the histamine control. The current trend is to record the measurement of the largest diameters of the wheal and to note whether there is surrounding erythema (F for flare) or the presence of another wheal (P for pseudopod) or both. The presence of a pseudopod is a sign of greater sensitivity. Therefore, a response to ragweed may read 5 × 5FP, meaning a 5 × 5-mm wheal with surrounding erythema (F) and the presence of a pseudopod (P). To ensure proper interpretation, positive (histamine) and negative (saline or 50% glycerinated human serum albumin [HSA]-saline), controls should be performed at the same time as the allergen tests. The positive histamine control is performed to make sure the patient's skin is normally reactive. In most patients, the skin prick for histamine usually produces 3 × 3F–6 × 6F. If a patient does not have a positive histamine control, then skin prick testing is unlikely to demonstrate any positive allergen tests because it is primarily histamine that is released at the site of the positive allergen skin prick test.

The most common cause of a negative histamine control finding is the concomitant use of antihistamines or medications with antihistaminic properties. Antihistamine medications need to be discontinued before allergy skin prick testing. The number of days the medications need to be stopped beforehand depends on the antihistamine. Representative antihistamines and other medications that interfere with the histamine response are outlined in Table 3.1. Other medications that can commonly interfere with the skin tests include tricyclic antidepressants and tranquilizers. H_2 antagonists may cause mild suppression and should be discontinued for 24 hours before testing. Short-term oral corticosteroids do not suppress skin tests. However, long-term oral corticosteroids (>20 mg per day) may have a suppressive effect. Skin testing should not be performed in areas where potent topical corticosteroids have been applied long term.

The negative controls (saline or glycerinated HSA-saline) are helpful to check for dermatographism and to identify the amount of response needed to constitute a

Table 3.1 Drugs that suppress skin prick and intradermal tests[a]

Generic name	No. of days medication should be discontinued before skin testing
Antihistamine, first generation	
Chlorpheniramine	3
Diphenhydramine	2
Hydroxyzine	5
Antihistamine, second generation	
Cetirizine	4
Fexofenadine	4
Loratadine	6
Tricyclic antidepressants	
Desipramine	3
Imipramine	10
Doxepin	7
H_2 Antihistamines	
Ranitidine	1

[a] Leukotriene antagonists and topical antihistamines azelastine (nose), levocabastine (eye), and topical nasal corticosteroids do not affect skin prick and intradermal tests

positive test. Patients with dermatographism may form a significant wheal and flare from the pressure caused by the instrument on the skin. Skin prick devices should not be used that produce a 3-mm wheal or more for the negative control. The negative control should have no response. A general rule for a positive skin test is the formation of a wheal with erythema that is at least 3 mm larger in diameter than the negative control (negative control 0, allergen 3 × 3F).

The reliability and interpretation of the skin prick test depend on the skill and interpretation of the individual tester, the reliability of the test instrument, the potency and stability of the test extracts, and skin reactivity on the day of the test. If these quality controls are not used, the interpretation of the test will vary. Correct procedure, taking into account the force, duration, depth, and angle of the prick, and positive and negative controls help ensure reliability. Standardized allergen extracts should be used when possible to provide consistency in testing. The extraction process for nonstandardized and standardized products is essentially the same. The allergen extracts are derived from cultures or natural sources, for example, collected pollen, and represent complex heterogeneous mixtures of allergenic and nonallergenic proteins and macromolecules. Nonstandardized extracts, with their designated labels of extraction ratio (w/v) or PNU do not convey specific information about their allergenic potency, and this may result in considerable lot-to-lot variability. Mold and insect extracts have greater lot-to-lot variability than pollen and mite extracts. Standardized extracts are measured in bioequivalency allergy units per milliliter (BAU mL^{-1}) based on titrated intradermal skin testing of highly allergic individuals. These extracts standardized by biologic activity yield the most reproducible, accurate results. Standardized extracts are now commercially available for rye, timothy, meadow fescue, and Bermuda grass; short ragweed; cat epithelium, and dust mites *Dermatophagoides farinae* and *D pteronyssinus*. One example in which extract potency can decrease significantly over time is commercial extracts with fruits. Testing for fresh fruits should be performed with freshly made fruit extracts or by the prick/prick method in which the tester first pricks the fresh food and then the skin. The composition of nonstandardized extracts varies from manufacturer to manufacturer. Stability of the extracts is preserved by glycerin and storage at 4°C.

Skin prick tests can be performed on the upper back or volar surface of the forearm. Tests should not be placed within 5 cm of the wrist or within 3 cm of the antecubital fossa. Skin reactivity varies with location. The upper and middle portions of the back are more reactive than the lower portion, and the back is more reactive than the forearm. Each allergen should be placed at least 2 cm from the next allergen to prevent the reaction from one allergen interfering with that from the adjacent allergen. Skin tests should not be performed in areas of active dermatitis. Skin prick tests may be performed in infants as young as 1 month, although positive reactions tend to have a smaller diameter in infants and young children than in adults.

The diagnostic validity of skin prick tests has been confirmed not only in patients exposed to allergens under natural conditions but also in patients undergoing controlled organ challenge tests. Many studies have verified the sensitivity and specificity of skin prick tests for both inhalant and food allergens when correlated with nasal and oral challenge tests. A recent meta-analysis that compared skin prick tests with nasal challenge showed positive likelihood ratios of 4.93, 16.17, 3.23, and 4.06 for cat, tree pollen, grass pollen, and house dust mite, respectively; the corresponding negative likelihood ratios were 0.08, 0.03, 0.04, and 0.03. Overall, the correlation between a positive skin prick test and response to aeroallergens is approximately 70–90%.

The diagnostic accuracy of skin prick tests in food allergy has been compared in patients who have positive open or double-blinded controlled positive reactions to specific foods. In some of these studies, it was possible to determine cutoff levels of skin prick wheal diameters that were 100% diagnostic for a positive reaction for several foods. These values included >8 mm for milk, >7 mm for egg, and >8 mm for peanut. These findings help obviate the need for provocative challenges. However, commercial reagents for food allergy skin testing have not been standardized and may have varying concentrations of relevant proteins. Sensitivity of food skin prick tests typically exceeds 85%, but specificity is lower, usually in the range of 40–80%. These test findings generally indicate that a negative test is able to "rule out" an IgE-mediated reaction to the food tested, but a positive test may not be a true positive. Therefore, large screening panels of food allergy tests should not be performed without a clear history of suspicion, because of the possibility of irrelevant positive results. This is especially a problem with patients who have high total IgE, such as those with atopic dermatitis.

The question often arises, "How many skin tests should be performed?" This can be difficult, considering that hundreds of commercially prepared allergenic extracts are available for skin testing. A detailed clinical and environmental history can usually limit the need for extensive testing. For airborne allergens, the number of skin prick tests performed is guided by the following:

- Local aerobiologic data (pollen counts) obtained by a qualified counting station – it is important to be familiar with the pollens of the region. It would not be prudent to test to pollens that are not found in the region.
- Correlation between patients' symptoms and aerobiologic data – obtain information about which months of the year the patient has the most trouble. For example, springtime symptoms usually are due to tree pollens and molds, whereas fall symptoms more commonly are due to weed pollens and molds. Knowledge of whether the symptoms are strictly seasonal or perennial is also helpful.
- Knowledge about the clinical significance of pollens in the region – some pollens may be found in abundance but have low allergenicity, for example, pine pollen.
- Knowledge of the cross-reactivity patterns between allergens – because of the extensive cross-reactivity among some pollens, particularly the prairie grasses, even if rye, blue, and orchard are present, only one may be required for skin testing. This is discussed in more detail below in Sect. 3.2 and in Chap. 2.
- Knowledge of fungi prevalent in the outdoor and indoor air – in addition to the outdoor pollens and molds, perennial indoor allergen testing to house dust mite, indoor molds, cockroach, and animals is often indicated. The major clinically relevant aeroallergens are listed in Table 3.2. This list can be increased or decreased depending on the region and the patient's exposure history.

Table 3.2 The major clinically relevant aeroallergens of North America[a]

Tree Pollen
  Chinese elm (*Ulmus parvifolia*);[b,c] Siberian elm (*Ulmus pumila*);[b,c] elm (*Ulmus americana*)[b,c]
  Red oak (*Quercus rubra*);[b] white oak (*Quercus alba*)[b]
  Paper birch (*Betula papyrifera*)
  Alder (*Alnus rubra*)
  Box elder (*Acer negundo*);[b] red maple (*Acer rubra*)[b]
  Eastern cottonwood (*Populus deltoids*)
  Sycamore (*Platanus occidentalis*)
  White ash (*Fraxinus americana*);[b] olive (*Olea europaea*)[b,c]
  Black walnut (*Juglans nigra*)
  Mulberry (*Moras rubra*)
  Mountain cedar (*Juniperus ashei*)
  Pecan (*Carya illinoensis*)

Grass pollen
  Rye (*Lolium perenne*)[d,e]
  Timothy (*Phleum pretense*)[d,e]
  Meadow fescue (*Festuca elatior*)[d,e]
  Bermuda (*Cynodon dactylon*)[e]
  Johnson (*Sorghum halepense*)
  Bahia (*Paspalum notatum*)

Weed pollen
  Short ragweed (*Ambrosia artemisiifolia*)[e,f]
  English (narrow leaf); plantain (*Plantago lanceolata*)
  Mugwort (*Artemisia vulgaris*)
  Russian thistle (*Salsola kali*)
  Burning bush (*Bassia scoparia*)
  Sheep (red) sorrel (*Rumex acetosella*)
  Red root pigweed (*Amaranthus retroflexus*)

Indoor aeroallergens
  Cat epithelium (*Felis domesticus*)[e]
  Dog epithelium (*Canis familiaris*)
  Arthropods (domestic mites: *Dermatophagoides farinae*;[e] *D pteronyssinus*[e])
  Insects (German cockroach: *Blattella germanica*)

Fungi
  Alternaria alternata[g]
  Cladosporium (*C cladosporioides*, *C herbarum*)[g]
  Penicillium (*P chrysogenum*, *P expansum*)[g]
  Aspergillus fumigatus[g]
  Epicoccum nigrum
  Drechslera or *Bipolaris* type (e.g., *Helminthosporium solani*)[g]

From Li, J. T., Lockey, R. F., Bernstein, I. L., et al., Joint Task Force on Practice Parameters, American Academy of Allergy, Asthma and Immunology; American College of Allergy, Asthma and Immunology; Joint Council of Allergy, Asthma and Immunology. (2003) Allergen immunotherapy: a practice parameter. Ann Allergy Asthma Immunol. 90, 12. Used with permission

[a] Compiled and selected in collaboration with the American Academy of Allergy, Asthma, and Immunology Immunotherapy committee and Allergen subcommittee for the identification of 35 key allergens in North America

[b] Extensive cross-reaction of spp. within the genus

[c] Apart from regional prevalences, are limited to local sites with substantial stands of these trees

[d] Extensively cross-react with one another and bluegrass, orchard, red top, and sweet vernal

[e] Allergens for which standardized extracts are commercially available

[f] Like all ragweeds, extensively cross-react with other spp. within their genus

[g] Spp. that are widely distributed and clinically important

Because of the number of false positives, skin prick tests to foods should not be performed unless the history is suspicious for an IgE-mediated reaction. The testing should be limited to the most likely foods. Testing a large number of foods without sufficient reason for suspecting a food allergy is rarely helpful. Food diaries can be helpful, particularly for patients who have the potential for food-induced anaphylaxis. The number of tests performed will vary with the clinical situation. Skin tests are not available for food preservatives. In many cases, it is not known if food preservatives cause an IgE-mediated reaction.

Skin prick testing is safe. Adverse effects are infrequent; if one occurs, it is primarily a large, localized skin reaction. Systemic reactions are rarely caused by skin prick tests because of the low exposure to the allergen. Occasionally, patients may have a late phase reaction. This is manifested as erythema and edema at the site of the skin test approximately 6–12 hours after the test and resolves over 24–48 hours. The pathophysiology and clinical significance of the late phase reaction are not clear. The majority occur in patients who had an immediately positive test, but this is not always the case. For those with negative immediate skin prick tests, a late phase reaction does not appear to be predictive of their subsequent clinical course.

Skin prick tests in conjunction with an appropriate history and physical examination are still considered the first line of allergy testing for airborne allergens and food allergens.

3.1.2   Skin Intradermal Testing

Intradermal tests generally are used when increased sensitivity is the main goal of testing. Intradermal tests are performed by injecting 0.02–0.05 mL of allergen extract with a 26–30 gauge needle, almost parallel to the skin surface and under the skin just enough to cover the beveled portion. The allergen extract is then injected as superficially as possible, raising a small wheal usually 2–3 mm in diameter. Because of the increased sensitivity of the test and exposure of the patient, more dilute extracts are used for testing. Intradermal tests are usually performed at 1:500–1:1,000 dilution of the extract used for skin prick tests. After the extract is placed, the patient is observed for 15 minutes and the skin test site read and recorded. The final reading is compared with the initial size of the wheal. As with skin prick testing, a standard grading system has not been devised. Qualitative grading systems have been used, grading from 0–4+, where 0 is no response, 2+ is erythema with a wheal <3 mm, and 4+ is erythema with a pseudopodial wheal >3 mm. This can cause confusion, because a 2+ response is actually negative. For accuracy, the diameters of the wheal and erythema both should be measured in millimeters and recorded. Any reaction larger than the negative control may indicate the presence of specific IgE antibody; however, because of the increased sensitivity, very small positive reactions may not be clinically significant. Most allergists use the criterion of an increase in diameter of the wheal >3 mm than that of the initial wheal or negative control to define a positive test. The reliability of intradermal tests is affected by the same variables as for the skin prick tests: correct procedure, interference by medications, and potency and stability of the allergen test extracts.

The primary value of intradermal skin testing is in the assessment of medication and Hymenoptera sensitivity. The diagnostic accuracy of intradermal tests is greater than that of skin prick tests when testing for penicillin, insect venoms, and other drug classes. The use of intradermal skin testing for food or airborne allergens is discouraged because of the high percentage of false-positive tests. The correlation between a positive test and clinical response to aeroallergens is only 30–40%. Intradermal testing to foods also adds the potential risk of a systemic reaction. In these situations (food and airborne allergens), the use of an intradermal test is usually restricted to a single dose (1/1,000 w/v), which is often an irritant. The use of end-point titrations (serial threshold dilutions performed until the lowest dose that produces a positive response is obtained) intradermally are associated with a better positive predictive value at lower concentrations of extracts (10^{-5}, 10^{-6}), but the end-point titrations are time consuming and generally do not add more clinical relevancy than the skin prick tests. Intradermal tests are helpful for Hymenoptera and medication assessments. Before the intradermal tests are performed, skin prick tests should be used to detect highly sensitive patients who may be at risk for a systemic reaction from the intradermal tests. If the skin prick tests are negative, then intradermal tests can be performed.

Skin testing to venoms should be performed only in patients with a previous history of a systemic reaction after a sting. The tests should not be used to screen for venom allergy without a history of a reaction. Theoretically, there is a risk of inducing sensitization if performed only for screening purposes. Skin testing should begin with skin prick testing to the clinically pertinent stinging insects, depending on the clinical situation. For example, fire ants leave a characteristic vesicular pattern and are confined to the southern states; they do not need to be included when testing for a stinging insect reaction in nonendemic areas. Typically, fire ants are tested separately from apids and vespids. Venom extracts are used for honeybee, yellow jacket, *Polistes* wasp, yellow hornet, and white-faced hornet. Whole body extract is used for fire ant. If skin prick tests are negative, they are followed by intradermal testing, with concentrations of 0.2 µg mL^{-1}, followed by 1 µg mL^{-1}. Cross-reactivity does occur with the stinging insects. The most extensive cross-reactivity occurs among the yellow jacket and hornets. Typically, skin tests are positive to white-faced hornet and yellow hornet in patients allergic to yellow jacket. *Polistes* wasp is not as closely related to the other vespids. Approximately 50% of patients allergic to yellow jacket have positive skin tests to wasp. Inhibition testing shows that in this group, half of the patients are allergic to both the yellow jacket and wasp separately. There is very little cross-reactivity between the bees and vespids and between the vespids and fire ants.

For antibiotics, skin testing has been validated only for penicillin. Penicillin testing should be performed only if there is a history of a possible allergic reaction. It is important that both the major and minor determinants of penicillin are covered in skin testing. The major determinant, penicilloyl (a product of the major metabolic pathway), is positive in approximately 80% of penicillin-sensitive patients. The minor penicillin determinants (products of the minor metabolic pathway) are also capable of producing anaphylactic reactions in penicillin-sensitive patients.

The testing is initiated with skin prick testing to the penicillin components, followed by intradermal testing. A negative test denotes that the patient may receive penicillin without risk of a significant IgE-mediated reaction. If the test is positive, the patient requires a desensitization protocol to receive the penicillin. Skin testing with nonirritating concentrations of other antibiotics is not standardized. Most importantly, when testing nonpenicillin antibiotics, a negative skin test does not rule out the possibility of an IgE-mediated sensitivity. A positive test suggests IgE-mediated sensitivity, but the positive predictive value is unknown. Intradermal testing has also been helpful in the evaluation of cancer chemotherapeutic agents, muscle relaxants, insulin, and heparin. Although standardization of these agents is limited compared with that of penicillin, their positive and negative predictive values appear to be similar.

Immediate systemic reactions are more common with intradermal tests than with skin prick tests, but they still are rare. Six fatalities attributed to intradermal tests were reported by the Committee on Allergen Standardization of the American Academy of Allergy, Asthma, and Immunology. Five of these patients had asthma and were tested without preceding skin prick tests. No fatalities associated with intradermal testing were reported in the most recent 12-year survey (1990–2001).

Despite the sensitivity of skin prick and intradermal tests, challenge tests with allergens occasionally have shown end-organ sensitivity despite negative skin prick and intradermal tests. The underlying pathophysiology of these reactions has not been defined, but it may be due to locally secreted IgE or an IgE-independent mechanism.

3.1.3 In Vitro Testing

Many in vitro allergen-specific IgE tests have been developed over the past 30 years to help identify IgE-mediated disease. The first assays for allergen-specific IgE were performed in the 1960s and termed radioallergosorbent test (RAST). The current various allergen-specific in vitro tests are based on the same principles. The patient's serum, containing allergen-specific IgE (if allergic), is mixed with bound solid-phase allergen. The specific IgE that binds to the allergen is insolubilized onto a solid phase and the rest is washed away. The bound specific IgE is detected and quantified by adding labeled anti-IgE antibody. This binds the solid-phase specific IgE-allergen complex. The labeled anti-IgE can be measured with a gamma counter (radioactive anti-IgE, Phadebas RAST, modified RAST), with colorimetry or fluorometry (enzyme-labeled anti-IgE antibody), or with monoclonal and polyclonal anti-IgE antibodies. Progress has been made in expressing the results of in vitro tests. Initially, results were expressed relative to that of nonallergic patients with no specific IgE (e.g., 3 SD greater than the mean of the negative control) or expressed as a ratio of the mean of the negative control (e.g., three times greater than negative control).

Second-generation methods had improvements such as greater speed, higher binding capacity, and the use of nonisotopic labels. Third-generation systems have even faster turnaround times and use chemiluminescence. The second- and third-generation assays for allergen-specific IgE antibody use a scheme in which a total serum IgE calibration curve is used to report results as International Units of IgE per mL ($kIU\ mL^{-1}$). In this system, 1 IU = 2.4 ng of protein. Multiple dilutions of reference and test sera are analyzed simultaneously, and their dose response curves are plotted in parallel. Allergen IgE specificity should be confirmed for each allergen used in the control sera. Ideally, this implies that each allergen has a homologous internal control positive reference-specific IgE serum (test serum specific for timothy vs. internal control timothy-specific IgE serum). The difficulty obtaining a sufficient quantity of serum from IgE antibody–positive individuals has caused some manufacturers to adopt a heterologous calibration approach. This results in less agreement between test specimen dilutions, and it lessens the assay's working range.

Several factors can affect the accuracy of in vitro allergen-specific IgE tests. Standard curves are not always formulated for each allergen-specific IgE and may not be a valid representation of different allergens. Tests for unusual allergens may be limited by the unavailability of a positive control. The process of binding the allergen to the solid phase may alter the allergen and not allow adequate recognition by the circulating IgE. The solid phase attempts to be as allergen rich as possible to help ensure that all the allergen-specific IgE present can be bound to the allergosorbent. IgG antibodies in the test serum can block the binding of IgE. Patients with high total IgE levels, such as those with atopic dermatitis, could have nonspecific binding that produces positive tests.

The IgE-specific antibody test, as mentioned above, is complex. The physician who orders the test needs to ensure that the blood sample is sent to a clinical laboratory that performs accurate measurements in the most quantitative manner. The laboratory should be certified under the Clinical Laboratory Improvement Amendments of 1988 and should participate successfully in external proficiency testing to ensure accuracy of the test results.

Because of a wide overlap in total serum IgE between nonatopic and atopic populations, persons with normal levels of total serum IgE can still have IgE antibody specific to a given allergen and, consequently, have allergic disease. Mean serum IgE levels progressively increase in healthy children up to 15 years of age and then decrease through the eighth decade of life. The total IgE level typically is not helpful in the evaluation of clinical allergy for routine airborne, food, and medication allergens. Total serum IgE is used primarily in assessing the activity of allergic bronchopulmonary aspergillosis and in determining the dosage of omalizumab.

Several in vitro allergen-specific IgE tests have been studied more rigorously recently to determine sensitivity, specificity, and positive and negative predictive values. Previously, the effectiveness of the tests were measured against a gold standard of medical history and questionnaire-derived diagnoses of allergic rhinitis. Identifying patients who have both a positive skin prick test and a clinical history of allergy to grass pollen, cat epithelium, and birch pollen as the standard, the Phadezyme assay exhibited optimal sensitivity and specificity with class 2 binding (0.7–3.5 Phadebas units [PRU] mL^{-1}). In the Pharmacia CAP specific IgE assay, the optimal cutoff values that distinguished between symptomatic and asymptomatic patients who had positive skin prick tests for the relevant allergens were 10.7 kU L^{-1} for seasonal allergens and 8.4 kU L^{-1} for perennial allergens. In studies with cat dander, in which symptom scores and FEV$_1$ changes were used as the standard, in vitro testing with the Phadezyme RAST and CAP RAST had specificity similar to that of skin prick tests (95%), but slightly lower sensitivity (69% vs 79%). Of the in vitro tests, ImmunoCAP technology has been considered the quasistandard because of its widespread use, analytical reliability, and the generally reasonable correspondence of its results with those of skin prick testing. Overall, with regard to inhalant allergens, in vitro testing has improved, but overall sensitivity is still considered slightly lower than that of skin prick tests. Validated specific IgE assays can be useful in confirming clinical sensitization to certain allergens. Because skin prick tests generally have a higher sensitivity, a negative in vitro specific IgE test cannot definitely exclude an allergy to inhalant allergens.

In vitro allergen-specific food testing has been performed to initially diagnose food allergy and also to predict the likelihood to a positive food challenge in persons with known food allergy. With regard to initial diagnosis of food allergy, in vitro allergen testing has limitations, as do the skin prick tests. The sensitivity generally is good, but the specificity is questionable. Because no test is 100% specific and 100% sensitive, it is imperative that a good history be obtained. Clearly, if the patient has a history suspicious for a severe anaphylactic event to a certain food but in vitro testing is negative, the food likely should still be avoided. Because of the possible severity of a reaction to a food allergen, it is important to consider the prior probability of a reaction in combination with the sensitivity and specificity of the test. Obtaining a detailed diet history, identifying a probable food, and assessing the potential immunopathophysiology are paramount. Age is important because the epidemiology of food allergy indicates a higher probability of reactions to cow's milk, egg, wheat, and soy in infants and to peanut, tree nuts, seafood, and raw fruits in older children and adults. Increasingly higher concentrations of food-specific IgE antibodies correlate with an increasing risk for a clinical reaction. Using the Pharmacia CAP System FEIA, Sampson reported that levels of IgE antibody ≥7 kIU L^{-1} for egg, 15 kIU L^{-1} for milk, and 14 kIU L^{-1} for peanut reflect a >95% chance of a reaction. When reviewing this type of data, it is important to note the characteristics of the tested population. In the example above, the subjects were atopic children with a median age of 3.8 years. Studies of younger children (<2 years) have shown a 95% reaction rate to challenge when egg values were >2 kIU L^{-1} and milk values were 5 kIU L^{-1}. Therefore, lower values can result in significant reactions in a younger age group. Even undetectable food-specific IgE testing can produce a reaction in up to 20% of high-risk children. In those at risk who have a negative in vitro test, skin prick testing should be performed.

Specific in vitro IgE testing is not recommended solely as a definitive confirmatory test for venoms or penicillins because of low sensitivity. Also, although penicilloyl can be conjugated to polylysine or to a protein carrier that can be coupled to a solid phase, analogous reagents are not available for the

Table 3.3 Current recommendations for in vitro IgE specific antibody, skin prick, and intradermal testing

Allergens	Clinical symptoms/ diagnosis	Specific serum IgE antibody	Skin prick test	Intradermal skin test
Venom and drug allergens	Urticaria, angioedema, nausea, vomiting, abdominal cramping, diarrhea, wheezing, anaphylaxis	Complementary to intradermal tests	Not sufficient alone	Preferred (prick tests done first)
Airborne allergens	Allergic rhinitis, asthma	Acceptable	Preferred	Not needed
Food allergens	Urticaria, angioedema, nausea, vomiting, abdominal cramping, diarrhea, wheezing, anaphylaxis	Acceptable	Acceptable	Not needed

minor determinants. The specificity for venoms and penicillin is comparable to that of the skin tests; therefore, a positive test is likely a true positive. Unexpectedly, up to 15% of patients who are allergic to insects and who have negative venom skin tests have positive results with the latest specific IgE in vitro tests; therefore, both tests should be used if either is negative in patients with a suspected clinical sensitivity.

Potentially, immunoassays for allergen-specific IgE also can be used to examine cross-reactivity between allergens by the use of soluable allergen inhibition. These assays are performed chiefly at research centers. The clinical utility of this could be seen with venom sensitivity. If a patient is found to be positive to yellow jacket at a low concentration and positive to *Polistes* wasp at a higher concentration, it is difficult to know if the patient is sensitive to both or whether the sensitivity to the wasp venom is due to cross-reactivity. An inhibition assay can be performed, and if it is found that all the reactivity to the *Polistes* wasp venom could be inhibited by yellow jacket venom, then it is likely that the positivity to the wasp venom was due to cross-reactivity. With this knowledge, immunotherapy would only have to be given to yellow jacket instead of to both yellow jacket and wasp.

Specific IgE immunoassays should be considered preferentially when a skin disease precludes skin tests, the patient is unable to discontinue medications that inhibit the histamine response, or when the history suggests an exquisite sensitivity. The next generation of in vitro tests will likely include multiplex allergen assays that are able to measure multiple allergens simultaneously. This should result in decreased cost and increased patient comfort. With the use of array technology, quantitative measurements of specific IgEs to numerous allergens are made simultaneously. Approaches include using glass slides with microdot placement of allergens or allergens covalently attached to microspheres that have been dyed and are spectrally distinguishable. One assay has been used for simultaneously measuring specific IgEs to house dust mite, cat, birch, grass, and mugwort. Compared with the CAP System, cat, birch, and grass detection was similar; sensitivity was slightly lower for house dust mite but did not reach statistical significance; however, mugwort sensitivity was significantly low. The specificity for the test was good. The allergen microarray is a promising option, requiring only 20 μL of serum; however, the clinical relevance of each allergen needs to be validated separately before multiallergen panels are used for routine diagnosis.

The current recommendations for skin prick, intradermal, and in vitro IgE specific antibody testing are summarized in Table 3.3.

3.2   Allergen Immunotherapy

Allergen-specific immunotherapy (SIT) is highly effective in the treatment of IgE-mediated diseases such as rhinitis, conjunctivitis, asthma, and venom sensitivity. First introduced in 1911 for treatment of allergic rhinitis due to grass pollen, it is a technique by which increasing amounts of allergen extract are injected subcutaneously over several months until a maintenance dose is reached. The maintenance dose is given monthly for several years to lessen clinical symptoms that arise on exposure to allergens. SIT is the only treatment that potentially leads to a life-long tolerance against previously disease-causing allergens because of the restoration of normal immunity. It also has been shown to prevent the onset of new sensitizations and to reduce the development of asthma in patients with allergic rhinitis.

3.2.1   Clinical Effectiveness of Allergen Immunotherapy

3.2.1.1   Allergic Rhinitis and Asthma

Many double-blind, placebo-controlled, randomized clinical trials have found that immunotherapy has a beneficial effect for the treatment of allergic rhinitis, including ocular symptoms, and allergic asthma in both children and adults. Efficacy has been confirmed for the treatment of inhalant allergy attributable to tree, grass, and weed pollens; fungi; animal allergens; dust mites; and cockroaches. Outcomes used to measure the efficacy of immunotherapy include symptom and medication scores, organ challenge, immunologic change in cell markers, and cytokine profiles. The magnitude of the effect depends on the outcome measure used. For example, studies with dust mite have shown a several fold improvement in symptom score and reduction in medication use and more than a tenfold reduction in bronchial hyperresponsiveness. Studies of other allergens, besides dust mites, have shown an approximately fivefold improvement in symptom score and reduction in bronchial hyperresponsiveness. Importantly, seasonal pollen immunotherapy has been shown to be effective even for patients who have severe seasonal rhinitis and conjunctivitis resistant to conventional drug therapy. The benefits of SIT for house dust mite perennial rhinitis are less than for seasonal rhinitis. This may be due to the contribution of vasomotor mechanisms to perennial rhinitis. Of interest, perennial rhinitis due to cat allergen has shown marked improvement in tolerance of cat exposure after SIT, as confirmed with both challenge tests and natural exposure.

Some studies have shown limited clinical effectiveness of SIT, particularly in asthma, but they were only marginally powered to show efficacy. To increase statistical power, meta-analyses of the efficacy of SIT for rhinitis and asthma have been performed. According to the most recent meta-analysis of 16 double-blind, placebo-controlled prospective studies of 759 patients with allergic rhinitis, immunotherapy was effective in 94% of studies, with improvement in symptoms and a reduction in medication use. In the 2000 meta-analysis of 24 double-blind, prospective, controlled studies of allergen immunotherapy in 962 patients with asthma, immunotherapy was effective in 71% of the studies, as shown by improvement in the symptoms of asthma, a reduction in medication, improved pulmonary function, and protection against bronchial challenge. These meta-analyses strongly support the efficacy of immunotherapy for allergic rhinitis and asthma.

Patient selection is important. The allergic basis of the rhinitis and asthma should be assessed carefully with exposure history and then objectively shown on skin tests or in vitro tests.

3.2.1.2 Venom Hypersensitivity

Venom immunotherapy has been found to be very effective in preventing subsequent systemic reactions from a Hymenoptera sting in patients with a history and confirmation of IgE sensitivity to stinging insects. However, the frequency of systemic reactions to stings in children and adults with a history of large local reactions to stinging insects is only 5–10%; the risk in patients with previous systemic reactions ranges from 20–70%, depending on the severity of the initial reaction. Venom immunotherapy decreases the risk in those with a history of systemic reaction to honeybee to 5–10% and to vespids (yellow jacket, white-faced hornet, yellow hornet, and wasp) to <5%. After 5 years of venom immunotherapy, stings years later cause a systemic response approximately 10% of the time.

3.2.2 Immunologic Changes in Immunotherapy

The initial event responsible for the development of allergic diseases is the generation of allergen-specific CD4+ T-cells. Antigen is presented to the T-cell by an antigen-presenting cell (APC) such as a B-cell, dendritic cell, or macrophage. Under the influence of interleukin (IL)-4, naïve T-cells activated by APCs differentiate into Th2 cells. The Th2 response, an allergic-type response, results in the release of IL-4, IL-5, and IL-13. IL-4 and IL-13 stimulate B-cell production of specific IgE, and IL-5 stimulates eosinophil activation and survival. Once specific IgE is formed to an allergen, subsequent allergen exposure results in the degranulation of mast cells by IgE-mediated cross-linking, with the subsequent release of histamine, leukotrienes, and prostaglandins. This is the key event in a type I hypersensitivity reaction and results clinically in watery, itchy eyes; itchy nose; sneeze; rhinorrhea; nasal congestion; cough; wheeze; vomiting; diarrhea; and possibly anaphylaxis (with systemic exposure). In contrast to a Th2 response, a Th1 response is characterized by the release of interferon (IFN)-γ and IL-2, but not IL-4 or IL-5. Hence, neither IgE antibody synthesis nor eosinophilic inflammation is induced. The Th1 response has been considered the "nonallergic" response.

Because of the central role of T-cells in either initiating or not initiating an allergic response to an antigen, multiple studies have been performed to address changes in the T-cell in response to immunotherapy. Initial studies of allergic patients receiving SIT have shown a reduction in proliferative responses to allergen and a shift in the cytokine release pattern from a Th2 profile to a Th1 profile when in vitro T-cell responses to allergen were measured from peripheral blood. However, these studies have not been uniformly reproducible, and recent studies have demonstrated that peripheral T-cell tolerance is crucial for a healthy immune response and successful treatment of allergic disorders. The tolerant state of specific cells results from increased secretion of IL-10. The cellular origin of IL-10 is the antigen-specific T-cell population and activated CD4$^+$CD25$^+$ T-cells as well as monocytes and B cells. An increase of IL-10 both during SIT and natural allergen exposure has been demonstrated. Healthy subjects and those with allergy exhibit subsets of allergen-specific CD4$^+$ cells that secrete IFN-γ (Th1), IL-4 (Th2), and IL-10 (Tr1), but in different proportions. In healthy subjects, Tr1 cells are the dominant subset for common environmental allergens, whereas a high frequency of allergen-specific IL-4-secreting cells is found in allergic individuals. Immunotherapy increases allergen-specific Tr1 cells, which suppress both the Th1 and Th2 types of responses by IL-10. It appears these allergen-specific Tr1 cells keep normal subjects from becoming allergic. The generation of Tr1 cells restores the normal immune response to these allergens. This may explain why the beneficial results of SIT can be long lasting.

SIT also has an effect on serum antibody isotypes. Although peripheral T-cell tolerance is induced during SIT, it does not appear that B-cell tolerance occurs. SIT frequently induces a transient increase in serum-specific IgE, followed by a gradual decrease over months or years of treatment. The changes in IgE do not seem to explain the diminished responsiveness to specific allergen in SIT, because the decrease in serum IgE is small and correlates poorly with the clinical response. Even though tolerance does not occur in the B-cell lineage, SIT induces blocking antibodies.

Early studies focused on the development of allergen-specific IgG4. It was thought that this antibody would capture the allergen before it could cross-link IgE and, thus, prevent the activation of mast cells. Several studies demonstrated a correlation between allergen-specific IgG4 levels and clinical improvement. Further work has shown that the blocking antibodies not only inhibit allergen-induced release of mast cell mediators but also inhibit allergen presentation to T-cells and prevent an increase in memory IgE production during exposure to high levels of allergen. IgG4 antibodies can be considered to have the ability to modulate the immune response to allergen and, thus, to influence the clinical response. SIT increases IgG4 allergen-specific antibodies. This has also been found to correlate with IL-10 production. IL-10 is a suppressor of both total and allergen-specific IgE and increases IgG4 production.

SIT is associated with a significant reduction in not only the immediate response to allergen provocation but also the late phase reaction in the nasal and bronchial mucosa. The late phase reaction, which typically occurs 6–12 hours after allergen exposure, is characterized by the recruitment and activation of eosinophils and activated T-cells. The inflammation in the late phase response is similar to the changes in the mucosal tissues of patients chronically exposed to inhalant allergens. Because the late phase response to inhaled allergens is associated with increased hyperresponsiveness and results in chronic allergic inflammation, the effect of SIT on the late phase reaction has been studied. SIT has been shown to increase the amount of allergen necessary to elicit the late phase response. Similarly, SIT decreases bronchial, nasal, and conjunctival hyperreactivity to nonspecific stimuli, which reflects a decrease in underlying inflammation. Biopsy specimens from patients receiving grass SIT showed a decrease in eosinophil and mast cell infiltration into nasal and bronchial mucosa; these changes correlated with the clinical effect. Therefore, in addition to tempering the acute reaction, SIT decreases the chronic inflammation associated with allergic exposure. This likely occurs by inducing peripheral T-cell tolerance to allergens, which results in decreased production of cytokines by T-cells and, thus, lack of stimulation for the priming, survival, and activation of mast cells and eosinophils. A summary of the effects of SIT on immunologic parameters is shown in Fig. 3.1.

3.2.3   Practical Considerations in Allergen Immunotherapy

3.2.3.1   Patient Selection

Allergen immunotherapy is appropriate for patients who have symptoms of allergic rhinitis or allergic asthma with natural exposure to the allergens and who demonstrate specific IgE antibodies by skin tests or in vitro tests to the relevant allergens. Allergen immunotherapy is also used in patients who have a systemic reaction and evidence of IgE sensitivity to stinging insects. The pattern of symptoms must conform to the pattern of exposure. Patients are not candidates for immunotherapy unless either skin tests or in vitro allergy testing show a positive result to the relevant allergens. Specific immunotherapy has not been shown to be effective in treating food allergy. Patients particularly suited to allergen immunotherapy

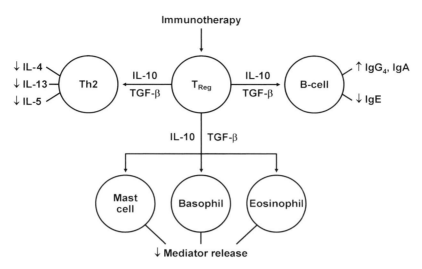

Fig. 3.1 Effects of allergen-specific immunotherapy on immunologic parameters. Allergen-specific immunotherapy upregulates T-regulatory cells. This appears to be the primary effect that results in suppression of Th2 cells and Th2 cytokines; decreased mediator release from mast cells, basophils, and eosinophils; and increased serum specific IgG_4 and IgA and decreased serum specific IgE from B-cells. *IL* interleukin; *TGF* transforming growth factor

are those whose allergic rhinitis and asthma symptoms are not controlled adequately by pharmacotherapy and avoidance measures or those who wish to reduce long-term use of pharmacotherapy or to avoid adverse effects of pharmacotherapy. Hymenoptera immunotherapy is used to help prevent the occurrence of an anaphylactic reaction to a sting. The clinical indications for allergen immunotherapy are outlined in Table 3.4.

3.2.3.2 Formulation of an Extract for Specific Immunotherapy

In formulating an immunotherapy extract, the following factors must be considered: (1) optimal dose of each constituent, (2) cross-reactivity of the allergens, and (3) possible enzymatic degradation of the allergens.

Adequate Dosing of Immunotherapy

The highest concentration of an immunotherapy extract projected as the therapeutically effective dose is called the maintenance concentrate. The maintenance concentrate should be selected to deliver a dose considered to be therapeutically effective for each of its constitutive components. Allergen extracts are commercially available for most of the commonly recognized allergens. Whenever possible, standardized

Table 3.4 Indications for allergen immunotherapy

Allergic rhinitis

Symptoms of allergic rhinitis after natural exposure to aeroallergens with demonstrable evidence of IgE sensitivity by skin prick testing or in vitro specific IgE to the relevant allergen(s)
Particularly helpful for those with:
   Poor response to pharmacotherapy and allergen avoidance
   Coexisting allergic rhinitis and asthma
   Poor tolerance of medications

Allergic asthma

Symptoms of asthma after natural exposure to aeroallergens with demonstrable evidence of IgE sensitivity by skin prick testing or in vitro specific IgE to the relevant allergen(s)
Stable asthma with FEV_1 >70% predicted
Particularly helpful for those with:
   Poor response to pharmacotherapy and allergen avoidance
   Coexisting allergic rhinitis and asthma
   Poor tolerance of medications

Hymenoptera stings
History of a systemic reaction to a Hymenoptera sting and demonstrable evidence of IgE sensitivity by skin prick testing or in vitro specific IgE History of a systemic reaction to imported fire ant and demonstrable evidence of IgE sensitivity by skin prick testing or in vitro specific IgE

Modified from Li, J. T., Lockey, R. F., Bernstein, I. L., et al., Joint Task Force on Practice Parameters, American Academy of Allergy, Asthma and Immunology; American College of Allergy, Asthma and Immunology; Joint Council of Allergy, Asthma and Immunology. (2003) Allergen immunotherapy: a practice parameter. Ann Allergy Asthma Immunol. 90, 15. Used with permission

extracts should be used to prepare the immunotherapy treatment set. Standardized extracts are available for cat hair, cat pelt, *D pteronyssinus*, *D farinae*, short ragweed, Bermuda grass, Kentucky bluegrass, perennial ryegrass, orchard grass, timothy grass, meadow fescue, red top, sweet vernal grass, and Hymenoptera venoms (yellow jacket, honeybee, wasp, yellow hornet, and white-faced hornet). Many allergens are not yet standardized. The labeling of the extracts can be confusing because allergen extracts are quantified in several ways with different unitage systems. Potency can be measured practically in different ways: skin test end-point titration, radioimmunoassay inhibition, or content of a known major allergen. Standardized extracts in the United States were first labeled in potency units (AU) on the basis of the major allergen content. The extracts subsequently have been labeled on the basis of comparative skin test potency (BAU). This standard can then be applied to all allergen extracts and have equal meaning. Nonstandardized extracts are labeled as either weight to volume (w/v) or in protein nitrogen units (PNU). Note that PNU or weight per volume (w/v) are not necessarily reliable indicators of potency. Weight to volume indicates how the extract was produced; a weight to volume of 1:100 indicates that 1 g of dry allergen was added to 100 mL of buffer for extraction. Extracts with a particular weight to volume may have widely varying biologic activities. One PNU equals 0.01 µg of protein nitrogen (phosphotungstic acid precipitable nitrogen). The true allergenicity is difficult to decipher because the source material can contain various proteins that contribute to the PNU without being allergenic.

Many of the double-blind, placebo-controlled studies report the allergen dose administered. Occasionally, more than one dose is tested to establish not only an effective dose but also to generate a dose-response curve and to determine an ineffective dose. Generally, the noneffective doses have been about one-fifth to one-tenth the effective dose, indicating a narrow dosing window. Effective doses of the standardized extracts have often been defined on the basis of their major allergen content. However, the current method of standardization in the United States does not always use this information on dosing. Representative lots of standardized extracts have been assessed for their major allergen content, allowing an approximation of proven doses. The major allergen content and effective maintenance doses for common allergens are outlined in Table 3.5.

Among the US standardized extracts, pollens are generally 5–10 times as potent as indoor allergens. In the majority of US extracts that are not standardized, the pollen extracts tend to be of good quality, comparable to the standardized pollen extracts. Extracts of the nonstandardized indoor allergens, however, such as cockroach and molds, tend to be weak and of highly variable potency.

Patterns of Cross-Allergenicity

Knowledge of allergen cross-reactivity is important in the selection of allergens for immunotherapy because the number of allergens that can be optimally placed in a treatment vial is limited. The use of one allergen that has significant cross-reactivity with other clinically relevant allergens saves volume when formulating an immunotherapy mix. Because cross-allergenicity is variable for many grass and weed pollens, their intrinsic allergenicity, prevalence, and aerobiologic distribution within a specific region should be considered. The general pattern of cross-allergenicity shows rare significant cross-allergenicity between families, variable cross-allergenicity between tribes or genera of a family, and a high degree of cross-allergenicity between species of the same genus. Many of the temperate pasture grasses of the subfamily Poaceae, such as fescue, rye, timothy, blue, and orchard, share major allergens. Therefore, the use of one of the grasses, such as rye, fescue, or timothy, provides protection against the entire group. Grasses in other subfamilies show greater diversity and should be evaluated separately. Bermuda, Bahia, and Johnson, important grasses in U.S. southern states, are not closely related and should be evaluated separately. Tree pollen generally has limited cross-allergenicity, although some cross-allergenicity does occur. Pollen from members of the cypress family, such as juniper, cedar, and cypress, strongly cross-react; therefore, only one would be required for the immunotherapy mix. The birch (birch, alder, hazel, hornbeam, top hornbeam) and beech (beech, oak, chestnut) have strong cross-allergenicity. The use of one of the locally prevalent pollens should be adequate. A single oak should provide coverage for other oaks. Although maple and

Table 3.5 Expressed concentration, major allergen content, and effective dosing of common allergen extracts

Extract	Major allergen	Expressed concentration	Mean major allergen content ($\mu g\ mL^{-1}$)	Effective dosing ($\mu g\ mL^{-1}$)	Add to 5-mL vial (assuming 0.5 mL maintenance injection) (mL)	Maintenance concentration	Maintenance dose (0.5 mL of maintenance concentration)
Short ragweed	Amb a 1	1:10 w/v	424	6–24	0.4	1:125 w/v	1:125 w/v
Timothy grass	Phl p 5	100,000 BAU mL^{-1}	680	15–20	0.3	6,000 BAU mL^{-1}	3,000 BAU
D pteronyssinus	Der p 1	10,000 AU mL^{-1}	76	7–12	1.1	2,200 AU mL^{-1}	1,100 AU
D farinae	Der f 1	10,000 AU mL^{-1}	56	10	1.5	3,000 AU mL^{-1}	1,500 AU
Cat dander	Fel d 1	10,000 BAU mL^{-1}	43	11–17	3	6,000 BAU mL^{-1}	3,000 BAU
Dog dander (AP)	Can f 1	1:100 w/v	180	15	1	1:500 w/v	1:500 w/v

Modified from Nelson, H. S. (2007) Allergen immunotherapy: where is it now? J. Allergy Clin. Immunol. 119,770–771. Used with permission

AP acetone precipitated; *AU* allergy units; *BAU* bioequivalent allergy units

box elder trees are in the same genus, they have little similarity and should be considered separately. In the genus *Carya*, pecan and hickory have strong cross-allergenicity, and in the genus *Populus*, poplar, cottonwood, and aspen show significant cross-allergenicity. The common ragweed species, short, giant, false, and western, have strong cross-allergenicity, and a single pollen can be used for these allergens. Weeds other than ragweeds, such as marsh elders, sages, and mugworts, need to be treated separately from the ragweeds. The sages and mugwort are strongly cross-reactive. Among the chenopod-amaranth family, the *Amaranthus* spp. (redroot pigweed, spiny pigweed, and careless weed) require only one member, as do the *Atriplex* spp. (saltbushes, allscales, and lenscales). Among the chenopods, Russian thistle appears to have the most cross-allergenicity.

The most prevalent house dust mites, *D pteronyssinus* and *D farinae*, are members of the same family and genus. Despite this, they have unique allergenic epitopes and should be considered separately.

Mixing Allergen Extracts

Allergen extracts contain mixtures of proteins and glycoproteins. There have been reports of interactions between extracts when mixed together. When mixed together, extracts such as those of *Alternaria* spp. have been shown to decrease the IgE-binding activity of timothy grass extract but not ragweed. All the possible interactions between extracts have not been fully delineated. Generally, extracts that have higher proteolytic enzyme activity, such as fungi, dust mites, and insects, should be kept separate from those with less proteolytic activity, such as the tree, grass, and weed pollen extracts. *Alternaria* is most frequently responsible for the loss of potency of other allergens, followed by cockroach and *Cladosporium*. Although proteolytic, *D farinae* does not appear to significantly alter the potency of other allergens. Short ragweed appears to be relatively resistant to the effects of proteases. This can be summarized as follows:

- Allergens with high protease activity (may be mixed together): arthopods (dust mites), fungi (mold spores), and insects (cockroaches)
- Allergens with low protease activity (may be mixed together): tree, grass and weed pollens, and animals (cat and dog)
- Ragweed likely can be mixed with either group above.
- Hymenoptera venoms require a separate vial and injection.

Writing an Allergen Extract Prescription

Once the decision has been made about which allergen extracts to include based on potency and the maintenance dose required for symptom control, patterns of cross-allergenicity, and ability or inability of the allergen extracts to be mixed with each other, an allergen immunotherapy prescription can be written. See the examples in clinical vignette 1. The maintenance doses for each allergen in each vial should be listed. This should start with the amount of extract used from the commercially supplied extract and the concentration of the allergen in the extract. For example, if 0.2 mL of standard timothy extract (100,000 BAU mL^{-1}) from the supply is used this should be listed first. This amount provides 20,000 BAU. At our institution, this is diluted in 5 mL, giving a maintenance vial concentration of 4,000 BAU mL^{-1}. Serial dilutions of the maintenance concentrate should be made in preparation for the buildup phase of the immunotherapy (see below). At full maintenance, the patient normally receives 0.5 mL from the maintenance concentration vial (4,000 BAU mL^{-1}), resulting in the patient receiving 2,000 BAU per injection at full maintenance dosing. The amount of allergen received at each point in the buildup process is listed in parentheses in Table 3.6, based on using 0.2 mL timothy extract (100,000 BAU mL^{-1}) with a maintenance concentration of 4,000 BAU mL^{-1}.

Injection Schedules

The immunotherapy schedule is divided into a buildup phase and a maintenance phase. The initial buildup to maintenance is conventionally achieved by twice-weekly to weekly injections of the immunotherapy extract. It is essential that the patient maintain a regular schedule during this time. Alternative schedules such as cluster and rush protocols have also been used. An example of a conventional buildup schedule is shown in Table 3.6. The immunotherapy schedule is basically a stepwise increase in allergen concentration that starts from the most dilute concentration vial and proceeds to the maintenance concentration vial. The first dose is from the most dilute vial (typically 1:1,000 dilution of maintenance concentration); 0.05 mL is administered, followed by increasing volumes from that vial (0.1, 0.2 mL, etc.) with the subsequent injections. Once the patient receives the 0.5-mL dose from the vial, he or she advances to the lowest dose of the next vial and continues in that manner until reaching the maintenance concentrate. Clinical experience has shown that the 1:1,000 dilution of the maintenance dosage is generally a safe starting concentration. For those exquisitely sensitive, particularly if there is underlying asthma, a 1:10,000 dilution can be used for the initial concentration. For uniformity, the 1:1,000 vial is colored green, the 1:100 blue, the 1:10 yellow, and the concentrate red. When the patient has reached a maintenance dose, the interval between injections can be increased to every 4 weeks (aeroallergens) to 6 weeks (Hymenoptera venom). The more dilute the allergen in the vial, the faster the potency of the mixture decreases. It has been estimated that the 1:1,000 dilution remains potent for approximately 6 weeks, the 1:100 and 1:10 dilutions for 6 months, and the concentrate for 6 months to 1 year.

Hymenoptera dosing differs from the dosing for airborne allergens. A common dosage schedule for Hymenoptera venoms is shown in Table 3.7. A commercially available mixed vespid regimen combines yellow jacket, white-faced hornet, and yellow hornet into one injection; hence, the concentration is three times that for a single Hymenoptera venom. Despite the higher concentrations, the mixed vespid immunotherapy regimen is well tolerated. It is important to note that *Polistes* wasp is not included in the mixed vespid regimen.

Table 3.6 Immunotherapy schedule[a]

Bottle #	Dose #	Dose (mL)	BAU per dose[b]
#1	1	0.05	0.2
	2	0.10	0.4
	3	0.20	0.8
1:1,000	4	0.30	1.2
	5	0.40	1.6
	6	0.50	2
#2	7	0.05	2
	8	0.10	4
	9	0.20	8
1:100	10	0.30	12
	11	0.40	16
	12	0.50	20
#3	13	0.05	20
	14	0.10	40
	15	0.20	80
1:10	16	0.30	120
	17	0.40	160
	18	0.50	200
#4	19	0.05	200
	20	0.10	400
	21	0.20	800
Concentrate	22	0.30	1,200
	23	0.40	1,600
	24	0.50	2,000

After reaching last dose, begin "stretch." Repeat last dose in 1 week, 2 weeks, and 3 weeks. Then maintain at this dose once every 4 weeks

[a]Injections given no less than 3 days and no more than 8 days apart

[b]The amount of allergen received with each dose based on using 0.2 mL timothy extract (100,000 BAU mL), with maintenance concentration of 4,000 BAU mL^{-1}

Dosage adjustments are made if a patient misses scheduled dosages of immunotherapy or if there are reactions to the immunotherapy. General guidelines can be given for missed dosages during the buildup phase and during the maintenance phase. During the buildup phase, if >8 days but <20 days have elapsed since the last dose, the same dose as the last injection should be given. If >20 days but <40 days have elapsed since the last injection, give half of the last dose given, followed by a repeat half dose in 1–5 days, then continue to build according to schedule. If >40 days have elapsed since the last injection, individual recommendations should be made. During the maintenance phase, if >36 days but <75 days have elapsed, half of the last dose should be given, followed by a repeat half dose in 1–5 days, then a full dose in 1 week, another full dose in 2 weeks, and then back to the every 4-week schedule. If >75 days have elapsed, individual recommendations should be made. Dosage changes are customized for maintenance Hymenoptera venom because they are often given every 6 weeks during the maintenance phase. If >50 days but <90 days have elapsed since the last injection, give half of the maintenance dose, repeat

Table 3.7 Schedule for venom immunotherapy

	Venom	
Bottle #1	1 µg mL^{-1}	0.05 mL
		0.10 mL
		0.20 mL
		0.40 mL
Bottle #2	10 µg mL^{-1}	0.05 mL
		0.10 mL
		0.20 mL
		0.40 mL
Bottle #3	100 µg mL^{-1}	0.05 mL
		0.10 mL
		0.20 mL
		0.40 mL
		0.60 mL
		0.80 mL
		1.00 mL
	Mixed vespid	
Bottle #1	3 µg mL^{-1}	0.05 mL
		0.10 mL
		0.20 mL
		0.40 mL
Bottle #2	30 µg mL^{-1}	0.05 mL
		0.10 mL
		0.20 mL
		0.40 mL
Bottle #3	300 µg mL^{-1}	0.05 mL
		0.10 mL
		0.20 mL
		0.40 mL
		0.60 mL
		0.80 mL
		1.00 mL

Repeat last dose in 1 week, 2 weeks, 3 weeks, and
every 4 weeks for 6 months, then maintain at once
every 6 weeks

the half dose in 1–5 days, full dose in 1 week, full dose in 2 weeks, full dose in 4 weeks, and then back to an every 6-week schedule.

Reactions to immunotherapy require individualized adjustment based on the patient's allergy history, compliance with the immunotherapy, and history of previous reactions. In general, local reactions <3 cm and lasting <24 hours do not require change in dosing. Large local reactions may require repeating the previous dose or returning to the dose for which there was no reaction, depending on the history. Large local reactions are not predictive of a subsequent systemic reaction. Any history of systemic reactions to immunotherapy requires close physician review to determine dosage adjustment and whether immunotherapy should be continued.

Cluster immunotherapy is characterized by administration of immunotherapy one or two times weekly, with two or more buildup injections given per visit. Typically, injections are given at 30–120-minutes intervals. This scheduling allows the patient to reach the maintenance dose in less time. However, compared with conventional dosing, the cluster schedule has the potential to induce a systemic reaction. Another dosage option is rush immunotherapy. Rush schedules are more rapid than cluster immunotherapy. Accelerated schedules have been described for inhalant allergens in which up to eight injections have been given over the course of 6 hours. Hymenoptera rush immunotherapy schedules have been reported in which maintenance levels are achieved in as little as 90 minutes. The accelerated schedules, however, are associated with a significantly increased risk of local and systemic reactions. These schedules are labor intensive and can be difficult for both the patient and medical staff. Close observation and the ability to treat effectively a severe, life-threatening anaphylactic reaction are required.

In general, because of the complexity of immunotherapy, which involves appropriate patient selection, allergen strength, and cross-reactivity, and the potential of a severe anaphylactic reaction, immunotherapy should be formulated and administered only by those with expertise in this area.

Storage of Allergen Extracts

Many allergen extracts are heat sensitive. It is thought that the loss in potency when allergen extracts are exposed to high temperatures may be due to the heat-labile proteins, whereas the loss of potency due to prolonged exposure at room temperature may be due to the proteases in the extract. Allergenic extracts exposed to room temperature over time may lose potency. Therefore, allergen extracts should be kept at refrigerator temperature at all times except when in use. Also, repeated freezing and thawing can decrease the potency of some allergens and should be avoided. Preservatives for allergen extracts are designed to preserve potency as well as to provide antibacterial activity. The three most common preservatives used are glycerin, phenol, and HSA. Glycerin is an effective stabilizer of extract potency and appears to inhibit proteolytic enzyme activity. At high concentrations, glycerin can be associated with skin irritation at the site of injection. In some studies, but not others, glycerin in 50% solution has been associated with irritation. Solutions of 25% glycerin or less for immunotherapy appear to be well tolerated by most patients. Ten percent glycerin is as effective as 0.03% HSA, and the preservative effects of the 10% glycerin and 0.03% HSA are additive. Phenol is used as an antibacterial agent, but at high concentrations may be associated with allergen breakdown. Phenol will denature proteins, including allergen extracts, preserved in 50% glycerin. This seems to occur primarily when very dilute allergen concentrations are used. HSA is thought to decrease the adsorption of the allergen to the vial surface. It is a less potent stabilizer than glycerin. Because HSA does not have antimicrobial activity, it is often combined with phenol. HSA is more protective than 50% glycerin against the deleterious effects of phenol on allergens.

3.2.4   Duration of Immunotherapy

The optimal duration of inhalant allergen immunotherapy has not been studied extensively. Inhalant allergy immunotherapy is usually effective within the first year, and studies have suggested that a 3–5-years treatment produces long-term symptom relief for the majority of patients. In this situation, some patients experience a prolonged remission after discontinuation of therapy, but others may have disease relapse. From the available evidence, it appears that immunotherapy for <3 years results in significant relapse within 1–2 years compared with immunotherapy of longer duration. No adequate diagnostic tests are available for identifying which patients will experience a sustained clinical improvement and which ones will experience relapse. General guidelines are that the course of allergen immunotherapy should be continued until the patient has been symptom-free or has had reduced symptoms for 3–5 years. Longer duration of treatment should be determined by the physician and patient after considering the risks and benefits associated with continuing or discontinuing immunotherapy. Treatment may be considered for a longer period depending on the patient's exposure and previous and current response to treatment. If immunotherapy is discontinued and then started at a later time, the patient needs to start at the buildup phase and cannot immediately resume treatment using the monthly maintenance dosing.

The duration of allergen immunotherapy has been studied more extensively for Hymenoptera immunotherapy. Although studies have suggested that a 5-year treatment course should be sufficient for most allergic individuals, relapse rates ranging from 5 to 15% in the 10-year period after discontinuation of immunotherapy have been reported. Higher relapse rates are associated with honeybee sensitivity, significant reactions to immunotherapy injections, allergic reactions to stings while receiving immunotherapy, and a severe initial anaphylactic reaction to the sting. The duration of venom immunotherapy should be individualized on the basis of risk factors for relapse, the likelihood of exposure, and the patient's comfort level.

3.2.5   Safety of Allergen Immunotherapy

The rate of severe reactions in the United States from immunotherapy is very low. Reported rates of systemic reactions vary from 1 to 2.9%. The reactions occur more frequently during the initial buildup phase. It was anticipated that systemic reactions would occur more commonly during a patient's relevant pollen seasons, but this has not been the case in large studies. Local reactions, although annoying and sometimes painful, are not predictive of a systemic reaction. Modification of the immunotherapy dosage regimen for local reactions is based primarily on patient comfort. The interval between injection of the allergen extract and development of a systemic reaction is important. The more severe reactions tend to occur earlier, with most of them occurring within 30 minutes. Fatal reactions rarely occur with immunotherapy. Based on surveys, it is estimated that one fatal reaction occurs for every 2.5 million injections. There are clear risk factors for the fatalities. These include asthma that is labile or symptomatic at the time of injection, cardiovascular disease, first injection from a new vial of extract, dosage errors, concomitant treatment with β-adrenergic blocking agents, and home administration or unsupervised administration of immunotherapy. Precautions that should be undertaken to decrease the risk of a severe systemic reaction or a fatality include the following:

- Observing the patient for 30 minutes after the immunotherapy injection
- Not administering immunotherapy to patients with symptomatic asthma
- Performing peak expiratory flow measurements before administering immunotherapy and not administering immunotherapy if peak flow is <80% of the patient's customary level
- Splitting the first dose of a new immunotherapy vial, for the patient to receive one-half the dose of the new vial, followed by the second half 1–5 days later
- Using a check system to ensure correct dosage
- Avoiding β-adrenergic blocker therapy for patients receiving immunotherapy
- Having the equipment, medication, and expertise to treat a severe anaphylactic reaction

3.2.6   Allergen Immunotherapy in Children

Specific immunotherapy is safe and effective for children. The dosing of immunotherapy is the same for children as for adults. Immunotherapy may be even more effective for children and young adults than for older adults. Specifically, in addition to symptom control of allergic rhinitis and allergic asthma, immunotherapy decreases the development of new allergens in monosensitized persons and reduces the development of asthma in children with allergic rhinitis. Studies have shown that administering immunotherapy to a child, adolescent, or young adult who has a single positive skin prick test reduces the likelihood of additional positive skin prick tests developing during the duration of immunotherapy and for 3 years after immunotherapy has been discontinued. It is not known whether new sensitization is similarly prevented in those initially with multiple positive skin prick tests. The Preventive Allergy Treatment Study (PAT) has shown that in children with allergic rhinitis, but initially no asthma, approximately 45% develop asthma over a 5–10-year period when treated without immunotherapy; however, of those who receive immunotherapy, only 20% develop asthma at 5 years and 25% at 10 years.

There is some disagreement about the role of allergen immunotherapy for children younger than 5 years. Some studies have shown benefit for this age group, but there is a concern about the ability for the child and physician to quickly recognize the symptoms of a systemic reaction. Typically, inhalant immunotherapy is not considered necessary for those younger than 5 years, because pollen sensitivities usually do not develop during infancy or when the child is a toddler. For children younger than 5 years who have a history of anaphylaxis to Hymenoptera, the benefits of venom therapy may outweigh the risks and should be addressed on an individual basis.

3.2.7 Allergen Immunotherapy in Pregnancy

Allergen immunotherapy is effective treatment for pregnant patients. The general rule of management is that maintenance dosing can be continued during pregnancy; however, neither a buildup program nor any increase in dose is given during pregnancy because of the possible increased risk of a systemic reaction. Possible complications of a systemic reaction in the pregnant patient include spontaneous abortion, premature labor, and fetal hypoxia.

3.2.8 Future Allergen Immunotherapy

Our current understanding and approach to the improvement of immunotherapy is focused on two concepts: (1) the effectiveness of allergen immunotherapy is secondary to T-cell modification, and (2) the adverse reactions to allergen immunotherapy are mediated by injected allergens that combine with IgE on mast cells, triggering an allergic reaction. On the basis of these concepts, extracts are being modified to reduce their allergenicity without reducing their immunogenicity. Various approaches being studied include modification of current allergen extracts by mode of delivery (sublingual), concomitant administration of anti-IgE, or by adjustment of the vehicle in which the extract is injected. Other approaches use recombinant and peptide technology to produce immunotherapy that provides a T-cell modifying, yet nonallergic, response.

3.2.8.1 Current Extract Adjustment

Vehicle Adjustment and Anti-IgE

A common approach is to decrease the rate of dissemination of the allergen extract from the injection site, thus reducing systemic reactions. Adsorption of the allergen extract to alum has been used for this purpose. Although often used in Europe, alum-adsorbed extracts are available for only a small number of allergens in the United States and are not available for house dust mites and animal danders. Other substances that have been used to decrease systemic uptake include L-tyrosine and encapsulation in liposomes. These measures continue to be studied.

The monoclonal anti-IgE antibody omalizumab has been studied in conjunction with rush immunotherapy. Theoretically, the binding of free IgE would be expected to decrease the risk of a systemic reaction during immunotherapy. In one study, patients who were given omalizumab for 9 weeks before a single day of rush immunotherapy with ragweed extract experienced a fivefold decrease in the number of systemic reactions during the 1-day protocol and a reduction in systemic reactions during the subsequent buildup phase. Further studies will be helpful to delineate the role of omalizumab in cluster schedules and in treating patients with high sensitivity.

Sublingual Immunotherapy

Sublingual immunotherapy (SLIT) is delivered by two methods. With sublingual spit, the extract is kept under the tongue for a short period then spat out. More often, however, the sublingual swallow method is used. With this method, the extract is kept under the tongue for 1–2 minutes, then swallowed. SLIT has been used with increasing frequency in Europe and is being viewed with increased interest by allergists in the United States. Fifty clinical SLIT studies were reviewed for efficacy analysis by the ACAAI/AAAAI task force. Although the majority of SLIT studies reviewed showed some evidence of clinical efficacy improved symptom scores, medication scores, or both – approximately one-third of the randomized double-blind, placebo-controlled studies did not show efficacy in either symptom score or medication score. Dosage was extremely variable throughout the studies and a consistent relation among allergen dose, treatment duration, and clinical efficacy has not been established. Many studies of SLIT have shown a decrease in circulating eosinophils, a decrease in serum levels of eosinophil cation protein, and an increase in allergen-specific IgG4 and IgA levels. Peripheral blood lymphocytes have been shown to have a reduced proliferative response to allergen and enhanced secretion of IL-10, IL-12, and IFN-γ. Both immediate and late phase cutaneous responses to allergen are decreased. Like subcutaneous SIT, SLIT also has been shown to decrease the development of new skin test reactivity and progression of rhinitis to asthma. The expected primary advantage of SLIT is safety. The most common adverse effects with SLIT, by far, are local symptoms (itching and swelling) in the oral cavity; however, abdominal complaints, urticaria, and asthma have been reported, although rarely. Severe anaphylactic reactions with hypotension, although rare, have recently been reported. Fatal reactions have not been reported. The general lack of life-threatening side effects has allowed SLIT to be routinely administered by the patient at home. Of note, SLIT usage has not been reported for patients with severe asthma, and multiple allergen SLIT has not been reported.

Many questions have not been answered about SLIT. The main areas of concern are dosing and scheduling. Cumulative dosage regimens have varied by 500-fold without a clear dose response. The treatment schedule and overall duration of treatment are unknown. It is not clear if this therapy results in long-term improvement after it has been discontinued. From the standpoint of individual patients, it is not known whether SLIT can be administered to high-risk asthma patients or to those requiring a mixture of noncross-reacting allergens. These questions will need to be addressed to assess the cost:benefit ratio. Currently, no sublingual allergy extract has been approved for use in the United States.

3.2.8.2 Allergen Modification

Recombinant Allergens in Immunotherapy

Recombinant allergens may be the future of immunotherapy. Allergens from most relevant sources have been identified, characterized, and produced as recombinant proteins with biologic activity comparable to that of their natural counterparts.

Sequences and structural features of more than 500 allergens derived from various sources have been described. The majority of the allergens have been cloned for research purposes, but few have been used in clinical studies. Recombinant allergens have several advantages over natural allergen extracts. The natural allergen extracts contain allergens with widely varying potencies and undefined components, they may contain low amounts of important allergens, and they are difficult to compare between different products and batches. Recombinant allergens are molecules with defined physiochemical and immunologic properties that can be modified to allow for immunologic tolerance (preserved T-cell epitopes) yet not produce an IgE-mediated response. Also, recombinant allergens can be compared precisely to provide consistent and reproducible products.

Two types of recombinant allergen-based immunotherapy regimens have been developed and tested in clinical trials. The first type is based on the use of recombinant allergens that equal the natural allergens (recombinant wild type-based immunotherapy), and the second type is based on genetically engineered or modified hypoallergenic recombinant allergens. Studies of recombinant wild-type allergen with timothy and birch allergens have shown clinical improvement of symptoms and robust development of IgG4. Studies with modified hypoallergenic birch recombinant allergens have shown clinical improvement, increased development of IgG4, and blunting of seasonal pollen exposure-induced increases in allergen-specific IgE. Because of the hypoallergenic nature of the modified recombinant allergen, a higher allergen dose could be used and tolerated by patients. These initial results of recombinant allergen immunotherapy are encouraging. Future work will focus on the identification of the relevant allergens in allergen extracts, with the development of recombinant wild-type allergens and modified hypoallergenic recombinant allergens.

Allergen-derived peptides are also being studied. Because the T-lymphocyte epitopes are short segments of adjacent amino acids, it is possible to devise allergen peptides too small to react with the 3-dimensional structure of IgE yet still able to produce a T-cell response. This approach is being studied with the major cat allergen Fel d 1.

Conjugation with Immunostimulatory Sequences of DNA

Immunotherapy attempts to redirect the underlying immune dysfunction that elicits and maintains immediate hypersensitivity reactions, particularly by attempting to establish a more balanced Th1/Th2 response. In animal studies, immunostimulatory DNA sequences (unmethylated cytosine phosphorothionate guanosine segments-CpG) induce Th1-biased immune responses and inhibit the development of Th2 immunity when administered before antigen exposure by reacting with toll-like receptor 9 of antigen-presenting cells. Initial studies in humans linked purified Amb a 1 (primary ragweed allergen) to an immunostimulatory phosphorothioate oligooxydeoxyribonucleotide forming the Amb a 1-immunostimulatory DNA sequence conjugate (AIC). AIC injections led to a prolonged shift from Th2 immunity toward Th1 immunity and were tolerated. Subsequent studies in adults receiving six weekly injections of AIC before ragweed season noted better peak season rhinitis scores, peak season daily nasal symptom scores, and midseason overall quality of life scores compared with placebo. This modality will continue to be studied.

3.3 Summary

Allergen immunotherapy is effective treatment for allergic rhinoconjunctivitis, asthma, and Hymenoptera sensitivity in appropriately selected patients. By modifying the immune response to allergen, immunotherapy not only treats the disease while treatment is being administered, but also results in disease modification after therapy is discontinued. Immunotherapy can prevent new sensitizations in monosensitized persons and prevent the development of asthma in those with only allergic rhinitis. Immunotherapy is being refined further to increase the immune-modifying effects of allergen administration and to decrease allergic reactions to the therapy. New approaches to immunotherapy under study include modified recombinant allergens, peptides, and immunostimulatory DNA sequences bound to allergenic proteins.

3.4 Clinical Vignettes

3.4.1 Vignette 1

A 23-year-old midwestern (US) woman presents with allergic rhinitis and mild persistent asthma. She remains symptomatic despite adequate pharmacologic treatment with regularly dosed nonsedating H_1-blocker, topical nasal corticosteroid, low-dose inhaled corticosteroid, and inhaled β_2-agonist, used as needed. Her symptoms are perennial, with marked worsening seasonally in the spring, late summer, and fall. Symptoms consist of watery, itchy eyes; nasal congestion; nasal itch; rhinorrhea; and intermittent wheezing. She lives in an old house (approximately 100 years old); she does not have air conditioning and does not have any pets or animal exposure. The physical examination findings are consistent with allergic rhinoconjunctivitis. She inquires about allergy testing and "allergy shots."

Comment: The patient is symptomatic despite reasonable treatment. Allergen skin prick testing should be performed to the possible aeroallergens that contribute to her symptoms. This will help in making recommendations about environmental modification and would form the basis for possible immunotherapy. Her perennial symptoms may be due to molds and dust mites, her spring symptoms may be due to outdoor molds and trees, and her late summer and fall symptoms may be due to outdoor molds and weeds. The tree, mold, and weed allergens should be selected on the basis of regional pollen and mold counts and also on their cross-reactivity patterns. Allergen skin prick tests are the preferred method of testing in this situation based on sensitivity and cost.

Allergen skin prick testing shows a negative histamine control. The patient states she mistakenly continued her nonsedating antihistamine, although she was instructed to discontinue the medication 5 days before the appointment.

Comment: This scenario is not uncommon. Many patients are not sure what antihistamines are. When instructing the patient to discontinue antihistamines, it is important to also supply a list of commonly used antihistamine medications, both prescription and nonprescription. It is also helpful to inform the patient that it is okay to continue topical nasal corticosteroids and lung inhalation medications. At this point, skin prick testing can be performed at a later date or in vitro specific IgE testing can be performed. The use of antihistamines does not interfere with the in vitro specific IgE testing.

The patient discontinued her antihistamine, and allergen skin prick testing was performed 1 week later. This time, there was a normal positive response to the histamine control (6 × 6F) and a negative response to the glycerin negative control (0). Skin prick testing showed positive responses to *D farinae* (6 × 6F), birch tree (10 × 10F), ragweed (9 × 11F), and *Alternaria* (8 × 8F).

Comment: These findings are consistent with her history of perennial symptoms (*D farinae*) and worsening symptoms in the spring (birch, *Alternaria*) and late summer and fall (ragweed, *Alternaria*). Allergen avoidance recommendations should be made for dust mite. Avoidance measures for tree, weed, and outdoor mold exposures are not particularly helpful. The patient would be a good candidate for immunotherapy. Her pulmonary function should be assessed before immunotherapy is initiated.

Spirometry was performed. The FEV_1/FVC ratio was slightly decreased at 78% (normal ≥80%). FEV_1 was 3.6 L, which was 88% of predicted.

Comment: The spirometry results are within normal limits. If FEV_1 showed a significant reduction (<70% predicted), she likely would not be a good candidate for immunotherapy because she would be at higher risk for a severe reaction. The risks, benefits, and scheduling of immunotherapy should be reviewed in detail with the patient.

The risks, benefits, and scheduling of immunotherapy were reviewed with the patient, and she wished to proceed.

Comment: The next step is making the immunotherapy. There is no cross-reaction between the relevant allergens: *D farinae*, birch, *Alternaria*, and ragweed. *D farinae* and *Alternaria* contain proteases; they can be mixed together in an injection but should not be mixed with the other extracts. The birch and ragweed extracts do not contain proteases and can be mixed together. (Some studies also support the mixing of ragweed with protease-containing extracts.) Next, the amount of each allergen to be used needs to be calculated. The dosage should be based on the amount of allergen in the extract that has been shown to be clinically effective. These are as follows:

D farinae	500–2,000 AU (10 μg)	Supplied as 10,000 AU mL^{-1} (56 μg mL^{-1})
Birch	800–2,000 PNU	supplied as 40,000 PNU mL^{-1}
Alternaria	2,000 PNU	supplied as 40,000 PNU mL^{-1}
Ragweed	1/150 w/v	supplied as 1/10 w/v

Some general rules for calculating the dose and how many allergens can be mixed in one vial are listed below:

1. Most commercially available extracts are concentrated so that 0.3–1.5 mL of supply extract is used to make the formulation (cat may require larger amounts).
2. The total amount of the supply extracts cannot exceed the total volume for one mix; in these calculations, it is 5 mL.
3. The volume of the supplied extract from one allergen can serve as "diluent" for another allergen when mixed together.
4. When the final concentration of allergen extract is made with 5 mL (as in these calculations), the volume of the supplied extracts is subtracted from 5 mL to determine the amount of diluent added to the final concentration.

Thus, in this formulation (Note that *D farinae* extracts are expressed in both AU and μg of mean major allergen content.):

D farinae	1.5 mL of supply = 15,000 AU (84 μg) Final concentration (supply diluted in 5 mL) = 15,000 AU per 5 mL = 3,000 AU per mL^{-1} (16.8 μg $^{-1}$) Maintenance dose is 0.5 mL of final concentration = 1,500 AU (8.4 μg)
Birch	0.5 mL of supply = 20,000 PNU Final concentration (supply diluted in 5 mL) = 20,000 PNU per 5 mL = 4,000 PNU mL^{-1} Maintenance dose is 0.5 mL of final concentration = 2,000 PNU
Alternaria	0.5 mL of supply = 20,000 PNU Final concentration (supply diluted in 5 mL) = 20,000 PNU per 5 mL = 4,000 PNU mL^{-1} Maintenance dose is 0.5 mL of final concentration = 2,000 PNU
Ragweed	0.3 mL of 1:10 w/v supply diluted in 5 mL = 3/10 × 1/10 × 1/5 = 1/166 w/v

Therefore, the final patient prescription report would read as follows:

Mite/mold mix

Extract used	Volume (mL)	Concentration used	Final concentration	Maintenance dose
D farinae	1.5	10,000 AU mL^{-1} (56 µg mL^{-1})	3,000 AU mL^{-1} (16.8 µg mL^{-1})	1,500 AU (8.4 µg)
Alternaria	0.5	40,000 PNU mL^{-1}	4,000 PNU mL^{-1}	2,000 PNU
Subtotal	2.0			
Diluent	3.0			
Total amount	5			

Dosage is started by diluting the final concentration dose by 1,000 (3 AU mL^{-1} [0.0168 µg mL^{-1}]) *D farinae* and (4 PNU mL^{-1}) *Alternaria* and administering 0.05 mL as shown in Table 3.6, then increasing accordingly.

Tree/weed mix

Extract used	Volume (mL)	Concentration used	Final concentration	Maintenance dose
Ragweed	0.3	1:10 w/v	1:166 w/v	1:166 w/v
Birch	0.5	40,000 PNU mL^{-1}	4,000 PNU mL^{-1}	2,000 PNU
Subtotal	0.8			
Diluent	4.2			
Total amount	5			

Dosage is started by diluting the final concentration dose by 1,000 (1/166,000 w/v). Ragweed and (4 PNU mL^{-1}) birch and administering 0.05 mL as shown in Table 3.6, then increasing accordingly

3.4.2 Vignette 2

A 30-year-old woman started specific allergen immunotherapy for seasonal allergic rhinitis and extrinsic asthma 6 weeks ago. She has been receiving 1–2 injections weekly, as outlined by her buildup immunotherapy schedule. She has been tolerating the injections well; she has not had any reactions to the injections. Currently, she is scheduled to receive 0.3 mL of the 1:100 concentration of the birch and maple tree, timothy grass, and short ragweed immunotherapy formulation. She has learned that she is pregnant.

Comment: The patient is currently in the buildup phase of her immunotherapy. She has received 9 of the 24 doses required to attain the maintenance concentration. Although she has tolerated the immunotherapy well to this point, the immunotherapy should be discontinued. The primary rule pertaining to immunotherapy and pregnancy is that dose escalation (buildup) should not be performed during pregnancy. Because it is early in the immunotherapy course, it is difficult to know if she may have an adverse reaction to the immunotherapy. Also, adverse reactions tend to be more common during the buildup phase than in the maintenance phase. If the immunotherapy is going to be restarted after her pregnancy, she would have to start at the first dose (0.05 mL of the 1:1,000 concentration); she would not be able to restart at her current dose. Immunotherapy can be continued during pregnancy if the patient is kept at the same dosage. For example, if this patient were receiving the maintenance dosage or near-maintenance dosage, the immunotherapy could be continued at the constant dosage during her pregnancy.

3.4.3 Vignette 3

A 37-year-old woman has a history of an anaphylactic reaction to a honeybee sting manifested by widespread urticaria, wheezing, and dyspnea. Evaluation showed a positive intradermal skin test to honeybee and negative intradermal skin tests to the vespids. She has been receiving honeybee immunotherapy for 1 month. During this time, she noted a small local reaction to the immunotherapy injection consisting of a 10–15-mm diameter raised "bump." The raised area disappeared by the following day. She had no other signs or symptoms such as urticaria, angioedema, pruritus, wheeze, or dyspnea.

Comment: The presence of a small local reaction to the immunotherapy injection is not uncommon. When the local reaction is not associated with any other signs or symptoms, the local reaction is not considered a risk factor for a systemic reaction to the immunotherapy injections.

The patient continued the buildup phase of her immunotherapy injections. Twenty-five minutes after receiving 0.4 mL of the 10 µg mL^{-1} concentration, she developed widespread urticaria and pruritus and wheezing.

Comment: The patient is having an allergic reaction to the injection. The majority, but not all, allergic reactions to immunotherapy occur within 30 minutes after the injection. Therefore, it is imperative that all patients remain at the provider's office for 30 minutes after the injection. In this situation, epinephrine should be administered immediately. The usual dosage for adults is 0.3 mg intramuscularly (0.3 mL of 1:1,000). Antihistamine, such as diphenhydramine 50 mg intramuscularly, can also be given with the epinephrine. Corticosteroids are also often used in this situation. Although they do not take effect immediately, they may help ameliorate future symptoms.

The patient was given epinephrine 0.3 mg intramuscularly, diphenhydramine 50 mg intramuscularly, and prednisone 60 mg orally. Within 15 minutes, there was marked improvement in her respiratory status and diminution of the urticaria. She was observed in the office for 3 hours and was asymptomatic during the last 2 hours of observation.

Comment: The response to treatment was rapid. A small percentage of patients may experience a late phase allergic reaction that can occur 12–36 hours after the original reaction. She should be educated about this possibility and instructed about the treatment of allergic symptoms. If she does not already have injectable epinephrine, she should be given an epinephrine kit and instructed in its correct use.

Anytime a reaction occurs to an immunotherapy injection, the entire immunotherapy process should be reviewed. The lot and vial of the immunotherapy extract should be studied to determine if the correct dosage was administered. Potency can vary from lot to lot, and it is important to note if a new vial was used (typically, if a new vial is used, the dose should be split).

The entire process was reviewed. The patient received the correct dosage from a previously used vial. The dosage was checked by two nurses before administration. The patient did not have any symptoms before the injection.

Comment: No abnormalities were noted in the immunotherapy procedure. Allergic reactions to immunotherapy can occur. In this situation, the risks and benefits of the immunotherapy injections would again need to be reviewed with the patient. Important points to consider would be her risk of subsequent honeybee sting and the risk of another systemic reaction to the immunotherapy. If the immunotherapy is to be continued, a dosage adjustment would be required. A common approach in this situation would be to decrease the dosage to the $1 \mu g \ mL^{-1}$ concentration and attempt to rebuild from the lower dose.

3.4.4   Vignette 4

A 7-year-old boy has a history of egg allergy and atopic dermatitis. At age 1 year, he developed hives, primarily around his mouth, and wheezing with the ingestion of egg. Skin testing at that time was positive to egg. Since that time, no other food allergies have developed. The family has been strictly avoiding egg and any egg-containing foods. Approximately 2 years ago, a few small hives developed on his face after he inadvertently took a bite of French toast at a neighbor's home. The family does not think he has had any egg exposure since that time. He has not had any significant problems with atopic dermatitis since age 2 years. The parents wonder whether he is still allergic to egg.

Comment: His history and subsequent testing are consistent with an IgE-mediated allergy to egg. He did have some reaction to egg ingestion 2 years ago. Unlike peanut, tree nut, fish, and shellfish allergy, most children outgrow egg allergy. His atopic dermatitis has been quiescent. The first step at this point would be a skin prick test to egg.

Skin prick test to egg showed a 4 × 4-mm wheal with flare. The histamine control was a 5 × 5-mm wheal with flare. The glycerin control showed no response.

Comment: His skin test is considered positive because the response was larger than 3 × 3 mm. Because the skin test is positive, although not markedly positive, a food challenge could be risky. Further information should be obtained with in vitro testing to egg.

IgE antibody to egg using the Pharmacia CAP System FEIA was 7 kIU L^{-1}.

Comment: This is a significantly positive test. According to the work of Sampson, this level of specific IgE results in a positive food challenge >95% of the time. This vignette emphasizes the importance of in vitro testing, especially when the skin prick testing is low-grade positive. In this instance, no further evaluation should be undertaken. The patient and parents should be counseled to continue the strict avoidance of eggs. The parents and child should also be instructed about the correct technique of epinephrine injection. Because there still is a chance the boy will outgrow the egg allergy, repeat egg skin prick and in vitro testing should be considered in another 2–3 years.

Suggested Reading

Abramson, M. J., Puy, R. M., Weiner, J. M. (1995) Is allergen immunotherapy effective in asthma? A meta-analysis of randomized controlled trials. Am. J. Respir. Crit. Care Med. 151, 969–974

Boyano Martinez, T., Garcia-Ara, C., Diaz-Pena, J. M., Munoz, F. M., Garcia Sanchez, G., Esteban, M. M. (2001) Validity of specific IgE antibodies in children with egg allergy. Clin. Exp. Allergy 31, 1464–1469

Casale, T. B., Busse, W. W., Kline, J. N., et al. (2006) Omalizumab pretreatment decreases acute reactions after rush immunotherapy for ragweed-induced seasonal allergic rhinitis. J. Allergy Clin. Immunol. 117, 134–140

Cox, L. S., Linnemann, D. L., Nolte, H., Weldon, D., Finegold, I., Nelson, H. S. (2006) Sublingual immunotherapy: a comprehensive review. J. Allergy Clin. Immunol. 117, 1021–1035

Graif, Y., Yigla, M., Tov, N., Kramer, M. R. (2002) Value of a negative aeroallergen skin-prick test result in the diagnosis of asthma in young adults: correlative study with methacholine challenge testing. Chest 122, 821–825

Hamilton, R. G. and Adkinson, N. F., Jr. (2003) 23. Clinical laboratory assessment of IgE-dependent hypersensitivity. J. Allergy Clin. Immunol. 111, S687–S701

Moller, C., Dreborg, S., Ferdousi, H. A., et al. (2002) Pollen immunotherapy reduces the development of asthma in children with seasonal rhinoconjunctivitis (the PAT-study). J. Allergy Clin. Immunol. 109, 251–256

Nelson, H. S. (2007) Allergen immunotherapy: where is it now? J. Allergy Clin. Immunol. 119, 769–779. Epub 2 March 2007

Pajno, G. B., Barberio, G., De Luca, F., Morabito, L., Parmiani, S. (2001) Prevention of new sensitizations in asthmatic children monosensitized to house dust mite by specific immunotherapy: a six-year follow-up study. Clin. Exp. Allergy 31, 1392–1397

Pastorello, E. A., Incorvaia, C., Ortolani, C., et al. (1995) Studies on the relationship between the level of specific IgE antibodies and the clinical expression of allergy: I. Definition of levels distinguishing patients with symptomatic from patients with asymptomatic allergy to common aeroallergens. J. Allergy Clin. Immunol. 96, 580–587

Ross, R. N., Nelson, H. S., Finegold, I. (2000) Effectiveness of specific immunotherapy in the treatment of asthma: a meta-analysis of prospective, randomized, double-blind, placebo-controlled studies. Clin. Ther. 22, 329–341

Ross, R. N., Nelson, H. S., Finegold, I. (2000) Effectiveness of specific immunotherapy in the treatment of allergic rhinitis: an analysis of randomized, prospective, single- or double-blind, placebo-controlled studies. Clin. Ther. 22, 342–350

Sampson, H. A. (2001) Utility of food-specific IgE concentrations in predicting symptomatic food allergy. J. Allergy Clin. Immunol. 107, 891–896

Schafer, T., Hoelscher, B., Adam, H., Ring, J., Wichmann, H. E., Heinrich, J. (2003) Hay fever and predictive value of prick test and specific IgE antibodies: a prospective study in children. Pediatr. Allergy Immunol. 14, 120–129

Simons, F. E., Shikishima, Y., Van Nest, G., Eiden, J. J., HayGlass, K. T. (2004) Selective immune redirection in humans with ragweed allergy by injecting Amb a 1 linked to immunostimulatory DNA. J. Allergy Clin. Immunol. 113, 1144–1151

Sporik, R., Hill, D. J., Hosking, C. S. (2000) Specificity of allergen skin testing in predicting positive open food challenges to milk, egg and peanut in children. Clin. Exp. Allergy 30, 1540–1546

Wohrl, S., Vigl, K., Zehetmayer, S., et al. (2006) The performance of a component-based allergen-microarray in clinical practice. Allergy 61, 633–639

Wood, R. A., Phipatanakul, W., Hamilton, R. G., Eggleston, P. A. (1999) A comparison of skin prick tests, intradermal skin tests, and RASTs in the diagnosis of cat allergy. J. Allergy Clin. Immunol. 103, 773–779

Chapter 4
Allergic Rhinitis and Rhinosinusitis

Abbreviations AERD: aspirin-exacerbated respiratory disease; CSF: cerebrospinal fluid; CT: computed tomography; FESS: functional endoscopic surgery; HIV: human immunodeficiency virus; IL: interleukin; NARES: nonallergic rhinitis with eosinophilia syndrome; RAST: radioallergosorbent test.

4.1   Overview

Rhinitis and sinusitis are two of the most common health problems in the United States. Rhinitis affects nearly 100 million Americans. Sinusitis affects nearly 40 million Americans; costs nearly $6 billion in office visits, hospitalizations, and medications; and accounts for nearly one million lost work days. Rhinitis and sinusitis also significantly affect quality of life. In quality-of-life surveys, rhinitis and sinusitis have had lower scores than other chronic diseases, such as chronic obstructive pulmonary disease, angina, and back pain. *Rhinitis* is defined as an inflammation of the nasal lining characterized by nasal congestion, rhinorrhea, sneezing, and nasal itching. *Sinusitis* is defined as an inflammation of the paranasal sinuses. The term *rhinosinusitis* has been suggested to replace sinusitis because sinusitis is almost always accompanied by nasal airway inflammation. In addition, rhinitis and sinusitis frequently occur together, and the symptoms of nasal discharge and nasal obstruction are prominent in sinusitis. In this chapter, the term rhinosinusitis will be used instead of sinusitis. Because of the contiguous lining of the airway between the nose and the sinuses, it can be difficult to distinguish clinically between the signs and symptoms of rhinitis and those of rhinosinusitis.

The focus of this chapter is primarily diagnostic, with a discussion of the similarities and differences in the presentation of the various forms of rhinitis and rhinosinusitis. Many clinical presentations can be classified as a specific syndrome by the clinical pattern. An algorithm is presented to help clinicians place patients in the correct group of rhinitis and rhinosinusitis on the basis of the presenting signs and symptoms (Fig. 4.1). This is particularly important in the evaluation of patients who have chronic symptoms, because a delay in correct diagnosis can lead to significant morbidity.

G.W. Volcheck, *Clinical Allergy: Diagnosis and Management*
DOI: 10.1007/978-1-59745-315-8_4, © 2009 Mayo Foundation for Medical Education and Research

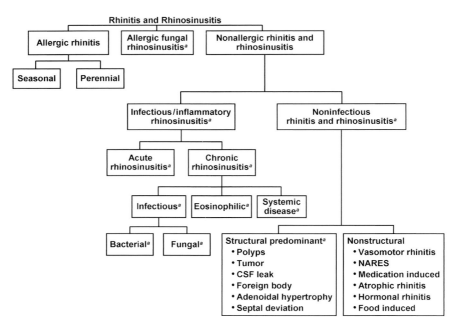

Fig. 4.1 Major classification of rhinitis and rhinosinusitis based on underlying pathophysiology.
[a]Significant changes on coronal computed tomographic scan of the sinuses. *CSF* cerebrospinal fluid; *NARES* nonallergic rhinitis with eosinophilia syndrome

4.2 Nasal Anatomy and Function

The nasal cavity is divided into two separate airways by the nasal septum. The two airways start at the anterior nares and then separate from each other until they reunite at the nasopharynx. The lateral wall of the nose is formed by the inferior, middle, and superior turbinates. The turbinates act to warm, humidify, and clean the inspired air. The superior, middle, and inferior meatus are air passageways located beneath the turbinate of the same name. The narrowest point of the nasal airway, 30 mm^2, occurs approximately 3 cm into the nostrils, at the anterior end of the inferior turbinate. This nasal valve is the major site of airway resistance. Beyond this, the nasal cavity expands to 130 mm^2. The main air stream is directed inferiorly around the inferior turbinate along the floor of the nasal cavity. With increased nasal pressure, as with sniffing, the air stream rises toward the middle and superior turbinates and the olfactory region of the upper part of the nasal cavity.

The four pairs of nasal sinuses are the frontal, maxillary, ethmoid, and sphenoid sinuses (Fig. 4.2). The maxillary sinus is the first to develop, with pneumatization beginning in the first year. The maxillary sinus reaches maturity at approximately age 12 years. Ethmoid sinuses reach adult size at age 12–14 years. The frontal and sphenoid sinuses develop later and reach adult size in mid to late adolescence.

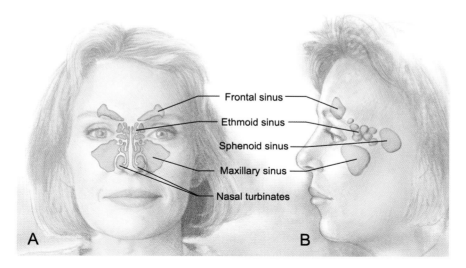

Frontal sinus

Ethmoid sinus

Sphenoid sinus

Maxillary sinus

Nasal turbinates

A   B

Fig. 4.2 (**a**) *Frontal* and (**b**) *side views* of the frontal, ethmoid, sphenoid, and maxillary sinuses

Because of the later development of the frontal and sphenoid sinuses, frontal and sphenoid sinusitis is uncommon in childhood. The frontal sinuses are located superior to the orbits; the maxillary sinuses are between the upper teeth and the inferior aspect of the orbit; the ethmoid sinuses are medial to the orbits; and the sphenoid sinuses are posterior to the ethmoid sinuses. Because of the location of the frontal and sphenoid sinuses, inflammation of these sinuses can potentially cause intracranial complications. Veins that pass through the posterior wall of the frontal sinus enable the spread of a frontal sinus infection intracranially. The optic nerve, cavernous sinus, and carotid artery are adjacent to the sphenoid sinus. Tumor and infection in the sphenoid sinus may present with involvement of these structures.

Each sinus has an opening that allows drainage and free exchange of fluid and air, and the mucous membrane lining the sinuses and that lining the nasal cavity are continuous through the openings. The anterior ethmoid, frontal, and maxillary sinuses all drain into the middle meatus through a narrow, convoluted, final common drainage pathway termed the *ostiomeatal unit*. The ostiomeatal unit is located primarily in the anterior third of the middle meatus and the superior part of the maxillary sinuses. Blockage of this critical area results in poor drainage from the sinuses, predisposing to infection and the accumulation of mucus. This is typically the first and most frequently involved region in chronic rhinosinusitis. The posterior ethmoid sinuses drain into the superior meatus. The sphenoid sinuses drain by separate ostia into the sphenoethmoidal recess on either side of the nasal septum posteriorly.

Respiratory mucus has the key role in the function of the nose and sinuses. The nose and sinuses act as an air conditioning system to warm, humidify, and filter the inspired air. The mucus provides the interface between the inhaled air and the delicate epithelium of the nasal cavity. On the surface of the respiratory epithelium, the nasal mucus consists of two layers: a lower layer with low viscosity in which the cilia beat freely and propel the overlying layer of viscous, thick mucus. The nasal fluid is derived primarily from the seromucous glands within the nasal mucosa and the goblet cells distributed along the surface of the nasal mucosa. The cilia sweep mucus to the ostial opening for drainage.

The nose is lined by three distinct types of epithelia: stratified squamous epithelium in the most anterior part of the nose and in the nasopharynx, pseudostratified ciliated columnar epithelium in the main respiratory area of the nasal cavity, and specialized olfactory epithelium in the superior olfactory area. In the anterior region, the stratified squamous epithelium has sensory properties similar to those of facial skin and contains thermoreceptors that detect temperature change. This "skin" is covered with short stiff hairs that are extremely sensitive to mechanical stimuli, and when stimulated, they cause itch and sneezing. Just past the nasal valve area, the skin is transformed into the ciliated columnar respiratory mucosa. At this transition is Kiesselbach's plexus, a region of capillary loops that are a common source of nasal bleeding. The respiratory epithelium is primarily a columnar, pseudostratified, ciliated epithelium that includes basal cells, goblet cells, and nonciliated columnar cells. The density of goblet cells increases as the epithelium goes posteriorly. The ciliated columnar cells move the mucus that covers the nasal mucosa, allowing secretions to be cleared.

The sensory innervation of the nose is supplied primarily by the olfactory and trigeminal nerves. The olfactory nerves traverse the cribriform plate. These nerves not only provide our sense of smell but also contribute to our sense of taste. The sensory nerves to the nose are primarily the ophthalmic and maxillary branches of the trigeminal nerve, serving the sensations of hot, cold, itch, and touch and also the sensation of nasal airflow, which is perceived as a cool sensation on inspiration. The trigeminal nerves initiate the sneezing and secretion associated with infection and allergy. Neurovascular homeostasis is maintained by a balance of parasympathetic and sympathetic tone. Parasympathetic nerve stimulation induces the release of acetylcholine and neuropeptides. This produces mucus secretion, resulting in nasal congestion and watery rhinorrhea. Sympathetic nerve stimulation causes the release of norepinephrine and neuropeptide Y. These substances constrict the nasal vasculature, resulting in nasal decongestion.

The nasal blood supply is complex and consists of resistance vessels and large venous sinuses, or capacitance vessels. The resistance vessels are primarily small arteries and arterioles innervated by sympathetic nerves. Under normal conditions, nasal blood flow appears to be controlled by local mediators because the vessels have little sympathetic vasoconstrictor tone and nerve blockade causes only a slight increase in blood flow. The venous sinuses, however, have an important role in nasal airway resistance. These sinuses have a dense sympathetic innervation, and congestion and constriction are regulated by the sympathetic supply to this area. The airway resistance of the nasal passage is normally asymmetrical, with the nasal venous tissue exhibiting congestion on one side of the septum and less congestion on the other side. This is termed the *nasal cycle*. The average length of this cycle is 1–4 hours. The cycle results in the reciprocal increase and decrease in functional nasal airflow. The function of the nasal cycle has not been clearly established.

Various physical maneuvers can affect the nasal cycle. Nasal airway resistance decreases on exercise. It is not uncommon for a patient with chronic rhinitis to note that the nose "clears" with vigorous exercise, but congestion returns after exercise. Nasal airway resistance increases when the patient is supine. With the head lying in the lateral position, reflex changes occur that produce congestion in the dependent (lower) nasal passage and decongestion in the upper nasal passage.

4.3 Clinical Overview

This chapter categorizes the various forms of rhinitis and rhinosinusitis on a clinical basis. By emphasizing key points in the history and physical examination, the clinician can place the patient in an appropriate category for treatment or further evaluation (or both). The first division is between allergic rhinitis, allergic fungal rhinosinusitis, and nonallergic rhinitis and rhinosinusitis (Fig. 4.1). Nonallergic rhinitis and rhinosinusitis is subdivided into infectious/inflammatory rhinosinusitis and noninfectious rhinitis and rhinosinusitis. The infectious/inflammatory rhinosinusitis subgroup includes acute rhinosinusitis that is primarily infectious and chronic rhinosinusitis. Chronic rhinosinusitis has been defined poorly. In an effort to include all patient presentations, chronic rhinosinusitis is subdivided into an infectious subgroup (subdivided further into bacterial and fungal rhinosinusitis subgroups), the newly defined eosinophilic subgroup (i.e., chronic eosinophilic fungal or hyperplastic rhinosinusitis subgroup), and the systemic disease subgroup. Although the eosinophilic and systemic disease subgroups do not represent a classic infectious process, their clinical presentations are similar to those of the infectious subgroup because of the underlying inflammation and often concomitant infection. Noninfectious rhinitis and rhinosinusitis is divided into structural-predominant causes and nonstructural causes. The structural causes are characterized typically by unilateral symptoms and anosmia and include primarily septal deviation, adenoidal hypertrophy, nasal and sinus polyps, and tumors. The nonstructural causes include various syndromes, for example, vasomotor rhinitis, nonallergic rhinitis with eosinophilia syndrome (NARES), hormonal rhinitis, rhinitis due to medications, rhinitis due to food, and atrophic rhinitis. These conditions are characterized by predominantly nasal symptoms as opposed to nose and sinus symptoms (Fig. 4.2). Although there is overlap between nasal symptoms alone and nasal and sinus symptoms, the latter are characterized by significant nasal congestion, postnasal drainage, facial pressure, and recurrent infection.

4.4 Allergic Rhinitis

Allergic rhinitis is the most common atopic disease in the United States and is estimated to affect up to 25% of adults and 40% of children. Approximately 80 million individuals experience symptoms for >7 days per year. Allergic rhinitis accounts for 2 million lost school days annually, 6 million lost work days, and medication expenditure of more than \$3 billion annually.

Symptoms of allergic rhinitis include watery rhinorrhea, paroxysms of sneezing, nasal congestion, itchy palate, and itchy, watery eyes. These symptoms are reproducible on exposure to allergens to which the patient has been sensitized. Nasal congestion alone, particularly in children, may be the sole or major complaint. Allergic rhinitis is divided into seasonal allergic rhinitis, which is induced by tree, grass, and weed pollens and fungal spores, and perennial allergic rhinitis, which is induced by dust mites, fungal spores, animals, and cockroaches. With seasonal allergic rhinitis, symptoms recur at the same time each year, corresponding to the pollinating season of the plants and molds. The symptoms of perennial allergic rhinitis tend to be less severe than those of seasonal allergic rhinitis. Nasal congestion is often the primary symptom, but sneezing, clear rhinorrhea, and itching of the eyes, nose, and throat may also occur.

The prevalence of allergic rhinitis is lowest among children younger than 5 years and peaks in early schoolhood years and early adult years. The onset of allergic rhinitis can occur at any age, but it is less common in patients older than 50 years.

4.4.1   Pathophysiology

The symptoms of allergic rhinitis are due to inflammation induced by an IgE-mediated immune response to an airborne allergen. The complex immune response consists of the release of inflammatory mediators and the activation and recruitment of inflammatory cells to the nasal mucosa (Fig. 4.3).

Allergen exposure leads to presentation of the allergen by antigen-presenting cells to T-lymphocytes. These T-lymphocytes, sometimes called Th2 lymphocytes, release cytokines, particularly interleukin (IL)-4 and IL-13, which induce the production of IgE antibody specific for the allergen. This general process has been termed the *sensitizing phenomenon*. Once the patient is sensitized, subsequent exposure to the allergen causes IgE-bound allergen to trigger a cascade of events that result in the symptoms of allergic rhinitis. The allergic response is divided into two phases: the early phase and the late phase.

The early phase, or immediate, response begins within minutes after exposure to the allergen. The allergen is inhaled, taken into the mucosa, and binds to IgE, which triggers mast cell degranulation. The mast cell releases several preformed and newly synthesized mediators that lead to the characteristic symptoms of allergic rhinitis. The primary preformed mediators that are released include histamine, tryptase, chymase, and kininogenase. The newly formed mediators include prostaglandin D_2, cytokines, leukotrienes C_4, D_4, and E_4. In addition to directly causing symptoms, mediators also serve to recruit inflammatory cells into the nasal mucosa, setting up the late phase response. Mucosal glands are stimulated to secrete conjugates and compounds that dilate the nasal venous vasculature, leading to sinusoidal filling and nasal congestion. The mediators also stimulate sensory nerves, producing the symptoms of nasal itch.

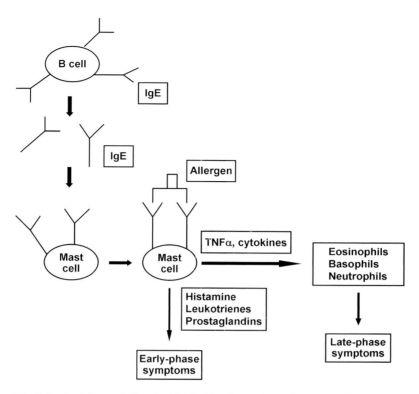

Fig. 4.3 Pathophysiology of allergic rhinitis. B-cells produce allergen-specific IgE. Allergen-specific IgE binds to mast cells in the nasal mucosa. Inhaled allergens bind to allergen-specific IgE on mast cells, triggering release of mast cell mediators. These mediators produce (1) early-phase symptoms (rhinorrhea, sneezing, itching, and nasal obstruction) and (2) recruit eosinophils, basophils, and neutrophils for the late-phase response. *TNF* tumor necrosis factor

In the late phase response, nasal congestion becomes more prominent. The mast cell-derived mediators act on endothelial cells to promote the expression of vascular cell adhesion molecules that facilitate the adhesion of circulating leukocytes to the endothelial cells. In addition, chemoattractants such as IL-5 promote the infiltration of eosinophils, neutrophils, basophils, lymphocytes, and macrophages. The leukocytes then migrate into the nasal mucosa. These inflammatory leukocytes further sustain the nasal inflammatory reaction.

Eosinophils are the predominant cell in the chronic inflammatory process of allergic rhinitis. Eosinophils release several proinflammatory mediators, including cationic proteins, eosinophil peroxidase, major basic protein, and cysteinyl leukotrienes. They also release inflammatory cytokines such as IL-3, IL-5, IL-13, granulocyte-macrophage colony-stimulating factor, platelet-activating factor, and tumor necrosis factor.

The allergic rhinitis cascade is quite complex and reflects an interplay of numerous inflammatory cells and the mediators they release. This cascade results in chronic inflammation and likely produces a priming effect (i.e., after repeated exposure, the amount of allergen necessary to produce an allergic response decreases).

Nasal inflammation associated with allergic rhinitis can also cause obstruction of the sinus ostiomeatal unit, predisposing to viral and bacterial infections of the sinus. Other comorbidities of allergic rhinitis are otitis media, asthma, allergic conjunctivitis, and rhinosinusitis.

4.4.2 History

The history can be extremely helpful in categorizing allergic rhinitis. Initially, it is important to determine whether the presenting symptoms are indeed allergic (IgE mediated) in origin. A common misperception is to label all rhinitis as "allergic." The following questions are helpful in initially categorizing rhinitis:

1. Are nasal itch or sneezing episodes prominent symptoms of the rhinitis complex?
2. Are watery, itchy eyes associated with the rhinitis?
3. Is wheeze associated with the rhinitis?

Positive answers to these questions point strongly to an allergic origin for the rhinitis. However, these symptoms are not required for the rhinitis to have an allergic origin. For example, dust mite-induced allergic rhinitis may present with only chronic nasal congestion, with the absence of prominent itch, sneezing, or eye symptoms. If an allergic origin is strongly suspected because of positive answers to the three questions or mildly suspected because of chronic nasal congestion, the next step is to identify the timing of the symptoms. Broadly, this can be approached by answering the following questions:

1. Are the symptoms prominent year-round or are they present only at certain times of the year? If present only during certain months of the year, which months?
2. Do the symptoms occur with certain exposures?

This places the rhinitis in either the perennial or seasonal category. If the symptoms are perennial and allergy is suspected, the major allergens are dust mites, cockroaches, household pets such as cats and dogs, and molds. Typically, tree, grass, and weed pollens would not be expected to cause perennial symptoms, except in a multisensitive patient who lives in a warm climate where pollens are present year-round. If the patient's symptoms are limited to certain months, the main possibilities are tree, grass, and weed pollens and molds. These have regular patterns of release, with tree pollens released primarily in the spring, grass pollens in the summer, and weed pollens in late summer and autumn. Molds are present throughout the warmer months of the year. Episodic symptoms can occur with certain exposures. Reproducible symptoms in the setting of cat, dog, horse, or mouse exposure point to a specific allergen. The specific characteristics of perennial and seasonal allergens are discussed in Chap. 2.

A thorough environmental history is helpful in assessing possible exposures in allergic rhinitis. The environmental history should include the following:

1. Age, location, and type of home
2. History of dampness or water problems in the home
3. Type of heating and air-conditioning system
4. Presence or absence of smoking in the home
5. All indoor and outdoor pets
6. Occupational exposure

There are also screening questions that can help rule out allergies as the primary cause of chronic rhinitis. Positive answers to the following questions would not be considered typical for allergic rhinitis alone:

1. Are the nasal symptoms exclusively one sided?
2. Is there purulent nasal discharge?
3. Is facial or teeth pain associated with this?

A positive answer to any of these questions requires further evaluation for other causes, particularly infectious/inflammatory rhinosinusitis and predominantly structural forms of rhinosinusitis.

4.4.3   Physical Examination

Physical examination findings can vary in allergic rhinitis. The classic findings on nasal examination include a pale or bluish, boggy nasal mucosa with a thin, clear, watery nasal discharge. The turbinates are swollen. In the setting of obstruction and posterior nasal drainage, the drainage can cause lymphoid hyperplasia in the posterior pharynx that resembles cobblestones. Allergic facies demonstrate dark infraorbital swollen semicircles, "the allergic shiner." The eyes have varying degrees of conjunctival erythema. Children may exhibit a transverse nasal crease caused by constant nose itching or Morgan–Dennie lines, accentuated horizontal skin folds on the lower lid that are parallel with the lower lid margin. The physical examination findings can vary depending on the severity and chronicity of the allergic rhinitis and the presence of complicating conditions such as infection and polyposis. No features detected on physical examination are exclusive to allergic rhinitis.

Overall, the history and physical examination are helpful in the assessment of allergic rhinitis. However, because of the variability of the findings and the overlap of signs and symptoms with other causes of rhinitis and rhinosinusitis, particularly entities in the group of noninfectious nonstructural rhinitis and rhinosinusitis, further testing is often indicated.

4.4.4   Testing

Allergy testing is performed to confirm which allergens contribute to the patient's symptoms. Identification of the allergen is critical for establishing the diagnosis, counseling on environmental avoidance measures, and identifying allergens for use in allergen immunotherapy. Allergy testing is performed by skin prick testing or in vitro testing. Skin prick testing is the most commonly performed testing because of its low cost, the immediacy of results, and its higher sensitivity. For seasonal symptoms, skin prick tests are performed to the environmentally relevant tree, grass, and weed pollens and molds. For perennial symptoms, the tests are performed to dust mites, household pets or other animals, cockroaches, and molds. To ensure accuracy, a positive histamine control is placed on the skin with the skin testing. Patients are to refrain from taking second-generation antihistamines (fexofenadine, loratadine, desloratadine, cetirizine) for 4 days before the test and refrain from first-generation antihistamines (diphenhydramine, chlorpheniramine) for 2 days before the test. In some patients, other classes of medications, including benzodiazepines, H_2 blockers, and tricyclic antidepressants, can interfere with the skin test. This varies from person to person.

In skin prick testing, a drop of the allergen is placed on the skin and the skin is pricked. The area is observed for 15 min and then measured for wheal and flare. A wheal larger than 3 mm is generally considered positive. An intradermal skin test, in which a small amount of allergen is injected just under the skin, can also be conducted; however, the specificity of this test is low in airborne allergen testing and should only be performed in special situations. If skin testing cannot be performed, in vitro tests for serum IgE antibody to allergens can be conducted. These include the radioallergosorbent test (RAST) and enzyme-linked immunosorbent assay. These estimate the amount of allergen-specific IgE antibody in a patient's serum. Medications do not interfere with this type of testing.

The measurement of total serum IgE alone is not useful in screening for allergic rhinitis.

Nasal smear for cytology generally is not indicated in this setting. The finding of eosinophils on a nasal smear is suggestive but nonspecific for allergy. A predominance of neutrophils suggests an infectious process.

4.4.5   Treatment

4.4.5.1   Avoidance

Allergen avoidance should be recommended as a primary treatment for allergic rhinitis. Preventing the allergen from triggering an IgE-mediated response basically stops the allergic condition before it starts. Unfortunately, avoidance is difficult and can be accomplished only partially, particularly in the case of seasonal tree, grass, and weed pollen and mold allergy. Knowledge of the specific outdoor seasonal allergens can help identify the weather conditions, the months, and the time of day of peak exposure. With this information, plans for outdoor activities can be made accordingly. Details of strategies for avoiding pollen and mold allergens are provided in Chap. 2.

Avoidance of indoor allergens involves environmental modifications to decrease exposure to dust mites, animal dander, and molds. Several recommendations have been made for decreasing exposure to improve symptoms; these are outlined in detail in Chap. 2.

4.4.5.2 Pharmacotherapy

The complex pathophysiology of allergic rhinitis allows multiple interventions at various stages in the disease pathway. A wide spectrum of medications is available for the treatment of allergic rhinitis. Therapy can be tailored to specific clinical symptoms (Table 4.1). A treatment regimen can involve a single medication or multiple medications, depending on the severity of the disease. The severity of the disease can be classified as *intermittent* or *persistent* and the symptoms as *mild* or *moderate-severe*. Intermittent rhinitis is defined as symptoms that are present for <4 days per week or <4 weeks in duration. *Persistent rhinitis* is defined as symptoms that are present for >4 days per week and are present for >4 weeks. Mild symptoms do not affect sleep, interfere with work or school, or impair daily activities and, although present, are not considered troublesome. Moderate-severe symptoms, however, impair these activities. The agents used to treat allergic rhinitis include antihistamines, decongestants, corticosteroids, mast cell stabilizers, anticholinergics, leukotriene antagonists, and immunotherapy. An algorithm for treatment of allergic rhinitis is shown in Fig. 4.4.

Antihistamines

Antihistamines are the mainstay of treatment for mild intermittent allergic rhinitis. As competitive inhibitors of histamine, antihistamines reduce the effect of histamine even in the presence of continued histamine release. Antihistamines can be divided into the older, or first-generation, agents and newer, or second-generation, agents.

The older (first-generation) antihistamines were first produced and made available in the late 1930s and 1940s. The most commonly used first-generation antihistamines include chlorpheniramine, brompheniramine, hydroxyzine, and diphenhydramine. Although they are effective in the treatment of allergic rhinitis, use has been limited by adverse effects due to the lack of selectivity for the H_1 receptor and a propensity to cross the blood-brain barrier and thus affect the central nervous system. Because of the lack of selectivity, first-generation antihistamines cause anticholinergic effects such as dry mouth, headache, and urinary retention. By crossing the blood-brain barrier and binding to H_1 receptors in the brain, these agents produce sedation and cognitive impairment. Recent studies have shown that first-generation antihistamines can significantly affect sensorimotor coordination, attention span, memory function, ability to process information, and psychomotor performance. These changes can occur without drowsiness and may not be perceived by the patient. Therefore, patients need special counseling about the use of these medications and the potential for decreased performance, particularly with

Table 4.1 Medications commonly used in the treatment of allergic rhinitis

Class of agent	Indication	Medication (trade name)	Dose	
			Pediatric	Adult
Second-generation antihistamine	Reduces sneezing, rhinorrhea, ocular and nasal itching	Fexofenadine (Allegra)	2–11 years: 30 mg twice daily 12 years: adult dose	180 mg once daily
		Cetirizine (Zyrtec)	6–23 months: 2.5 mg once daily 2–5 years: 2.5–5 mg once daily 6–11 years: 5–10 mg once daily 12 years: adult dose	5–10 mg once daily
		Levocetirizine (Xyzal)	6–11 years: 2.5 mg once daily 12 years: adult dose	5 mg once daily
		Loratadine (Claritin, Alavert)	2–5 years: 5 mg daily 6 years: 10 mg daily	10 mg once daily
		Desloratadine (Clarinex)	6–11 months: 1 mg daily 12 months to 5 years: 1.25 mg daily 6–11 years: 2.5 mg daily 12 years: 5 mg daily	5 mg once daily
		Azelastine (Astelin)	5–11 years: 1 spray twice daily 12 years: adult dose	2 sprays/nostril twice daily
Nasal corticosteroid	Reduces sneezing, rhinorrhea, ocular and nasal itching, and nasal congestion	Beclomethasone (Beconase aq, 42 µg)	6 years: 1–2 sprays/nostril twice daily	1–2 sprays/nostril twice daily
		Beclomethasone (Vancenase double strength, 84 µg)	6 years: same as adults	1–2 sprays/nostril once daily
		Budesonide (Rhinocort aq)	6–12 years: 1–2 sprays/nostril once daily 12 years: same as adult	1–4 sprays/nostril once daily
		Fluticasone propionate (Flonase)	4 years: 1 spray/nostril daily	2 sprays/nostril once daily
		Fluticasone furoate (Veramyst)	2–11 years: 1 spray/nostril daily	2 sprays/nostril once daily
		Mometasone (Nasonex)	2–11 years: 1 spray/nostril daily	2 sprays/nostril once daily

Class	Description	Drug	Pediatric dose	Adult dose
		Flunisolide (Nasalide)	12 years: adult dose; 6–14 years: 1 spray/nostril twice daily or 2 sprays/nostril twice daily	2 sprays/nostril once daily
		Ciclesonide (Omnaris)	12 years: 2 sprays/nostril once daily	2 sprays/nostril once daily
		Triamcinolone (Nasacort Aq)	6 years: 1 spray/nostril once daily	2 sprays/nostril once daily
Leukotriene receptor antagonist	Reduces mucosal inflammation	Montelukast (Singulair)	2–5 years: 4 mg daily; 6–14 years: 5 mg daily; 15 years: adult dose	10 mg once daily
Anticholinergic agent	Reduces rhinorrhea	Ipratropium (Atrovent)	6 years: 0.03% 2 sprays/nostril 2–3 times daily; 5 years: 0.06% 2 sprays/nostril four times daily for up to 3 weeks	0.03% 2 sprays/nostril 2–3 times daily; 0.06% 2 sprays/nostril 4 times daily up to 3 weeks
Mast cell stabilizer	Reduces sneezing, rhinorrhea, and nasal itch	Cromolyn (Nasalcrom)	2 years: same as adult	1–2 sprays/nostril 3–4 times daily
α-Adrenergic agonist	Reduces nasal congestion	Pseudoephedrine (Sudafed)	Not FDA-approved for children 12 years; 12 years: 30 mg every 6 hours	30–60 mg every 4 hours; Slow-release 120 mg every 12 hours; 240 mg every 24 hours
		Phenylephrine (Neosynephrine)[a]	6–12 years: (0.25%) 2 drops or 2 sprays every 6 hours	2–3 sprays each nostril every 6–8 hours
		Oxymetolazone (Afrin)[a]	>6 years: 2 sprays each nostril twice daily	2–3 sprays each nostril twice daily

[a] Not for long-term use. Can use for up to 3 days

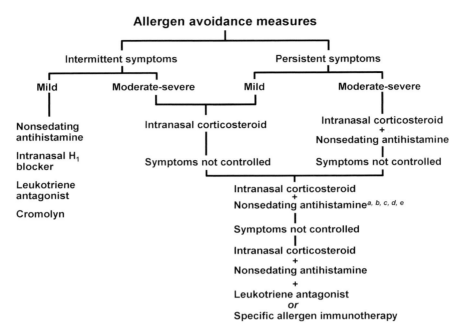

Fig. 4.4 Algorithm for treatment of allergic rhinitis. [a]Decongestants can be added for nasal congestion. Topical decongestants can only be used for ≤3 days. [b]Intranasal ipratroprium can be used for recalcitrant rhinorrhea. [c]Cromolyn is not likely to ameliorate symptoms acutely but may be helpful preventively with continual allergen exposure. [d]Systemic corticosteroids (short course) can be used for severe allergic rhinitis. [e]Although typically considered after a medication trial, specific allergen immunotherapy can be considered at any point (moderate-severe intermittent or persistent allergic rhinitis)

driving or performing a job that requires considerable physical coordination. Compared with second-generation antihistamines, first-generation agents appear to offer similar improvement in allergic rhinitis.

The newer (second-generation) antihistamines were developed in the 1980s, with the aim of their being more specific for the H_1 receptor and overcoming the anticholinergic and sedative adverse effects of first-generation antihistamines. The second-generation agents available in the United States include fexofenadine, desloratadine, loratadine, levocetirizine, and cetirizine. All these medications have been shown to be effective in relieving the majority of symptoms of allergic rhinitis. Antihistamines substantially reduce symptoms of nasal itching, watery eyes, rhinorrhea, and sneezing. However, they have minimal effect on the symptom of nasal congestion. In a few controlled studies, second-generation antihistamines have been compared directly and no evidence-based data demonstrate the superiority of one agent over another in the treatment of allergic rhinitis. However, patients often report significant symptom relief with one antihistamine but not another. Therefore, if one antihistamine is not helpful, consideration could be given to a trial of another antihistamine. Second-generation agents have better sedative profiles than first-generation agents; however, at higher-than-recommended doses, sedation and impairment can become evident. In several studies, it appears that fexofenadine has the least sedative-impairment properties, followed by loratadine and desloratadine, with cetirizine having the most. All these agents with the exception of fexofenadine have the potential to cross the blood-brain barrier, primarily at higher-than-recommended doses. Although cetirizine is less sedating than first-generation antihistamines, the US Food and Drug Administration has classified it as a sedating rather than a nonsedating antihistamine, and the product carries the full sedation precaution.

Azelastine is an intranasal second-generation antihistamine. It is approved for treatment of seasonal allergic rhinitis and vasomotor rhinitis and has been found to improve the symptoms of rhinorrhea, sneezing, and itchy nose. Overall, it appears that the improvement in symptoms is similar to that of oral second-generation antihistamines. The most common adverse effects are bitter taste and sedation.

Decongestants

Decongestants or vasoconstrictors are available in oral and intranasal forms. Oral decongestants relieve nasal obstruction through the vasoconstrictor activity of α-adrenergic receptors present on nasal capacitance vessels, which decrease mucosal swelling and associated nasal congestion. They relieve nasal obstruction but do not have an appreciable effect on other symptoms of rhinitis. Oral decongestants are primarily the catecholamines pseudoephedrine and phenylephrine. Pseudoephedrine is a commonly used decongestant that is available over the counter and is short acting. Decongestant medications are also combined with an antihistamine in both prescription and nonprescription medications. Oral decongestants can produce troubling adverse effects such as nervousness, insomnia, irritability, headache, increased blood pressure, palpitations, and tachycardia. They are contraindicated in patients with severe hypertension or coronary heart disease. Because of concerns about the use of pseudoephedrine in the illegal production of methamphetamine, pseudoephedrine is now kept behind the pharmacy counter and identification is required for purchase. Care should be taken with the long-term use of decongestants because of their considerable side effect profile.

Decongestants or vasoconstrictors are also available in topical nasal preparations. Topical decongestants include catecholamines and imidazaolines (e.g., oxymetazoline). Topical decongestants provide faster and greater relief of congestion. The systemic adverse effects of topical decongestants are less marked than those of the oral agents. However, tolerance and rebound congestion can develop when intranasal decongestants are used for more than 4 days. The rebound congestion appears to be due to obliteration of the normal nasal cycle, leaving the nasal vessels dilated, causing obstruction. Prolonged use leads to hypertrophy of the nasal turbinates, termed *rhinitis medicamentosa*. Topical decongestants are contraindicated for patients with narrow-angle glaucoma. Topical decongestants should never be used for long-term treatment. If used, patients need to be counseled about the importance of limited usage of the medication. Other adverse effects include nasal burning, stinging, and dryness.

Intranasal Corticosteroids

Because of the broad anti-inflammatory activity of intranasal corticosteroids, they are highly effective in the treatment of allergic rhinitis. They are recommended as first-line therapy for intermittent moderate to severe allergic rhinitis and persistent allergic rhinitis. Intranasal corticosteroids improve sneezing, nasal itch, rhinorrhea, and congestion. Compared with antihistamines and cromolyn, intranasal corticosteroids consistently provide a greater decrease in sneezing and nasal congestion.

Although intranasal corticosteroids are effective for allergic rhinitis, approximately 50% of patients may require additional medication to control allergic rhinitis. Because various medications influence different inflammatory mechanisms, multiple medications may be used. Oftentimes, patients are treated with an antihistamine and an intranasal corticosteroid, but data showing superiority of this regimen over intranasal corticosteroid alone are lacking. Once symptoms are controlled, the number of medications can often be decreased to a single agent. Intranasal corticosteroids have a delayed onset of action. Efficacy may appear 7 hours after administration, but full efficacy may take up to 2 weeks. These agents are most effective when used daily or prophylactically rather than intermittently. When given before the allergy season, intranasal corticosteroids can prevent nasal symptoms and reduce the severity of subsequent symptoms.

Nasal corticosteroids are considered safe and have few adverse effects. However, some patients dislike using nasal sprays, and compliance can be a problem. The most common adverse effect is epistaxis, which can occur in up to 10% of patients. It is important to educate the patient about the proper application of the nasal spray. Patients should avoid pointing the spray toward the septal wall. Also, keeping the nose well humidified with saline gel may help alleviate this problem. Other adverse effects include nasal burning, stinging, and dryness. With increasing indications for prolonged use of intranasal corticosteroids, studies have shown that they are safe, in that the histologic appearance of the nasal mucosa and ciliary function are preserved with long-term daily use of these agents. The nasal mucosa does not atrophy. Potential systemic safety concerns with intranasal corticosteroids include a transient effect on growth velocity in children, increased intraocular pressure, and subcapsular cataracts. However, studies have found that intranasal corticosteroids used in prescribed doses did not restrict skeletal growth in children. Also, the eye findings were very uncommon, and the risk is considered minimal for those using correctly prescribed dosages.

Overall, there are no significant clinical differences among the various nasal corticosteroid preparations. To optimize compliance, the favored preparations have once-daily dosing. These include triamcinolone acetonide, budesonide, fluticasone propionate, and mometasone furoate. Clinicians should become comfortable with several intranasal corticosteroids because each has its advantages and disadvantages in relation to patient acceptance based on smell, taste, and irritation. Also, different intranasal corticosteroids may or may not be covered by the patient's insurance or formulary. The various intranasal corticosteroids and their dosage are outlined in Table 4.1.

Systemic corticosteroids are not considered for chronic treatment of allergic rhinitis because of their side effect profile. Occasionally, patients with severe symptoms that are uncontrolled with other medications may be treated with systemic corticosteroids for the short term. These agents can be given in a depot injection or orally. The depot injection should be equivalent to 80–100 mg of prednisone. Oral dosing should use at least 20 mg of prednisone to be effective. Various dosing strategies have been used. A steroid burst of 40–50 mg per day for 5 days is used in adults and 1 mg kg^{-1} daily for 5 days in children. Further dosing depends on the patient's response to the overall management plan.

Anticholinergics

Anticholinergics are effective in treating rhinorrhea because the glandular secretion in the nose is under cholinergic control. However, they have little effect on nasal congestion, nasal itch, or sneezing. Because of the adverse effects, anticholinergics are administered only intranasally. Ipratropium bromide is the primary topical anticholinergic medication, and it is available in two strengths, 0.03% and 0.06%. For effectiveness, the medication should be used 3–4 times daily. Overall, ipratropium appears safe with long-term use. The main adverse effects are nasal irritation, crusting, and occasional mild nosebleed. No rebound hypersecretion occurs with this medication. Systemic anticholinergic symptoms may be apparent in sensitive patients, especially the elderly. Ipratropium should be administered primarily when rhinorrhea is not well controlled.

Mast Cell Stabilizer (Cromolyn)

Cromolyn, an intranasal mast cell stabilizer, inhibits the degranulation of sensitized mast cells. This medication is available over the counter. Although it helps reduce the symptoms of allergic rhinitis, the effects are modest. Cromolyn is more effective if given before exposure to the allergen, for example, with preseasonal treatment. Once symptoms are severe, treatment with cromolyn produces little acute improvement. Cromolyn requires dosing four times daily, making compliance difficult. Its safety profile is excellent, and no significant adverse effects have been noted.

Leukotriene Receptor Antagonists

Antileukotriene medications target the cysteinyl leukotrienes, which are part of the inflammatory cycle in allergic rhinitis. These medications were used initially in the treatment of asthma, but they also have demonstrated efficacy in reducing the symptoms of allergic rhinitis. Their efficacy seems to be similar or slightly less than that of antihistamines and significantly less than that of intranasal corticosteroids. The main indications for use are in patients who are unable to use intranasal corticosteroids or antihistamines or possibly as an additional medication for patients whose allergic rhinitis is not controlled with intranasal corticosteroids.

Currently, montelukast has been approved for treating allergic rhinitis, and zafirlukast has been approved only for treating asthma. Overall, the medication is considered safe; there have been concerns about the use of leukotriene antagonists and the development of Churg–Strauss syndrome. There is not thought to be an association.

Immunotherapy

Allergen immunotherapy has proved highly effective for controlling the symptoms of allergic rhinitis due to various aeroallergens, including dust mites, cats, trees, grasses, and weeds. Efficacy has also been shown for mold allergen, but this is less consistent than that for the other allergens. Allergen immunotherapy should be considered for patients who remain symptomatic despite therapy, who require systemic corticosteroids, or who have a coexisting condition such as sinusitis or asthma.

The mechanism of action of immunotherapy has been characterized only recently despite this treatment being available since the 1940s. Allergen immunotherapy increases allergen-specific IgG, which is thought to function as a blocking antibody. It also decreases allergen-specific IgE and allergen-induced mediator release and shifts the cytokine release profile of T-cells from a Th2 pattern to a Th1 pattern. The shift in cytokine release decreases the levels of IL-4 and IL-5 and decreases activation of eosinophils and mast cells. Immunotherapy also increases IL-10, which serves as a regulatory cytokine and dampens the inflammatory response.

Immunotherapy is the only intervention for allergic rhinitis that alters the natural history of the disease. A typical course of immunotherapy is 3–5 years. Termination of the immunotherapy results in continued symptom improvement for at least 3 years in the majority of patients. Recent studies have shown that children with allergic rhinitis receiving immunotherapy have a lower rate of development of asthma than those not receiving immunotherapy. Furthermore, for children sensitized only to dust mites, immunotherapy resulted in the development of fewer new allergens than in children not given immunotherapy. The mechanism for this has not yet been elucidated.

The main risk of immunotherapy is a systemic allergic reaction. Approximately 0.6–5% of patients undergoing immunotherapy have a systemic reaction, depending on the study. For this reason, immunotherapy should be given only in a physician's office or clinic where a health care provider is present to treat an allergic reaction. It is recommended that patients wait 30 min in the office or clinic after the injection because most reactions occur within that time. Allergen immunotherapy injections should not be given to patients whose asthma is not well controlled. Immunotherapy generally is safe when administered by competent specialists.

Allergen immunotherapy can also be administered sublingually. Currently, this formulation is not available in the United States but is in Europe. It appears that the overall efficacy of sublingual immunotherapy is less than that of subcutaneous immunotherapy, but it has fewer systemic reactions. Allergen immunotherapy is reviewed in detail in Chap. 3.

4.5   Nonallergic Rhinitis and Rhinosinusitis

The first branch point in the algorithm in Fig. 4.1 is the separation of rhinitis and rhinosinusitis into allergic vs. nonallergic forms. The nonallergic forms can be classified as infectious/inflammatory or noninfectious. The infectious/inflammatory forms include acute and chronic rhinosinusitis. The noninfectious forms are divided into the structural-predominant causes, which include polyps, cerebrospinal fluid (CSF) leak, adenoid hypertrophy, tumor, septal deviation, and foreign body, and the nonstructural forms, which include vasomotor rhinitis, NARES, atrophic rhinitis, hormonal rhinitis, rhinitis induced by medication, and rhinitis induced by food.

4.6   Infectious-Acute Rhinosinusitis

The clinical presentations of rhinosinusitis and allergic rhinitis can be similar, and the two conditions share certain underlying mechanisms, including mucociliary dysfunction, tissue edema, and increased mucus production. The most common factors that contribute to acute rhinosinusitis are local. Acute rhinitis of either an infectious or allergic origin results in edema that obstructs the nasal ostia, decreases paranasal sinus ciliary action, and increases mucus production. During a common cold, nasal fluid containing viruses, bacteria, and inflammatory mediators may be blown into the sinuses, causing infection or inflammation or both.

Distinguishing between acute viral rhinosinusitis and bacterial rhinosinusitis is difficult. In most patients, viral rhinosinusitis improves in 7–10 days; therefore, a diagnosis of acute bacterial sinusitis requires the persistence of symptoms for longer than 10 days or a worsening of symptoms after 5–7 days. The diagnosis is also considered when symptoms of an upper respiratory tract infection are disproportionate to symptoms typical of a viral upper respiratory tract infection, that is, localized pain or fever. Classically, in viral rhinosinusitis, the nasal discharge is clear and thin instead of yellow-green and thick as in bacterial sinusitis. The division between acute and chronic rhinosinusitis is based on the duration of symptoms. Acute rhinosinusitis has acute onset of symptoms that resolve in 4 weeks. Chronic rhinosinusitis is defined as the presence of sinus symptoms for at least 8 weeks.

Various criteria have been proposed for clinically diagnosing acute rhinosinusitis, but the correlation with computed tomographic (CT) findings and rhinolaryngoscopy has been disappointing. Symptoms associated with acute rhinosinusitis include a combination of nasal congestion, purulent nasal discharge, postnasal drainage, headache, facial pain or pressure, olfactory disturbance, dental pain, fever, or cough. In children, cough and nasal discharge are the most common symptoms, and facial pain is unusual. Adults more commonly report unilateral facial pain and headache in addition to symptoms of rhinitis. The distribution of facial pain and pressure may help to localize the infection to a particular sinus. Maxillary sinusitis typically causes discomfort in the cheek or upper teeth, whereas frontal sinusitis causes pain in the forehead. Ethmoid involvement may present with tenderness over the medial canthal region, and pain from the sphenoid sinus is often retro-orbital but can radiate to the occiput. In all age groups, less frequent symptoms associated with acute rhinosinusitis are nausea, irritability, and halitosis.

4.6.1   Physical Examination

Physical examination of the nose can be performed in the office with an otoscope or nasal speculum. The structures that usually can be visualized are the inferior and middle turbinates, the inferior and middle meatus, and the nasal septum. Findings include erythematous, swollen turbinates; nasal crusts; and purulent secretions on the floor of the nose or the back of the throat. However, the absence of purulent secretions does not rule out infection because sinus drainage may be intermittent. Tenderness may be elicited by percussion over the sinuses, but this sign is unreliable because it lacks both sensitivity and specificity. Children often have middle ear effusions; this is less common in adults.

Transillumination of the sinuses has been performed by placing a light source against the skin overlying the infraorbital rim and directing the light inferiorly. The patient is asked to open the mouth so the hard palate can be examined. Possible results are an opaque or normal palate. This procedure has low sensitivity and specificity because of anatomical variability and subjective interpretation of the findings.

Patients with obvious acute sinusitis should be evaluated carefully for evidence of possible complicating factors such as osteitis and orbital cellulitis. The patient should be examined for the presence of facial swelling or erythema over an involved sinus, visual changes, proptosis, periorbital inflammation, and involvement of the central nervous system.

4.6.2   Microbiology

Bacteria can be isolated from two-thirds of patients with acute infection of the maxillary, ethmoid, frontal, or sphenoid sinuses. The paranasal sinuses are believed to be sterile under normal circumstances; however, the nose and nasopharynx are colonized with flora consisting of coagulase-negative staphylococci, *Corynebacterium* spp., and *Staphylococcus aureus*. The responsible organisms in acute rhinosinusitis are the common respiratory pathogens: *Streptococcus pneumoniae*, *Moraxella catarrhalis*, *Haemophilus influenzae*, and β-hemolytic streptococci. Both *M. catarrhalis* and *H. influenzae* can produce β-lactamase, thereby being resistant to penicillin and its derivatives. The prevalence of penicillin-resistant *S. pneumoniae* is increasing. There is wide geographic variation in the resistance patterns. The infection is polymicrobial in approximately one-third of cases. Enteric bacteria are rarely found. Anaerobic bacteria are recovered when acute sinusitis is associated with dental disease, primarily as an extension of the infection from the roots of the upper premolars or molars. *Pseudomonas aeruginosa*, *Klebsiella pneumoniae*,

Enterobacter spp., *Proteus mirabilis*, and other gram-negative rods are common in sinusitis of nosocomial origin and in immunocompromised patients, patients with human immunodeficiency virus (HIV) infection, and patients with cystic fibrosis.

4.6.3   Testing

Nasal cultures are not reliable for establishing the diagnosis of rhinosinusitis or for determining a specific causative organism. Obtaining cultures of the middle meatus through endoscopically directed culture may be helpful in adults but not in children. A definitive diagnosis can be made by aspiration of the maxillary antrum for culture, but because this is invasive, it is indicated only when microbial identification is essential.

   Plain radiographs have significant false-positive and false-negative results in acute rhinosinusitis and generally are not indicated. Occasionally, radiographs may be useful in supporting the diagnosis or providing evidence of the degree of involvement. Plain radiographs that show more than 6 mm of mucosal thickening in the maxillary sinuses of adults and 4 mm of thickening in children are compatible with the diagnosis of bacterial rhinosinusitis. Other findings compatible with bacterial rhinosinusitis are opacification and air–fluid levels in any of the paranasal sinuses or more than 33% loss of air space within the maxillary sinuses. The ethmoid and sphenoid sinuses are poorly visualized on plain radiographs. CT of the sinuses is indicated if orbital involvement is suspected. Because of cost and radiation exposure, CT is not indicated for untreated, uncomplicated acute rhinosinusitis.

4.6.4   Treatment

Antibiotics are the primary treatment for acute rhinosinusitis. The goals of antibiotic therapy are to decrease the severity and duration of symptoms and to preclude the development of complications. Several options are available for antibiotic treatment of acute rhinosinusitis (Table 4.2). The antibiotic of choice for uncomplicated rhinosinusitis is ampicillin or amoxicillin because the organisms that are usually responsible are sensitive to this antibiotic and adequate levels of the drug are achieved in the sinus mucosa. Many antibiotics are effective for acute rhinosinusitis and care needs to be taken in using them in a stepwise fashion to help prevent the emergence of resistant bacteria. The other major first-line antibiotic is trimethoprim-sulfamethoxazole. Bacterial resistance can pose a problem, particularly the production of β-lactamase. β-Lactamase enzymes destroy the β-lactam ring of the penicillins and cephalosporins. Clavulanic acid inhibits β-lactamase activity and is effective when used in combination with amoxicillin as amoxicillin–clavulanic acid (Augmentin). This combination serves as a second-line antibiotic. In addition to amoxicillin–clavulanic acid, other second-line antibiotics include the cephalosporins,

Table 4.2 Antibiotics commonly used in the treatment of rhinosinusitis

Antibiotic (trade name)	Dose	
	Pediatric	Adult
Penicillins		
Amoxicillin (Amoxil, Trimox)	25–50 mg kg^{-1} per day divided every 8 hours	875 mg every 12 hours 500 mg every 8 hours
Amoxicillin/clavulanate potassium (Augmentin, Augmentin XR)	<3 months: 30 mg kg^{-1} per day divided every 12 hours	250–500 mg per 125 mg every 8 hours
	3 months: 45 mg kg^{-1} per day every 12 hours	875 mg per 125 mg every 12 hours
	40 kg: adult dosing	2,000 mg per 125 mg every 12 hours
Folate inhibitor		
Trimethoprim/ sulfamethoxazole (Septra, Bactrim)	8 mg kg^{-1} trimethoprim and 40 mg kg^{-1} sulfamethoxazole per 24 hours in 2 divided doses every 12 hours	800 mg per 160 mg twice daily
Cephalosporins		
Cefuroxime axetil (Ceftin)	3 months to 12 years: 30 mg kg^{-1} per day divided twice daily (maximum dose 1,000 mg) >12 years: 250 mg twice daily	250 or 500 mg twice daily
Cefpodoxime proxetil (Vantin)	2 months to 12 years: 5 mg kg^{-1} per 12 hours (maximum dose 200 mg) >12 years: adult dose	200 mg every 12 hours
Cefprozil (Cefzil)	6 months to 12 years: 7.5 mg kg^{-1} every 12 hours >12 years: adult dose	250 or 500 mg every 12 hours
Cefixime (Suprax)	6 months to 12 years: 8 mg kg^{-1} per day once daily or divided twice daily >12 years: adult dose	400 mg daily
Ceftibuten (Cedax)	9 mg kg^{-1} per day (maximum dose 400 mg)	400 mg daily
Cefdinir (Omnicef)	6 months to 12 years: 7 mg kg^{-1} every 12 hours	300 mg twice daily
Macrolides		
Erythromycin ethylsuccinate/ sulfisoxazole (Pediazole)	12.5/37.5 mg kg^{-1} per dose four times daily	…
Azithromycin (Zithromax)	6 months 10 mg kg^{-1} daily (3 days)	500 mg daily (3 days)
Clarithromycin (Biaxin)	7.5 mg kg^{-1} per every 12 hours	500 mg twice daily

(continued)

Table 4.2 (continued)

Antibiotic (trade name)	Dose	
	Pediatric	Adult
Fluoroquinolones		
Ciprofloxacin (Cipro)	10–20 mg kg^{-1} per every 12 hours (maximum dose 750 mg)	500 mg every 12 hours
Levofloxacin (Levaquin)	…	500 mg daily
Moxifloxacin (Avelox)	…	400 mg daily
Gatifloxacin (Tequin)	…	400 mg daily
Clindamycin (Cleocin)	8–16 mg kg^{-1} per day divided into 3 or 4 doses	300 mg every 6 hours
Metronidazole (Flagyl)	20–40 mg kg^{-1} per day divided into 3 or 4 doses	500–750 mg 3 times daily
Ketolide		
Telithromycin (Ketek)[a]	…	800 mg daily

[a] Associated with hepatic failure or severe hepatic injury during or immediately after treatment

macrolides, ketolides, and fluoroquinolones. These antibiotics should be considered when patients have clinically significant coexisting illnesses or more potentially serious disease such as frontal or sphenoidal sinusitis or when initial treatment has failed.

Cephalosporins are commonly prescribed for acute rhinosinusitis. First-generation agents have poor coverage for *H. influenzae* and, thus, should be avoided. Cefuroxime axetil and cefprozil are second-generation agents appropriate for acute sinusitis. These medications have activity against β-lactamase-producing *H. influenzae*, *M. catarrhalis,* and *S. aureus.* Third-generation agents appropriate for treatment include cefpodoxime proxetil and cefdinir. Cefixime and ceftibuten have poor activity against *S. pneumoniae* and so are not an ideal choice for acute sinusitis when gram-negative bacteria are unlikely. Azithromycin and clarithromycin are relatively weak against penicillin-resistant *H. influenzae* and *S. pneumoniae*. If a patient does not have an appropriate response to these medications, a substitution should be made to cover penicillin-resistant organisms. The new ketolide telithromycin covers the common respiratory pathogens, including macrolide- and penicillin-resistant strains. Telithromycin has caused severe hepatotoxicity, and its use should be limited to rare instances. Fluoroquinolones are effective against the primary organisms but are reserved for treating adults.

These agents should be used in situations where resistance is high or if the patient's condition has not improved within 3–5 days after receiving a first-line antibiotic. Clindamycin and metronidazole should be used with a broad-spectrum antibiotic if the suspicion for an anaerobic infection is high. The duration of treatment for acute bacterial rhinosinusitis is debated. Most patients receive treatment with antibiotics for 10–14 days, but few studies have been conducted to support or refute this approach. Antibiotic therapy should continue for 7 days beyond the point of symptomatic improvement.

Other adjunctive treatments have been used for acute rhinosinusitis but have not been studied rigorously. Topical and oral decongestants are often prescribed because they decrease nasal resistance and theoretically should increase ostial drainage. However, prospective studies have not been done. Before recommending these modalities, physicians should review the adverse effects. Topical decongestants can cause rebound congestion and rhinitis medicamentosa when used more than a few days. Oral decongestants can be associated with increased blood pressure, insomnia, and urinary retention. A few studies have shown that intranasal corticosteroids used adjunctively with antibiotics are modestly beneficial. The use of systemic corticosteroids has not been studied.

Many nonpharmacologic measures are used for symptomatic relief of acute sinusitis; however, data on efficacy are lacking. Saline is commonly used to aid drainage of mucus and to prevent crusting. Studies have shown benefit when hypertonic saline is used. The optimal delivery system for the saline has not been clarified. The options include bulb syringe, Neti Pot, squeezable plastic bottle with nasal adaptor, and a pulse irrigator combined with a nasal adaptor. Steam inhalation is used to liquefy and soften crusts while moisturizing the dry inflamed mucosa. This may provide some short-lived symptomatic relief but likely does not affect the overall course. Mentholated preparations in combination with steam produce a subjective sensation of increased air flow. However, no data support objective improvement even though patients often feel that these agents help.

4.7   Chronic Rhinosinusitis

Chronic rhinosinusitis affects more than 14% of the population annually, resulting in millions of dollars in health care expenditure. Chronic rhinosinusitis has been shown to have a significant effect on patients' quality of life and can lead to substantial physical and functional impairment. The criteria for making the diagnosis of chronic rhinosinusitis are a matter of considerable controversy. Chronic rhinosinusitis is a group of disorders characterized by sinus symptoms that persist for 8 weeks or longer. Symptoms in chronic rhinosinusitis are typically less prominent than in acute rhinosinusitis and consist primarily of a combination of nasal congestion, postnasal drainage, facial pressure, fatigue, cough, and dental pain. Purulent nasal secretions or purulent postnasal drainage may or may not accompany these symptoms. Some patients with chronic rhinosinusitis may present with vague or insidious symptoms. These symptoms are nonspecific, and nasal endoscopy or CT is usually required to make the diagnosis. In chronic rhinosinusitis, findings on sinus CT are generally abnormal. On physical examination, patients have mild or moderate turbinate swelling, watery congestion, and occasionally purulent drainage.

Part of the difficulty in finding uniformity of signs and symptoms is that chronic rhinosinusitis likely has multiple causes and more than one cause can be present at any time. The notion that all chronic rhinosinusitis can be explained on the basis of obstruction of sinus ostia and bacterial infection is gradually being abandoned.

Chronic rhinosinusitis has a significant inflammatory component that may be caused by various factors. Possible causes of chronic rhinosinusitis are still being elucidated, and the mechanisms are not fully characterized. Currently, the main causes include chronic infectious rhinosinusitis, chronic allergic fungal sinusitis, chronic fungal or hyperplastic eosinophilic rhinosinusitis, and systemic disease. The role of infection is unclear. Certainly, bacteria have an important role in a subset referred to as *infectious chronic rhinosinusitis.*

The role of fungi in the etiology of chronic rhinosinusitis is more problematic. Fungal sinusitis can take multiple forms: fulminant infection, chronic eosinophilic fungal rhinosinusitis, allergic fungal sinusitis, and mycetoma. In chronic eosinophilic fungal rhinosinusitis and allergic fungal sinusitis, it is surmised that the fungi, instead of acting as an infectious agent, trigger an inflammatory eosinophilic response that results in chronic rhinosinusitis. However, in mycetoma, a "fungal ball" is present in the sinuses, but there does not appear to be any invasion.

Although classified under noninfectious, structural-predominant rhinosinusitis, nasal and sinus polyposis can complicate all these processes. Polyposis is particularly prominent in chronic fungal or hyperplastic eosinophilic rhinosinusitis.

4.8   Infectious Chronic Rhinosinusitis

Central to the pathogenesis of chronic rhinosinusitis is impaired patency of the ostiomeatal complex. This obstruction impairs drainage, which results in the accumulation of mucus, foreign material, and bacteria in the sinuses. The obstruction causes oxygen levels to decrease, thus creating an environment that promotes secondary bacterial growth and inflammation. The decrease in oxygen levels allows the proliferation of anaerobic bacteria. In adults, anaerobic bacteria account for nearly 50% of cases of infectious chronic rhinosinusitis compared with <10% of cases of acute rhinosinusitis. The microorganisms of chronic rhinosinusitis consist of the anaerobes such as gram-positive streptococci, *Bacteroides* spp., and *Fusobacterium* spp. and aerobic bacteria such as *S. aureus* and *Pseudomonas aeruginosa* and the organisms of acute sinusitis. In children, even in chronic rhinosinusitis, isolation of anaerobic bacteria is rare and found only with the more severe and protracted symptoms. In children, the microorganisms are predominately *S. pneumoniae, H. influenzae,* and *M. catarrhalis.*

Fungal sinus infections can take various forms. Fungal infection can occur in both immunocompromised and immunocompetent patients, although it typically is more common in the immunocompromised. Factors that predispose to fungal infections include radiotherapy, diabetes mellitus, immunosuppressive treatment, and long-term systemic corticosteroid therapy. *Aspergillus fumigatus* is the most commonly found fungus. Other fungi associated with an infectious form of rhinosinusitis include *Nocardia, Mucor,* and *Alternaria.* Fulminant fungal sinusitis occurs exclusively in immunocompromised patients and is characterized by fever, headache, and mental status changes. Urgent aggressive treatment is warranted. In comparison, a mycetoma or fungus ball is noninvasive. Fungus ball occurs in the maxillary or sphenoid sinuses and is usually unilateral. Symptoms are chronic and include headache and obstruction. Surgical removal is usually indicated.

The presentation and microbiology of infectious chronic rhinosinusitis of immunocompromised patients differ from those of immunocompetent patients. Most immunodeficient patients with recurrent sinusitis have defects in humoral immunity, primarily selective IgA deficiency and common variable immunodeficiency (hypogammaglobulinemia). Other types of immunodeficiencies can present with recurrent sinusitis, including acquired immunodeficiency syndrome (AIDS). Suspicion for immunodeficiency is heightened when the patient also has a history of recurrent bronchitis, pneumonia, or bronchiectasis (or a combination of these). Patients with humoral immunodeficiency have a more prevalent and severe chronic rhinosinusitis that responds poorly to treatment. The organisms usually are not markedly different from those encountered in immunocompetent patients. In patients with cystic fibrosis, sinusitis is nearly ubiquitous because of the retention of viscous tenacious sinus secretions that predispose to bacterial infection. The sinus pathogens in patients with cystic fibrosis are similar to those that cause recurrent respiratory infection in these patients: *P. aeruginosa*, *H. influenzae*, *Streptococcus* spp., *Burkholderia cepacia*, *S. aureus*, and anaerobes.

4.8.1 Testing

Nasal cultures typically are not helpful for determining the cause of chronic rhinosinusitis because of nasal contamination, and they do not provide an accurate picture of the organisms responsible for the sinusitis. Antral puncture and sterile culture give an accurate picture of the microbiology, but this test is difficult and generally performed by an otolaryngologist. This test is performed when rhinosinusitis is associated with signs of severe toxicity and identification of the exact organism and antimicrobial susceptibilities are required.

A nasal smear is obtained by fixing the nasal secretions on a slide. Hansel staining is used to highlight eosinophil granular proteins. Additional stains can be used to identify other elements. The presence of polymorphonuclear cells suggests bacterial infection. An abundance of eosinophils suggests allergic rhinitis, NARES, or chronic eosinophilic rhinosinusitis. The results are most useful clinically when there is a predominance of neutrophils or eosinophils.

Imaging studies of the sinuses are helpful in the evaluation of chronic rhinosinusitis, but the specific indications are not well defined. Plain film radiographs include an occipitomental view (Waters view) taken with the head tilted back, to help view the maxillary sinuses. The occipitofrontal view (Caldwells view) helps demonstrate the ethmoid and frontal sinuses. The sphenoid sinus is seen in the lateral view. Opinions differ about what constitutes radiographic sinusitis. Generally, there is a good correlation with the results of antral puncture culture when there are air–fluid levels or opacification in any of the sinuses. In adults, mucosal thickening of 6 mm or more (4 mm or more in children) correlates with bacterial sinusitis. Because of poor overall specificity and sensitivity, plain sinus films are not generally helpful in diagnosing chronic rhinosinusitis.

CT has been helpful in the diagnosis of chronic rhinosinusitis. CT should be performed on patients who have persistent symptoms of rhinosinusitis despite medical treatment. Coronal CT scans can demonstrate the ostiomeatal complex and show membrane inflammation, particularly in the ethmoid and sphenoid sinuses, not seen well on plain films. CT is particularly helpful in the evaluation of patients who have had previous sinus surgery. Mucosal defects and bony changes are well delineated, which helps to differentiate the components of the opacification. Positive CT findings usually are not specific for clearly distinguishing between bacterial, fungal, or noninfectious rhinosinusitis. Differentiating the cause of the inflammation requires clinical correlation based on the history and physical examination findings.

Immunodeficiency should be considered in any patient with recurrent or chronic sinusitis in whom aggressive medical or surgical management has failed. Appropriate laboratory assessment of the immune system might include quantitative determination of immunoglobulins (IgG, IgA, IgM) and specific antibody responses (tetanus toxoid and pneumococcal vaccine) to measure the humoral immune response. Flow cytometry of T-cells (for determining T-cell number) and delayed hypersensitivity skin tests (for determining T-cell function) can be used to measure the cell-mediated immune response.

Flexible fiberoptic rhinolaryngoscopy is a safe, effective way to visualize the inside of the nose, the eustachian tube openings, the adenoids and tonsils, and the throat and vocal cords. This procedure assesses for the presence of purulent discharge, blockage of the sinus ostia, polyps, tumor, and septal deviation. It is indicated in the evaluation of chronic rhinosinusitis, nasal polyps, epistaxis, snoring, sinus discomfort, chronic postnasal drainage, nasopharyngeal pain, and nasal obstruction of unknown cause. The entire procedure takes 10–15 min and is well tolerated. It can be performed in conjunction with coronal CT scanning of the sinuses to further define the anatomy in patients with chronic symptoms or those who do not have a response to conventional treatment.

4.8.2 Treatment

Antibiotic treatment is required for chronic infectious rhinosinusitis. Typically, the specific pathogen is not identified and treatment is empiric, based on the usual pathogens encountered. The length of therapy has not been well defined for chronic rhinosinusitis, but 21 days is considered standard treatment. The choice of antibiotic follows the same algorithm as for acute rhinosinusitis; however, amoxicillin usually is not the first choice. Alternatives include amoxicillin–clavulanic acid, cephalosporins, ketolides, macrolides, and fluoroquinolones (Table 4.2). If symptoms persist despite treatment and infection seems the likely cause, it may be appropriate to obtain a culture specimen.

This is invasive and requires an otolaryngologist. Consideration could be given to using an antibiotic with more anaerobic coverage, for example, amoxicillin–clavulanic acid, clindamycin, or metronidazole. If symptoms persist, the patient should be evaluated for other underlying causes.

In addition to antibiotics, other agents can help decrease congestion associated with chronic rhinosinusitis. Saline nasal spray, saline irrigation, or saline gel is helpful in humidifying the nasal airway and preventing crusting. Saline is helpful in thinning secretions, decreasing nasal blood flow, and improving sinus symptoms. Saline irrigation can be performed with warm saline solution and a bulb syringe or other device. The saline is prepared by adding one-fourth teaspoon of salt to two cups of warm water. The saline is squirted gently into the nose with the bulb syringe or other device, with the patient bending over a sink. The solution drains from the nostrils, carrying excess mucus with it. Topical decongestants help reduce nasal swelling. However, these agents can be used only for 3–4 days consecutively because of development of rhinitis medicamentosa. Oral decongestants can also help with decongestion, but they have not been studied in chronic rhinosinusitis and the adverse effects need to be considered. Evidence supporting the use of intranasal corticosteroids is equivocal. They are indicated for treatment of patients with concomitant allergic rhinitis. Systemic corticosteroids generally are not indicated except for patients with concomitant nasal polyp disease.

When maximal medical treatment fails, referral for consideration of surgical treatment is appropriate. The goal of sinus surgery is to restore ventilation and drainage by removing debris and inflammation. The most common type of surgery is functional endoscopic surgery (FESS). This is performed with endoscopes passed through the nostrils, where, under direct visualization, the ostiomeatal complex is opened and the sinus ostia enlarged. Debris trapped within the sinuses can be evacuated and cultured. Complications of FESS include bleeding, infection, and, rarely, orbital injury, intracranial injury, or CSF leak.

4.9 Allergic Fungal Rhinosinusitis

Allergic fungal rhinosinusitis is a specific form of rhinosinusitis that occurs in immunocompetent hosts. It is characterized by nasal polyposis, "allergic mucin" within the sinuses, fungal identification by histology or culture, positive skin prick test or in vitro testing to common airborne fungi, and characteristic CT findings. CT shows a speckled pattern of high attenuation within the inflammation caused by a collection of high-density materials. This "allergic mucin" is a rubbery, tenacious mucus that is primarily eosinophilic. It is surmised that it represents an exaggerated IgE response to airborne fungi. The most common fungi to cause this clinical syndrome are *Bipolaris*, *Curvularia*, and *Aspergillus* spp. The clinical presentation is essentially identical to that of other forms of chronic rhinosinusitis, with chronic nasal obstruction and congestion as primary symptoms. Because of the underlying inflammation and drainage problems, recurrent infections are frequent. In the United States, allergic fungal rhinosinusitis is most common in the south, southwest, and western regions of the country.

Treatment of allergic fungal rhinosinusitis often involves surgical removal of the allergic mucin, which consists of thick secretions with concretions containing a large number of fungal hyphae and eosinophils. Systemic corticosteroids help reduce the symptoms of rhinosinusitis, particularly when used postoperatively. Intranasal corticosteroids are also frequently prescribed postoperatively for these patients. The role of fungi immunotherapy and antifungal antibiotics administered topically or systemically has not been well delineated.

4.10 Chronic Eosinophilic (Fungal or Hyperplastic) Rhinosinusitis

Eosinophilic fungal or hyperplastic rhinosinusitis is similar to allergic fungal rhinosinusitis except that the patients do not show any IgE sensitivity to airborne fungi. It has been theorized by some investigators that the fungi contribute to the eosinophilic inflammation through a non-IgE-mediated mechanism. Investigators who favor fungi as the stimulus for the eosinophilic inflammation use the term *eosinophilic fungal rhinosinusitis* and those who question the role of fungi use the term *eosinophilic hyperplastic rhinosinusitis*. Currently, investigators are considering further dividing these groups into those with polyps and those without polyps. The patients have a clinical presentation of chronic rhinosinusitis manifested by chronic nasal congestion, drainage, difficulty breathing through the nose, and often recurrent infections. Sinus tissue sampling shows an allergic mucin similar to that of allergic fungal rhinosinusitis, with eosinophilic inflammation and the presence of fungi. However, patients have negative findings on skin and in vitro testing to common airborne fungi. In vitro studies in these patients show a striking eosinophilic degranulation with exposure to *Alternaria*, as compared with normal controls. CT of the sinuses shows mucosal thickening or partial or complete opacification of two or more sinus cavities.

The treatment of chronic eosinophilic rhinosinusitis is problematic. Studies of treatment with antifungal irrigation solutions and systemic antifungal medication to remove the stimulus (the fungi) have been conflicting, and no definitive studies have been performed. However, patients typically have a response to treatment with systemic corticosteroids. The response is short-lived unless systemic corticosteroids are continued. Topical intranasal corticosteroids can be helpful after a surgical procedure but are of limited value when the disease is fulminant. Saline irrigations, although not vigorously studied, appear to help symptom improvement. The overall medical management plan consists of a combination of systemic corticosteroids, intranasal corticosteroids, saline irrigations, and possibly antifungal preparations and judicious use of decongestants. Antihistamines typically are not helpful in this process. Sinus surgery is often required.

4.11   Systemic Disease

Systemic disease can present with significant sinus symptoms. In addition to cystic fibrosis and primary immunodeficiency described above, other entities associated with rhinosinusitis include sarcoidosis, Wegener granulomatosis, and ciliary dyskinesia. Sarcoidosis is a relatively common multisystem disease. The hallmark of sarcoidosis is the presence of noncaseating granulomas. The nasal mucosa is involved in up to 20% of patients. In addition to nasal sinus involvement, other signs and symptoms are typically present, particularly involving the lungs. The most common nasal finding is nasal congestion. Sarcoidosis should be considered in patients with multisystem disease or those with disease recalcitrant to standard treatment measures.

Wegener granulomatosis is a systemic autoimmune disease characterized by a necrotizing vasculitis of the upper and lower respiratory tracts. Patients present with epistaxis, refractory sinusitis, serous otitis, nodular pulmonary infiltrates, and focal necrotizing glomerulonephritis. Chronic sinusitis can precede pulmonary and renal manifestations for years before the disease becomes fulminant. The diagnosis should be considered in patients with chronic rhinosinusitis recalcitrant to conventional therapy. Diagnosis can be confirmed by the presence of c-ANCA. Biopsy specimens show vasculitis of small arteries and veins with granuloma formation.

Ciliary dyskinesia typically presents with persistent or recurrent sinusitis. Because the ability to clear mucus and bacteria is impaired, upper and lower respiratory tract infections are protracted. Patients often have productive cough with underlying bronchiectasis. A specific subgroup is Kartagener syndrome, which is characterized by recurrent sinusitis, nasal polyps, situs inversus, infertility, and bronchiectasis. A screening test for ciliary function is the saccharin test, which measures the amount of time it takes for a patient to taste the saccharin after it is placed on the inferior turbinate. The usual time is 15–20 minutes. Delayed perception of saccharin is suggestive of disordered motility. Electron microscopic examination of the cilia obtained by a brush sample is the only way to document abnormal ciliary structure.

4.12   Noninfectious Structural Rhinosinusitis

Noninfectious, structural rhinosinusitis is typically characterized by the presence of unilateral symptoms and anosmia. Congestion, nasal blockage, and postnasal drainage that is primarily one-sided are the most prominent symptoms. Whenever symptoms are primarily one-sided, further evaluation is required to determine the cause, because of the potential for tumor or involvement of the surrounding orbital or cranial structures. The primary entities in this classification are nasal and sinus polyposis, tumors, CSF rhinorrhea, adenoidal hypertrophy, foreign body, and septal deviation.

4.12.1 *Nasal and Sinus Polyposis*

Nasal polyps are smooth, pale, gelatinous outgrowths of the nasal mucosa that resemble a peeled grape. Most polyps are located in the middle meatus and originate from the ethmoid sinuses. Histologic sections of nasal polyp tissue exhibit eosinophils, plasma cells, lymphocytes, and mast cells. The pathogenesis of nasal and sinus polyps is not known. It has been postulated that a combination of allergic, infectious, environmental, genetic, and metabolic factors result in the formation of nasal polyps. These polyps occur equally in atopic and nonatopic patients. Of note, nasal polyps are twice as likely to occur in men as in women. The diagnosis of nasal and sinus polyposis is made most often in the third and fourth decades of life. A subgroup of patients with nasal polyposis also have aspirin sensitivity and asthma. Nasal polyps are much less common in children than adults. If nasal polyps are diagnosed in a child, cystic fibrosis must be excluded.

Most patients with nasal and sinus polyps have a long history of symptoms of perennial rhinitis. Nearly all patients report nasal obstruction and congestion, and most have a decrease in or absence of the sense of smell. Other common symptoms include rhinorrhea, sneezing, postnasal drainage, and facial pain. Nasal polyps are often seen in association with chronic fungal or hyperplastic eosinophilic rhinosinusitis. The major complication of nasal polyps is infectious sinusitis. In severe polyposis, enlargement of the nasal polyps may lead to broadening of the nasal bridge or encroachment into the orbit, causing compression of ocular structures.

Nasal polyps appear as bulbous translucent or opaque growths. They are best visualized when they extend from the middle and inferior nasal turbinates. Hypertrophied or polypoid nasal turbinates can sometimes be confused with nasal polyps. One distinguishing characteristic of polyps is insensitivity to pain on direct manipulation. Polyps are only minimally vascular and, thus, do not tend to bleed. In addition to turbinates, tumors may also be mistaken for nasal polyps. Friability or bleeding should alert the physician to a tumor.

The management of nasal polyps is difficult. Antihistamines, decongestants, and leukotriene receptor antagonists are of little benefit. The primary medical approach for the management of nasal polyps is the judicious use of corticosteroids. Corticosteroids are effective in reducing polyp size and can be administered intranasally or systemically. Intranasal corticosteroids decrease nasal congestion and rhinorrhea and increase nasal air flow. With severe polyposis, they are less effective because of the blockage of the nasal airway, which prevents entrance of the drug. In this situation, aggressive treatment of nasal polyps helps decrease the requirement for nasal surgery. Commonly used regimens include intramuscular injection of corticosteroid, such as triamcinolone 60–100 mg in an adult or a 10–14-day course of oral prednisone, beginning with 60 mg and tapering by 5 mg daily. Once nasal polyps have been reduced in size with systemic corticosteroid therapy, intranasal corticosteroids are more likely to prevent or delay regrowth of the polyps. However, because of side effects, long-term management with systemic corticosteroids is not ideal. Often, coexistent infectious rhinosinusitis is encountered in patients. Appropriate antibiotic therapy should be used to improve the overall situation.

In the setting of marked mechanical obstruction despite aggressive medical management, simple polypectomy or FESS can be performed. Neither of these surgical procedures is curative, and the recurrence rate is high. Systemic corticosteroids are often administered preoperatively to decrease the polyp load and also to help manage asthma, which is often concomitant.

4.12.1.2 Polyposis with Aspirin Sensitivity

A subset of patients has the triad of asthma, nasal or sinus polyps, and aspirin sensitivity. The aspirin sensitivity is manifested by an exacerbation of nasal sinus symptoms or asthma (or both) with the ingestion of aspirin or other nonsteroidal anti-inflammatory medication. This condition is termed *aspirin-exacerbated respiratory disease* (AERD). These patients have a respiratory dose-dependent reaction to all nonsteroidal anti-inflammatory medications. Although the mechanism has not been clearly delineated, it appears that the blockade of cyclooxygenase results in decreased production of protective prostaglandins and increased production of inflammatory leukotrienes, resulting in nasal congestion, rhinorrhea, and bronchospasm. Only one-third of the patients have positive skin tests to aeroallergens; therefore, IgE is not thought to be important in the pathogenesis. Patients with AERD generally have more extensive sinus disease and more severe asthma than those without aspirin sensitivity (Fig. 4.5). Even without ingestion of nonsteroidal anti-inflammatory drugs, the patients have chronic nasal congestion, obstruction, anosmia, and persistent asthma.

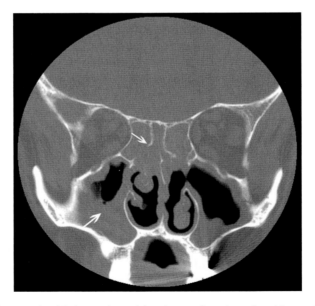

Fig. 4.5 Diffuse pansinusitis in a patient with asthma, polyposis, and aspirin sensitivity. Despite previous medial antrostomies and uncinectomies, ethmoid air cells (*top arrow*) and frontal sinuses are completely opacified bilaterally. There is diffuse membrane thickening and inflammation (*bottom arrow*) within the maxillary sinuses

Over the past 20 years, a unique treatment has been used for patients with AERD. Aspirin desensitization followed by daily aspirin treatment has been beneficial for the majority of patients in reducing the number of episodes of sinusitis, the amount of systemic corticosteroids required for symptom control, and requirements for polypectomies and sinus surgery. Improvements have also been seen in the general assessment of nasal sinus and asthma symptoms. Because respiratory symptoms are induced with aspirin desensitization, this procedure must be performed in a controlled environment with resuscitation materials available. Aspirin desensitization should be performed by a subspecialist and considered only for patients whose condition is refractory to conventional therapy.

4.12.2 Tumors

Sinus tumors are relatively rare but must be considered in the differential diagnosis of chronic rhinosinusitis. The presentations of sinus tumor vary; however, the most common presenting symptoms are *unilateral* nasal stuffiness and discharge (Fig. 4.6).

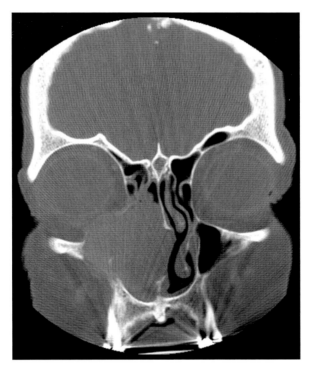

Fig. 4.6 A 71-year-old woman had an 18-month history of exclusively right-sided nasal congestion and pressure. Note the 4-cm soft-tissue mass in the right maxillary sinus and right nasal cavity, with right-to-left bowing and erosion of the nasal septum and destruction of the right orbital floor. Pathology examination showed an adenoid cystic carcinoma

Approximately one-fourth of patients have eyelid swelling, unilateral tearing, diplopia, and proptosis. With progression of the tumor, involvement of the infraorbital nerve results in numbness or paresthesia of the cheek and involvement of cranial nerves VII and VIII causes facial paralysis and unilateral deafness. Most sinus tumors emanate from the maxillary sinuses, followed by the ethmoid and frontal sinuses. Squamous cell carcinoma is the most common cell type. Other important tumors and cancers are inverting papilloma, sarcoma, and angiofibroma. Metastatic cancer to the sinuses is less common but most often associated with renal cell tumor. Furniture and nickel workers have a higher incidence of sinus carcinoma than the general population.

The key to treatment is early detection. Inverting papillomas can resemble nasal polyps but are more friable and vascular. Angiofibromas are most common in young boys. They are highly vascular tumors that bleed excessively with manipulation. Any patient with unilateral symptoms requires further examination with rhinolaryngoscopy or CT of the sinuses. Treatment depends on the cell type and extent of spread of the carcinoma. Multiple modalities, including chemotherapy, radiation, and surgery, are often required for treatment.

4.12.3   Foreign Body

Foreign bodies placed in the nose can present with symptoms of rhinosinusitis. This is found most commonly in young children, psychiatric patients, and senile patients. Common presenting symptoms include unilateral nasal blockage with nasal bleed or purulent discharge. The foreign object usually can be detected on nasal examination or with a radiographic study. Depending on the location of the object, otorhinolaryngology consultation may be required for removal.

4.12.4   Adenoidal Hypertrophy

The adenoids are lymphatic tissue located high on the posterior wall of the pharynx, superior and posterior to the tonsils. Adenoids typically stop enlarging between ages 4 and 7 years and then start decreasing in size, so they are hardly present during the teen years. Adenoidal hypertrophy is seen primarily in young children and presents with any combination of mouth breathing, halitosis, persistent runny nose or nasal congestion, ear infections, and snoring. The adenoids cannot be seen on a routine throat examination, but they are easily visualized with nasal endoscopy or a mirror placed at the back of the throat. Depending on the size of the adenoids and the clinical scenario, they may require removal. After age 1 year, the adenoids are not an important part of the immune system and removal is not associated with an increase in upper respiratory tract infections.

4.12.5   Cerebrospinal Fluid Rhinorrhea

CSF rhinorrhea is a rare cause of rhinorrhea that may follow head trauma or sinus or intracranial surgery. Nontraumatic CSF rhinorrhea due to anatomical abnormalities accounts for 10% of the cases. CSF rhinorrhea results from a defect in the anterior, middle, or posterior cranial fossa. The typical defective sites include the cribriform plate, sella turcica, and frontal and sphenoid sinuses. CSF is a clear, watery fluid that resembles the watery discharge seen in allergic and vasomotor rhinitis. A patient with CSF rhinorrhea typically presents with unilateral watery rhinorrhea that worsens when the patient bends forward and produces a sensation of postnasal drip when the patient is supine. On physical examination, the internal and external appearance of the nose is unremarkable. There is no inflammation or congestion.

Diagnosis is made by testing the nasal discharge with a glucose oxidase test strip or B2 transferrin immunofixation. A glucose measurement of more than 30 mg per 100 mL is a positive result. False positives can occur when there is contamination by lacrimal fluid, which has a high concentration of glucose. B2 transferrin is highly specific for CSF and is preferred over the glucose oxidase test. If the test result is positive, imaging studies are needed to localize the site of the leak. Neurosurgery consultation should be arranged quickly to help avoid the development of meningitis or brain abscess.

4.12.6   Septal Deviation

Deviation of the septum to one side can be congenital or induced by trauma. Unless severe, septal deviation usually does not result in pronounced symptoms unless a concomitant rhinosinusitis process is present. Septal deviation can intensify and lateralize the congestion and drainage of all the nasal sinus processes. Septal deviation can be detected on nasal physical examination. Radiographic or CT imaging and rhinolaryngoscopy can help quantitate the extent of the deviation and assess for impingement on the ostiomeatal unit. Septal deviation can be corrected surgically when the deviation is thought to significantly obstruct drainage.

4.13   Noninfectious Nonstructural Rhinitis and Rhinosinusitis

Noninfectious, nonstructural rhinosinusitis is characterized by the presence of bilateral nasal symptoms. Symptoms are limited primarily to the nose instead of the nose and sinus. Purulent drainage, sinus pressure, headache, and copious postnasal drainage are not present. The primary symptoms are bilateral nasal congestion with intermittent rhinorrhea. The primary entities in this group are vasomotor rhinitis, NARES, atrophic rhinitis, hormonal rhinitis, medication-induced rhinitis, and food-induced rhinitis.

4.13.1 Vasomotor Rhinitis

Vasomotor rhinitis is the most common form of chronic nonallergic rhinitis. It is an idiopathic condition diagnosed in the absence of allergy, polyposis, NARES, rhinosinusitis, infection, or drug exposure. For this reason, this condition is sometimes referred to as *idiopathic rhinitis*. Patients with this disorder present with chronic nasal congestion with intermittent rhinorrhea and sneezing. Vasomotor rhinitis is characterized by the presence of nasal symptoms for ≥9 months each year. The condition is often exacerbated by exposure to irritants such as smoke or dust, wind, rapid changes in temperature or atmospheric pressure, and smells. It is difficult to distinguish between perennial allergic rhinitis and vasomotor rhinitis on the basis of symptoms alone. Generally, allergic rhinitis is associated more commonly with itching, clear rhinorrhea, and eye symptoms than is vasomotor rhinitis. Vasomotor rhinitis has a later age of onset and lack of atopic comorbidities, as opposed to allergic rhinitis. *Mixed rhinitis* refers to the presence of both allergic and nonallergic rhinitis. This is thought to occur in approximately 35% of all patients with chronic rhinitis. In a study of nearly 1,000 patients with rhinitis from a variety of allergy practices, approximately 40% had pure allergic rhinitis, 25% had pure nonallergic rhinitis, and 35% had mixed rhinitis. It is important for the clinician to be aware of the possible overlap.

The pathophysiology of vasomotor rhinitis has not been clearly defined; however, this condition is thought to represent a dysfunction of the autonomic nervous system. It has been postulated that vasomotor rhinitis is more likely the result of a hypoactive sympathetic nervous system than a hyperactive parasympathetic nervous system. Other possible contributing mechanisms include an overexpression of the tachykinin response, heightened sensory nerve ending response with neuropeptide release, and epithelium abnormalities.

On physical examination, the nasal turbinates are often erythematous and boggy in appearance as opposed to a pale or bluish hue found in allergic rhinitis. Purulence is not seen unless there is concurrent infection. Nasal eosinophilia is unusual with vasomotor rhinitis.

To diagnose vasomotor rhinitis, allergic rhinitis should be ruled out with allergy skin prick testing or in vitro allergy testing. NARES can be ruled out with nasal wash cytology or nasal brushing.

Treatment of vasomotor rhinitis is not standardized, and there are considerably fewer reports on the treatment of vasomotor rhinitis than on allergic rhinitis. According to the reports available, it appears that intranasal corticosteroids help improve nasal congestion in vasomotor rhinitis. In two studies, azelastine nasal spray reduced all nasal symptoms, including congestion, as compared with placebo. Intranasal ipratropium helps improve rhinorrhea but does not appear to help congestive symptoms. No clinical trials have been performed on leukotriene antagonists or oral decongestants in this group. In clinical practice, typically little or no response is seen to oral antihistamines as compared with their effect in allergic rhinitis. Although there is no clear role for oral antihistamines in vasomotor rhinitis, patients who have sneezing as a primary symptom may have a favorable response.

Although not rigorously studied, symptomatic improvement is often seen with saline irrigations, especially when they are administered two or more times daily. An algorithm for the treatment of vasomotor rhinitis is shown in Fig. 4.7.

4.13.2 Nonallergic Rhinitis with Eosinophilia Syndrome

The presentation of this condition is similar to that of vasomotor rhinitis, with paroxysms of sneezing, profuse watery rhinorrhea, and occasional loss of the sense of smell. Nasal cytology or smear, however, shows significant eosinophilia. It is generally accepted that nasal scrapings from the nasal turbinate that show 5–25 eosinophils per high-power field is compatible with the diagnosis. Despite the eosinophilia, neither skin prick testing to allergens nor in vitro allergy testing is positive. The onset of NARES is typically later than that of allergic rhinitis or vasomotor rhinitis. Some researchers believe NARES represents an early stage of the process leading to nasal polyposis or chronic eosinophilic rhinosinusitis. Patients should be followed closely for subsequent development of polyps, aspirin sensitivity, and asthma. Although the treatment of NARES has not been studied extensively, intranasal corticosteroids are considered standard treatment.

4.13.3 Atrophic Rhinitis

Atrophic rhinitis is a syndrome of progressive atrophy of the nasal mucosa in elderly patients. The primary symptoms are chronic nasal congestion and the sensation of

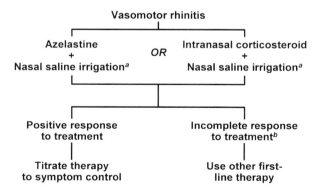

Fig. 4.7 Algorithm for treatment of vasomotor rhinitis. [a]Saline irrigation can be performed with bulb syringe, squeezable plastic bottle with nasal adaptor, Neti Pot, or a pulse irrigator combined with a nasal adaptor. Saline irrigations should be performed at least twice daily. Home saline solution can be made by dissolving 1/8 teaspoon salt in 1 cup of warm water. [b]Intranasal ipratropium can be added for rhinorrhea

an unpleasant odor. The etiology can be idiopathic, but atrophic rhinitis usually is seen in conjunction with chronic nasal inflammation or multiple nasal and sinus surgical procedures. Physical examination shows crusting and loss of nasal mucosa. In severe cases, there is loss of underlying bone. There is no effective treatment, but supportive treatment with nasal humidification may decrease symptoms.

4.13.4 Hormonal Rhinitis

The most common hormonal causes of rhinitis are pregnancy, oral contraceptives, conjugated estrogens, and hypothyroidism. During pregnancy, rhinitis symptoms, primarily congestion, begin in the second month and continue to term. This is relatively uncommon, and nonhormonal causes of rhinitis should also be assessed in a pregnant patient. Rhinitis of pregnancy abates soon after delivery. Hypothyroidism has been associated with increased nasal secretions and nasal congestion, but the evidence for an association is limited. Symptoms of hypothyroidism such as fatigue, hair thinning, doughy skin, and constipation should also be sought.

4.13.5 Medication-Induced Rhinitis

Medication-induced rhinitis can occur with various medications. It is associated most commonly with the use of intranasal over-the-counter decongestant products containing α-adrenergic agonists (i.e., oxymetazoline or phenylephrine). Use of these medications for more than 4 days induces a rebound nasal congestion. This often sets off a vicious cycle in which the patient uses more and more of the medication to decongest the nose as the normal nasal cycle becomes obliterated. Extensive use leads to hypertrophy of the nasal mucosa, called *rhinitis medicamentosa*. Rhinitis medicamentosa occurs most commonly in young and middle-aged adults of both sexes. The nasal mucosa appears inflamed and erythematous. Similar features are seen in intranasal cocaine users. The appearance of the nasal mucosa cannot be used to distinguish between rhinitis medicamentosa and other types of rhinitis. Patients note primarily marked nasal obstruction.

Although other medications can induce symptoms of nasal congestion and rhinorrhea, the symptoms generally are not as intense as with topical α-adrenergic decongestants. Antihypertensive medications associated with nasal symptoms include β-blockers, angiotensin-converting enzyme inhibitors, and α-receptor antagonists. Other medications most frequently cited include chlorpromazine, aspirin, and nonsteroidal anti-inflammatory agents.

Treatment involves discontinuation of the offending medication. Treatment of rhinitis medicamentosa can be difficult. Complete abstinence from the topical decongestant is required, and this can be uncomfortable for the patient. Topical intranasal corticosteroids appear to help relieve symptoms until the patient's normal nasal cycle returns. Normal function returns in 7–28 days.

4.13.6 Rhinitis from Food Ingestion

Ingested food allergens rarely produce isolated IgE-mediated rhinitis without other signs of an allergic reaction such as urticaria, angioedema, bronchospasm, or gastrointestinal symptoms. If other signs are also present, allergen testing to foods based on the patient's history may be helpful. However, in the absence of systemic symptoms, food allergy testing is not indicated. Gustatory rhinitis refers to watery rhinorrhea that occurs immediately after the ingestion of foods, particularly spicy foods. This is vagally mediated and responds to treatment with intranasal ipratroprium.

4.14 Clinical Vignettes

4.14.1 Vignette 1

A 50-year-old woman reports she has had nasal symptoms over the last 10 years. The symptoms consist primarily of constant nasal congestion and the sensation that she is not able to breathe well out of her nose. The symptoms are bilateral. She has also noticed a "nasal voice." She states that she does not have chronic rhinorrhea, facial pain, fever, or purulent discharge, but she has had sinus infections twice a year described as episodes of purulent discharge and low-grade fever that responded to antibiotic treatment. She notes postnasal drainage, sometimes with thick, white sputum. Her sense of smell is decreased. Her symptoms seemed to start after her basement was flooded when the garden hose was inadvertently left on. After the flooding, sheetrock was removed from the basement, the furnace deckboard was cleared, and the entire basement was bleached professionally. It was believed that all water-damaged areas and all potential mold growth had been treated. A dehumidifier continues to be used in the basement in the summer, but she rarely goes into the basement. She does not have any pets, and she does not work outside the home. Her symptoms are the same throughout the year, without seasonal variation.

She says she does not have a history of asthma or other respiratory disease. She has not had other infections. She has never had nasal or sinus surgery. She is otherwise healthy except for a history of hypertension, for which Toprol (metoprolol) is currently prescribed. She has been taking this medication for 3 years.

Treatment with H_1 blockers and intranasal corticosteroids has been tried intermittently without any significant relief. She did have some benefit from a combination H_1 blocker–decongestant medication, but this increased her blood pressure. She says that for the past few months she has used a topical decongestant, oxymetazoline, 2–4 times daily. She has received two injections of corticosteroid in the past year, which produced significant improvement for approximately 6 weeks on both occasions.

Physical examination revealed normal vital signs. The eye examination was normal. Anterior rhinoscopy showed mildly erythematous nasal mucosa with scant clear and whitish discharge. The middle turbinates were congested bilaterally. Airflow was

diminished but present bilaterally. No purulence was noted, and no polyps were identified. The throat, neck, and lung examinations were unremarkable.

Comment: The patient describes chronic perennial symptoms of nasal congestion,
decreased nasal airflow, nasal voice, and decreased sense of smell, with infections
twice a year. In approximately half the cases of this type of situation, allergens have
a role. On the basis of her environmental history, the main considerations would be
dust mites and fungi. It appears her house was thoroughly cleaned after the flooding; however, the potential for mold growth remains. With mold and dust mite sensitivities, there generally is no significant seasonal variation.

Other factors include the recent use of topical decongestants and the addition of
the β-blockers. In both instances, her symptoms preceded the use of these medications. Certainly, the current use of the topical decongestant can contribute to her
symptoms. Although β-blockers can cause rhinitis symptoms, they do so less commonly than topical decongestants.

At this point, allergy skin prick testing is indicated to determine if there is an
underlying allergic diasthesis.

Further evaluation was performed with allergen skin prick testing to the
Dermatophagoides farinae and *D. pteronyssinus* (dust mites) and the common
indoor and outdoor molds. The skin tests were entirely negative, with a normal
histamine control.

Comment: The negative skin tests make an IgE-mediated cause of her nasal and sinus
symptoms unlikely. Further review of her symptoms, particularly the "nasal voice,"
decreased sense of smell, and decreased nasal airflow, make it hard to distinguish
between purely nasal involvement and nose and sinus involvement. Her current symptoms and previous lack of improvement with intranasal corticosteroid therapy raise
suspicion about both nasal and sinus involvement. Further evaluation with either rhinoscopy or coronal CT of the sinuses would help classify this as an infectious/inflam-
matory rhinosinusitis or a noninfectious, nonstructural rhinitis or rhinosinusitis.

Further evaluation was performed with coronal sinus CT, which showed moderate inflammation of both the maxillary and ethmoid sinuses, with only mild inflammation of the frontal and sphenoid sinuses. The ostiomeatal unit was opacified on
the left side.

Comment: The CT scan showed significant inflammation throughout the sinuses.
This likely explains her lack of improvement with intranasal corticosteroids alone.
Her history did not describe symptoms usually associated with bacterial infection,
such as persistent purulent discharge, sinus tenderness, cough, or fever. The role of
bacterial infection in this type of situation is not well known. Fungal involvement
is even more difficult to discern. Clearly, chronic allergic fungal rhinosinusitis is
not the cause because skin testing to the molds was negative. CT findings are not
consistent with mycetoma. The patient's clinical presentation was not consistent
with invasive fulminant fungal infection. Polyps were not seen on CT scan, and she
said she did not have a history of aspirin sensitivity. Because she is otherwise well,
immunodeficiency or systemic disease seems unlikely. The other major consideration

is chronic eosinophilic fungal or hyperplastic rhinosinusitis. Often, a peripheral eosinophil count is increased in these patients, but the sensitivity or specificity is not known. Nasal cytology can also be helpful.

An eosinophil count was obtained. It was 0.7×10^9 L^{-1}, which is slightly above the normal range (0.05–0.5×10^9 L^{-1}). Nasal cytology showed a predominance of eosinophils.

Comment: Although the eosinophil count helps confirm the likely underlying etiology, a normal count would not have ruled out the working diagnosis. Management of these patients is difficult, with no clear consensus about overall treatment. At this time, consideration could be given to an otorhinolaryngologic consultation for consideration of surgery to open the ostiomeatal unit, to remove inflammation from the sinuses, and to obtain a pathology specimen to study the inflammation. In chronic eosinophilic fungal or hyperplastic rhinosinusitis, the disease has a high rate of recurrence after surgery, similar to polyposis. Another option is aggressive medical management consisting of systemic corticosteroids, an empiric 21-day course of antibiotics, intranasal corticosteroids, and nasal irrigations with antifungal solution and normal or hypertonic saline.

The patient did not elect to have a surgical procedure but wanted to try medical management. The topical decongestant was discontinued. The patient received an intramuscular injection of 60 mg triamcinolone and was placed on a regimen of Levaquin (levofloxacin) 500 mg per day for 21 days, intranasal mometasone 2 squirts in each nostril daily, nasal irrigation with itraconazole (100 mg per 1 L, 20 mL each nostril) daily, and nasal irrigation with normal saline twice daily.

Comment: This type of regimen has not been subject to controlled trials, but noncontrolled trials of antifungal irrigation have shown promise for this difficult disorder. The patient should be followed closely to assess clinical and CT improvement. Once symptoms are controlled, the medication regimen should be tailored to the symptoms.

4.14.2 Vignette 2

A 19-year-old man presents with a 2-year history of perennial symptoms of daily nasal congestion and intermittent mild rhinorrhea, itchy nose, and sneezing. The symptoms are bilateral. He states that he does not have any notable eye or throat symptoms, sinus infections, sinus pain, loss of sense of smell, or history of nasal or sinus surgery. There is no prominent seasonality to his symptoms. For treatment, he has tried over-the-counter antihistamine-decongestant combination medications on occasion, with some symptom relief, but he has never used them regularly. He does not use any nasal sprays.

Comment: His symptoms are consistent with chronic rhinitis without typical sinus symptoms. There do not appear to be any red flags such as unilateral symptoms, loss of sense of smell, recalcitrant severe disease, or recurrent infections that would raise suspicion for a structural problem or underlying systemic disease. At this point, the main considerations would be allergic rhinitis, vasomotor rhinitis, or NARES. His history is not suggestive of medication-induced rhinitis, atrophic rhinitis, or hormonal- or food-induced rhinitis. Further information in regard to his home and occupational environment would be helpful.

The patient is a college student. During the school year, he lives in a ground-level apartment with two roommates. The apartment is in an old building and is carpeted throughout except for the kitchen. He is not aware of any water damage. There are no animals in the apartment. He does not get exposure to animals at other people's homes. In addition to going to school, he works at the local supermarket, primarily unloading inventory and stocking shelves. When discussing this, he recalls that his symptoms worsen when he is opening boxes in the storage area, but the symptoms occur whether he is at home, work, or school.

Comment: The patient does not describe any markedly unusual type exposures. Worsening of symptoms at work in the storage area can be due to dust mites, mold, or nonspecific irritants in the air. To make a diagnosis, further evaluation with skin testing would be helpful.

Skin testing was performed. Positive responses were noted to *D. pteronyssinus* and *D. farinae* mites. Skin testing was negative to molds, cat, and dog.

Comment: The positive skin tests are diagnostic for allergic rhinitis. This is helpful information in formulating an effective management strategy. The first rule in allergic disease is allergen avoidance. In this situation, dust mite avoidance measures should be used. At home, dust mite recommendations would include use of mite-impermeable encasements for the bed mattress and pillow and washing of sheets and pillowcases in hot water weekly. In addition, a room HEPA air filtration unit may help decrease dust mite exposure. At work, consideration could be given to wearing a mask when opening boxes in the storage area to help decrease inhaled dust and the corresponding dust mites. From a medication standpoint, it is known that antihistamines are more effective in allergic rhinitis than in vasomotor rhinitis or NARES. They are first-line treatment for mild intermittent allergic rhinitis and are often used as an adjunct for persistent allergic rhinitis. Therefore, the use of antihistamines can be considered for treatment. In this case, intranasal corticosteroids would be a good option because of the daily symptoms of nasal congestion. Immunotherapy is another option but would not likely be considered before a medication trial.

The patient was counseled on environmental allergen control and started receiving daily intranasal corticosteroid therapy. After 1 month, he noticed some improvement in his daily nasal congestion, but he continued to be bothered by intermittent rhinorrhea, nasal itch, and sneezing, particularly at work. He had not started the environmental control measures.

Comment: Although improved, he continues to have symptoms. On the basis of his current symptoms, the addition of a second-generation daily antihistamine should be helpful. Antihistamines are most effective for nasal itch, sneezing, and mild rhinorrhea. The patient was again encouraged to implement environmental measures.

Fexofenadine 180 mg once daily was added to treatment with intranasal corticosteroid. The patient obtained mite encasements for his mattress and pillows and washed his sheets and pillow case once a week but was not always compliant with wearing a mask at work. However, he did make an effort to avoid particularly dusty areas at work. He felt his symptoms were well controlled with the environmental measures used and the addition of the fexofenadine.

Comment: The patient made an effort to lessen his daily environmental exposures, and his knowledge of dust mite allergy helped him to avoid large exposures. He has responded to treatment with intranasal corticosteroid and antihistamine and has implemented environmental measures.

4.14.3   Vignette 3

An 11-year-old girl presents during the spring season with watery, itchy eyes; bilateral nasal congestion; sneezing; runny nose; and nasal itch of 3-weeks duration. The symptoms have been occurring daily and have interfered with her participation in track. She feels miserable when outdoors and has had difficulty breathing through her nose. These symptoms have also interfered with her sleep. She states that she does not have shortness of breath, wheeze, or cough. She also states that she does not have any fever, facial pain, or purulent nasal discharge. She had similar, but milder, symptoms the previous spring and fall. The previous spring and fall, her symptoms responded partially to treatment with an over-the-counter antihistamine. She has not been taking medication this year.

Comment: Her symptoms certainly suggest moderate-severe persistent allergic rhinitis. She does not have symptoms suggesting asthma or rhinosinusitis accompanying this. It is important to inquire about asthma symptoms because bronchial involvement is frequently found. This is her second season with symptoms in the spring. At this point, it would be helpful to delve further into her symptoms during the rest of the year and obtain information about her home environment.

She lives in 15-year-old two-story house on a wooded 1-acre lot. She has lived there her entire life. She lives with her parents and a younger sister age 7 years. They do not have any pets at home and the parents are nonsmokers. Her bedroom is on the top floor of the house. The family leaves the bedroom windows open at night because they like the night air and only rarely use air conditioning. Her symptoms are confined strictly to 2 months in the spring and 2 months in the fall. During the rest of the year, she is symptom free.

Comment: Her home environment history does not suggest other provocateurs such as pets or cigarette smoke exposure. However, she does get significant exposure to seasonal allergens, as does nearly everyone. Her exposure is increased by having the bedroom windows open. Her lack of symptoms at other times of the year makes any other cause of nonallergic rhinitis unlikely.

Physical examination findings of the eyes included mild hyperemia of the palpebral conjunctiva bilaterally. Her nasal examination showed nearly complete nasal occlusion bilaterally because of pale, boggy congestion of the middle turbinates. Clear discharge surrounded the turbinates. No polyps were visible. Throat examination did not show any postnasal drainage. Her lungs were completely clear to auscultation bilaterally.

Comment: The physical examination findings are consistent with allergic rhinitis. The timing of the symptoms suggests tree pollen sensitivity in the spring and weed pollen sensitivity in the fall. Allergen skin prick testing could be performed to confirm this. Because she does not have symptoms at any other time of year and has not had a good trial of medical therapy, allergen skin prick testing is not critical at this point unless specific allergen immunotherapy is being considered. The various treatment options should be reviewed with the patient and parents.

The patient and parents were concerned about the amount of difficulty the allergic rhinitis was causing her. She was having difficulty participating in track and sleeping at night, and she generally felt miserable. The parents were particularly interested if there were any treatments that could help her quickly.

Comment: All treatment options should be reviewed with the patient and parents. Allergen avoidance measurements should be reviewed. However, it is nearly impossible to avoid seasonal tree and weed pollens. Measures that could help include (1) immediately shower upon entering the house for the evening after spending time outdoors, (2) keep the windows of the house closed and use air conditioning during the troublesome months, and (3) try to exercise outdoors in the morning before the main pollen dispersal. From the medication standpoint, a short course of prednisone could be used 20–40 mg per day for 3–5 days, for her severe signs and symptoms. This would help decrease her marked nasal congestion and other symptoms of allergic rhinitis. In the meantime, treatment with a nasal corticosteroid and nonsedating antihistamine should be started to help control the symptoms through the allergy season. Immunotherapy should be considered if her symptoms do not respond well to treatment, she does not tolerate treatment, she continues to require systemic corticosteroids, or she wants immunotherapy.

4.14.4 Vignette 4

A 71-year-old woman presents with an 18-month history of nasal congestion and sinus pressure that is right sided. She says she does not have any itchiness of the eyes, nasal itchiness, sneezing, or purulent rhinorrhea. She occasionally notes some clear discharge, just from the right side. Initially, she received treatment with an antibiotic and nonsedating antihistamine, but without any change in her symptoms. Because of the persistence of symptoms, she subsequently received treatment with three more courses of antibiotics, another nonsedating antihistamine, and intranasal corticosteroids. She reports that she was compliant with these medications but had no improvement. She stated that she did not use any topical decongestant medication. She has no history of previous sinus surgery or significant nasal injury. No further studies, such as coronal CT of the sinuses or rhinoscopy, had been performed. She said she did not have a history of asthma or aspirin sensitivity.

Comment: The most important part of this history is the presence of chronic one-sided symptoms. Whenever chronic nasal or sinus symptoms are one sided, the structural causes need to be evaluated. In addition, she had no response to numerous treatments with antibiotics, antihistamines, and intranasal corticosteroids, raising further concern about the underlying process. The physical examination should be helpful to assess airflow of the nose and any abnormalities of the head and neck.

Findings on physical examination of the eyes and ears were normal. Nasal examination showed a patent left nasal airway. A large, pinkish variegated, vascular, soft, obstructing mass was noted in the right nasal airway. The appearance was not consistent with a nasal polyp, which has a white, opaque nonvascular appearance. The throat was clear. The neck examination did not disclose any masses or adenopathy.

Comment: The patient has an obstructing mass in the right nasal airway. This emphasizes the importance of searching for a structural cause when a patient has one-sided symptoms. In the situation in which nothing is found on nasal examination in the office, further evaluation should be performed with coronal sinus CT or rhinoscopy. In this patient, further evaluation of the mass would include coronal sinus CT, otolaryngologic evaluation, and staging.

Sinus CT was performed (see Fig. 4.6). A biopsy specimen from the lesion showed adenoid cystic carcinoma. She underwent right lateral rhinotomy, medial maxillectomy, and debulking of the tumor along the medial and inferior orbit. Tumor was noted to be coming through the ethmoid area onto the periorbita and to involve the lacrimal sac and globe. The maxillary sinus was filled with tumor except for the posterolateral and inferior aspects of the bony maxilla. Gross total removal of the tumor within the maxillary and ethmoid sinuses was accomplished. Although the periorbita appeared normal, biopsy specimens were positive for tumor. Further treatment included radiation and chemotherapy. The goal of treatment was tumor control to prevent neurologic sequelae.

Comment: Because of the length of time between symptom onset and diagnosis, there had been significant spread of the tumor. Although the majority of sinus tumors are diagnosed within 8 months after the onset of symptoms, approximately 20% are diagnosed >1 year after symptom onset. Unilateral nasal stuffiness and discharge is the most common presentation of nasal or sinus tumor, occurring in approximately 50–85% of patients. Other symptoms that usually indicate more widespread disease include tooth pain, uncomfortable dentures, unilateral tearing, proptosis, and diplopia.

4.14.5   Vignette 5

A 52-year-old man presents with a 15-year history of nasal congestion. The bilateral nasal congestion is present every day, and there is no seasonal variation. He does not have any eye symptoms with this. He states that he does not have other significant nasal symptoms; there is no itchiness or sneezing. However, he has intermittent clear rhinorrhea. His sense of smell is intact. He has not had sinus pressure or pain or a history of acute sinus infection. He does not have a history of nasal or sinus surgery or facial trauma. He says he does not have any cough, wheeze, or shortness of breath.

The symptoms are troubling to the patient, and he is tired of always having a "stuffy nose." He notes that the congestion improves while exercising, then returns after he exercises. He does think that strong odors, wind, and smoke exposure make his symptoms worse and induce some rhinorrhea.

Previous evaluation included coronal CT of the sinuses 2 years ago that was normal. At that time, allergen skin prick testing to pertinent perennial and seasonal aeroallergens was negative. He has never received a prolonged course of treatment. He has been prescribed nonsedating antihistamines and intranasal corticosteroids, which he has taken at various times for up to 2 or 3 weeks without having significant improvement in his symptoms. He thinks that his congestion has been worse over the past year.

Comment: The patient describes symptoms of chronic rhinitis. The lack of eye symptoms, nasal itch, and sneeze and previous negative results on allergy testing make allergic rhinitis unlikely. There does not seem to be a significant sinus component because of the normal sense of smell, lack of sinus infections, and lack of postnasal drainage. His symptoms are most consistent with nonstructural rhinitis. The primary differential diagnosis includes vasomotor rhinitis, NARES, and medication-induced rhinitis. Additional information should be obtained about his medications, especially with his symptoms worsening in the last year.

His medication list was reviewed. Treatment with atorvastatin (Lipitor) and valsartan (Diovan) was started approximately 2 years ago for hyperlipidemia and hypertension. He said he was not taking any other medications.

Comment: Atorvastatin and valsartan are not associated with rhinitis. Further evaluation should include physical examination and nasal scraping for eosinophils.

Physical examination of the nose showed large, erythematous, and boggy nasal turbinates bilaterally. The septum was midline. Airflow was symmetric bilaterally. There were no polyps or secretions. After the examination, the patient pulled oxymetazoline (Vicks nasal spray) from his pocket and immediately took 2 sprays.

Comment: This was a rather unusual turn of events. The patient should be questioned further about the use of the nasal spray.

The patient did not consider the nasal spray a medication and did not list it with his medications because he obtained it without a prescription. He states that he has been using the nasal spray 3–4 times daily for the past 8 months and that if he went without it for more than half a day, the nasal congestion became markedly worse.

Comment: The patient's history and examination are consistent with rhinitis medicamentosa due to the nasal decongestant spray. Patients often do not mention over-the-counter products on their list of medications. They need to be asked directly whether they are using any over-the-counter medications or nasal sprays. The first goal in the treatment of rhinitis medicamentosa is the immediate discontinuation of the topical decongestant. Because abrupt cessation can result in increased congestion, various treatment programs have been suggested. Intranasal corticosteroids are the most effective. If this is not effective, a brief 5–days burst of systemic corticosteroid can be instituted. Although rhinitis medicamentosa contributed to the patient's worsening symptoms over the last year, the underlying cause of his nasal congestion needs to be addressed. On the basis of his history and physical examination findings, vasomotor rhinitis or NARES is most likely. A nasal cytology examination can distinguish between the two conditions.

A nasal smear was performed, and no eosinophils were identified.

Comment: Vasomotor rhinitis is the most likely underlying condition. Treatment should be commenced with an intranasal corticosteroid (which also treats the rhinitis medicamentosa) and twice daily nasal saline irrigations. Because both rhinitis medicamentosa and vasomotor rhinitis are being treated, it may take 4–6 weeks before significant improvement is noted.

The patient returned in 6 weeks with notable improvement. After an initial increase in nasal congestion after discontinuing the topical nasal decongestant, his symptoms improved. Currently, he only notes a minimum of symptoms using the intranasal corticosteroid and saline irrigations (1 cup each nostril twice daily) via a plastic bottle with nasal adaptor.

Comment: The patient has had marked improvement. He can adjust the amount of nasal saline irrigations and intranasal corticosteroid needed to control symptoms.

Suggested Reading

Bernstein, D. I. (2002) Nasal polyposis, sinusitis, and nonallergic rhinitis. In: Grammer, L. C., Greenberger, P. A., eds. Patterson's Allergic Diseases, 6th ed. Philadelphia: Lippincott Williams and Wilkins. pp. 403–414

Casale, T. B., Blaiss, M. S., Gelfand, E., et al. (2003) First do no harm: managing antihistamine impairment in patients with allergic rhinitis. J. Allergy Clin. Immunol. 111, S835–S842

Greiner, A. N. and Meltzer, E. D. (2006) Pharmacologic rationale for treating allergic and nonallergic rhinitis. *J. Allergy Clin. Immunol.* 118, 985–996

Moller, C., Dreborg, S., Ferdousi, H. A., et al. (2002) Pollen immunotherapy reduces the development of asthma in children with seasonal rhinoconjunctivitis (the PAT-study). J. Allergy Clin. Immunol. 109, 251–256

Pajno, G. B., Barberio, G., De Luca, F., Morabito, L., and Parmiani, S. (2001) Prevention of new sensitizations in asthmatic children monosensitized to house dust mite by specific immunotherapy: a six-year follow-up study. Clin. Exp. Allergy 31, 1392–1397

Piccirillo, J. F. (2004) Clinical practice: acute bacterial sinusitis. N. Engl. J. Med. 351, 902–910

Plaut, M. and Valentine, M. D. (2005) Clinical practice: allergic rhinitis. N. Engl. J. Med. 353, 1934–1944

Sasama, J., Sherris, D. A., Shin, S. H., Kephart, G. M., Kern, E. B., and Ponikau, J. U. (2005) New paradigm for the roles of fungi and eosinophils in chronic rhinosinusitis. Curr. Opin. Otolaryngol. Head Neck Surg. 13, 2–8

Schubert, M. S. (2000) Medical treatment of allergic fungal sinusitis. Ann. Allergy Asthma Immunol. 85, 90–97

Settipane, R. A. and Lieberman, P. (2001) Update on nonallergic rhinitis. Ann. Allergy Asthma Immunol. 86, 494–507

Shehata, M. A. (1996) Atrophic rhinitis. Am. J. Otolaryngol. 17, 81–86

Simons, F. E. (2004) Advances in H1-antihistamines. N. Engl. J. Med. 351, 2203–2217

Slavin, R. G., Spector, S. L., Bernstein, I. L., Joint Task Force on Practice Parameters, American Academy of Allergy, Asthma and Immunology; American College of Allergy, Asthma and Immunology; Joint Council of Allergy, Asthma and Immunology. (2005) The diagnosis and management of sinusitis: a practice parameter update. J. Allergy Clin. Immunol. 116(Suppl. 1), S13–S47

Zlab, M. K., Moore, G. F., Daly, D. T., and Yonkers, A. J. (1992) Cerebrospinal fluid rhinorrhea: a review of the literature. Ear Nose Throat J. 71, 314–317

Chapter 5
Allergic Eye Disease

Abbreviation IL: interleukin

5.1 Overview

Allergic conjunctivitis occurs in approximately 20% of the population worldwide, and prescription costs for ocular allergy products in the United States cost almost $200 million a year, not including the vast cost of over-the-counter products. The eye may be the only organ that is involved in an allergic reaction or the eye can be involved in conjunction with associated allergic disorders, including rhinitis, sinusitis, asthma, and eczema. Patients may not report eye symptoms spontaneously and often medicate with over-the-counter eye drops. It is imperative for practitioners to inquire specifically about eye symptoms and use of eye drops to help optimize care, especially when treating patients who have other allergic conditions.

There are five basic types of allergic and allergic-like ocular diseases. Each type has different historical presentations, symptoms, and signs. These diseases are seasonal allergic conjunctivitis, perennial allergic conjunctivitis, vernal keratoconjunctivitis, atopic keratoconjunctivitis, and giant papillary conjunctivitis. Differentiation of these is important for proper management and prevention of vision loss, which can complicate vernal keratoconjunctivitis and atopic keratoconjunctivitis. In addition to allergic eye diseases, "red eye" may include viral and bacterial conjunctivitis, chlamydial conjunctivitis, herpes simplex keratitis, contact dermatoconjunctivitis, blepharoconjunctivitis, and dry eye syndrome. These entities are also considered in this chapter because they can be confused with allergic eye diseases or complicate allergic eye disease.

5.2 Basic Eye Anatomy

In the evaluation of conjunctivitis, knowledge of basic eye anatomy is critical to correctly describe findings. The following anatomical terms are helpful for discussion of various eye diseases (Fig. 5.1):

G.W. Volcheck, *Clinical Allergy: Diagnosis and Management*
DOI: 10.1007/978-1-59745-315-8_5, © 2009 Mayo Foundation for Medical
Education and Research

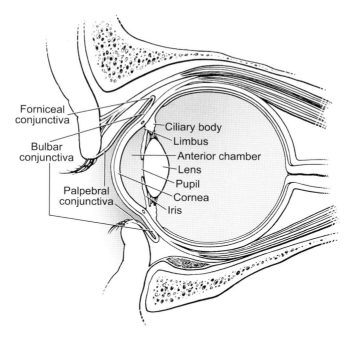

Fig. 5.1 Basic anatomy of the eye

1. Conjunctiva: thin, transparent tissue that lines the inner surfaces of the eyelids and folds back to cover the anterior surface of the eyeball, except for the cornea
2. Palpebral conjunctiva: the conjunctiva on the innerside of the eyelids
3. Bulbar conjunctiva: the conjunctiva covering the anterior sclera of the eyeball, "the white of the eye"
4. Forniceal conjunctiva: loose redundant conjunctiva that swells easily and is at the junction of the palpebral and bulbar conjunctivae
5. Limbus: the corneal–scleral junction
6. Cornea: transparent, dome-shaped window covering the anterior aspect of the eye
7. Sclera: with the cornea, it forms the rigid outer covering of the eye. It is fibrous and whitish to opaque

It is important to examine the skin around the eye, the eyelids, upper and lower palpebral and bulbar conjunctivae, limbus, and cornea. The skin around the eye is examined to assess for the presence of dermatitis (primarily atopic or contact) or angioedema. The eyelids, including the eyelashes, should be inspected for the presence of swelling or discharge. The conjunctiva should be examined for reddening, secretion, thickening, papillae, or scars. To examine the lower palpebral conjunctiva, the lower lid should be everted. This can be accomplished by having the patient look up while the examiner pulls the lower eyelid

downward, exposing the lower palpebral and bulbar conjunctiva. To examine the upper palpebral and bulbar conjunctiva, the upper eyelid is everted. This is performed by having the patient look down while the examiner places a swab on the upper eyelid and grasps the eyelashes of the upper eyelid between the thumb and forefinger, applies slight traction, and then everts the eyelid, using the swab as a fulcrum. The limbus should be assessed for ciliary flush. The cornea is examined with a pointed light source. The cornea should be smooth, clear, and reflective. Sensitivity to light, the pupillary response, and the presence of opacities should be assessed.

5.3   Approach to the Patient

The broad spectrum of the clinical signs and symptoms of allergic conjunctivitis can make the diagnosis difficult. First, when approaching a patient with "red eye," the practitioner should exclude diseases that can result in acute loss of vision or that warrant emergent treatment. Although many eye diseases may warrant emergent treatment, those that may bear some resemblance to the allergic and allergic-like ocular diseases include infectious keratitis, iritis, and acute angle-closure glaucoma. These diseases are differentiated from the allergic and allergic-like eye diseases by the presence of decreased visual acuity, pain, and photophobia. Patients with infectious keratitis are likely to have trouble keeping the eye open, suggesting an active corneal process. On penlight examination, the cornea is often opaque and the pupil is pinpoint. A white spot or opacity on the cornea suggests bacterial keratitis. This usually can be seen with or without the aid of fluoroscein. Angle-closure glaucoma causes marked distress to the patient, who complains of headache and malaise. With increasing intraocular pressure, nausea and vomiting may develop. The pain is typically a dull pain that often is described as a headache more than eye pain. Although the patients are photophobic, they do not complain of a foreign body sensation, as do those with infectious keratitis. Typically, the pupil is dilated. Iritis, the most frequent form of uveitis, causes dull pain in the eye or forehead, accompanied by impaired vision, photophobia, and excessive tearing. The perilimbal vessels may appear blue and red. Often, a reactive miosis is present. Another major physical examination finding in infectious keratitis, iritis, and angle-closure glaucoma is the pattern of eye redness. When ciliary flush occurs in these conditions, erythema is most marked at the limbus and then diminishes toward the periphery. In contrast, on physical examination of a patient with an allergic eye condition, the bulbar conjunctival erythema is more pronounced in the periphery and decreases as it approaches the cornea. A classic ciliary flush is not common; therefore, its absence does not rule out infectious keratitis, iritis, or angle-closure glaucoma. In general, allergic conditions do not present with a direct decrease in visual acuity (although perhaps indirectly because of copious discharge), photophobia, or pain.

After the practitioner has determined that the patient does not have an acutely threatening eye disease, the second step is to determine if the conjunctivitis is allergic or nonallergic. A few key historical questions can be extremely helpful in this regard:

1. Does the eye itch? It is important that the patient distinguish between itching and other sensations such as burning, grittiness, or dryness, which may be confused with itch. If itch is truly present, it points to an allergic cause. All the allergic eye conditions have itch as a prominent symptom; nonallergic eye conditions typically do not have itch.
2. Are other allergic conditions present? Although not required, the concomitant presence of rhinitis or asthma increases the likelihood of an allergic conjunctivitis. The presence of atopic dermatitis increases the likelihood of atopic keratoconjunctivitis.
3. What type of discharge is present? A clear, thin, watery discharge is typical of allergic rhinitis. This type of discharge can also be seen in viral conjunctivitis.

Table 5.1 Signs and symptoms of conjunctival inflammatory eye disease

	Pruritus	Gritty sensation	Photo-phobia	Visual acuity	Discharge	Cardinal feature
Allergic conjunctivitis	+	±	−	Nl	Watery/ mucoid	Pruritus, concomitant rhinitis symptoms
Vernal conjunctivitis	++	±	−	Nl	Stringy/ mucoid	Large upper palpebral conjunctival papillae
Atopic keratoconjunctivitis	+++	±	±	Nl	Stringy/ mucoid	Atopic dermatitis
Giant papillary conjunctivitis	++	+	−	Nl	Watery/ mucoid	Contact lens wearer
Viral conjunctivitis	−	+	−	Nl	Watery/ mucoid	None/concomitant URI symptoms
Bacterial conjunctivitis	−	+	±	Nl	Mucoid/ purulent	Persistent purulent discharge
Chlamydial conjunctivitis	−	+	±	Nl/↓	Mucoid/ purulent	Concurrent urogenital infection
Herpes simplex keratitis	−	+	+	Nl/↓	Mucoid	Branching corneal opacity
Contact dermatoconjunctivitis	+	−	−	Nl	Mucoid	Eyelid involvement
Blepharoconjunctivitis	±	++	−	Nl/↓	Mucoid	Lid margin inflammation
Dry eye syndrome	−	+++	±	Nl/↓	Mucoid	Decreased tearing

Nl normal; *URI* upper respiratory tract infection

A mucoid discharge is typical of vernal conjunctivitis. A purulent discharge suggests a bacterial cause.

4. What type, if any, of lid involvement is there? Dermatitic lid involvement is associated with atopic dermatitis, contact dermatitis, or other primary skin condition. The conjunctiva itself may or may not be affected. If the conjunctiva is also involved, atopic keratoconjunctivitis and contact dermatoconjunctivitis are primary considerations. Swelling of the eyelid, without a dermatitic component, in the presence of pruritic conjunctivitis is seen primarily in allergic conjunctivitis. Therefore, it is important to note the type and extent of involvement of the areas surrounding the eyes.

These questions help determine the presence or absence of a primary allergic eye process. In this chapter, the focus is on the differential diagnosis of the inflamed eye, with the emphasis on the spectrum of the five major allergic and allergic-like eye diseases and the eye disorders with which they can be confused (Table 5.1).

5.4   Allergic and Allergic-Like Eye Disease

5.4.1   Seasonal Allergic Conjunctivitis

5.4.1.1   Pathophysiology

Seasonal allergic conjunctivitis is the most common form of allergic conjunctivitis and accounts for about 50% of all cases seen. It is a bilateral, self-limited conjunctival inflammatory process. Because the eye is among the first organs to encounter environmental allergens, sensitivity to airborne allergens; to tree, grass, and weed pollens; and to fungal spores results in ocular inflammation triggered by IgE-mediated mast cell activation. As in allergic rhinitis, mast cells release histamine, kinins, leukotrienes, and prostaglandins that produce symptoms typical of allergic conjunctivitis. Also, the release of cytokines, chemokines, and chemoattractants recruit inflammatory cells into the conjunctiva, increasing the inflammation. Although allergic conjunctivitis has been less studied than allergic rhinitis, patients with allergic conjunctivitis have increased amounts of total IgE, allergen-specific IgE, histamine, tryptase, Th2 cytokines, and interleukin (IL)-4 and IL-5 in their tears. Eosinophils are present in ocular scrapings and are the predominant inflammatory cell. It appears they are recruited to the conjunctiva as part of the late phase reaction, mimicking allergic rhinitis.

5.4.1.2   Clinical Presentation

The typical symptoms of seasonal allergic conjunctivitis are itch, tearing, redness, and burning of the eyes. The symptoms are almost always bilateral and follow a typical seasonal pattern of exposure to tree, grass, and weed pollens and fungal spores, as outlined in allergic rhinitis (see Chap. 4). Patients usually have concomitant symptoms of allergic rhinitis. The ratio of the presence of allergic rhinitis symptoms alone to those of allergic rhinitis and conjunctivitis is approximately 5:3. There is not always a clear-cut correlation between the severity of the allergic eye symptoms and the allergic rhinitis symptoms, and the eye symptoms may be more prominent. However, complete absence of any symptoms of rhinitis casts doubt on the diagnosis of allergic conjunctivitis.

Physical examination findings include diffuse injection involving the palpebral and bulbar conjunctivae (Fig. 5.2). Erythema of the bulbar conjunctiva is more pronounced in the periphery, as opposed to centrally around the cornea. The conjunctiva may be edematous and have a mushy appearance. With severe symptoms, the lid can swell. A watery discharge can be seen in the eye; there is no purulent discharge. There is no corneal involvement.

5.4.1.3 Testing

Laboratory testing for the allergic component of allergic conjunctivitis is performed with skin prick tests or in vitro tests to the suspected airborne allergens. The details for this are outlined in Chap. 4. The conjunctival surface can be scraped for eosinophils, but this is not often performed. In patients without eye disease, no eosinophils are present. The presence of eosinophils is associated with allergic eye disease; the greater the number of eosinophils, the more severe and longer standing the ocular allergy. The absence of eosinophils on the scraping does not rule out an allergic process.

5.4.1.4 Treatment

As with allergic rhinitis, the treatment of allergic conjunctivitis consists of allergen avoidance, medications for symptom control, and immunotherapy. Allergen avoidance

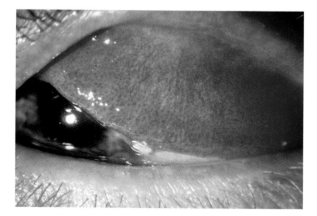

Fig. 5.2 Chronic allergic conjunctivitis. With repeated exposure, the palpebral conjunctiva can change from pale pink to deep red, making it difficult to differentiate from other inflammatory causes

is difficult for seasonal allergens. To reduce exposure to tree, grass, and weed pollens and to fungal spores, patients should be instructed to keep windows closed at home, particularly bedroom windows, during the pollen season. Also, taking a shower and washing the hair and changing clothes on entering the home after being outdoors helps decrease indoor exposure to seasonal pollens. Outdoor activities should be performed in the early morning before maximal pollen dispersion. Knowledge of the seasonal pattern of the allergen is helpful so outdoor activities and vacations can be scheduled at a time when the specific allergen pollen count traditionally is lower.

5.4.1.5 Medications

A plethora of medications are available for the treatment of seasonal allergic conjunctivitis. Available treatments include over-the-counter preparations such as artificial tears, topical vasoconstrictors, topical combination antihistamine-vasoconstrictor preparations, and topical mast cell stabilizers. Prescription medications include topical antihistamines, topical mast cell stabilizers, topical combination antihistamine–mast cell stabilizers, topical nonsteroidal anti-inflammatory medication, and topical corticosteroids (Table 5.2).

Table 5.2 Common agents used in the treatment of allergic eye disease

Classification	Drug (trade name)	Age: dosage
Vasoconstrictors	Tetrahydrozoline (Visine)	≥6 years: 1–2 drops 4 times per day
	Naphazoline (Allerest, Opcon-A)	≥13 years: 1 drop 4 times per day
Combination vaso-constrictor and H$_1$ receptor antagonists	Antazoline-naphazoline (Vasocon-A)	≥6 years: 1–2 drops 4 times per day
	Pheniramine-naphazoline (Visine-A, Naphcon-A)	≥6 years: 1–2 drops 4 times per day
Histamine H$_1$ receptor antagonists	Emedastine (Emadine)	≥3 years: 1 drop 4 times per day
	Levocabastine (Livostin)	≥12 years: 1 drop 4 times per day
Mast cell stabilizers	Cromolyn (Crolon, Opticrom)	≥4 years: 1–2 drops 4–6 times per day
	Lodoxamide (Alomide)	≥2 years: 1–2 drops 4 times per day
	Nedocromil (Alocril)	≥3 years: 1–2 drops twice daily
	Pemirolast (Alamast)	≥3 years: 1–2 drops 4 times per day
Combination H$_1$ receptor antagonist and mast cell stabilizers	Olopatadine (Patanol)	≥3 years: 1–2 drops twice daily
	Ketotifen (Zaditor)	≥3 years: 1 drop twice daily
	Azelastine (Optivar)	≥3 years: 1 drop twice daily
	Epinastine (Elestat)	≥3 years: 1 drop twice daily
Nonsteroidal anti-inflammatory drug	Ketorolac (Acular)	≥3 years: 1 drop 4 times per day
Corticosteroid	Loteprednol etabonate 0.2%, 0.5% (Alrex, Lotemax)	Adult: 1 drop 4 times per day
	Rimexolone (Vexol)	Adult: 1–2 drops 4 times per day

Artificial tears (e.g., ReFresh, Hypotears) can help soothe the eyes, especially if they are cooled before being administered. They help moisturize the eye and flush aeroallergens and irritants from the eye. The use of the drops with a cold compress can help decrease symptoms.

Topical vasoconstrictors constrict ocular blood vessels and decrease conjunctival hyperemia and erythema. Hence, they get the red "out." This improves cosmetic results but does not affect itch or the allergic cascade. Oxymetazoline has a faster onset and longer duration of action than naphazoline and tetrahydrozoline. Rebound hyperemia can occur with frequent use of these preparations. These agents are contraindicated in patients with narrow-angle glaucoma.

Topical antihistamine-vasoconstrictor preparations are effective in mild allergic conjunctivitis by combining a decrease in hyperemia (vasoconstrictor effect) with a decrease in pruritus (antihistamine effect). These medications are available over the counter, for example, pheniramine maleate-naphazoline (Naphcon-A, Opcon-A). These medications have a short duration of action and can be applied four times daily. Because of the vasoconstrictor component, they are contraindicated in patients with narrow-angle glaucoma.

Topical mast cell stabilizers are available both over the counter and by prescription. The primary over-the-counter preparation is cromolyn (Crolom, Opticrom). Cromolyn has been in clinical use for many years. It is surmised that it helps impede mediator release from mast cells, but its exact mechanism of action is unknown. Cromolyn is most effective when used for a few weeks before exposure to the allergen, for example, before the seasonal onset of symptoms due to pollens or before exposure to an animal. It also is most effective when used four times daily, making compliance difficult. Once the allergic conjunctivitis is full blown, cromolyn is only minimally effective in reducing symptoms. Nedocromil (Alocril), another mast cell stabilizer, has a longer duration of action and can be given every 12 hours. When administered twice daily, nedocromil has been shown to be as effective as cromolyn administered four times daily. Like cromolyn, it is most effective when given before exposure to the allergen. Lodoxamide (Alomide) is another mast cell stabilizer. Like cromolyn, it is dosed four times daily. It has the same limitations as other mast cell stabilizers.

Topical antihistamines alone are prescription medications. The three major topical antihistamines levocabastine (Livostin), azelastine (Optivar), and emedastine (Emadine) are more potent than over-the-counter topical antihistamines. They are effective for pruritus and hyperemia. Most topical antihistamines are short-acting and require dosing four times daily to be effective. Azelastine can be given twice daily. Adverse effects for this class of medications include eye burning and stinging and headache. Patients should be warned, particularly if their eyes are already irritated, that these medications may cause a burning sensation the first few times the medication is applied. As a group, topical antihistamines are more effective than mast cell stabilizers for acute symptoms, but they, too, are most effective if given before exposure to the allergen.

Topical antihistamine–mast cell stabilizers use other mechanisms in addition to their antihistamine properties. Overall, these medications provide the best control of mild to moderate allergic conjunctivitis by their ability to provide both immediate relief from pruritus, tearing, and hyperemia, with long-term mast cell stabilization. They also reduce eosinophil activity and downregulate the expression of chemotactic molecules. The available preparations are olopatadine (Patanol) and ketotifen (Zaditor), which can be given twice daily and are approved for ages 3 years and older.

Ketorolac (Acular) is the only available topical nonsteroidal anti-inflammatory medication. It is most effective at reducing ocular itch. This effect comes from the inhibition of prostaglandin synthesis; the prostaglandins cause itch when acting on the conjunctiva. This medication is short-acting and is given four times daily. Initial stinging and burning on administration is a frequent side effect. To increase compliance, the patient should be counseled about this effect. Ketorolac should not be administered to patients with a history of aspirin- or nonsteroidal anti-inflammatory-exacerbated respiratory disease or ketorolac sensitivity.

Topical corticosteroids are highly effective in the treatment of allergic conjunctivitis. These can be considered when other topical treatments such as antihistamines, mast cell stabilizers, and vasoconstrictors are ineffective. However, the use of these medications involves serious potential adverse effects, including increased intraocular pressure, cataract formation, and risk of viral or fungal infection. Because of these potential adverse effects, patients who use topical corticosteroids should be closely monitored in conjunction with an ophthalmologist. Two modified topical corticosteroids commonly used are rimexolone and loteprednol.

Allergen immunotherapy has been clearly shown to be beneficial for allergic rhinoconjunctivitis. In a large number of studies, however, many of the end points have involved nasal symptoms, not eye symptoms. More recent studies have focused on improvement in ocular signs and symptoms, with most of the subjects having a positive result. With conjunctival provocation tests, other studies have shown an increase in allergen tolerance, demonstrating the benefits of immunotherapy. The effect of immunotherapy in allergic rhinoconjunctivitis occasionally varies in nose versus eye symptom improvement. In some situations, eye symptoms are more responsive to immunotherapy. The role of immunotherapy as a primary treatment option for isolated allergic conjunctivitis has not been studied definitively. Overall, immunotherapy has been shown to be effective in allergic conjunctivitis and is a reasonable alternative if topical treatments with antihistamines, mast cell stabilizers, and nonsteroidal anti-inflammatory medications are not beneficial.

5.4.2 Perennial Allergic Conjunctivitis

Perennial allergic conjunctivitis, like seasonal allergic conjunctivitis, is typically associated with symptoms of rhinitis. Perennial allergic conjunctivitis occurs less frequently than seasonal allergic conjunctivitis. Perennial allergic conjunctivitis is present year-round and is caused primarily by dust mite and pet allergy. The clinical presentation typically is less dramatic than that of seasonal allergic conjunctivitis. Patients note chronic injected, itchy, watery eyes. Although the symptoms are primarily bilateral, unilateral allergic conjunctivitis can occur with manual contamination of the eye with allergens such as animal dander.

The pathophysiology of perennial allergic conjunctivitis is the same as for seasonal allergic rhinoconjunctivitis. Testing is focused on measuring specific IgE to the perennial allergens: dust mite, animals (particularly pets and occupational exposures), and molds.

Allergen avoidance has a primary role in treatment because environmental modifications for dust mite and animal exposures can markedly improve symptoms. These measures are outlined in Chap. 2. The topical medications are the same as those used for the treatment of seasonal allergic conjunctivitis, as described above.

5.4.3   Atopic Keratoconjunctivitis

Atopic keratoconjunctivitis is a bilateral, chronic inflammation of the conjunctiva and lids associated with atopic dermatitis. Approximately 15–40% of patients with atopic dermatitis have ocular involvement, primarily as atopic keratoconjunctivitis. Other eye conditions associated with atopic dermatitis include lid dermatitis, blepharitis, and cataracts. Atopic keratoconjunctivitis usually does not appear until the late teen years, with a peak incidence between ages 30 and 50 years. Males are affected more commonly than females. Atopic keratoconjunctivitis is more severe and threatening to sight than seasonal and perennial allergic conjunctivitis. Complications include decreased vision and blindness from corneal epithelial defects, cataracts, corneal scarring, and superficial punctate keratitis. Herpes keratitis is more common in patients with atopic dermatitis.

The inflammation in atopic keratoconjunctivitis is directed primarily by T cells. The T-cell cytokine release profile includes Th2 cytokines IL-4, IL-5, and IL-13. Of interest, T-cells also produce interferon-γ and IL-2 or Th1-type cytokines. This indicates that a delayed hypersensitivity response is involved in the chronic inflammation. In addition, a greater number of mast cells and eosinophils are found in the conjunctival epithelium than in seasonal and perennial allergic conjunctivitis.

Patients with atopic keratoconjunctivitis usually have a notable history of atopic diseases such as atopic dermatitis, asthma, and allergic rhinitis. The major eye symptoms are pruritus, burning, tearing, blurry vision, and photophobia. The eyelids are often swollen, erythematous, and eczematous. Papillary hypertrophy is often seen on the lower palpebral conjunctiva. Corneal involvement is common and usually presents as pinpoint defects.

Although no confirmatory diagnostic tests are easily accessible for atopic keratoconjunctivitis, it usually is easy to diagnose. The appearance of the eyelids and skin surrounding the eye differentiates it from seasonal and perennial allergic conjunctivitis (Figs. 5.3 and 5.4). In addition, the hypertrophy of the papillae is small compared with that in vernal conjunctivitis, in which the increased hypertrophy, resulting in "giant papillae," involves primarily the upper palpebral conjunctiva.

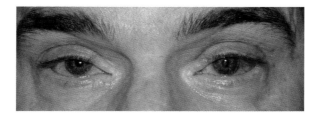

Fig. 5.3 Atopic keratoconjunctivitis, showing edematous, coarse, and thickened eyelids. Similar changes can also be seen in contact dermatitis

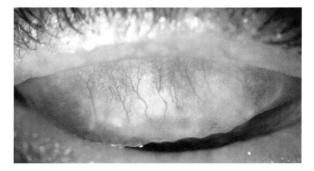

Fig. 5.4 Atopic keratoconjunctivitis. Chronic changes include cicatrizing conjunctivitis with fibrosis. Papillary hypertrophy of the palpebral conjunctiva is also present

However, almost any inflammatory disease of the conjunctiva has the potential to cause the formation of small papillae.

Blepharitis, or inflammation of the lid margin, can complicate this disorder because of orbital eczema. Chronic inflammation can obstruct meibomian glands, resulting in decreased lubrication, dry eye symptoms, and predisposition to infection. The prominent symptoms of blepharitis are burning, redness, and irritation, as opposed to pruritus. *Staphylococcus* blepharitis is often found in moderate to severe atopic keratoconjunctivitis. This is characterized by irritation and mucopurulent discharge, with matting of the eyelids. Over time, signs include yellow crusting of the eyelid margins and small ulcerations of the lid margin. When corneal involvement is suspected, it is important to stain the cornea to examine for tiny corneal ulcerations.

Treatment of atopic keratoconjunctivitis consists of the avoidance of allergen triggers, treatment of symptoms, and prevention of complications. The allergen triggers are the same as those listed for seasonal and perennial allergens. Food allergy does not appear to have an important role in atopic keratoconjunctivitis. Symptomatic treatment includes the entire arsenal of topical medications used in seasonal and perennial allergic conjunctivitis. Topical corticosteroids are often needed to control the marked inflammation. Treatment for gland complications includes lid cleansing, warm compresses, and antibiotics. Because of the severity of the inflammation and complications, atopic keratoconjunctivitis is difficult to treat. Ophthamologic consultation is often required.

5.4.4   Vernal Conjunctivitis

Vernal conjunctivitis is a chronic allergic inflammatory disorder that affects primarily children during the warm weather seasons. The symptoms can be perennial in those with severe disease. Onset typically occurs in the preadolescent years and the condition resolves after puberty. When onset is during preadolescence, vernal conjunctivitis has a male predominance. When onset occurs later, the disease tends to be milder and has a female predominance. The incidence is higher in warm weather regions.

The primary symptom is an intense pruritus that may be associated with burning and photophobia. Several physical examination findings help differentiate vernal conjunctivitis from other allergic eye disorders. Large papillae, ranging in size from one to several millimeters, are found on the upper palpebral conjunctiva, as opposed to smaller papillae in atopic keratoconjunctivitis (Fig. 5.5). These papillae have a large cobblestone appearance and can be seen when the upper lid is everted. Trantas dots are large clumps of cellular infiltrates, particularly eosinophils, that appear as white raised dots at the limbus, the cornea–sclera junction. This can be a subtle finding and may require slit-lamp examination and diagnosis by an ophthalmologist. The eye discharge is often a thick, white, ropelike discharge that is highly elastic. This discharge can string out over an inch when removed from the eye.

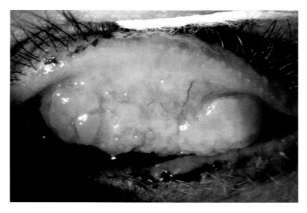

Fig. 5.5   Vernal keratoconjunctivitis. Large, irregular papillary hypertrophy of the upper palpebral conjunctiva in severe vernal conjunctivitis

Biopsy specimens of the papillae show the presence of increased neovascularization, fibrosis, mast cells, lymphocytes, and eosinophils. The tears contain increased levels of IgE, tryptase, eosinophil cationic protein, IL-4, and IL-5. These suggest Th2 cell activity in the pathogenesis of this condition. Unlike in atopic keratoconjunctivitis, increased levels of Th1-type cytokines, such as interferon-γ and IL-2, are not found. In severe cases, corneal ulcers may develop with the accumulation of inflammatory infiltrates; this may impede reepithelialization and lead to the formation of corneal scars.

The treatment for vernal keratoconjunctivitis is more difficult than for regular allergic conjunctivitis. Symptoms can be decreased somewhat with conservative measures such as cold compresses, avoidance or elimination of environmental allergens, eye washing, and the use of artificial tears. If these measures do not provide adequate relief from the symptoms, the commonly prescribed topical ophthalmic preparations such as mast cell stabilizers and antihistamines are indicated. Because the complications of vernal keratoconjunctivitis can be quite serious, topical corticosteroids are often required. The possible adverse effects of topical corticosteroids, including increased intraocular pressure and posterior subscapular cataract, require close observation and the expertise of an ophthalmologist. Currently, immunomodulation of T cells is being studied in the treatment of vernal conjunctivitis. Cyclosporine and other calcineurin inhibitors may be another treatment option for this difficult condition.

5.4.5   Giant Papillary Conjunctivitis

Giant papillary conjunctivitis is an inflammatory disorder of the conjunctiva involving both mechanical and immunologic mechanisms. This condition occurs primarily in contact lens wearers, but it also can occur in those with ocular prostheses or exposed sutures that come into contact with the conjunctiva. Several factors are important in the development of giant papillary conjunctivitis, including contact lens chemistry, edge design, surface properties, protein deposits on the lens, fitting characteristics, and the lens replacement cycle. Giant papillary conjunctivitis generally is more common in wearers of soft hydrogel lenses than wearers of rigid gas-permeable lenses, but it is found in patients who wear soft, hard, and rigid gas-permeable lenses. People who sleep wearing disposable lenses are more likely to be affected that those who remove the lenses daily. Patients who replace a soft contact lens at intervals of every 4 weeks or more instead of every 3 weeks or less have a greater chance of developing giant papillary conjunctivitis.

Several immune processes may contribute to giant papillary conjunctivitis. Inflammatory cells, including mast cells, eosinophils, basophils, and plasma cells, are found in the palpebral conjunctiva in patients with this condition. Increased levels of tear immunoglobulins, IgG, and IgE are also found. Lens trauma to the conjunctiva causes the release of neutrophil chemotactic factor, which augments the inflammation. A specific antigen trigger for this cascade has not been identified. It is postulated that giant papillary conjunctivitis represents a delayed hypersensitivity response.

The onset of symptoms can vary from a few weeks to years after a person begins to wear contact lenses. Often, eye symptoms precede the development of the papillae. The primary symptoms are foreign body sensation in the eye, pruritus, discomfort on insertion of the lenses, mucus production, and blurry vision. The most specific finding on physical examination is giant papillae, 1 mm large, on the palpebral conjunctiva lining the upper eyelids (Fig. 5.6). The papillae tend to be spread more evenly and to be more uniform and smaller than those in vernal conjunctivitis. Other findings include conjunctival hyperemia and excessive mucus production. In typical giant papillary conjunctivitis, the cornea is not involved.

The diagnosis is made by obtaining a history of contact lens use and identifying characteristic findings on physical examination. It is important to note that the presentation can vary markedly. The physical examination findings can range from mild mucus discharge, mild itching, and no papillae to severe mucus discharge, severe itching, and large papillae. There are no confirmatory laboratory tests, and conjunctival scraping is not usually helpful.

The primary treatment is discontinuation of the use of contact lenses. Once the lenses are removed, the symptoms typically resolve within a week. However, long-term elimination of contact lens use can be a problem for most patients. Most patients can resume wearing contact lenses after a "contact lens holiday" of 2 weeks or more. If the patient changes the polymer of the contact lens and is refitted with new lenses, the condition likely will not recur. Patients should be changed to a frequent replacement (<3 weeks) or disposable contact lens plan that does not include overnight wear. Mast cell stabilizers can be added to help in symptom relief.

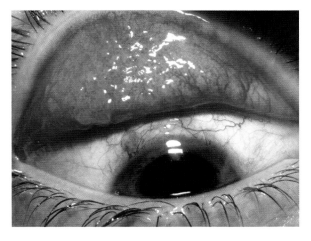

Fig. 5.6 Giant papillary conjunctivitis. Note upper palpebral papillary hypertrophy "cobblestoning"

5.4.6   Infectious Conjunctivitis

Infectious causes of conjunctivitis can often mimic allergic types of conjunctivitis. Infectious conjunctivitis can vary from mild and almost inapparent disease to severe infection with significant morbidity. Most cases of infectious conjunctivitis appear to be viral, but bacterial conjunctivitis appears to be more prevalent among children than among adults.

5.4.6.1   Viral Conjunctivitis

Typically, viral conjunctivitis is caused by multiple serotypes of adenovirus. The conjunctivitis may be part of upper respiratory tract viral symptoms or may be the only manifestation of the disease. Viral conjunctivitis is highly contagious. The incubation period is 4–10 days. After the onset of conjunctivitis, the virus is shed for about 12 days. It is shed by respiratory or ocular secretions, and transmission can occur through contaminated objects and surfaces.

The symptoms of viral conjunctivitis include watery or seromucus discharge, redness, and a burning, sandy, or gritty discomfort in the eye. Often one eye is affected initially, with the second eye becoming involved 24–48 hours later. Though matting of the eye can occur, this typically is present only in the morning. The crusting subsides throughout the day. A watery discharge occurs intermittently throughout the day. A thick, purulent discharge is not seen in viral conjunctivitis.

On physical examination, the bulbar and palpebral conjunctivae are injected. A mild follicular reaction may occur. This appears as multiple, slightly elevated lesions that resemble small grains of rice and are most prominent in the inferior palpebral conjunctiva. These lesions are caused by expansion of the subepithelial lymphoid tissue. Prominent tearing or thin discharge is usually present. There may be an enlarged and tender preauricular node. Bacterial conjunctivitis is almost never associated with preauricular adenopathy; therefore, this can be a differentiating feature.

Simple viral conjunctivitis is a self-limited process. There is no specifically recommended treatment. The overall course is similar to that of an upper respiratory tract viral infection. Typically, symptoms peak over the first 3–4 days, gradually resolving over 2 weeks.

Epidemic keratoconjunctivitis is a severe subtype of viral conjunctivitis caused by adenovirus types 8, 19, and 37. In addition to conjunctivitis, the viral infection causes inflammation of the cornea or keratitis. Patients present with a foreign body sensation in the eye, difficulty opening the eye, and decreased visual acuity in addition to the primary symptoms of conjunctivitis. On physical examination, the keratitis is categorized into three stages. The first stage occurs within 10 days after the onset of symptoms and is characterized by punctate epithelial lesions on the cornea. These lesions resolve within 2 weeks. The second stage is characterized by focal, white subepithelial opacities thought to represent an immune response to the virus. The third stage includes stromal infiltrates that can last

from months to years. Treatment depends on the stage of the disease. Topical corticosteroids are used for stage 2 and 3 lesions. Treatment of stage 1 depends on the severity of the symptoms. Whenever the cornea is involved, full ophthalmologic evaluation is recommended.

5.4.6.2 Bacterial Conjunctivitis

Simple bacterial conjunctivitis is a common and usually a self-limited condition. The most frequent causative organisms are *Staphylococcus aureus*, *S. epidermidis*, *Streptococcus pneumoniae*, *Haemophilus influenzae*, and *Moraxella catarrhalis*. Like viral conjunctivitis, bacterial conjunctivitis is highly contagious and is spread by direct contact with eye or respiratory secretions or contact with contaminated objects and surfaces. "Pink eye" is the name given to this type of acute purulent conjunctivitis that tends to spread rapidly through families and classrooms.

Patients present with eye redness, grittiness, burning, and discharge. A key point in the presentation is the type of discharge. As in allergic conjunctivitis and viral conjunctivitis, the patients frequently note difficulty opening their eyes in the morning because the eyelids are stuck together. In this condition, however, the discharge is purulent, typically green or yellow, and thick, as opposed to watery, and results in a thicker crusting. Also, the purulent discharge continues throughout the day.

On examination, the eyelids are crusted and often edematous. Purulent discharge is present at the lid margins and in the corners of the eye. Even after the lids are cleared, the discharge recurs within minutes, in contrast to that in allergic or viral conjunctivitis. The palpebral conjunctiva has a velvety, beefy-red appearance.

Bacterial conjunctivitis is usually self-limited and generally resolves within 14 days even if untreated. Appropriate choices for treatment include erythromycin ophthalmic ointment or sulfa ophthalmic drops. The ointment is applied to the inside of the lower lid twice daily, and the drops are given as 1–2 drops four times daily for 5–7 days. Patients should have clinical improvement within 2 days. The ointment is generally preferred for children and those with poor compliance. Because the ointments blur vision for approximately 20 min after being applied, drops are preferable for adults who need to drive or perform other tasks that require clear vision immediately after dosing. Numerous other topical antibiotics are available, including gentamicin, tobramycin, neomycin, polymyxin B, tetracyclines, and ofloxacin. Fluoroquinolones are the treatment of choice for corneal ulcers and are effective against *Pseudomonas* infections. They should not be used as first-line therapy for routine cases of bacterial conjunctivitis because of concern about emerging resistance. The exception is contact lens wearers, who have a high incidence of *Pseudomonas* infection.

5.4.6.3 Chlamydial Conjunctivitis

Adult inclusion (or chlamydial) conjunctivitis can present as acute conjunctivitis or chronic indolent conjunctivitis. It is caused by certain serotypes of *Chlamydia*

trachomatis. Patients typically have a concurrent asymptomatic urogenital infection from the organism. The eye infection presents as unilateral or bilateral follicular conjunctivitis with mucopurulent discharge that does not respond to treatment with topical antibiotics. The diagnosis can be confirmed with Giemsa or direct fluorescent antibody staining of conjunctival smears. Systemic therapy with doxycycline, tetracycline, erythromycin, or azithromycin is required to eradicate the infection.

5.4.6.4   Herpes Simplex Keratitis

Herpetic infection of the eye may occur with or without skin involvement. Patients present with tearing, ocular irritation, blurred vision, and photophobia. Milder cases can sometimes resemble allergic conjunctivitis. The absence of pruritus in the setting of eye irritation should raise suspicion for a nonallergic process. The diagnosis can be confirmed by the presence of a linear branching ulcer on corneal staining. Treatment consists of antiviral agents or débridement.

5.4.7   *Contact Dermatoconjunctivitis*

Contact dermatitis can involve the skin of the eyelid, and when the conjunctiva is also involved, dermatoconjunctivitis can occur. Dermatoconjunctivitis is more common in women because of their use of cosmetics. However, a wide variety of agents can cause dermatoconjunctivitis. The most common agents are those applied directly to the eyes, for example, eyebrow pencil, eyebrow brush-on products, eye shadow, eye liner, mascara, artificial lashes, and lash extenders. Other agents are aerosolized or airborne products such as hair spray; volatile substances contacted at work; airborne pollens; cosmetics applied to areas of the body other than the eyes, such as nail polish, soaps, and face creams; and any medication or contact lens solution applied to the eye.

The typical presentation is an extremely pruritic dermatitis involving the eyelids. Small vesicles and weeping may be seen early in the course. The lids are red, inflamed, and swollen. Rubbing the eyes intensifies the itching. The conjunctiva is erythematous with tearing. This can be difficult to distinguish from atopic keratoconjunctivitis. In contact dermatoconjunctivitis, the skin lesions usually only involve the eyelid area in contrast to atopic keratoconjunctivitis. A previous history of atopic dermatitis, even if remote, also favors atopic keratoconjunctivitis. Papillae on the lower lid favor atopic keratoconjunctivitis over contact dermatoconjunctivitis.

To evaluate for the offending substance, patch testing can be performed. However, patch tests can have a substantial false-negative rate because of the sensitivity of the eyelid skin and high local concentrations of the substance on the conjunctiva. Testing should be performed to standard allergens and to the patient's own cosmetics. Another method for identifying the offending substance is an elimination-provocation procedure. In this procedure, the patient removes from the environment all substances under suspicion. This is difficult because it requires the complete removal of all topically applied substances, including cosmetics, hair sprays, and spray deodorants, and changing to a bland soap and formalin-free shampoo. Contact lenses should not be worn. After the dermatoconjunctivitis has cleared, the different substances can be returned at a rate of one a week, monitoring for any recurrence of symptoms.

The primary treatment is removal of the offending agent. If this agent cannot be identified, treatment is symptomatic. This consists primarily of topical corticosteroid creams, ointments, and drops. Because of the possible adverse effects of these medications, particularly if used long term, consultation with an ophthalmologist is recommended.

5.4.8 Blepharoconjunctivitis

Blepharoconjunctivitis is a general term for conjunctivitis in conjunction with inflammation of the lid margin. Three distinct types of blepharitis may occur: (1) seborrhea- or rosacea-associated blepharoconjunctivitis, (2) staphylococcal blepharoconjunctivitis, and (3) meibomian gland dysfunction blepharoconjunctivitis. Seborrheic blepharitis is seen as part of seborrheic dermatitis and is often associated with dandruff of the eyelid, brows, and scalp. The irritation results in erythema of the conjunctiva (Figs. 5.7 and 5.8). Symptoms include the sensation of eye irritation and burning without marked pruritus. Rosacea can similarly cause blepharitis. Patients present with classic rosacea findings, that is, malar hyperemia and telangiectasias, and similar findings on the eyelids. As with seborrheic blepharitis, pruritus is not prominent. The primary symptoms are redness, burning, and irritation. Staphylococcal infection is often associated with styes (hordeola). Meibomian gland dysfunction is often associated

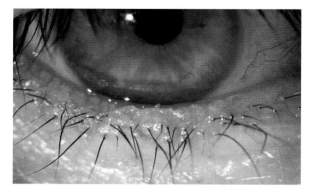

Fig. 5.7 Seborrheic blepharitis. Magnified view of the lid showing exudative material around the base of the eyelashes

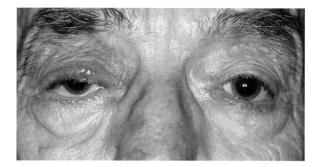

Fig. 5.8 Seborrheic blepharitis

with a firm, well-demarcated nodule just below the lid margin (chalazion). The therapy for these conditions consists primarily of treating the underlying disorders. Blepharitis can be controlled by scrubbing the lid margins daily with a cotton-tipped applicator dipped in dilute baby shampoo to remove exudates, scales, and bacteria. Massage of the lid margins may help express the abnormal meibomian secretions. Antibiotic treatment can be used if the lid scrubs are ineffective.

5.4.9 Dry Eye Syndrome

Dry eye syndrome is due to decreased tear production, increased tear evaporation, or an abnormality in the specific components of the tear film. This may be idiopathic or associated with an underlying autoimmune or connective tissue disease. Dry eye syndrome is often confused with a mild infectious or allergic process because of the symptom overlap. Patients present with foreign body sensation, dryness, burning, mild conjunctival injection, and mucoid discharge. The lack of pruritus helps to differentiate dry eye syndrome from an allergic eye disorder. Although dry eye syndrome can occur as a distinct disorder, it is associated more often with other ocular and systemic disorders, including allergy and blepharitis. Dry eye syndrome and ocular allergy conditions are not exclusive, especially in the older population in which the likelihood of dry eye complicating ocular allergy increases. A more systemic form of dry eye syndrome associated with autoimmune diseases such as Sjögren syndrome and rheumatoid arthritis is commonly termed keratoconjunctivitis sicca. Other common causes of dry eye syndrome include medications with anticholinergic properties. The diagnosis of dry eye syndrome can be confirmed by inadequate wetting of a Shirmer test strip. This commonly shows decreased tearing (0–1 mm at 1 min and 2–3 mm at 5 min, with normal values of 4 mm at 1 min and 10 mm at 5 min). Treatment consists of addressing any underlying disorders and wetting of the eye with artificial tears and lubricants.

5.5 Clinical Vignettes

5.5.1 Vignette 1

A 24-year-old woman complains of watery, itchy, red eyes with swollen lids. In addition, she has had sneezing and rhinorrhea. Her symptoms worsened after she mowed the lawn. She said she had no change in visual acuity and no photophobia. On physical examination, the eyelids were slightly swollen, but without erythema or dermatitic changes. The facial skin surrounding the eyes was normal. Eye examination showed injection of both the lower palpebral and bulbar conjunctivae, with watery discharge. No purulence was noted. Examination of the upper palpebral conjunctiva by eversion of the upper lid was notable only for injection and mild swelling. No papillae were present. Pen light examination of the cornea showed normal pupillary response to light. No corneal opacities were present.
Comment: This case is classic for seasonal allergic conjunctivitis. The eye symptoms worsened with exposure to outdoor pollens. She has concomitant allergic rhinitis. The physical examination is complete because it describes the skin surrounding the eye, the eyelids, bulbar and palpebral conjunctivae, and cornea. Examination of the upper palpebral conjunctiva by eversion is necessary to assess for papillae and the presence of vernal conjunctivitis.

The patient relates that she has been using over-the-counter naphazoline-pheniramine eye drops, but they have not been effective in relieving her symptoms.
Comment: The combination antihistamine-decongestant preparations often are not successful in relieving the symptoms of seasonal allergic conjunctivitis. In this situation, allergen avoidance would be recommended. This consists of limiting exposure to outdoor pollens by keeping outdoor activities to a minimum and keeping the windows to the home closed. Changing clothes and showering on entering the home after outdoor activities helps prevent further exposure. Medication treatment would be changed to an antihistamine–mast cell stabilizer combination such as olopatadine (Patanol) or ketotifen (Zaditor), two drops in each eye twice daily. Topical corticosteroids are not required in this situation.

5.5.2 Vignette 2

A 35-year-old man who does not wear contact lenses has a 3-month history of bilateral itchy, red eyes. He also notices a thick, ropelike mucus discharge. He has mild photophobia and the sensation of "something" in his eyes. His vision is unchanged.
Comment: The presence of itch suggests an allergic eye disorder. The symptoms of photophobia and the sensation of a foreign body in the eye are worrisome for

potential corneal involvement. In taking the history, it is very important to specifically delineate the sensation of "something in the eye." If this refers to "grittiness" or a sensation like "sand in the eye," it is not specific for corneal involvement because these symptoms can also occur with viral and allergic conjunctivitis. However, if "something in the eye" refers to the patient having trouble keeping the eye open or difficulty opening the eye, the likelihood of corneal involvement is high. Overall, the patient here is more symptomatic than would be expected with simple allergic conjunctivitis. The physical examination should help to further delineate the process.

On physical examination, an eczematous rash is noted around the eye and eyelids. There is crusting around the eyelashes. The palpebral conjunctiva is erythematous, with small papillae on the lower lid.

Comment: The physical examination findings show dermatitis around the eye and eyelids. Further history elicited from the patient reveals a history of asthma and atopic dermatitis. The constellation of symptoms and physical findings is consistent with atopic keratoconjunctivitis. The other main entity in the differential diagnosis is contact dermatoconjunctivitis. Because of the symptom of photophobia, the cornea should be examined closely for corneal neovascularization, superficial punctate keratopathy, ulcers, or cataracts. A patient with this condition should be managed in conjunction with an ophthalmologist.

The patient received treatment with the combination of a topical antihistamine–mast cell stabilizer and topical corticosteroids. Initially, his condition improved, but then the photophobia increased and visual acuity decreased. This occurred in the setting of a recent cold sore.

Comment: Patients with atopic keratoconjunctivitis are prone to herpes simplex infections, particularly when receiving treatment with corticosteroids. In this situation, staining of the cornea shows a dendritic ulcer diagnostic for herpes keratitis. Treatment includes topical antiviral drops and possibly systemic antiviral agents. The patient should be managed under the guidance of an ophthalmologist.

5.5.3   Vignette 3

A 15-year-old boy who wears contact lenses who has a history of seasonal allergic rhinitis presents with a 2-week history of watery, itchy, red eyes. Five days earlier, he began experiencing a thick purulent discharge, primarily from the right eye. He says he does not have photophobia, fever, visual changes, or other systemic symptoms. Physical examination shows normal facial skin and normal eyelids. The upper and lower bulbar and palpebral conjunctivae are injected, without evidence of papillae. A thick yellow discharge emanates from the medial aspect of the right eye and recurs after it is wiped away. The pupil reacts normally to light. No corneal opacities are seen.

Comment: The patient has a history of allergic rhinitis and, initially, likely had allergic conjunctivitis. Because he wears contact lenses, giant papillary conjunctivitis is a consideration, but the lack of papillae makes it less likely. However, the development of a purulent discharge is highly suggestive of a bacterial infection. Because of the absence of corneal symptoms (no photophobia or visual change), the presentation likely represents simple bacterial conjunctivitis. *Pseudomonas* infection is a concern in someone who wears contact lenses. The patient should receive treatment with a topical fluoroquinolone and be advised to obtain new contact lenses and a new contact lens case.

5.5.4 Vignette 4

A 75-year-old woman complains of red eyes that tear. Itch is not prominent. She also notes a foreign body sensation, and her vision varies with eye blinking. She feels that this has worsened over the last couple years. On physical examination, the skin surrounding the eye and the eyelids appears normal. The bulbar and palpebral conjunctivae are reddened. There is scant mucuslike discharge. No papillae are seen. The cornea is clear, and the pupils are normally reactive to light.

Comment: Because itch is not a prominent symptom, an allergic eye disorder is unlikely. In this situation, the major possibilities are dry eye syndrome, infection, or sensitivity to eye drops.

Additional history is obtained. The patient states that she does not use eye drops. She has not had any purulent discharge. She says she does not have inflammatory arthritis, dry mouth, or skin lesions. Her medication list is reviewed. Approximately 1 year ago, she began taking diphenhydramine 50 mg at night for sleep. She is not receiving hormone replacement therapy, anticholinergic agents, β-blockers, or a phenothiazine.

Comment: The patient likely has dry eye syndrome. She is not using any type of eye drops. All eye drops have the potential to cause a sensitivity response, and it is important to review this in the history. Keratoconjunctivitis sicca can be associated with collagen vascular disease, particularly rheumatoid arthritis and Sjögren syndrome. She does not have other symptoms that suggest this. Dry eye syndrome can be idiopathic or associated with other eye conditions or with medications. She is not taking medications associated with dry eye except for diphenhydramine. Diphenhydramine and other first- and second-generation antihistamines have the potential to increase drying of the eye. Other medications that can be associated with dry eye syndrome include β-blockers, phenothiazines, tricyclic antidepressants, atropine, and scopolamine.

A Shirmer test can be performed to quantify her tearing. The cornea should be stained to examine for any defects. Treatment is aimed at increasing the tear film, primarily through the use of artificial tears and ointments. Punctal occlusion can be performed to keep tears in the eye longer if the artificial tears are not effective.

Suggested Reading

Bielory, L. (2006) Allergic diseases of the eye. Med. Clin. North Am. 90, 129–148.

Bielory, L. and Mongia, A. (2002) Current opinion of immunotherapy for ocular allergy. Curr. Opin. Allergy Clin. Immunol. 2, 447–452.

Donshik, P. C. (2003) Contact lens chemistry and giant papillary conjunctivitis. Eye. Contact Lens 29(Suppl. 1), S37–S39.

Lieberman, P. and Blaiss, M. S. (2002) Allergic diseases of the eye and ear. In: L.C. Grammer and P.A. Greenberger (Eds.), Patterson's Allergic Diseases, 6th ed. Philadelphia: Lippincott Williams & Wilkins. pp. 195–223.

Stahl, J. L. and Barney, N. P. (2004) Ocular allergic disease. Curr. Opin. Allergy Clin. Immunol. 4, 455–459.

Tabbara, K. F. (2003) Immunopathogenesis of chronic allergic conjunctivitis. Int. Ophthalmol. Clin. 43, 1–7.

Chapter 6
Asthma

Abbreviations ABPA: allergic bronchopulmonary aspergillosis; AERD: aspirin-exacerbating respiratory disease; ANCA: antineutrophilic cytoplasmic antibody; BAL: bronchoalveolar lavage; CBC: complete blood count; COPD: chronic obstructive pulmonary disease; COX: cyclooxygenase; CT: computed tomography; D_{LCO}: diffusing capacity for carbon monoxide; DPI: dry powder inhaler; ECP: eosinophilic cationic protein; EDN: eosinophil-driven neurotoxin; EPO: eosinophil peroxidase; FEV_1: forced expiratory volume in 1 s; FVC: forced vital capacity; GERD: gastroesophageal reflux disease; GM-CSF: granulocyte-macrophage colony-stimulating factor; ICAM: intercellular adhesion molecule; IFN: interferon; IL: interleukin; MBP: major basic protein; MDI: metered dose inhaler; MRI: magnetic resonance imaging; NAEPP: National Asthma Education and Prevention Program; NSAIDs: nonsteroidal anti-inflammatory drugs; p-ANCA: perinuclear anti-neutrophilic cytoplasmic antibody; PEFR: peak expiratory flow rate; PGD_2: prostaglandin D_2; PGE_2: prostaglandin E_2; PGF_{2a}: prostaglandin F_{2a}; RADS: reactive airways dysfunction syndrome; RANTES: regulated on activation, T-cell expressed and secreted; RSV: respiratory syncytial virus; STAT: signal transducer and activator of transcription; TGF: transforming growth factor; TNF: tumor necrosis factor; VCAM: vascular cell adhesion molecule.

6.1 Overview

Asthma is a complex genetic disorder characterized by airway inflammation and reversible airflow obstruction resulting in a symptom complex of wheezing, dyspnea, or cough (or some combination of these). It is characterized further by multiple phenotypes that may differ on the basis of the age at onset, triggering factors, response to treatment, and variable patterns of reversibility both during acute exacerbations and with long-standing disease.

G.W. Volcheck, *Clinical Allergy: Diagnosis and Management*
DOI: 10.1007/978-1-59745-315-8_6, © 2009 Mayo Foundation for Medical Education and Research

6.2   Epidemiology

Asthma is a common disease that is increasing in prevalence worldwide, with the highest prevalence in industrialized countries. It is estimated that nearly 300 million people in the world have asthma. In the United States, more than 20 million people report symptoms consistent with the diagnosis of asthma, including 5 million younger than 18 years, and nearly 5,000 people die each year with asthma reported as the underlying cause of death. People who have asthma account for nearly 500,000 hospitalizations annually. Because the prevalence and morbidity of asthma have been increasing worldwide, there is concern that asthma patients are not always readily identified and may not receive optimal treatment for their disease.

6.3   Pathophysiology

6.3.1   Genetics

As commonly observed clinically, atopic diseases such as allergic rhinitis, atopic dermatitis, and asthma occur in families. Subsequent familial aggregation, twin, and gene linkage studies have provided evidence to support this. Studies of twins allow comparisons between monozygotic twins who share 100% of their genes and dizygotic twins who share approximately 50% of their genes. The greater occurrence of asthma in monozygotic twins, even those raised in different environments, is evidence for a genetic component. In family studies, asthma is more common in children of allergic asthmatic parents than in those of nonallergic asthmatic parents, underscoring the importance of atopy. Asthma occurs less frequently in the children of parents who are nonasthmatic and nonallergic. Applying a specific risk ratio for a given family is difficult because of the different environmental variables that can contribute to the development of asthma and also the differences in the population prevalence of asthma. Generally, in the United States, if one parent has allergic asthma, the child has approximately a 20% chance of developing asthma, and if both parents have allergic asthma, the child has approximately a 40% chance.

The inheritance pattern of asthma is a "complex genetic disorder" similar to hypertension and diabetes mellitus. Asthma cannot be classified as simply having an autosomal dominant, recessive, or sex-linked mode of inheritance. It is polygenic. Several gene linkages have been shown with asthma. These are summarized in Table 6.1. The primary chromosomes and regions that have been identified include chromosome band 5q31 (total IgE and eosinophils, interleukin [IL]-4, IL-5, IL-13, CD14), chromosome 6 (major histocompatibility complex, tumor necrosis factor [TNF]), chromosome band 11q13 (β-chain of the high-affinity IgE receptor), chromosome 12q (interferon [IFN]-γ, nitric oxide synthetase, leukotriene A_4 hydrolase, signal transducer and activator of transcription [STAT]-6), and chromosome 13q (cysteinyl leukotriene 2 receptor). Recently, the *ADAM33* gene on chromosome 20,

Table 6.1 Genetic linkages associated with asthma

Chromosome	Candidate genes or products
1p	Interleukin (IL)-12 receptor
5q23-25	IL-3, IL-4, IL-5, IL-9, IL-13, granulocyte macrophage colony-stimulating factor (GM-CSF)
	LTC4S
	GM-CSF receptor
	β_2-Adrenergic receptor
	Glucocorticosteroid receptor
6p21-23	Major histocompatibility complex
	Tumor necrosis factor
	Transporters involved in antigen processing and presentation (TAP1 and TAP2)
7q11-14	T-cell receptor γ chain, IL-6
11q13	High-affinity IgE receptor (FcϵRI) β chain
	Fibroblast growth factor 3
12q14-24	Interferon-γ
	Stem cell factor
	Nitric oxide synthetase (constitutive)
	Leukotriene A$_4$ hydrolase
13q21-24	Cysteinyl leukotriene 2 receptor
14q11-13	T-cell receptor α and δ chains
	Nuclear factor $\kappa\beta$ inhibitor
16p11-12	IL-4 receptor
17p12-17	CC chemokine cluster
19q13	CD22, transforming growth factor β_1
20p13	*ADAM33*

Modified from Steinke, J. W., Borish, L., and Rosenwasser, L. J. (2003) Genetics of hypersensitivity. J. Allergy Clin. Immunol. 111, S495–S501. Erratum in: J. Allergy Clin. Immunol. 112, 267. Used with permission

which encodes a protein-processing enzyme (a metalloprotease) that is expressed in lung fibroblasts, myofibroblasts, and smooth muscle cells, has been found to be commonly associated with asthma. In addition to the effect of the gene itself, the interaction between the gene and the environment may also have a role. Once specific sequences are identified for genetic susceptibility, the gene–environment interaction will need to be studied to help understand the importance of the relationship of the gene and the environment on the overall asthma process.

Pharmacogenetics is another key area in the gene–asthma relationship. Pharmacogenetics uses the variation in drug response in different individuals as a result of genetic differences. Genetic variations in drug target genes can be used to predict clinical responses to treatment. In asthma, alterations in the β_2-adrenoceptor, cysteinyl leukotriene synthesis, the glucocorticoid receptor, muscarinic receptors, and phosphodiesterases may all affect the response to treatment with different classes of drugs.

The gene for the β_2-adrenoceptor has received extensive attention as a candidate gene for asthma risk and severity and response to treatment with β-agonists. Two important coding variants at position 16 and position 27 appear to be functionally important. Because of linkage disequilibrium, however, individuals with polymorphisms at one genetic locus may or may not have changes at another position. Therefore, a "bad" polymorphism at one site may be countered by a "good" polymorphism at another site. At this point, however, it appears that chromosome 5 arg16/arg16 homozygous asthma patients have an increase in asthmatic exacerbations and decrease in peak expiratory flow when taking albuterol regularly. If these results are confirmed, they could have a significant effect on how one-sixth of asthma patients in the United States with the arg16/arg16 phenotype are treated. Another example of this is the lipoxygenase pathway, which results in the synthesis of the cysteinyl leukotrienes. The promoter region of 5-lipoxygenase has variants labeled "wild type" and "non-wild type." The wild type variant is the more common and more effective enzyme and, thus, produces more leukotrienes. Because of less effective enzymatic activity, the non-wild type produces fewer leukotrienes. Consequently, blockage of the leukotriene pathway would be expected to result in better clinical outcomes in the wild type than in the non-wild type. This was borne out when the use of leukotriene inhibitors was found to increase forced expiratory volume in 1 s (FEV_1) in the wild-type asthma patients compared with the non-wild type. Clinical screening for these and other polymorphisms are in their infancy. In the near future, it is likely that genetic testing will help guide therapy.

6.3.2 Airway Obstruction

6.3.2.1 Inflammation

Airway inflammation is the characteristic feature of asthma and contributes to many hallmarks of the disease, including airflow obstruction, bronchial hyperresponsiveness, and the initiation of remodeling. The classic microscopic features include infiltration of the airways by inflammatory cells, hypertrophy of the smooth muscle, and thickening of the lamina reticularis just below the basement membrane. Persistent airway inflammation is considered the characteristic feature of severe, mild, and even asymptomatic asthma. The pattern of inflammation varies with the severity and the chronicity of the disease and may also determine the responsiveness of the patient to treatment. Many inflammatory cells, cytokines, chemokines, and adhesion proteins contribute to airway inflammation in asthma.

One mechanism that initiates airway inflammation is antigen exposure in sensitized individuals. This results in the activation of the resident cells of the airways (mast cells) and the recruitment of inflammatory cells (lymphocytes, neutrophils, and eosinophils) into the airways (Fig. 6.1). The antigen binds with specific IgE antibody bound to mast cells. This binding activates mast cells to release preformed histamine and newly generated leukotrienes and prostaglandins along with transcription of numerous cytokines. Histamine and prostaglandin D_2 (PGD_2) and leukotriene C_4 induce bronchoconstriction, mucus secretion, and mucosal edema. The key proinflammatory cytokines include IL-4, IL-5, and IL-13. They regulate

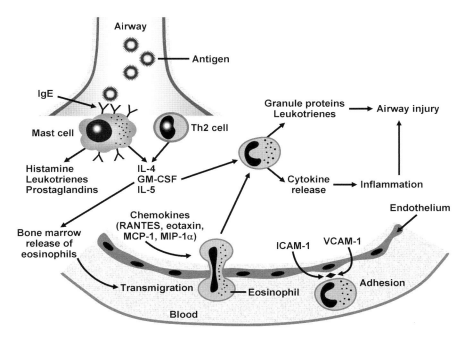

Fig. 6.1 Pathogenesis of allergic asthma. Antigen binds with mast cell-bound IgE, resulting in release of histamine, leukotrienes, prostaglandins, and cytokines. The cytokines induce the influx of inflammatory cells and their activation through the upregulation of chemokines, adhesion molecules, and bone marrow release. Inflammatory cells in the airway release granule proteins, leukotrienes, and cytokines, causing airway injury. *GM-CSF* granulocyte-macrophage colony-stimulating factor; *ICAM* intercellular adhesion molecule; *IL* interleukin; *MCP* monocyte chemotactic protein; *MIP* macrophage inflammatory protein; *RANTES* regulated on activation, T-cell expressed and secreted; *VCAM* vascular cell adhesion molecule. Modified from Busse, W. W. and Lemanske, R. F. (2001) Asthma. N. Engl. J. Med. 344, 344–362. Used with permission

IgE synthesis, Th2 lymphocyte differentiation, and the development of eosinophilic inflammation. The mast cell also produces other cytokines and proteases including TNF-α, transforming growth factor (TGF)-β, fibroblast growth factor, tryptase, and chymase, which may contribute to remodeling of the airway wall by activating myofibroblasts. T-lymphocytes are the primary effector cells in asthma by coordinating many of the actions of other inflammatory cells in the airways through the release of cytokines. Also, lymphocytes and epithelial cells generate chemokines, including RANTES and eotaxin, which enable the recruitment of eosinophils to the airway.

Another critical step in this process is the activation of endothelial adhesion proteins, such as intercellular adhesion molecule (ICAM)-1 and vascular cell adhesion molecule (VCAM)-1. These proteins combine with specific receptors on neutrophils, eosinophils, and lymphocytes to reduce the flow of these cells in blood vessels and to assist in cell movement from the vessels into the airway. Once in the airway, the inflammatory cells release various enzymes and proteins that damage the airway epithelium and contribute to the inflammation.

Eosinophils are considered the predominant and most characteristic cells in asthma, as observed with both bronchoalveolar lavage (BAL) and bronchial biopsy. The eosinophils contain several granules that are toxic to the airway. The four principal basic proteins are major basic protein (MBP), eosinophilic cationic protein (ECP), eosinophil peroxidase (EPO), and eosinophil-driven neurotoxin (EDN). These proteins are associated with the desquamated epithelium in asthmatic airways and enhancement of vagally mediated bronchoconstriction. Eosinophils also produce inflammatory cytokines, growth factors, and chemokines. Neutrophils likely have a role in certain subsets of asthma. Neutrophils can become activated and release myeloperoxidase, which is toxic to the respiratory epithelium. Neutrophil accumulation is a hallmark of patients who die suddenly of asthma and of patients with severe, corticosteroid-dependent asthma.

Cytokines are glycoproteins that are synthesized and released by many cell types after activation. Cytokines include interleukins, interferons, and growth factors. Their primary effect on inflammation includes regulation of IgE synthesis, mediation of eosinophil activation, and induction of cellular adhesion molecules that mediate the transendothelial migration of leukocytes. The primary cytokine airway profile in asthma patients includes IL-3, IL-4, IL-5, and granulocyte-macrophage colony-stimulating factor (GM-CSF). In patients with allergic asthma, IL-4 and IL-5 are increased, whereas in those with nonallergic asthma, primarily IL-5 is increased. The lack of increase in IL-4 in nonallergic asthma is likely due to lack of an IgE-mediated response, whereas both groups have eosinophil involvement, which is regulated by IL-5. Chemokines are another group of molecules that contribute to asthma inflammation through chemotactic activity. Chemokines are divided into two main families: A chemokines, which recruit neutrophils, and B chemokines, which recruit eosinophils and mononuclear cells. The latter includes RANTES and eotaxin, which work in conjunction with IL-5 by causing local tissue migration of eosinophils after they are released into the circulation. The relative contributions of A and B chemokines will emerge with the development of specific antagonists and their effect in various asthma models.

6.3.2.2 Airway Mucosal Edema

The thickness of the airway wall is increased in asthma and related to disease severity. The increase in thickness results from an increase in most tissue compartments, including the smooth muscle, epithelium, submucosa, adventitia, and mucosal glands. Inflammatory edema involves the entire airway, particularly the submucosal layer, with marked hypertrophy and hyperplasia of the submucosal glands and hyperplasia of goblet cells. Also, many of the same mediators that lead to contraction of bronchial smooth muscle, such as histamine and leukotrienes, can increase the permeability of the capillary membrane to cause mucosal edema. These changes combine to contribute to the obstruction of airway flow.

6.3.2.3   Mucus Hypersecretion

One of the characteristic features of severe asthma is the overproduction of mucus. Mucus can mechanically narrow the airway lumen and cause obstruction. In severe asthma, tenacious mucus plugs can cause airway obstruction that leads to ventilation-perfusion mismatch and hypoxemia. Mucus plugs are composed of mucus, serum proteins, inflammatory cells, and cellular debris, including desquamated epithelial cells and macrophages arranged in a spiral pattern (Curschmann's spirals). The development of mucus plugging occurs in severe, prolonged attacks of asthma or in patients with chronic disease. The end result is compromise of the airway lumen and impairment of mucociliary clearance.

6.3.2.4   Remodeling

Some patients with asthma develop irreversible airflow obstruction. This process has been labeled *airway remodeling* and represents an injury-repair process of the airway tissue. The remodeling occurs from a dysregulated attempt at tissue repair. Several components of airway remodeling have been identified, including hypertrophy of airway smooth muscle, hyperplasia of mucus glands and goblet cells, angiogenesis (vascular hyperplasia), and collagen deposition (fibrosis) in the airway. These features appear to be permanent and are not reversed by treatment. The processes that lead to this development have not been fully defined nor has the question been answered about why this process occurs in some asthma patients and not others. The process appears to be under the control of mediators distinct from those involved in the acute inflammatory response. The generation and presence of growth factors appear more critical and lead to structural changes in the airway tissue. The airway epithelium is likely a key regulator of the remodeling process. Bidirectional communication has been demonstrated between the epithelial and mesenchymal cells. In this system, damage to the epithelial layer stimulates a myofibroblast proliferative response associated with an increased level of growth factors. Overall, the transition to remodeling from inflammation suggests a new group of mediators with actions on smooth muscle growth, collagen deposition, blood vessel proliferation, and mucus gland hyperplasia. Although it has been theorized that adequate control of inflammation results in less remodeling, this has not been proved clinically and is currently a high-priority research subject.

6.3.3   Airway Hyperresponsiveness

Airway hyperresponsiveness is increased airway narrowing after exposure to constrictor-inducing agents. In asthma patients, it occurs with exposure to chemical and physical stimuli and allergens. Chemical stimuli include cholinergic agonists such as methacholine and carbachol and also histamine, leukotrienes C_4 and D_4, PGD_2, prostaglandin F_{2a} (PGF_{2a}), and adenosine. Physical stimuli include exercise, hyperventilation of cold dry air, and both hypotonic and hypertonic nebulized solutions. Airway hyperresponsiveness can be demonstrated in nearly all patients who have symptomatic asthma. Sometimes a specific trigger is needed to demonstrate it. Some subjects with normal methacholine responsiveness can still develop symptomatic asthma when exposed to appropriate stimuli such as specific allergens and occupational chemical exposures.

Airway hyperresponsiveness has been correlated directly with airway inflammation in asthma. Airway hyperresponsiveness improves in most children and adults with asthma treated with inhaled corticosteroids, which decrease inflammation. It appears that airway hyperresponsiveness is caused by inflammatory and structural changes in the airway, although the particular cells and mediators have not been fully identified. Structural changes associated with airway hyperresponsiveness include patchy desquamated epithelium, thickening of the reticular collagen layer of the basement membrane, and hypertrophy and hyperplasia of airway smooth muscle. Airway hyperresponsiveness itself, however, is not unique to asthma. A positive methacholine challenge test is diagnostic for airway hyperresponsiveness, which also can be seen in atopic disease, cystic fibrosis, rhinitis, and smokers and even in normal individuals for a few weeks after a viral respiratory infection.

6.3.4 Fatal Asthma

The pathologic changes seen in fatal asthma are generally similar to those seen in severe asthma but to a more significant extent. Multiple factors cause excessive airway narrowing in fatal asthma, including increased production of mucus, increased shortening of airway smooth muscle, alterations in the mechanics of the airway wall, loss of inflammatory inhibitory factors, and increased permeability from epithelial damage. One of the most common and characteristic findings is the occlusion of the bronchial lumen by mucus plugs. This occurs in airways of all sizes. Of interest, it has been calculated that the contents of the submucus glands alone cannot cause excessive narrowing; therefore, it is the accumulation of the mucus and the additional effects of smooth muscle shortening that cause excessive narrowing of the airway. The goblet cell hyperplasia that leads to excessive mucus production likely represents a reparative response to epithelial damage in an attempt to restore the normal protective barrier. The epithelial damage appears to have several sources. The inflammatory milieu results in the production of proteins, proteases, and chemicals toxic to the epithelium. Concomitant viral infections, often seen in fatal asthma, damage the epithelium. In addition to stimulating goblet cell hyperplasia, damaged epithelium results in easier access of irritants to nerve endings, enhanced penetration of allergen particles, loss of inactivation of proinflammatory peptides, and reduced mucociliary clearance.

The inflammatory pattern in fatal asthma is variable, with eosinophils and T-lymphocytes as the predominant cell types. Neutrophils have also been implicated in having a major role in a subset of patients with fatal asthma. Edema of the airway is regarded as an important feature of fatal asthma, but it is difficult to quantify. Edema contributes to the increased wall thickness in fatal asthma, causing a more pronounced decrease in the diameter of the airway lumen with the contraction of smooth muscle. Similarly, one of the hallmarks of severe and fatal asthma, the thickening of the subepithelial basement membrane zone with dense deposition of collagen fibrils, exponentially reduces airway diameter with smooth muscle contraction. Further studies of the clinical characteristics, with the histopathologic findings, will provide a better understanding of the mechanisms underlying the different clinical forms of asthma.

6.4   Clinical Presentation and Differential Diagnosis

Asthma can be manifested in several different ways. In some instances, it appears to be isolated, occurring only in the setting of upper respiratory infection, allergen exposure, or exercise. In others, particularly children, asthma may occur primarily as isolated chronic cough. More traditionally, asthma is manifested as repeated episodes of wheezing, cough, or dyspnea with varying levels of severity. The onset of asthma often occurs in childhood and has strong associations with other diseases, such as atopic dermatitis and allergic rhinitis. Asthma may also commence in adulthood in association with allergic disease or in the absence of allergic sensitization.

When obtaining a history, it is important to inquire specifically about what type of respiratory symptoms the patient is having. The patient or parent may not know what "wheeze" means and may use the term incorrectly to describe noisy breathing, snoring, or stridor. It is also important to quantify the frequency and duration of the asthma symptoms because the physician's interpretation of the history can significantly overestimate or underestimate the symptoms. Specific clues can be found in the timing, activities involved, and the environment in which symptoms occur; for example, symptoms triggered primarily at nighttime or by exercise, tobacco smoke, strong emotional expression, weather changes, aerosolized irritants, or cold air exposures are particularly helpful in establishing the diagnosis of asthma. There may be specific allergen triggers such as exposure to pollens, molds, dust mites, cockroaches, or pets. A frequent trigger for many asthma patients is a viral upper respiratory tract infection that can lead to an exacerbation of asthma and an increase in asthma symptoms that can persist for weeks after the infection has resolved. Because of the reversibility seen in asthma, the patient may be asymptomatic when evaluated, particularly if the asthma is mild. Key issues to globally address are the following:

1. Specific description of the respiratory difficulty
2. Details about the frequency of respiratory symptoms

- Length of time that symptoms persist (minutes, hours, days)
- Episodic or persistent
- Seasonal or perennial
- Time of day

3. Relationship to environment – home, work, indoors, outdoors, animals, temperature
4. Relationship to activity – exercise

On physical examination, the classic sign is expiratory wheezing or a prolonged expiratory phase. *Wheeze* is defined as a continuous musical sound heard during chest auscultation that lasts longer than 250 ms. Wheezes can originate from airways of any size and can be high or low pitched. In asthma, wheezes may vary in character as the degree of airway narrowing varies from place to place in the lung. Auscultation allows identification of the characteristics and location of the wheezing as well as variations in air entry among different lung regions. Wheezing requires sufficient airflow to produce the sound; hence, an asthma patient with a severely tight airway may not have a wheeze. Close attention should be paid to the chest examination. Findings that can suggest another process include a hyperexpanded chest, cyanosis, stridor, decreased inspiratory-to-expiratory ratio, and rhonchi. Crackles or other adventitious breath sounds suggest pulmonary parenchymal disease or pulmonary edema. The neck examination should include palpation for supratracheal lymphadenopathy or tracheal deviation. The cardiac examination should focus on the identification of congenital heart disease in children and congestive heart failure in adults. Nasal and skin evaluations are also helpful. The presence of pale, boggy nasal turbinates with clearish discharge is suggestive of allergic rhinitis, which likely contributes to allergic asthma. Nasal polyps are associated typically with a more severe underlying asthma and, in children, can be a clue to underlying cystic fibrosis. Skin findings of atopic dermatitis are consistent with an atopic diathesis, which often can include chronic rhinitis and asthma. The digits should be inspected for the presence of cyanosis or clubbing. The presence of these features suggests a process other than asthma.

In an acute attack, physical examination findings depend on the severity and may include an increased respiratory rate, use of accessory muscles, wheezing, tachycardia, and pulsus paradoxus. In an acute severe attack with pending respiratory arrest, the patient may appear drowsy or confused, the respiratory rate is often greater than 30 min^{-1}, wheezing is heard throughout inhalation and exhalation or may be absent if air movement is limited, and the initial tachycardia may revert to a bradycardia.

A definitive diagnostic test for asthma does not exist. The diagnosis of asthma requires the documentation of episodic airway obstruction and the reversibility of that obstruction. In older children and adults, spirometry is very helpful in quantifying the amount of airway obstruction and the presence of reversibility. In children younger than 5 years, repeat clinical evaluations are required. Testing performed in the diagnosis and assessment of asthma is outlined below in the chapter.

Wheezing is a common symptom in children. Up to 10–15% of infants wheeze during their first year of life, and up to 25% of children younger than 5 years wheeze. Most infants and children with recurrent wheezing are likely to have asthma; however, a wide variety of congenital and acquired conditions can have similar features. Several aspects of the medical history can raise questions about whether asthma is the correct or only diagnosis. These clinical features include the following:

- A history of persistent expiratory wheezing since birth suggests a congenital abnormality.
- Symptoms that vary with change in position may be caused by tracheomalacia or vascular rings.
- Failure to thrive and recurrent sinopulmonary infections suggest cystic fibrosis or immunodeficiency.
- Occurrence of wheezing with feeding can be associated with tracheoesophageal fistula or gastroesophageal reflux.
- Sudden onset of wheeze, followed by persistent wheeze, is consistent with foreign body aspiration.

These entities need to be considered particularly in patients who do not have a response to standard asthma treatment (Table 6.2).

Table 6.2 Differential diagnosis of asthma–airway diseases

Children

  Upper and middle respiratory tract
    Foreign body
    Laryngeal webs
    Tracheomalacia
    Tracheoesophageal fistula
    Vascular rings
    Vocal cord dysfunction

  Lower respiratory tract
    Bronchiolitis
    Cystic fibrosis
    Bronchiectasis
    Bronchopulmonary dysplasia
    Bronchiolitis obliterans

Adults

  Upper and middle respiratory tract
    Vocal cord dysfunction
    Vocal cord paralysis
    Laryngeal or subglottic stenosis
    Laryngotracheomalacia
    Foreign body

  Lower respiratory tract
    Chronic obstructive pulmonary disease
    Tumors
    Cystic fibrosis or immunodeficiency

6.4.1 Differential Diagnosis in Children

6.4.1.1 Cystic Fibrosis

Cystic fibrosis is an autosomal recessive disease with a frequency of one in approximately 2,500 births. Common presenting symptoms and signs include persistent sinopulmonary infections, pancreatic insufficiency, and failure to thrive. Respiratory symptoms include a persistent, productive cough; hyperinflation of the lung fields; and pulmonary function tests consistent with an obstructive airway disease. However, many patients demonstrate mild or atypical symptoms, including wheezing, and clinicians should remain alert to the possibility of cystic fibrosis even when only a few of the usual features are present. Particularly, the presence of nasal polyps in a child should alert the physician of the possibility of cystic fibrosis. The sweat chloride test can be performed to exclude cystic fibrosis. Even with the slightest suspicion of disease, this test should be performed because the diagnosis of cystic fibrosis has major implications for the patient.

6.4.1.2 Bronchopulmonary Dysplasia

Bronchopulmonary dysplasia is a chronic lung disease that occurs in premature infants and is characterized by impaired alveologenesis that leads to a global decrease in the number of alveoli and in gas-exchange surface area. It occurs infrequently in infants of more than 30 weeks' gestational age or birth weight more than 1,250 g. Most infants with bronchopulmonary dysplasia are ventilator-dependent from birth, with respiratory distress syndrome requiring surfactant therapy. However, bronchopulmonary dysplasia can develop in situations in which respiratory distress syndrome is mild or absent. The physical examination findings vary. The common findings are tachypnea, retractions, and, depending on the amount of atelectasis or pulmonary edema (or both), crackles. Expiratory wheezing may or may not be present. Chest radiographs can show various findings, including normal to low lung volumes, diffuse haziness due to inflammation or pulmonary edema (or both), atelectasis, and air trapping and hyperinflation. Most infants gradually improve over the first 4 months after initial instability during the first 6 weeks. Oxygen supplementation is gradually weaned until the infant can maintain adequate oxygenation on room air.

6.4.1.3 Foreign Body

Foreign body aspiration should be suspected in any patient who presents with sudden onset of wheezing, particularly if there is no previous history of wheezing. Approximately 80% of cases of pediatric foreign body aspiration occur in children younger than 3 years, with the peak incidence between 1 and 2 years of age. Commonly aspirated foreign bodies in children include peanuts, other nuts, seeds, hardware, and pieces of toys. The signs and symptoms of foreign body aspiration vary according to the location of the foreign body and the elapsed time since the event. In a severe acute event, the child presents with severe respiratory distress, stridor, hoarseness, and cyanosis. In this emergency situation, the object is usually lodged in the larynx or trachea. More commonly, the foreign body is located in the bronchi (right lung > left lung), and the situation is less emergent. Physical examination findings can include generalized wheezing or localized findings such as focal wheeze or decreased breath sounds. The classic triad of wheeze, cough, and diminished breath sounds are present in 50–60% of cases. Patients may also present days to weeks after the initial aspiration. In this situation, they often present with nonspecific symptoms of dyspnea, wheeze, chronic cough, or recurrent pneumonia. A careful history is required to inquire about an initial choking episode that may have been forgotten. A history of choking, when specifically sought, is found in approximately 80–90% of confirmed cases.

A plain chest radiograph is sometimes helpful in foreign body aspiration. Its usefulness depends on the degree of airway obstruction and whether the object is radiopaque. Most aspirated foreign bodies are radiolucent, such as foods, which limits the usefulness of radiographs. In bronchial foreign body aspiration, the most common radiographic findings are hyperinflated lung, atelectasis, mediastinal shift, and pneumonia. These findings are seen in approximately 1/3 of cases. In children who have a suggestive history and normal chest radiograph, expiratory chest radiography or fluoroscopy may be helpful. Computed tomography (CT) scans and magnetic resonance imaging (MRI) appear to be of limited use.

Rigid bronchoscopy should be performed if a foreign body is suspected. Although flexible bronchoscopy is also used for this purpose, rigid bronchoscopy is currently considered the procedure of choice for removal of aspirated foreign bodies in children.

6.4.1.4   Tracheoesophageal Fistula

Tracheoesophageal fistula is a common congenital anomaly, occurring in approximately 1 in 3,500 births. It typically occurs with esophageal atresia and occurs alone (H-type fistula) in only 5% of cases. In infants with tracheoesophageal fistula and esophageal atresia, symptoms develop immediately after birth, with excessive secretions, choking, drooling, respiratory distress, and inability to feed. Patients with the H-type fistula present with coughing and choking associated with feeding. Depending on the size of the fistula, the diagnosis can be delayed for months to years. With small fistulas, patients have a history of mild respiratory distress associated with feeding or recurrent episodes of pneumonia.

The diagnosis of tracheoesophageal fistula with esophageal atresia can be made by attempting to pass a catheter into the stomach and confirm coiling with a chest radiograph. Diagnosis of isolated tracheoesophageal fistula is more difficult. This sometimes can be confirmed with an upper gastrointestinal series, with use of a thickened water contrast material, but often esophageal endoscopy and bronchoscopy are required. Treatment is surgical ligation of the fistula and anastomosis of the esophageal segments. The prognosis is generally good, but close follow-up is required because esophageal stricture and tracheomalacia are reported complications.

6.4.1.5 Tracheomalacia

Tracheomalacia is characterized by a dynamic collapse of the trachea during respiration that results in airway obstruction. Most of the lesions are intrathoracic, causing airway collapse during expiration. Extrathoracic lesions are rare and lead to collapse during inspiration. There are three types of tracheomalacia. Type 1 is due to an intrinsic defect in the cartilaginous portion of the trachea that results in an increased proportion of membranous trachea and resultant airway collapse. Type 2 tracheomalacia is caused by extrinsic tracheal compression. This can be congenital or acquired and is associated with compression by cardiovascular structures, tumors, lymph nodes, or other masses. Type 3 lesions result from prolonged positive pressure ventilation or an inflammatory process that weakens the cartilaginous support of the trachea.

The signs and symptoms depend on the location and extent of the tracheal abnormality. Patients with intrathoracic tracheomalacia typically present with noisy breathing, a recurrent harsh, barking, or crouplike cough; in comparison, extrathoracic lesions cause inspiratory stridor. Symptoms may increase when the infant is supine. Wheezing can be present at birth but usually becomes apparent in the first 2–3 months of life. The wheezing becomes more prominent with upper respiratory tract infections and activity. Although chest radiographs are often normal, they are helpful in assessing for mediastinal masses and cardiomegaly. Changes in airway caliber during fluoroscopy can sometimes establish the diagnosis. Definitive diagnosis is usually made with bronchoscopy, with the observation of tracheal collapse with expiration. CT or MRI may help define the extent of the lesion. Most affected infants have spontaneous improvement by 12 months of age; however, patients can remain symptomatic into adulthood. Exercise intolerance may be seen in adults. In severe instances, treatment includes positive pressure ventilatory support, tracheal surgery, or placement of a tracheal stent.

6.4.1.6 Laryngeal Web

Laryngeal webs are a rare congenital abnormality caused by failure of resorption of the epithelial layer that covers the laryngeal opening. With failure of resorption, the vocal folds are incompletely separated, causing obstruction. Webs can occur anywhere along the anterior or posterior larynx and can also occur from trauma to the airway, as with intubation or injury. Patients with laryngeal webs usually present in infancy with respiratory distress and an unusual cry. In milder disease, symptoms may occur later and include a hoarse or weak voice, breathiness, and varying degrees of dyspnea and stridor, depending on the extent of the obstruction. Diagnosis is made with visualization of the web. The extent of surgical treatment required depends on the area of the lesion, and it can range from simple lysis of the web to laryngeal reconstruction.

6.4.1.7 Bronchiolitis

Bronchiolitis is a general term used to describe the presence of a nonspecific inflammatory response in the small airways. The term is confusing because it describes both a clinical syndrome and a constellation of histologic abnormalities that may occur from a number of various processes. In the published reports on bronchiolitis, there often is no tissue confirmation of the disease, which explains the many uncertainties about the epidemiology, pathophysiology, and therapy of the condition. The clinical syndromes associated with bronchiolitis include inhalation injury, drug-induced reactions, associations with connective tissue disease, idiopathic, and, most commonly, infections. In children, bronchiolitis has been referred to as "infectious asthma" and "wheezy bronchitis."

The diagnosis of bronchiolitis is based on a typical history and results of the physical examination. The key findings in infectious bronchiolitis include intermittent fever, runny nose, cough, tachypnea, abdominal pain, and crackles or wheezing. The presence or the severity of these findings has not been shown to distinguish reliably among viral, bacterial, or atypical organisms. Respiratory syncytial virus (RSV) is the most common viral cause of bronchiolitis in children younger than 2 years. Laboratory testing, including chest radiography, rapid viral panels or cultures, and complete blood count (CBC) are considered to have low utility in the evaluation of children who have mild airway disease. Reports are not clear about the benefits of the tests for children who have moderate to severe airway disease. Chest radiographs may be normal, although in some instances hyperinflation with peribronchial thickening or atelectasis may be present.

Although asthma and bronchiolitis share clinical manifestations and possible pathogeneses, it is important to try to distinguish between them on the basis of the past history and current presentation. Many children with bronchiolitis do not develop asthma and may be inappropriately labeled, particularly with the first episode. Risk factors identified for wheezing during viral infections in infancy and early childhood include maternal smoking, maternal history of asthma, and elevated IgE levels. Environmental history and overall review of systems can help distinguish between these entities and, thus, allow for implementation of avoidance techniques to prevent future exacerbations. Also, for a wheezing child younger than 3 years, risk for asthma is increased if one major criterion and two minor criteria are met:

- Major criteria – parental asthma, eczema
- Minor criteria – allergic rhinitis, eosinophilia, wheezing apart from viral upper respiratory tract illness

Children younger than 2 years frequently do not respond vigorously to inhaled or injected bronchodilators in a purely infectious setting, although there is a subset that does show improvement and a therapeutic trial should be considered.

6.4.1.8   Congenital Vascular Ring

Vascular ring abnormalities are caused by developmental failure of parts of the paired aortic arches during embryonic life. This may result in compression of the trachea or esophagus or both. Symptomatic vascular rings usually are diagnosed in early life, but the delay between the first appearance of symptoms and the time to diagnosis is significant. The diagnosis usually is made during the first year of life. Inspiratory stridor, wheezing, and dyspnea are prominent in cases of vascular ring, but other respiratory symptoms such as recurrent respiratory tract infections and cough may be associated with a vascular ring. Persistence of these symptoms should raise the question of a possible vascular ring.

   Clues to a vascular ring on chest radiography include a right-sided aortic arch or tracheal compression or both. However, these findings often are absent. Esophography is more sensitive and shows a double esophageal impression on the frontal view associated with a posterior notch on the side view. Other studies that can be performed to better define the anatomy include bronchoscopy, CT, MRI, and angiography. The treatment for symptomatic vascular rings is surgical correction.

6.4.1.9   Immunodeficiency

Immunodeficiency can present in myriad ways. Conditions that may be confused with asthma, particularly in the earlier stages, are humoral immune deficiencies. These result from impaired antibody production because of an intrinsic B-cell defect or dysfunctional interaction between B- and T-cells. Although T-cell defects underlie some of these diseases, cellular immunity is largely intact. The resultant antibody deficiency in humoral immune deficiencies leads to recurrent upper and lower respiratory tract infections with encapsulated bacteria such as *Streptococcus pneumoniae* and *Haemophilus influenzae*. The most common humoral primary immunodeficiencies are IgA deficiency, X-linked agammaglobulinemia, and common variable immunodeficiency. Most IgA-deficient individuals (nearly 90%) are asymptomatic. Those who are symptomatic often have a concurrent immunodeficiency. X-linked agammaglobulinemia and common variable immunodeficiency can be manifested in childhood or adulthood, although X-linked agammaglobulinemia typically becomes manifest between 6 and 18 months of age. The evaluation of patients with recurrent sinopulmonary infections should include IgA, IgM, and IgG immunoglobulin levels. IgG is markedly decreased in X-linked agammaglobulinemia and common variable immunodeficiency. For these conditions, treatment consists of immunoglobulin replacement. There is no immunoglobulin replacement therapy for IgA deficiency. These patients often have anti-IgA antibody and are at risk for an anaphylactic reaction when receiving blood products.

6.4.1.10 Bronchiolitis Obliterans

Bronchiolitis obliterans is a rare disease caused by epithelial injury to the lower respiratory tract that results in obstruction of the lower airways. It can be idiopathic or occur after infectious, chemical, or immunologic injury. Patients usually present with tachypnea, dyspnea, cough, and wheeze unresponsive to bronchodilator therapy. Physical examination shows diffuse wheezing and crackles. Chest radiographs typically show diffuse interstitial infiltrates and atelectasis. Pulmonary function testing shows airway obstruction without a response to bronchodilators.

6.4.2 Differential Diagnosis in Adults

The differential diagnosis of asthma in adults differs from that in children because congenital defects of the upper airway, heart, and lungs are rare. In adults, the primary distinctions need to be made between new-onset and acquired diseases of the upper airway, heart, and lungs (Table 6.2). Of primary importance is the distinction between upper and lower airway disease. Physical examination and pulmonary function testing can be helpful in this regard. Baughman and Loudon compared recorded sounds from the neck and chest in patients with upper airway obstruction, patients with asthma, and extubated patients with no airway obstruction. They found that the sound signal associated with asthma had a frequency similar to that of stridor. The musical sound in patients with stridor occurred during inspiration, but the sounds in those with asthma occurred predominantly during expiration. In addition, the signal was more intense over the neck than over the chest in those with stridor; for asthma patients, the reverse was true. Therefore, the major difference between upper respiratory airway obstruction and asthma was the inspiratory timing of the sound and the prominence of the sound over the neck. The differences in pulmonary function testing of these entities are reviewed below in the section on testing.

6.4.2.1 Obstructive Lung Disease

Chronic obstructive pulmonary disease (COPD) is characterized by air-flow limitation that (as opposed to typical asthma) is not fully reversible. The air-flow limitation is usually progressive and associated with an abnormal inflammatory response of the lungs to noxious particles or gases, primarily caused by cigarette smoking. The diagnosis of COPD should be considered for any patient who has cough, sputum production, or dyspnea or a history of exposure to risk factors, primarily smoking, for the disease. The diagnosis requires spirometry; a decreased FEV_1-to-forced vital capacity (FVC) ratio establishes an obstructive process. This alone though is not definitive, because the same pattern can be seen in asthma. The key differentiating features are the clinical presentation, lack of reversibility with treatment, exposure (primarily smoking) history, and the diffusing capacity for carbon monoxide (DLCO) with pulmonary function testing (Table 6.3). DLCO is normal or increased

Table 6.3 Differentiating asthma from chronic obstructive pulmonary disease (COPD)

Feature	Asthma	COPD
Age at onset	Child or adult	Fifth decade
Family history	Often positive	Noncontributory
Smoking role	Less significant	Highly significant
Respiratory symptoms	Vary daily	Slow, progressive decline
Inflammation	Th2 phenotype	Interleukin-8, tumor necrosis factor-α
	Eosinophils	Neutrophils
Response to corticosteroids	Highly responsive	Slightly responsive

in asthma and decreased in COPD. Some patients with asthma cannot be distinguished from those with COPD, and a subset of patients may have both asthma and COPD. The management of these patients should be similar to that of those with asthma. The primary treatment for COPD consists of bronchodilators, glucocorticoids, and oxygen therapy. The bronchodilators most commonly used are β-agonists, anticholinergic drugs, and, less commonly, methylxanthines. These medications can be used in combination in both short- and long-acting forms. For example, a patient with stage 2 COPD may use a long-acting anticholinergic agent in conjunction with a long-acting β-agonist agent daily, adding a short-acting anticholinergic or β-agonist as needed. The effect of glucocorticoids in COPD is less dramatic than in asthma. In some studies, inhaled corticosteroids cause a small increase in FEV_1, a small reduction in bronchial reactivity in stable COPD, and a reduction in COPD exacerbations. In other studies, no significant changes were noted. Currently, a trial of inhaled corticosteroids can be instituted in those with stage 3 COPD and continued if clinical improvement is noted over a 6-month period and withdrawn if no clinical improvement is noted.

Although neither chronic bronchitis nor emphysema is required in the definition of COPD, the terms are often used in describing patients with COPD. Chronic bronchitis, traditionally labeled as "blue bloater," is a clinical diagnosis defined by the presence of chronic productive cough for 3 months in each of two successive years. Emphysema, traditionally labeled as "pink puffer," is a pathology term that describes abnormal permanent dilatation of airspaces distal to the terminal bronchioles, which results in poor oxygen diffusion into the pulmonary vasculature. Patients can have COPD without falling into these two categories. Because obstruction is the primary manifestation, treatment for these groups is essentially the same as for COPD.

6.4.2.2 Mechanical Obstruction

Vocal Cord Paralysis

Vocal cord paralysis can cause respiratory symptoms that vary with the extent of the paralysis (paresis versus complete paralysis), exact location of the affected cord, and whether it is unilateral or bilateral. Unilateral vocal cord paralysis can be associated with breathy voice, ineffective cough, dysphagia, and aspiration. These signs and symptoms should be sought, particularly if there is any voice component to the symptoms. The paralysis is caused primarily by injury or inflammation of the vagus or recurrent laryngeal nerve. Common causes include surgery or procedures involving the thyroid gland, carotid artery, neck, chest, and base of the skull. Other causes include tumor, trauma, aneurysm, and neural disorders. However, bilateral vocal cord paralysis often is associated with preserved voice but more respiratory and aspiration signs. Bilateral vocal cord paralysis is usually caused by bilateral thyroid surgery but can also be caused by neurologic events.

Laryngeal and Subglottic Stenosis

Postintubation tracheal lesions are a common cause of upper airway obstruction and represent the principal indication for tracheal resection and reconstructive surgery in patients with subglottic stenosis. These injuries are caused by cuff-induced pressure necrosis, with subsequent formation of granulomas and fibrotic tissue. The main risk factor for development of the lesion is prolonged intubation. The obstruction can become manifest days to years after intubation. Therefore, if upper airway obstruction is suspected, it is imperative to inquire about a previous intubation history.

Several systemic diseases have been shown to cause upper airway obstruction. Wegener's granulomatosis is classically characterized by necrotizing granulomatous vasculitis of the upper and lower airway and, in most cases, involvement of the kidney. In a National Institutes of Health study of 158 patients with Wegener's granulomatosis, 16% had tracheal stenosis, with 2% presenting with this manifestation. Tracheal stenosis has also been reported in sarcoidosis and amyloidosis.

Idiopathic subglottic stenosis is a diagnosis of exclusion. It is not clear whether this group represents a distinctly separate group or a collection of different systemic illnesses that have not been identified. In general, there appears to be two groups of patients: those with mild disease that responds well to laser incision and dilatation, and those with more dense and complex scars that require resection and reconstruction. A disproportionate number of females are afflicted, the significance of which is unclear. The normal tracheal diameter ranges from 10–25 mm. With narrowing of the upper airway, dyspnea on exertion is typically the first symptom and becomes manifest when the airway diameter is narrowed to 8 mm. Symptoms at rest and decreased peak flow readings occur at 5 mm. Pulmonary function testing classically shows flattening of both the inspiratory and expiratory loop with a fixed upper airway obstruction.

Laryngotracheomalacia with Relapsing Polychondritis

Relapsing polychondritis can present in various ways depending on the severity and organ system involved. Auricular involvement is the most common feature, eventually appearing in approximately 85% of patients. Other areas that can be involved include the eye, nose, airways, cardiovascular system, skin, joints, kidney, and nervous system. The primary airway manifestations of relapsing polychondritis include glottic, subglottic, laryngeal, or tracheobronchial inflammation with luminal encroachment; fibrosis-induced luminal contracture; and loss of structural cartilaginous support resulting in laryngeal collapse during forced inspiration or tracheal collapse (or both) during expiration. Symptoms include hoarseness, aphonia, wheezing, inspiratory stridor, nonproductive cough, and dyspnea. Onset is most likely in the fifth and sixth decades, although all age groups can be affected. Relapsing polychondritis may coexist with various vasculitides or other autoimmune illnesses. Physical examination findings depend on the organs involved. Classic findings include a diffuse violaceous erythematous appearance to the cartilage-containing areas of the auricle and a saddle-nose nasal deformity. No test is diagnostically specific for relapsing polychondritis. The diagnosis is established by clinical findings, supportive laboratory data, and biopsy of an involved cartilaginous site. Pulmonary function testing may show varying degrees of inspiratory or expiratory obstruction (or both). Marked expiratory obstruction correlates well with bronchoscopic abnormalities in the upper airway.

Foreign Body Aspiration

Foreign body aspiration is more common in children than adults; approximately only 20% of recognized cases occur in patients older than 15 years. In adults, the nature of the foreign body is highly variable. Neurologic disorders, syncope, and alcohol or sedative abuse predispose to foreign body aspiration. Acute presentation in adults is rare. In a subacute or chronic presentation, the initial choking episode is often not recalled. Coughing is seen in approximately 80% of cases. Other associated symptoms include fever, hemoptysis, chest pain, or wheeze. Dyspnea is present only 25% of the time. The diagnosis is frequently overlooked unless the patient reports or is queried about a choking episode. Radiographically, a radiopaque foreign body can be seen on routine imaging. Unilateral hyperinflation can occur but is more common in the pediatric than in the adult population. Fiberoptic bronchoscopy is the diagnostic procedure of choice in adults, although rigid bronchoscopy may be required for extraction.

6.4.2.3 Cardiac Disorders

Atrial Myxoma

Myxomas are the most common primary cardiac tumor. The clinical manifestations depend on the anatomic location of the tumor. Approximately 80% of myxomas originate in the left atrium, and the majority of others are found in the right atrium. The tumors vary widely in size (range, 1–15 cm in diameter). The common respiratory symptoms are dyspnea and cough. Associated cardiovascular signs and symptoms often include orthopnea, paroxysmal nocturnal dyspnea, pulmonary edema, edema, and fatigue. Symptoms may worsen in certain body positions because of the location of the tumor in the atrium. Physical examination findings, in addition to evidence of right heart and left heart dysfunction, include diastolic murmur or evidence of embolization. Echocardiography is the test of choice for the initial evaluation; cardiac MRI or CT can also be performed to help distinguish the type of tumor. These studies provide the background regarding the need and type of surgical intervention.

Mitral Valve Prolapse

Mitral valve prolapse is a common disorder, occurring in 2–3% of the population. The cause of primary mitral valve prolapse is unknown. The classic auscultatory features are a midsystolic click or multiple clicks, sometimes followed by a midsystolic to late systolic murmur at the apex. Several nonspecific symptoms have been associated with mitral valve prolapse and termed the *mitral valve syndrome*. These include dyspnea, exercise intolerance, panic, anxiety, palpitations, and numbness. Controlled clinical studies suggest that patients with mitral valve prolapse and control subjects are equally symptomatic, although autonomic and neuroendocrine dysfunction may underlie some of the symptoms associated with mitral valve prolapse.

Congestive Heart Failure

Congestive heart failure may be manifested by symptoms similar to those of asthma: wheezing and worsening of respiratory symptoms at night and with physical activity. The main point is to be aware of the possibility of congestive heart failure, because the physical examination often provides the diagnosis. The major findings include an elevated jugular venous pulse, crackles on lung examination, and lower extremity edema. The cardiac examination may also show an abnormal rhythm, soft heart sounds, or murmur.

6.4.2.4 Vocal Cord Dysfunction

Vocal cord dysfunction, also known as functional upper airway obstruction, episodic paroxysmal laryngospasm, and paradoxic vocal cord movement, is an entity without a specific organic cause that may mimic asthma or organic upper airway obstruction. Normally during the respiratory cycle, the vocal cords are abducted during inspiration and expiration, allowing for maximal airflow. In vocal cord dysfunction, the vocal cords are inappropriately adducted on inspiration. This functional airway obstruction results in a marked inspiratory stridor that can be mistaken for asthmatic wheezing. During an attack, laryngoscopy shows a paradoxic inspiratory adduction of the anterior vocal cords with a posterior diamond-shaped glottic gap. At this time, spirometry demonstrates a flattened inspiratory flow-volume loop with a normal expiratory flow-volume loop. However, when the patient is asymptomatic, the results of laryngoscopy and spirometry are typically normal.

Vocal cord dysfunction appears to be psychogenic in nature. Patients are not considered to be malingering, because they do not intentionally produce their symptoms. Currently, it is thought to represent a conversion disorder associated with other conditions such as depression. Patients may present with significant respiratory distress and dramatic inspiratory stridor. On physical examination, harsh breath sounds are loudest above the sternal notch and less audible through the chest wall. Because of the suspicion of asthma, patients typically receive treatment with high-dose glucocorticoids and β-adrenergic agonists, which fail to relieve symptoms. The condition of these patients is often labeled as *refractory asthma*. Arterial blood gases are normal when the patient is symptomatic and asymptomatic. It is important to note that vocal cord dysfunction can coexist with true asthma. Up to 20% of asthma patients may have some degree of vocal cord dysfunction. Clues to help distinguish vocal cord dysfunction from asthma include the following:

- Minimal response to aggressive asthma treatment
- Flattened inspiratory flow-volume loop when symptomatic
- Stridor on physical examination when symptomatic
- Normal arterial blood gas measurements during a "severe" attack

Vocal cord dysfunction is difficult to treat. In most cases, the diagnosis is often delayed and it is difficult to taper or discontinue long-standing medications. It is difficult for patients to accept the diagnosis of a nonorganic disorder. There is no well-defined treatment protocol. No studies have been published on the effectiveness of psychodynamic or psychopharmacologic treatment. Some success has been reported with speech therapy, which uses breathing techniques and voice and neck relaxation exercises to eliminate the symptoms at their onset. These patients often have postnasal drainage and gastroesophageal reflux disease (GERD) that contribute to vocal cord dysfunction, and management of these disorders helps decrease the dysfunction.

6.4.2.5 Systemic Disorders

Cystic Fibrosis

Although cystic fibrosis is commonly thought of as a childhood disease, it is not uncommon for the initial diagnosis to be made during the adult years. The respiratory manifestations include a persistent productive cough, hyperinflation of the lungs seen on a chest film, pulmonary function tests consistent with an obstructive process, and concomitant sinus disease. With advancement of the disease, bronchiectasis appears. The sweat chloride test is the initial test of choice, but in adults, the results can sometimes be equivocal. Molecular diagnosis is usually made by

direct mutation analysis of specific known mutations in the cystic fibrosis transmembrane conductance regulator (*CFTR*) gene.

Carcinoid

Bronchial carcinoid tumors are rare, comprising less than 5% of the primary tumors
of the lung. They can occur at any age, but the mean age is between 43 and 60
years. The clinical presentation usually consists of recurrent pneumonitis, cough,
and hemoptysis. Of interest, dyspnea and the typical symptoms associated with
carcinoid syndrome (flush and diarrhea) are rare. Fiberoptic bronchoscopy and
tumor biopsy are the usual diagnostic procedures. The 10-year survival rate is
80–90%.

6.4.3 Testing

6.4.3.1 Spirometry

Pulmonary function testing can be used to detect airway expiratory flow obstruction and airway hyperresponsiveness. Pulmonary function testing has two components: spirometry and plethysmography. All patients who have asthma or are being
evaluated for asthma should have spirometry. Spirometry measures the maximal
volume of air forcibly exhaled from the point of maximal inhalation, the FVC, and
the volume of air exhaled during the first second of this maneuver, FEV_1. A flow-
volume curve is generated by plotting the flow rate (L s^{-1} on the *y*-axis) versus lung
volume (L on the *x*-axis). Expiratory flow obstruction is indicated by decreased
FEV_1 and decreased FEV_1/FVC ratio compared with the predicted values based on
age, height, sex, and race. In symptomatic asthma, FEV_1 typically is decreased,
whereas FVC remains relatively normal. Airway obstruction results in a characteristic appearance of the flow-volume loop – a scooped appearance of the expiratory
loop (Fig. 6.2).

These changes, however, are not specific for asthma, because they are also seen
in COPD. Spirometry is generally performed in children older than 5 years,
although many children cannot perform the maneuver until after age 7 years. In
younger children, management decisions about initiating and adjusting treatment
should be based primarily on the frequency and severity of past exacerbations and
symptom presentation, with spirometry used as a guide in the assessment and
response to treatment.

Another component of spirometry is the determination of reversibility as indicated
by a bronchodilator response to a β-adrenergic agonist such as albuterol. After a
bronchodilator is administered, the FEV_1 often improves. A significant improvement
in FEV_1 after a bronchodilator is administered is defined by the American Thoracic
Society as a 12% increase in FEV_1, which represents at least a 200-mL increase in

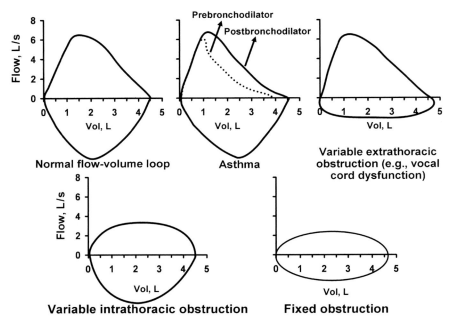

Fig. 6.2 Pulmonary function testing. Flow-volume loops

volume. Such a response is suggestive of a diagnosis of asthma. Some patients with asthma do not exhibit a significant bronchodilator response because of marked underlying inflammation. These patients often have a low baseline FEV_1 and may require anti-inflammatory treatment to demonstrate reversibility.

Methacholine bronchoprovocation testing can be performed to measure airway hyperresponsiveness. Methacholine is a cholinergic agonist that stimulates muscarinic receptors on airway smooth muscle and produces bronchoconstriction. In patients who have asthma, the airway smooth muscle is more sensitive to methacholine, resulting in bronchoconstriction at lower dosages, thus differentiating patients with asthma from those without asthma. Although different protocols are used for methacholine challenge, the results are often presented as the provocative concentration that results in a 20% decrease in FEV_1. One method for performing methacholine challenge uses a 0.25-mg mL^{-1} methacholine solution for inhalation. Two milliliters of this solution is placed in the nebulizer, and the patient is instructed to take one deep inhalation, followed by repeat spirometry. If FEV_1 has decreased less than 15%, four more breaths of methacholine are administered. If FEV_1 decreases 20% or more, the test is positive. A short-acting β-agonist should then be administered to ensure that FEV_1 returns toward the baseline value. This type of testing should not be performed in a patient known to have asthma, because some patients are very sensitive and can develop severe bronchospasm. This testing should be performed only if the patient has a normal baseline spirometry (FEV_1) and the diagnosis of asthma is in question. False-positive methacholine challenges can be seen in allergic rhinitis, cystic fibrosis, COPD, congestive heart failure, tobacco use, and upper respiratory tract infection.

Pulmonary function testing is also useful for diagnosing upper airway obstruction. The pattern of obstruction caused by upper airway lesions is determined by the level of the airway at which the obstruction occurs. Physiologically, the laryngotracheal airway can be divided into two levels: intrathoracic and extrathoracic. The intrathoracic airway is surrounded by pleural pressure and the extrathoracic airway, by atmospheric pressure. When the obstruction caused by a lesion changes with the respiratory cycle it is called a *variable lesion*. Variable extrathoracic obstruction, as with vocal cord paralysis and vocal cord dysfunction, is characterized by increased obstruction with inspiration. This increase is due to the negative pressure within the airway compared with the positive atmospheric pressure around the airway during inspiration. During expiration, however, the marked positive pressure within the airway decreases the obstruction so that the expiratory curve may be normal (Fig. 6.2). Conversely, variable intrathoracic obstruction, which is usually due to tumor, causes increased obstruction during expiration. This occurs because the positive pleural pressure during expiration causes compression of the airway at the site of the lesion. During inspiration, the negative pleural pressure lessens the obstruction, allowing a normal inspiratory loop (Fig. 6.2). In fixed obstruction, the airway diameter does not change with inspiration or expiration. Decreased airflow through the site of obstruction represented by a plateau will be seen in the expiratory and inspiratory curves (Fig. 6.2).

DLCO measures the ability of the lungs to transfer gas from the inhaled air to the red blood cells in the pulmonary capillaries, and this is helpful in distinguishing between asthma and emphysema, particularly in patients at risk for both illnesses, such as smokers and older patients. In asthma, DLCO is typically normal or increased, whereas in emphysema and other pulmonary parenchymal diseases in which gas exchange at the alveolar–capillary membrane is impaired, DLCO is decreased. Smokers with airway obstruction but normal DLCO values usually have chronic obstructive bronchitis, but not emphysema.

6.4.3.2 Peak Flow Measurement

Peak flow measurement is a simple and inexpensive way to monitor airflow in the office and at home. In this maneuver, patients expire forcefully into the peak flow meter, a hollow tube, which measures the peak expiratory flow rate (PEFR) in liters per second. Although PEFR is not as accurate as spirometry, it correlates well with the presence of bronchospasm and is a good estimate of the severity of asthma. It is particularly helpful in those with moderate-to-severe persistent asthma and with decreased awareness of asthma symptoms. A baseline measure should be obtained with which to compare future readings. The baseline value should be obtained when the patient is feeling well after a period of maximal asthma therapy; this represents the "personal best." Further monitoring can be performed on a scheduled or as needed basis depending on the patient's asthma history. The clinician should provide clear instructions for the patient to follow when the PEFR begins to decrease. This is outlined for the patient in the asthma action plan. An example of an asthma action plan and approximately normal values for PEFR are provided in Tables 6.4 and 6.5, respectively.

6.4.3.3 Sputum Eosinophils

Examination of the sputum for eosinophils is a noninvasive way to measure airway inflammation. Different induction and processing techniques can be used, but patients typically have sputum induction with aerosolized 3% hypertonic saline by way of a nebulizer. The patient then coughs sputum into a sterile container, which is processed and stained to obtain a total cell count and a differential cell count. The analysis of sputum eosinophils has provided results comparable to an analysis of specimens obtained with bronchoscopy. In mild and severe asthma, sputum eosinophils increase during exacerbations and increased baseline sputum eosinophil counts predict exacerbation with withdrawal of corticosteroid therapy. A recent study used sputum eosinophil counts to regulate the dosage of anti-inflammatory agents in patients with moderate to severe asthma. This approach resulted in significantly fewer exacerbations and fewer hospital admissions than in the guideline-based (clinical symptoms and spirometry) group at similar corticosteroid doses. This suggests that the measurement of sputum eosinophils is beneficial in selecting the appropriate amount of anti-inflammatory medication required to control asthma. Currently, this procedure is not widely available, but it is considered safe if performed in a controlled environment. Also, it potentially can be important in diagnosing and monitoring asthma.

6.4.3.4 Exhaled Nitric Oxide

Exhaled nitric oxide has been studied as another noninvasive measure of airway inflammation that increases with an acute exacerbation or loss of asthma control. The fraction of nitric oxide in the exhaled air increases in proportion to inflammation of the bronchial wall, induced sputum eosinophilia, and airway hyperresponsiveness. Increases in exhaled nitric oxide are associated with a deterioration in asthma control, and exhaled nitric oxide levels are decreased in a dose-dependent manner with anti-inflammatory treatment. Initial studies have shown that the use of exhaled nitric oxide measurements performed regularly in patients with moderate asthma resulted in a lower maintenance dose of inhaled corticosteroid needed to control asthma as compared with the use of a dose-adjustment strategy based on conventional guidelines. Exhaled nitric oxide has been proposed as a diagnostic tool for asthma, but the baseline levels of exhaled nitric oxide can vary significantly with age, sex, smoking, infection, allergic rhinitis, and genetic polymorphisms in the

Table 6.4 Asthma action plan

Name _____ Phone number _____ Date _____
Physician's name _____ Emergency phone number _____
Personal best peak flow _____

Green zone
    Peak flow between _____ to _____ (80–100% of personal best)
    Symptoms: no cough, wheeze, or shortness of breath during day or night
    Treatment plan: long-term controller medications – used daily
        1. _____
        2. _____
        3. _____
    : rescue medication
        1. _____

Yellow zone
    Peak flow between _____ to _____ (50–80% of personal best)
    Symptoms: cough, wheeze, shortness of breath, or waking at nighttime due to asthma
    Treatment plan: adjustment of long-term controller medications
        1. _____
        2. _____
        3. _____
    : rescue medication
        1. _____ 2 or 4 puffs or nebulizer every 20min up to 1h
    : if symptoms and peak flow do not return to green zone after 1h of treatment:
        Add _____ mg of _____ (oral steroid)
        Call physician

Red zone
(Medical alert)
    Peak flow <50% of personal best
    Symptoms: very short of breath or cannot do usual activities
      • Rescue medication   4 puffs or nebulizer
      • _____ mg prednisone
      • Seek emergent care

Table 6.5 Approximate normal peak flow rate values[a]

Children and adolescents

Height, inches	Males, L min⁻¹	Females, L min⁻¹	Height, inches	Males, L min⁻¹	Females, L min⁻¹
40	115	114	55	316	315
41	128	127	56	329	328
42	141	141	57	343	342
43	155	154	58	356	355
44	166	168	59	370	369
45	182	181	60	383	382
46	195	194	61	397	395
47	209	208	62	410	409
48	222	221	63	423	422
49	235	235	64	437	436
50	249	248	65	450	449
51	262	261	66	464	462
52	276	275	67	477	476
53	289	288	68	491	489
54	303	302	69	504	503

Males, L min⁻¹

Age, year	Height, inches				
	60	65	70	75	80
15	511	531	548	564	578
20	554	604	624	681	740
25	580	608	636	682	730
30	584	617	627	660	703
35	599	622	643	661	677
40	597	620	641	659	675
45	591	613	633	651	668
50	580	602	622	640	656
55	566	588	608	625	640
60	551	572	591	607	622
65	533	554	572	588	603
70	515	535	552	568	582
75	496	515	532	547	560

Females, L min⁻¹

Age, year	Height, inches				
	60	65	70	75	80
15	423	438	451	463	473
20	444	460	474	486	497
25	455	471	485	497	509
30	458	475	489	502	513
35	458	474	488	501	512
40	453	469	483	496	507
45	446	462	476	488	499
50	437	453	466	478	489
55	427	442	455	467	477
60	415	430	443	454	464
65	403	417	430	441	451
70	390	404	416	427	436
75	377	391	402	413	422

(Continued)

nitric oxide synthetase genes. Therefore, the usefulness of exhaled nitric oxide may be in monitoring asthma control, guiding therapy, and predicting response to corticosteroid therapy as opposed to making the diagnosis.

6.5 Classification of Asthma

6.5.1 Types

Asthma can be divided into various subtypes on the basis of the pathophysiologic mechanism of asthma. The two primary subtypes are allergic asthma and nonallergic asthma. Aspirin-induced asthma is another subtype.

6.5.1.1 Allergic Asthma

Allergic asthma is caused by the inhalation of a specific airborne allergen that triggers an IgE-mediated reaction. Allergic asthma implies a temporal relationship between allergen exposure and subsequent respiratory symptoms. The respiratory symptoms develop within minutes or up to an hour after allergen exposure. Allergic asthma occurs most commonly from ages 4–40 years but is also present in the older population. It is estimated that 75% of patients with persistent asthma have some component of allergic asthma.

Common allergens associated with allergic asthma include tree, grass, and weed pollens; molds; dust mites; animal dander; and cockroach. The diagnosis of allergic asthma should be suspected when the signs and symptoms of asthma correlate closely with the local patterns of pollen and mold release. When perennial symptoms of asthma are present, the temporal relationship may not be obvious because of continuous allergen exposure. Potential causes of perennial allergic asthma include animal dander, dust mite, cockroach, and, depending on the climate, pollens and molds.

6.5.1.2 Nonallergic Asthma

In nonallergic asthma, IgE-mediated sensitivity is not present. Nonallergic asthma occurs at any age but is more likely to occur in patients younger than 4 years and older than 50 years. The results of skin prick testing and in vitro allergen testing are

Table 6.5 (continued)

Data from National Asthma Education and Prevention Program: Expert Panel Report 3. (2007) Guidelines for the diagnosis and management of asthma. NIH publication No. 07-4051. Bethesda, MD: U.S. Department of Health and Human Services; National Institutes of Health; National Heart, Lung and Blood Institute

[a]These figures are a guideline only. The range of "normal" functions depends on many factors that cannot all be included in a table. These values represent average normal values with 100L min^{-1}

negative. Allergens do not trigger worsening of symptoms; the major triggers seem to be upper respiratory tract infections, GERD, and irritants. In addition, the underlying inflammation can wax and wane without obvious triggers. The respiratory inflammation is not IgE mediated, but it is still primarily eosinophilic. Nonallergic asthma generally appears to have a more severe and progressive course than allergic asthma, particularly if onset is late in life and requires more aggressive treatment.

The term *mixed asthma* refers to the presence of both allergic and nonallergic asthma. This likely represents the majority of asthma patients. A typical example is a patient with allergic asthma due to tree pollens who has a flare of asthma in the winter because of an upper respiratory tract infection. Other examples include patients with daily persistent asthma and positive skin tests that do not correlate with perennial asthma symptoms (skin tests positive only to tree and negative to dust mites, dog, cat, and molds).

6.5.1.3 Aspirin-Induced Asthma

Aspirin-induced asthma represents a small subset of asthma patients. These patients with underlying asthma, nasal polyposis, and chronic rhinosinusitis develop respiratory signs and symptoms with the use of aspirin or other nonsteroidal anti-inflammatory drugs (NSAIDs). This reaction is a class effect with the same respiratory symptoms produced with the use of any of the cyclooxygenase (COX)-1 inhibitors, including aspirin, ibuprofen, and naproxen. The respiratory reaction, consisting of rhinorrhea, nasal congestion, dyspnea, and wheezing, typically occurs within minutes and up to 3 hours after ingestion. Of interest, these patients typically have nonallergic asthma. This group is discussed in more detail in the medication-exacerbating asthma section and the chapter on rhinosinusitis (Chap. 4).

6.5.2 Initial Evaluation of Chronic Asthma Severity

The severity of asthma generally is considered a function of the intensity of the disease. However, it is difficult to easily define asthma severity because it can vary over time. The two primary measures used to define asthma severity are current impairment and future risk. These two measures do not correlate perfectly with each other, and both need to be considered to adequately address disease severity. Compounding the variables used in trying to define asthma severity are the measures used to define asthma control and the responsiveness of the asthma to treatment. Also, studies suggest that measures of health care use are an important addition to the traditional measures of asthma severity. Considering all this, the American Thoracic Society sponsored an expert workshop to develop a consensus definition for severe asthma that would apply not just to the initial evaluation but also to patients receiving treatment for asthma. The definition of the American Thoracic Society is based on a combination of major and minor criteria that aim to

Table 6.6 American Thoracic Society workshop consensus for definition of severe/refractory asthma[a,b]

Major characteristics
1. Treatment with continuous or near continuous (≥50% of year) oral corticosteroids
2. Requirement for treatment with high-dose inhaled corticosteroids

Minor characteristics
1. Requirement for additional daily treatment with a controller medication (e.g., long-acting β-agonist, theophylline, or leukotriene antagonist)
2. Asthma symptoms requiring short-acting β-agonist use on a daily or near-daily basis
3. Persistent airway obstruction (FEV$_1$ < 80% predicted, diurnal peak expiratory flow variability 20%)
4. One or more urgent care visits for asthma per year
5. Three or more oral corticosteroid bursts per year
6. Prompt deterioration with ≤25% reduction in oral or inhaled corticosteroid dose
7. Near-fatal asthma event in the past

From Moore, W. C. and Peters, S. P. (2006) Severe asthma: an overview. J. Allergy Clin. Immunol. 117, 487–494. Used with permission
[a]Definition requires one or both major criteria and two minor criteria
[b]Requires that other conditions have been excluded, exacerbating factors have been treated, and patient is generally compliant

identify subjects with inadequate control despite treatment with corticosteroids. According to this definition, subjects with severe asthma must meet one of two major criteria: (1) the use of high-dose inhaled corticosteroids or (2) the requirement for very frequent oral corticosteroid use (>50% of the year). Also, two of seven minor criteria must be met: (1) the use of additional controller medications besides inhaled corticosteroids, (2) the presence of daily symptoms requiring rescue inhaler, (3) reduced lung function (FEV$_1$ < 80% of predicted and diurnal PEF variability >20%), (4) one or more urgent care asthma visits per year, (5) recurrent (≥3) exacerbations requiring oral corticosteroids per year, (6) clinical deterioration with corticosteroid withdrawal, and (7) a history of a near-fatal asthma event (Table 6.6).

The "current impairment" in asthma is an evaluation of the frequency and intensity of symptoms and functional limitations the patient is experiencing. The goal is to achieve minimal or no chronic symptoms, including nocturnal awakenings; minimal or no need for acute rescue therapy, such as inhaled β$_2$-agonists; establishment of a normal lifestyle with no limitations on activities, including exercise; and normalization of pulmonary function. In 1997 and 2002, the National Asthma Education and Prevention Program (NAEPP) sponsored by the National Institutes of Health published comprehensive guidelines that classify asthma severity as mild intermittent or mild, moderate, or severe persistent asthma on the basis of symptoms and pulmonary function findings. Patients with mild intermittent asthma experience symptoms once or twice weekly and have normal or near-normal spirometry and PEFRs. Patients with symptoms 3 days of the week or more are classified as having persistent asthma. The degree of the asthma (mild, moderate, severe) then depends on daily symptoms, nighttime symptoms, frequency of exacerbations, and peak flow rates and spirometry readings. With the release of new information and the development of new therapies, an update of the NAEPP guidelines was released to the public for comment in February 2007, and the completed update was released in late 2007. One significant new concept is differentiating asthma "severity" from "control" and the incorporation of these areas as they relate to risk and impairment. Severity assessment is performed to initiate therapy, and control assessment is performed to adjust therapy. Separating the two concepts dispels the common misperception that well-controlled asthma is synonymous with mild asthma and poorly controlled asthma is synonymous with severe asthma. The classification of asthma according to severity for children ages 0–4, children ages 5–12, and for those older than 12 years according to the new guideline is shown in Tables 6.7, 6.8, and 6.9. Characterization of the severity is critical for outlining the initial treatment plan (see below). This is particularly important when separating patients with mild intermittent asthma from those with mild persistent asthma. For mild persistent asthma, a daily antiinflammatory medication is recommended, whereas mild intermittent asthma requires primarily a short-acting β-agonist to be used as needed.

Future risk is also critical in defining asthma severity and, thus, in outlining an overall management plan. Future risk considers the likelihood of future asthma exacerbations. This is important because exacerbations account for loss of time at work or school, decreased quality of life, and much of the cost of asthma care. The other primary future risk involved in asthma is the progressive loss of pulmonary function. Contrary to previous belief, asthma is not always a totally reversible process. Severe and irreversible airflow obstruction, accelerated loss of pulmonary function, and remodeling of all the tissue elements of the airway wall can be found in chronic "never smoker" asthma patients.

Of the future risks, the one that has been best assessed is asthma exacerbations. The strongest predictor of this risk is the history of previous exacerbations that resulted in emergency department visits, hospitalizations, or intubations. Also, assessment of the current severity with regard to increased day and nighttime symptoms, functional impairment, and frequent use of rescue therapy indicates an increased risk of exacerbations in the future. However, some patients with minimal symptoms for long periods can be prone to sudden and severe attacks. Therefore, a patient who currently has minimal symptoms but a past history of severe exacerbations would be considered to have a more severe form of asthma than a patient without a history of severe exacerbations.

Identifying possible markers for risk of exacerbations has been studied intensely. A decreased FEV_1 has been shown to be related to an increased risk of exacerbations. Measurement of bronchial reactivity, for example, to methacholine, has also been shown to be predictive of exacerbations. Patients receiving treatment with inhaled corticosteroids dosed to reduce bronchial reactivity were found to have fewer asthma exacerbations than those treated regularly. Markers of airway inflammation such as sputum eosinophils and exhaled nitric oxide have also been measured and used as the primary parameter for changing dosage of inhaled corticosteroids. Treatment in this fashion has shown a decrease in asthma exacerbations.

Table 6.7 Classifying asthma severity in children ages 0–4 years[a]

Components of severity	Classification of asthma severity (ages 0–4 years)[b]			
		Persistent		
	Intermittent	Mild	Moderate	Severe
Impairment				
Symptoms	≤2 days per week	>2 days per week but <1 time per day	Daily	Throughout the day
Nighttime awakenings	0	1–2 times per month	3–4 times per month	>1 time per week
Risk				
Exacerbations (requiring oral systemic corticosteroids)	0–1 per year	2–3 per year	4–5 per year	>5 per year
		Frequency and severity may fluctuate over time		
		Exacerbations of any severity may occur in patients in any severity category		
Recommended step for initiating treatment	Step 1	Step 2	Step 3	Step 3
			and consider short course of oral systemic corticosteroids	
	In 2–4 weeks, evaluate level of asthma control that is achieved, and adjust treatment accordingly			

From the National Asthma Education and Prevention Program: Expert Panel Report 3. (2007) Guidelines for the diagnosis and management of asthma. NIH publication No. 07-4051. Bethesda, MD: U.S. Department of Health and Human Services; National Institutes of Health; National Heart, Lung and Blood Institute

[a] Assessing severity and initiating therapy in children who are not currently taking long-term-control medication
[b] Level of severity is determined by both impairment and risk

Table 6.8 Classifying asthma severity and initiating treatment in children ages 5–11 years

Components of severity		Classification of asthma severity (ages 5–11 years)			
		Intermittent	Persistent		
			Mild	Moderate	Severe
Impairment					
Symptoms		≤2 days per week	>2 days per week but not daily	Daily	Throughout the day
Nighttime awakenings		≤2 days per month	3–4 per month	>1 per week but not nightly	Often 7 per week
Short-acting β_2-agonist use for symptom control (not prevention of exercise-induced bronchospasm)		≤2 days per week	>2 days per week but not daily	Daily	Several times daily
Interference with normal activity		None	Minor limitation	Some limitation	Extremely limited
Lung function		Normal FEV_1 between exacerbations $FEV_1 > 80\%$ predicted $FEV_1/FVC > 85\%$	$FEV_1 > 80\%$ predicted $FEV_1/FVC > 80\%$	$FEV_1 = 60$–80% predicted $FEV_1/FVC = 75$–80%	$FEV_1 < 60\%$ predicted $FEV_1/FVC < 75\%$
Risk					
Exacerbations (requiring oral corticosteroids)		0–1 per year	≥2 per year ⟶ Frequency and severity may fluctuate over time for patients in any severity category. Relative annual risk of exacerbations may be related to FEV_1		
Recommended step for initiating treatment		Step 1	Step 2	Step 3 medium-dose ICS option and consider short course of systemic oral corticosteroids	Step 3 medium-dose ICS option or Step 4

In 2–6 weeks, evaluate level of asthma control that is achieved, and adjust treatment accordingly

From the National Asthma Education and Prevention Program: Expert Panel Report 3. (2007) Guidelines for the diagnosis and management of asthma. NIH publication No. 07-4051. Bethesda, MD: U.S. Department of Health and Human Services; National Institutes of Health; National Heart, Lung and Blood Institute

FEV_1 forced expiratory volume in 1s; FVC forced vital capacity; ICS inhaled corticosteroid

Table 6.9 Classifying asthma severity and initiating treatment in adults and youths age ≥12 years

Components of severity		Classification of asthma severity (Age ≥12 years)			
		Intermittent	Persistent		
			Mild	Moderate	Severe
Impairment	Symptoms	≤2 days per week	>2 days per week but not daily	Daily	Throughout the day
	Nighttime awakenings	≤2 per month	3–4 per month	>1 per week but not nightly	Often 7 per week
Normal FEV₁/FVC: 8–19 years 85% 20–39 years 80% 40–59 years 75% 60–80 years 70%	Short-acting β₂-agonist use for symptom control (not prevention of exercise-induced bronchospasm)	≤2 days per week	>2 days per week but not >1 per day	Daily	Several times daily
	Interference with normal activity	None	Minor limitation	Some limitation	Extremely limited
	Lung function	Normal FEV₁ between exacerbations FEV₁ > 80% predicted FEV₁/FVC normal	FEV₁ > 80% predicted FEV₁/FVC normal	FEV₁ > 60 but <80% predicted FEV₁/FVC reduced 5%	FEV₁ < 60% predicted FEV₁/FVC reduced > 5%
Risk					
	Exacerbations (requiring oral corticosteroids)	0–1 per year	≥ 2 per year		
			Frequency and severity may fluctuate over time for patients in any severity category Relative annual risk of exacerbations may be related to FEV₁		
Recommended step for initiating treatment		Step 1	Step 2	Step 3	Step 4 or 5 and consider short course of systemic oral corticosteroids
		In 2–6 weeks, evaluate level of asthma control that is achieved, and adjust treatment accordingly			

Modified from the National Asthma Education and Prevention Program; Expert Panel Report 3. (2007) Guidelines for the diagnosis and management of asthma. NIH publication No. 07-4051. Bethesda, MD: U.S. Department of Health and Human Services; National Institutes of Health; National Heart, Lung and Blood Institute
FEV₁ forced expiratory volume in 1s; *FVC* forced vital capacity

However, the effect of inhaled corticosteroids dosed by various means to prevent the progressive loss of pulmonary function is not clear. Currently, no prospective study has shown that early treatment with an inhaled corticosteroid, despite preventing exacerbations, prevents the progression of asthma to a more severe form. Possibly, the ultimate answer to the question, "do inhaled corticosteroids alter the natural course of asthma?" will not be answered. Despite this lack of clarity, it is imperative to prescribe the most effective treatment and to prescribe it early. Recently, O'Byrne et al. have shown that daily low-dose anti-inflammatory treatment in patients with recent onset of persistent asthma decreased the loss of lung function over time, corroborating the earlier work of Agertoft and Pederson and Haahtela. Perhaps markers of inflammation or novel markers of remodeling will be helpful in the future to further assess this risk and, thus, help define the severity of the disease.

Clearly, the patient's current symptoms are not the only measurement of severity. Simple methods for assessing current impairment are available. Future risk, history of exacerbations, spirometry, and the amount of medication required to control the symptoms also contribute significantly. These areas need to be addressed during the initial evaluation. Because the severity of asthma fluctuates over time, repeated assessments are required. To summarize, the following information should be obtained on the initial evaluation. Positive answers on the risk assessment portion point to increased severity:

1. Current impairment

   - Symptoms
   - Nighttime awakenings
   - Need for rescue medication
   - Number of work/school days missed
   - Ability to participate in desired activities
   - Lung function: spirometry, peak flow

2. Risk Assessment

   - Amount of severe airflow obstruction on spirometry
   - Amount of persistent airflow obstruction despite maximal pharmacotherapy
   - History of two or more emergency department visits or hospitalizations for asthma in the past year
   - History of intubation or intensive care unit admission for asthma

6.6   Evaluation of Factors Contributing to Asthma Severity

Factors that exacerbate asthma should be identified and managed in all asthma patients, particularly in those with moderate or severe persistent asthma. Management of these factors results in better asthma control and the need for less pharmacotherapy to treat the asthma. In this chapter, the exacerbators of asthma are divided into

Table 6.10 Common exacerbators of and contributors to asthma

Common exacerbators of an acute asthma attack
   Infections
   Exercise
   Vocal cord dysfunction
   Allergens
   Medications

Common contributors to chronic asthma (airsmog)[a]
   *A*llergens
   *I*rritants/pollutants
   *R*hinitis/sinusitis
   *S*moking
   *M*edications
   *O*ccupational/obstructive sleep apnea
   *G*astroesophageal reflux

[a]These conditions should be assessed for and optimally managed in all patients with asthma

two groups: those that typically initiate an acute attack and those that contribute to ongoing chronic asthma. Although these groups overlap, the acute instigators most often include infections, allergens, exercise, vocal cord dysfunction, and medications. The chronic contributors can be remembered with the mnemonic "airsmog" (*a*llergens, *i*rritants/pollutants, *r*hinitis/sinusitis, *s*moking, *m*edications, *o*ccupational exposures, *o*bstructive sleep apnea, and *g*astroesophageal reflux) (Table 6.10).

6.6.1 Allergens

Allergen exposure can affect asthma in two critical ways: as a common precipitant of asthmatic symptoms and the inception of asthma through chronic airway inflammation. The airborne allergens (dust mites, pets, molds, trees, grasses, and weeds), as opposed to food allergens, contribute importantly to chronic asthma. The formation of IgE antibody to the airborne allergens does not usually occur until age 2–3 years. Therefore, aeroallergen-induced asthma is uncommon until that time. Allergens have the highest prevalence of involvement in asthma during later childhood and adolescence and peaks in the second decade of life. Airborne allergen-induced asthma can occur throughout adulthood; however, the prevalence decreases with increasing age.

   Indoor allergens, particularly cockroach, cat, and dust mite, clearly have a role in asthma provocation, and they appear to have a role in asthma inception. Decreasing the constant exposure to these allergens through environmental modifications diminishes the primary trigger for the chronic allergic and inflammatory response. This may result in marked relief from the symptoms of asthma and rhinitis and a reduction in airway hyperreactivity over time.

The same aeroallergens important in allergic rhinitis also contribute to asthma exacerbations. One aeroallergen in particular that appears to trigger severe asthma exacerbations is *Alternaria alternata*. *Alternaria* has been implicated as a risk factor for sudden respiratory arrest in adolescents and young adults with asthma. Tree, grass, and weed pollens can also trigger a seasonal asthma pattern. This is often associated with upper respiratory tract symptoms. Although food allergies can trigger bronchospasm, it is quite unusual for food to trigger bronchospasm without other concomitant symptoms. Typically, skin and gastrointestinal manifestations are present. This occurs within 1 hours after eating the food allergen.

6.6.2   Infections

Like allergens, infections can affect asthma by being a precipitant of an acute attack or having a role in asthma inception. Viruses, *Chlamydia* spp., and *Mycoplasma* spp. have been implicated in the pathogenesis of asthma. Viruses, particularly RSV, have been associated with the inception of the asthma phenotype. Because this virus is ubiquitous (nearly 100% of children are infected by age 2 years), additional genetic, environmental, sequential, or developmental factors must contribute to its linkage with asthma. Children who have persistent symptoms of asthma or develop asthma after an RSV infection usually have other risk factors such as a maternal history of asthma and increased IgE levels. Precisely how RSV infections pathogenically induce asthma has not been established. *Chlamydia* and *Mycoplasma* spp. are atypical bacteria associated with ciliary dysfunction and epithelial damage in airway cells. Their presence in the airway has been associated with chronic asthma. Although their presence does not provide a causal link to asthma, macrolide treatment of patients with chronic asthma, both with and without the presence of the bacteria, produced improvement only in those with the bacteria. Larger definitive studies are needed to determine whether antibiotic treatment in patients with chronic asthma and known infection with *Chlamydia* or *Mycoplasma* spp. alters the course of the disease.

In patients with established asthma, viral upper respiratory tract infections are important in producing acute exacerbations of airway obstruction. The increases in airway hyperreactivity that follow a respiratory viral infection usually occur within 48 hours after the cold symptoms and persist for at least 2 weeks. Possible mechanisms include direct epithelial damage, the production of virus-specific IgE antibodies, increased production of IgE antibodies specific for other antigens, and upregulation of inflammatory mediator release. Rhinovirus, the common cold virus, is the most frequent cause of exacerbations, but other viruses, including metapneumovirus, parainfluenza, RSV, influenza, and coronavirus, have also been implicated. The symptoms can include marked wheezing and shortness of breath or a prolonged cough, typically spasmodic, that is worse at night. Viral upper respiratory tract infections are the most common provocateur of asthma in children, particularly during the winter months. These asthma flares are at times resistant to

standard therapy of inhaled β-agonist and inhaled corticosteroids. Oral corticosteroids may be required and have been shown to decrease hospitalizations in viral-
induced asthma exacerbations.

Mycoplasma pneumoniae and *Chlamydia pneumoniae* are commonly associated
with severe exacerbations. These microbes can be causative in up to 20% of children with asthma exacerbations who require hospitalization.

However, infections may have the potential to actually prevent the development
of respiratory tract diseases, including asthma. The hygiene hypothesis purports
that an increased number of infections, particularly during early childhood, may
decrease the development of allergic sensitization or asthma. This is based on the
findings that lower rates of asthma and allergic diseases have been found in children
who are raised on farms, attend day care in the first 6 months of life, or have older
siblings. It is thought that the higher exposure to infectious agents or endotoxins
skews the immune system toward a vigorous Th1 system and a suppressed Th2
response to allergens. This hypothesis continues to be studied.

6.6.3 Exercise

Exercise is a common precipitant of asthma. The symptoms of exercise-induced
bronchospasm can include wheezing, coughing, shortness of breath, and, in children, chest pain or discomfort. The onset of symptoms is typically 10–15 min after
exercise begins or 5–15 min after exercise is completed. Sports most commonly
associated with precipitating the symptoms of asthma are aerobic in nature, such as
running or cross-country skiing, as compared with those that do not require a high
ventilatory rate, such as weight lifting or diving. The symptoms are most intense
for 5–10 min and usually resolve within 15–30 minutes. The degree of bronchoconstriction is rarely severe enough to be life threatening. If severe, there is often a
component of poorly controlled underlying disease or concomitant allergen or irritant exposure.

Exercise-induced bronchospasm can be confirmed with spirometry by showing
more than a 15% decrease in FEV_1 after exercise. In addition, peak flow readings
can be performed before and after exercise to document decreased airflow. The
diagnosis can also be suspected with alleviation of symptoms with use of a prophylactic
medication, such as a $β_2$-agonist before exercise. This phenomenon is discussed in
detail below in Sect. 6.7.7. Special Groups.

6.6.4 Vocal Cord Dysfunction

Vocal cord dysfunction, particularly diagnosis and management, is discussed above
in the section on Differential Diagnosis. Although vocal cord dysfunction can
present as an asthma masquerader, it is common for asthma and vocal cord

dysfunction to coexist. As many as 50% of patients with a diagnosis of vocal cord dysfunction also have airway hyperresponsiveness. It is estimated that 10–20% of asthma patients may have some component of vocal cord dysfunction. Of interest, other comorbidities for asthma are also associated with vocal cord dysfunction, including rhinitis and GERD. Rhinitis and GERD should be treated to minimize their contribution to irritation of the vocal cords. Coexisting vocal cord dysfunction should be considered in patients with known asthma that has become difficult to control, particularly if the clinical pattern features sudden onset and resolution of symptoms, a minimal response to increased asthma therapy, or symptoms localized to the vocal cords.

6.6.5 Irritants and Pollutants

Persons with asthma are more sensitive than those without asthma to air pollutants and irritants such as environmental cigarette smoke, traffic emissions, and photochemical smog components. Increased pollution levels, including particulates (<10 μm), sulfur dioxide, and nitric oxide, increase asthma symptoms. Ozone exposure and proximity to major roadways are associated with an increased incidence of the disease. Recently, complex organic molecules from diesel exhaust particles have been associated with worsening asthma and may also act, as other pollutants do, as allergic adjuvants through airway inflammation, which enhance the severity of immune-mediated lung disease.

Of the irritants and pollutants, cigarette smoke has been the most studied because it is likely the most important indoor pollutant that is harmful to human health. Tobacco smoke contains more than 4,000 chemical substances, many of which are carcinogenic, mutagenic, irritating, or toxic. Postnatal exposure to environmental tobacco smoke shows a causal link with the development of asthma in childhood. This is dose dependent, with the strongest effect detected in the youngest children. There is also evidence that environmental tobacco smoke exposure is related to an increased risk of adult-onset asthma, with the risk often most strongly related to workplace environmental tobacco smoke exposure as opposed to home exposure. There is evidence of a dose–response relationship. Although extensive evidence shows that ambient air pollution exacerbates existing asthma, the link with the development of asthma is less established, but it has been suggested. There are approximately 300 occupational asthmagens. Because exposures in the industrial workplace are often identifiable, the offending agent can usually be isolated. Occupational asthma has been prevented successfully through the identification and reduction of workplace exposure to enzymes in the detergent industry and the use of powdered natural rubber latex gloves in the health care industry.

It is important to inquire about the exposure to pollutants and irritants in both the home and work environment, particularly environmental cigarette smoke. Parents should be educated and encouraged not to smoke, or to quit if they are already smokers, to reduce childhood exposure. Once an asthmagen is recognized in the workplace, issues with respect to exposure, dose–response, and avoidance need to be addressed. Additional studies linking irritants and pollutants with asthma are needed to help determine the most effective way for individuals to be protected.

6.6.6   Rhinosinusitis (United Airway Hypothesis)

The link between upper airway and lower airway disease has long been of interest to clinicians. Recently, epidemiologic, immunologic, and therapeutic links have been established among rhinitis, sinusitis, and asthma. This has led to the concept of *united airways disease*, or *allergic rhinobronchitis*. The existence of the "united airways" was first deduced from epidemiologic studies. Several cross-sectional studies have shown the association between rhinitis and asthma: up to 50% of patients with rhinitis have asthma, and rhinitis occurs in up to 80% of patients with asthma. Longitudinal studies have confirmed this link and have shown that rhinitis usually precedes and is a risk factor for asthma, even independently of atopic status.

From the physiologic and immunologic standpoint, several studies have shown that the upper and lower respiratory airways behave as a single entity. It has been shown that a high percentage of patients with perennial allergic rhinitis alone without a clinical diagnosis of asthma have bronchial hyperreactivity and obstructive spirometric impairments. A direct correlation between the degree of nonspecific bronchial responsiveness (methacholine challenge) and the degree of nonspecific nasal responsiveness (histamine challenge) has been shown in patients with asthma and rhinitis. Bronchial mucosal inflammation mirrors changes seen in the nose with allergen challenge. These changes are bidirectional, whereby nasal challenge results in both nose and bronchial inflammation, and bronchial challenge also results in both nose and bronchial inflammation. This mechanism for the "cross-talk" between the nose and the lungs has not been clarified completely, but it has been hypothesized that these systemic events are mediated by a neurohumoral mechanism and the effect of cytokine release on the bone marrow.

The link between rhinitis and asthma has also been shown by the effect of medications on the nose and lung. Treatment of rhinitis with intranasal corticosteroids has a favorable effect on bronchial symptoms. Other studies have shown that correct treatment of rhinitis significantly reduces the rate of hospital admissions and emergency department visits for asthma exacerbation. Antihistamines have been shown to reduce asthma symptoms and bronchodilator use in patients with allergic rhinitis and asthma. Allergen immunotherapy has been shown to decrease the symptoms of asthma and to help prevent the development of asthma in adults and children who have seasonal or perennial rhinitis.

All asthma patients should be assessed carefully for rhinitis by environmental history, symptoms, and physical examination. Appropriate treatment of the rhinitis allows for better management of the asthma and may also favorably alter its course.

6.6.7 Smoking

In developed countries, approximately 25% of adults with asthma are current smokers and another 25% are former smokers. Asthma patients who smoke have worse symptom control, greater need for rescue medication, accelerated decrease in lung function, increased mortality rate at 6 years after a near-fatal asthma attack, alterations in the airway inflammatory cell milieu, and a decreased therapeutic response to corticosteroids.

There are numerous inflammatory changes in asthma patients who smoke compared with asthma patients who do not smoke. Of interest, the number of eosinophils is increased in sputum samples of asthma patients who smoke. In smokers, proinflammatory cytokines are increased, including IL-4, IL-8 and TNF-α, and anti-inflammatory cytokines, IL-10 and IL-18, are decreased. Exhaled nitric oxide levels are decreased in steroid-naïve smokers with mild asthma compared with those who are nonsmokers. Cigarette smoke may decrease exhaled nitric oxide by inhibiting inducible nitric oxide synthetase. In normal smokers, exhaled nitric oxide levels then increase after smoking cessation. Currently, it is not clear which of these effects is most important in causing asthma difficulty.

Cigarette smoking and asthma combine to accelerate lung function decline to a greater degree than either variable alone. The Copenhagen City Heart Study, performed over a 15-year period, found that the average annual decline in FEV_1 for asthma patients who were nonsmokers was 33 mL, whereas for asthma patients who smoked, it was 58 mL for males 40–59 years old. Perhaps most important for the long term is the reduced effectiveness of corticosteroids in asthma patients who smoke. In studies ranging from 3 weeks to 9 months, asthma patients who did not smoke had a significant increase in morning peak expiratory flow, mean FEV_1, and the mean provocative concentration required to elicit a 20% decrease in FEV_1 with methacholine compared with placebo, whereas no change was noted in asthma patients who smoked. Even oral prednisolone failed to provide a significant improvement in FEV_1, morning PEF, and asthma control score in asthma patients who smoked, whereas these parameters were improved in asthma patients who did not smoke.

The best treatment for smokers with asthma is smoking cessation. Former smokers, as opposed to current smokers, show improvement in morning PEF values after oral corticosteroid treatment. Smoking cessation in nonasthma subjects reduces respiratory symptoms and the frequency of respiratory infections. Over time, the rate of decline of lung function returns to that of never smokers. Few data are available of direct study of asthma patients who smoked but have quit. Nicotine replacement therapy or a medication such as bupropion in the setting of a structured smoking cessation program is most likely to be effective in smoking cessation. Smokers with asthma who are unable to stop may require alternative treatment or treatment in addition to corticosteroids. Cigarette smoke induces the CYP family of the cytochrome P-450 enzymes, which increases the clearance of theophylline. There is almost a twofold decrease in the half-life in smokers as compared with nonsmokers. Little information is available about the effects of other antiasthma drugs such as leukotriene antagonists or β_2-agonists. Theoretically, leukotriene antagonists may be of benefit for asthma patients who smoke because cigarette smoking induces higher levels of urinary leukotriene E_4.

6.6.8 Medications

Medications have the potential to exacerbate asthma. The most common medications implicated in exacerbating asthma are β-adrenergic blockers (β-blockers) and aspirin and other NSAIDs.

β-Blockers are useful in the treatment of numerous disease states, including hypertension, congestive heart failure, coronary artery disease, glaucoma, and migraine headache. They can be divided into multiple groupings, but the most practical classification is selective and nonselective β-blockers. Selective β-blockers are β_1 selective or cardioselective, preferentially blocking β_1-receptors in the heart. Common selective β_1-blockers include atenolol (Tenormin), metoprolol (Toprol), betaxolol (Kerlone), and bisoprolol (Zebeta). At higher doses, however, β_2 blockade also begins to occur and becomes more pronounced as the dosage is increased. Nonselective β-blockers block β_1 receptors in the heart as well as the β_2 receptors on bronchial smooth muscle cells. The commonly used nonselective β-agonists include propranolol (Inderal), sotalol (Betapace), timolol (Blocadren) and nadolol (Corgard). Timolol and betaxolol (Betoptic) are topical eye drop β-blockers used to treat glaucoma. Even though they are used topically, they have been reported to cause severe exacerbations of asthma. Patients often do not know the name of the eye drops they use; β-blockers usually have a yellow or blue cap on the bottle. Generally, nonselective β-adrenergic antagonists are more likely to induce bronchospasm in patients with known asthma than the selective β_1-blockers. However, severe exacerbations of asthma have been reported in both groups, with the exacerbations occurring in patients with mild, moderate, or severe asthma. The actual incidence of a severe asthma exacerbation with the use of a cardioselective or nonselective β-agonist is unknown. Certainly, some asthma patients are able to tolerate the use of cardioselective β-blockers without difficulty. According to a recent systematic review, a single dose of a cardioselective β-blocker produced a 7.46% reduction in FEV_1, whereas treatment for 3–28 days produced no change in FEV_1.

In determining the use of a β-blocker in treating an asthma patient, the benefit-to-risk ratio requires review. For strictly migraine prophylaxis, hypertension, or glaucoma, other medication options should likely be considered for asthma patients. For patients with severe angina, coronary artery disease, or congestive heart failure, for which β-blockers have been shown to decrease morbidity and mortality, a cardioselective β-blocker can be considered, particularly for a patient with mild, well-controlled asthma. However, there is no test or clinical pattern that predicts an asthma flare with the use of a β-blocker. If a cardioselective β-blocker is to be used, the patient should be counseled on the possibility of an asthma exacerbation and appropriate measures should be instituted to manage a possible exacerbation. Nonselective β-blockers should be avoided.

Aspirin and other NSAIDs can induce rhinorrhea and bronchospasm in a subset of patients with underlying rhinosinusitis, nasal polyps, and asthma. Various terms have been used to describe this phenomenon, including aspirin intolerance, aspirin sensitivity, aspirin-induced asthma, and aspirin idiosyncrasy. Currently, it is called *aspirin-exacerbating respiratory disease* (AERD). Aspirin and other NSAIDs that inhibit COX-1 cause this reaction. Because these reactions are dose dependent, small doses may not induce the reaction, but large doses may. Although aspirin and NSAID exposure trigger a respiratory reaction, sometimes very severe, the underlying asthma and rhinosinusitis continue in the absence of exposure to aspirin or NSAIDs. Except for sensitivity to aspirin and NSAIDs, these patients cannot be differentiated from other patients with asthma and sinus disease. The prevalence of aspirin and NSAID sensitivity among asthma patients with associated rhinosinusitis and nasal polyps is approximately 30–40%. In asthma patients without nasal polyposis, aspirin and NSAID sensitivity is approximately 10%. There is no skin test or in vitro test to identify these patients because the reaction is not IgE mediated. The reaction is mediated by COX-1 inhibition, which results in a decrease in the protective prostaglandin E_2 (PGE_2) and an increase in the production of inflammatory leukotrienes and prostaglandins. All the NSAIDs that inhibit COX-1 cross-react with aspirin, inducing the respiratory reaction. These include the most commonly used NSAIDs such as indomethacin, ibuprofen, and naproxen. Weak inhibitors of COX-1 such as acetaminophen and salsalate can produce respiratory reactions in patients with AERD, but this typically occurs only with large doses and only in a small proportion of these patients. Selective COX-2 inhibitors such as celecoxib and rofecoxib do not appear to cross-react with aspirin and appear to be safe for patients with AERD.

For patients with AERD for whom aspirin or NSAID therapy is critical, such as patients with coronary artery disease who need aspirin prophylaxis, patients with severe arthritis unresponsive to other treatments, or patients with AERD with intractable nasal polyp formation and rhinosinusitis, aspirin can be given through a supervised, graded, desensitization protocol. This protocol is outlined in the chapter on rhinosinusitis. The pathogenesis of aspirin desensitization is largely unknown, but it results in aspirin and NSAID tolerance when continued daily and, over time, down-regulation of leukotriene production.

6.6.9   Occupational

Occupational asthma, an often overlooked cause for asthma, is reviewed at the end of this chapter in the section Special Groups.

6.6.10   Obstructive Sleep Apnea

Obstructive sleep apnea is characterized by intermittent partial or total (or both) airway occlusion during sleep and is associated with serious health consequences, including insulin resistance, hypertension, cardiovascular diseases, and worsening of asthma control. It is estimated that 20% of adults have mild obstructive sleep apnea, and in nearly 7%, it is moderate to severe. The majority of patients, 50–90%, with nighttime asthma symptoms or severe asthma, have obstructive sleep apnea. Treatment with continuous positive airway pressure significantly improves nighttime symptom control but little change in baseline spirometry.

6.6.11 Gastroesophageal Reflux Disease

The true incidence of GERD in asthma and as a causative factor in asthma severity has not been fully established. It has been estimated that 45–65% of asthma patients have GERD. Epidemiologic evidence has established an association between GERD and asthma, and some evidence supports a causative role. The proposed mechanisms by which GERD may affect asthma include microaspiration of gastric refluxate or a vagally mediated esophagobronchial reflex mechanism with subsequent bronchospasm. Although no unique clinical identifiers establish whether GERD is contributing to asthma, it should be considered in difficult-to-control asthma, nonallergic asthma, asthma with moderate to severe GERD, and nocturnal asthma. Clinical suspicion is a critical component in the diagnosis of GERD-induced asthma. In patients with a history suggestive of the condition, an empiric trial of a high-dose proton pump inhibitor for 3–6 months is a reasonable strategy. Appreciable changes in spirometry in the short term are not typically seen. Esophageal pH monitoring should be performed in asthma patients with GERD symptoms that do not respond to an empiric trial of proton pump inhibitors and in patients in whom asymptomatic GERD (silent GERD) may have a role. Silent GERD may be present in up to one-third of asthma patients. Surgical therapy for GERD-triggered asthma may hold promise. Thus far, data consist mainly of uncontrolled studies. Additional large randomized studies in subgroups of patients with asthma treated with proton pump inhibitors or surgical intervention will help clarify the role of GERD treatment in asthma.

6.7 Treatment

The overall treatment of asthma is multifactorial, with the general goal of disease control. The key components to obtaining asthma control are patient education, evaluation, and management of all the asthma-exacerbating factors and the use of appropriate pharmacotherapy. All these components – not just pharmacotherapy – are integral to patient management.

6.7.1 Patient Education

In asthma as in other chronic diseases, education serves as the foundation to be built upon to obtain disease control. Key points that should be emphasized in asthma education include understanding (1) the basics of asthma, (2) the rationale for the use of the different medications, (3) the importance of compliance with the medications, (4) the correct use of the various inhalers and peak flow meters, (5) environmental modification of triggers of asthma, (6) recognizing and responding to asthma symptoms, and (7) knowing when to call a physician or to seek emergency department care. These seem to be self-evident; however, if they are not addressed with the patient repeatedly, as with other chronic diseases, compliance becomes poor, resulting in poor disease control.

Asthma education is not a one-time experience. To be effective, asthma education needs to be an ongoing experience that builds over time. This requires time and dedication by the health care team. Communication with the patient is needed to establish treatment goals that result in the patient living a normal lifestyle with minimal to no symptoms and reduce the risk of asthma exacerbations.

6.7.2   Pharmacologic Therapy

Medications for asthma can be divided into two major categories: medications for as-needed use, termed *quick-relief medications*, and medications for daily use, termed *long-term control* or *maintenance medications*. All patients with asthma should have a short-acting bronchodilator for as-needed use. All patients with persistent asthma, whether mild, moderate, or severe, should be using at least one long-term daily asthma controller medication with anti-inflammatory properties. Even though long-acting β-agonists such as salmeterol and formoterol are considered long-term control medications, they should only be prescribed in conjunction with a daily anti-inflammatory agent. The usual dosages for long-term control medications are listed in Table 6.11 and the dosages for the quick-relief medications, in Table 6.12. Although asthma medications are available in multiple forms, they are administered primarily by the inhalation route.

6.7.2.1   Inhalation Devices

The inhalation of therapeutic aerosols is an effective method of drug delivery in the management of asthma. Three principal types of devices are used to generate aerosols: metered dose inhalers (MDIs), dry powder inhalers (DPIs), and nebulizers. All three use different mechanisms to generate aerosols, and the differences among them are important for discerning the most appropriate device for drug delivery, depending on characteristics of the patient and the therapeutic agent used.

Metered Dose Inhaler

Most inhaled medications currently used for asthma are available as MDIs. MDI technology has used primarily chlorofluorocarbons as propellants. Chlorofluorocarbons

Table 6.11 Usual dosages for long-term control medications

Medication	Dosage form	Adult dose	Child dose
Systemic corticosteroids			
Methyl prednisolone	2-, 4-, 8-, 16-, 32-mg tablets	7.5–60 mg per day in single dose in am or qod as needed for control	0.25–2 mg kg^{-1} daily in single dose in am or qod as needed for control
Prednisolone	5-mg tablets, 5 mg per 5 mL, 15 mg per 5 mL	Short-course "burst" to achieve control: 40–60 mg per day as single or 2 divided doses for 3–10 days	Short-course "burst": 1–2 mg kg^{-1} per day, maximum 60mg per day for 3–10 days
Prednisone	1-, 2.5-, 5-, 10-, 20-, 50-mg tablets, 5 mg mL^{-1}, 5 mg per 5 mL		
Long-acting inhaled β$_2$ agonists[a]			
Salmeterol	MDI 21 μg per puff	2 puffs q12h	1–2 puffs q12h
	DPI 50 μg per blister	1 blister q12h	1 blister q12h
Formoterol	DPI 12 μg per single-use capsule	1 capsule q12h	1 capsule q12h
Combined medication			
Fluticasone-salmeterol	DPI 100, 250, or 500 μg per 50 μg	1 inhalation bid; dose depends on severity of asthma	1 inhalation bid; dose depends on severity of asthma
	MDI 45, 115, or 230 μg per 21 μg	2 puffs bid; dose depends on severity of asthma	2 puffs bid; dose depends on severity of asthma
Budesonide-formoterol	MDI 80 or 160 μg per 4.5 μg	2 puffs bid; dose depends on severity of asthma	2 puffs bid; dose depends on severity of asthma
Cromolyn and nedocromil			
Cromolyn	MDI 0.8 mg per puff	2–4 puffs tid–qid	1–2 puffs tid–qid
	Nebulizer 20 mg per ampule	1 ampule tid–qid	1 ampule tid–qid
Nedocromil	MDI 1.75 mg per puff	2–4 puffs bid–qid	1–2 puffs bid–qid
Leukotriene modifiers			
Montelukast	4- or 5-mg chewable tablet	10 mg qhs	4 mg qhs (1–5 years)
	4-mg granule packets		5 mg qhs (6–14 years)
	10-mg tablet		10 mg qhs (>14 years)

(Continued)

Table 6.11 (Continued)

Medication	Dosage form	Adult dose	Child dose
Zafirlukast[b]	10- or 20-mg tablet	40 mg daily (20-mg tablet bid)	20 mg daily (7–11 years) (10-mg tablet bid)
Zileuton[b]	300- or 600-mg tablet	2,400 mg daily (give tablets qid)	
Methylxanthines[c]			
Theophylline	Liquids, sustained-release tablets, and capsules	Starting dose 10 mg kg^{-1} per day; usual max 800 mg per day	Starting dose 10 mg kg^{-1} per day; usual max: <1 year of age: 0.2 (age in weeks) + 5 = mg kg^{-1} per day ≥1 year of age: 16 mg kg^{-1} per day

From the National Asthma Education and Prevention Program, Expert Panel Report (2002) Guidelines for the management and diagnosis of asthma – update on selected topics 2002. NIH Publication No. 02-5075. Bethesda, MD: US Department of Health and Human Services; National Institutes of Health; National Heart, Lung and Blood Institute and from the National Asthma Education and Prevention Program: Expert Panel Report 3. (2007) Guidelines for the diagnosis and management of asthma. NIH publication No. 07-4051. Bethesda, MD: U.S. Department of Health and Human Services; National Institutes of Health; National Heart, Lung and Blood Institute

bid twice daily; *DPI* dry powder inhaler; *MDI* metered-dose inhaler; *max* maximum; *q12h* every 12h; *qhs* at bedtime; *qid* 4 times daily; *qod* every other day; *tid* 3 times daily

[a]Should not be used for symptom relief or for exacerbations. Use with inhaled corticosteroids

[b]Monitor liver function tests

[c]Serum monitoring is important (serum concentration of 5–15 μg mL^{-1} at steady state)

Table 6.12 Usual dosages for quick-relief medications

Medication	Dosage form	Adult/adolescent dose	Child dose	Comments
Short-acting inhaled β₂-agonists				
	MDI			An increasing use or lack of expected effect indicates diminihed control of asthma; not generally recommended for daily long-term treatment
Albuterol	90 µg per puff	2 puffs q4h as needed and 15 min before exercise (applies to all four medications)	1–2 puffs q4h as needed and 15 min before exercise (applies to albuterol and levalbuterol for ages 5–11 years and albuterol for ages <5 years)	Use for symptom relief >2 times weekly indicates need for additional therapy
Albuterol HFA	90 µg per puff			Differences in potency exist so that all products are essentially equipotent on a per-puff basis
Pirbuterol	200 µg per puff			May double usual dose for significant exacerbations
Levalbuterol HFA	45 µg per puff			Nonselective agents (e.g., epinephrine, isoproterenol, metaproterenol) are not recommended
	DPI			
Albuterol Rotahaler	200 µg per capsule	1–2 capsules q4–6h as needed and before exercise	1 capsule q4–6h as needed and before exercise	
	Nebulizer solution			
Albuterol	5 mg mL^{-1} (0.5%) multi-dose vial	1.25–5 mg (0.25–1 mL) in 2–3 mL of saline q4–6h	0.1–0.2 mg kg^{-1} (minimum 1.25 mg, max. 2.5 mg) in 2–3 mL	May mix with cromolyn or ipratropium nebulizer solutions or saline q4–6h
	2.5 mg per 3 mL (0.83%) unit-dose vial 0.63 mg per 3 mL and 1.25 mg per 3 mL	1 vial q4–6h	1/2–1 vial q4–6h	May double dose for significant exacerbations
Levalbuterol	0.31 mg, 0.63 mg, or 1.25 mg per 3 mL	0.63–1.25 mg q6–8h	0.31–0.63 mg q6–8h (ages 5–11 years) 0.31–1.25 mg q4–6h (age <5 years)	

(Continued)

Table 6.12 (Continued)

Medication	Dosage form	Adult/adolescent dose	Child dose	Comments
Anticholinergics				
	MDI			
Ipratropium	18 µg per puff	2–3 puffs q6h	1–2 puffs q6h	Evidence is lacking for producing added benefit to β$_2$-agonists in long-term asthma therapy
Ipratropium with albuterol	18 µg per puff of ipratropium bromide and 90 µg per puff of albuterol	2–3 puffs q6h	...	
	Nebulizer solution			
Ipratropium	0.25 mg mL^{-1} (0.02%)	0.25–0.5 mg q6–8h	0.25 mg q6–8h	
Ipratropium with albuterol	0.5 mg per 3 mL ipratropium bromide and 2.5 mg per 3 mL albuterol	3 mL q4–6h	1.5 mL q4–6h	
Systemic corticosteroids Methylprednisolone	2-, 4-, 8-, 16-, 32-mg tablets	Short-course "burst"; 40–60 mg per day as single or 2 divided doses for 3–10 days	Short-course "burst"; 1–2 mg kg^{-1} per day, maximum 60 mg per day, for 3–10 days	Short courses or "bursts" are effective for establishing control when initiating therapy or during a period of gradual deterioration. Burst should be continued until patient achieves 80% PEF personal best or symptoms resolve. Usually achieved in 3–10 days, may require longer treatment periods. No evidence that tapering the dose after improvement prevents relapse
Prednisolone	5-mg tablets, 5 mg per 5 mL, 15 mg per 5 mL			
Prednisone	1-, 2.5-, 5-, 10-, 20-, 25-, 50-mg tablets; 5 mg mL^{-1}, 15 mg per 5 mL solutions			

Modified from the National Asthma Education and Prevention Program. Expert Panel Report (2002) Guidelines for the management and diagnosis of asthma – update on selected topics 2002. NIH Publication No. 02-5075. Bethesda, MD: US Department of Health and Human Services; National Institutes of Health; National Heart, Lung and Blood Institute and the National Asthma Education and Prevention Program: Expert Panel Report 3. (2007) Guidelines for the diagnosis and management of asthma. NIH publication No. 07-4051. Bethesda, MD: U.S. Department of Health and Human Services; National Institutes of Health; National Heart, Lung and Blood Institute

DPI dry powder inhaler; *HFA* hydroxyfluoroalkane; *max* maximum; *MDI* metered-dose inhaler; *q4h* every 4h; *q4–q6h* every 4-6h; *PEF* peak expiratory flow

constitute approximately 95% of the formulation released from an MDI. However, they have been found to deplete the stratospheric ozone, and, following adoption of the Montreal protocol, an international agreement has been placed to ban chlorofluorocarbons. The alternatives include MDIs with other propellants, such as hydrofluoroalkane and the DPIs. The U.S. Food and Drug Administration (FDA) approval process for new inhalers requires that the replacement products demonstrate comparability with the corresponding chlorofluorocarbon-containing inhalers so that clinicians and patients can anticipate similar effectiveness and safety with the new products. Currently, fluticasone, levalbuterol, and albuterol are available in hydrofluoroalkane formulations.

Spacers and valved holding chambers are accessory devices that reduce oropharyngeal deposition of the drug, enhance lung delivery, and minimize the importance of the hand–breath coordination. A spacer device is an open-ended tube that allows the MDI plume to slow down and the propellant to evaporate before inhalation. A valved holding chamber incorporates a one-way valve that traps the plume and allows the aerosol to be delivered from the chamber only during inspiration. A valved holding chamber can incorporate a mask for patients who are unable to use a mouthpiece because of age, poor coordination, or impaired mental status. The accessory devices should be washed with dishwashing detergent and allowed to air dry to remove residue from the medication and to eliminate static charge.

Dry Powder Inhaler

DPIs function by drawing air through a dose of powdered medication. This requires an inspiration at relatively high inspiratory flow rates. Larger carrier particles impact in the oropharynx, giving the patient the sensation of having inhaled the dose. However, this impaction is less than with an MDI, and patients may feel that they are not receiving any medication. DPIs are breath actuated; thus, coordination between manual inhaler actuation and inspiration is not required. However, because the magnitude and duration of the patient's inspiratory effort influence the aerosol generation from the DPI, these devices should be used cautiously in the very young, elderly, and those with neuromuscular weakness. Some DPIs require manual manipulation to load the dose, and this may be difficult for patients with limited dexterity. DPIs do not require the use of spacing devices.

Nebulization

Nebulization requires a pressurized gas supply that allows liquid atomization of the medication. Several factors contribute to the efficiency of the nebulization, including the respirable dose, nebulization time, dead volume, and patient interface. The respirable dose is a function of the total output of the nebulizer and the size of the particles produced. Droplet size should be 2–5 μm for airway deposition and 1–2 μm for parenchymal deposition. The nebulization time is an important determinant of patient compliance in the outpatient setting. This is a function of the volume of drug to be delivered and the flow rate of the driving gas. The treatment is complete when the nebulizer begins sputtering. Although nebulizers typically are used intermittently, continuous nebulizations can be administered in the emergency department or during hospital treatment of acute asthma. The volume of the medication trapped inside the nebulizer is referred to as the dead volume of the device. This volume is typically in the range of 1–3 mL. Increasing the fill volume helps to decrease the proportion of the dose lost as dead volume. This maneuver increases nebulization time. Considering these factors, a nebulizer fill volume of 4–6 mL is generally recommended. During nebulization, the solution within the nebulizer becomes increasingly concentrated as water evaporates from the solution; therefore, per breath, more medication is delivered late in the course of treatment. Nebulized aerosols can be administered with a mouthpiece or face mask. Because significant facial and eye deposition can occur when a face mask is used, a mouth piece is usually favored. Generally, for home use, MDIs or DPIs are recommended, and nebulizations are reserved for severe acute exacerbations. For patients unable to tolerate MDIs or DPIs, a nebulizer is an option.

6.7.2.2 Inhaled Corticosteroids

Corticosteroids are the most potent and effective long-term control medications for asthma. Their anti-inflammatory properties include the suppression of airway eosinophil recruitment, the suppression of cytokine production, and the suppression of inflammatory mediator release. Their clinical effects include reduction in the severity of symptoms, improvement in PEFR and spirometry, diminished airway hyperresponsiveness, prevention of exacerbations, and possibly the prevention of airway remodeling. Inhaled corticosteroids should be considered a first-line treatment for patients with mild, moderate, or severe persistent asthma. As a single agent, inhaled corticosteroids are more effective than theophylline, salmeterol, nedocromil, and leukotriene modifiers in the management of asthma.

The choice of a specific inhaled corticosteroid depends on the potency of the corticosteroid required and the delivery device. There is a significant difference in the potency among the various inhaled corticosteroids (Table 6.13). Realization of these differences is important in initiating or adjusting therapy. For example, for a patient with moderate-to-severe persistent asthma, a more potent corticosteroid such as budesonide or fluticasone (220 μg) would be used instead of triamcinolone or beclomethasone in an effort to minimize puffs. In contrast, for a patient with mild persistent asthma, lower potency corticosteroids could be prescribed, such as fluticasone (44 μg), triamcinolone, or beclomethasone. In principle, each patient should receive the lowest effective dose required to achieve good asthma control. On the basis of an evaluation of symptoms, supplemental bronchodilator use, exacerbations, peak flow, spirometry, and possibly sputum eosinophils and exhaled nitric oxide, the dose of inhaled corticosteroid can be adjusted so that the lowest effective dose is used.

Table 6.13 Estimated comparative daily dosages for inhaled corticosteroids

Drug	Low daily dose		Medium daily dose		High daily dose	
	Adult	Child[a]	Adult	Child[a]	Adult	Child[a]
Beclomethasone CFC 42 or 84 µg per puff	168–504 µg	84–336 µg	504–840 µg	336–672 µg	>840 µg	>672 µg
Beclomethasone HFA 40 or 80 µg per puff	80–240 µg	80–160 µg	240–480 µg	160–320 µg	>480 µg	>320 µg
Budesonide DPI 90, 180, or 200 µg per inhalation	180–600 µg	180–400 µg	600–1,200 µg	400–800 µg	>1,200 µg	>800 µg
Inhalation suspension for nebulization (child dose)		0.5 mg		1.0 mg		2.0 mg
Flunisolide 250 µg per puff	500–1,000 µg	500–750 µg	1,000–2,000 µg	1,000–1,250 µg	>2,000 µg	>1,250 µg
Flunisolide HFA 80 µg per puff	320 µg	160 µg	320–640 µg	320 µg	>640 µg	≥640 µg
Fluticasone						
MDI: 44, 110, or 220 µg per puff	88–264 µg	88–176 µg	264–440 µg	176–352 µg	>440 µg	>352 µg
DPI: 50, 100, or 250 µg per inhalation	100–300 µg	100–200 µg	300–500 µg	200–400 µg	>500 µg	>400 µg
Triamcinolone acetonide 75 µg per puff	300–750 µg	300–600 µg	750–1,500 µg	600–900 µg	>1,500 µg	>900 µg
Mometasone DPI 200 µg per puff	200 µg	NA	400 µg	NA	>400 µg	NA

From the National Asthma Education and Prevention Program, Expert Panel Report (2002) Guidelines for the management and diagnosis of asthma – update on selected topics 2002. NIH Publication No. 02-5075. Bethesda, MD: US Department of Health and Human Services: National Institutes of Health; National Heart, Lung and Blood Institute and the National Asthma Education and Prevention Program: Expert Panel Report 3. (2007) Guidelines for the diagnosis and management of asthma. NIH publication No. 07-4051. Bethesda, MD: U.S. Department of Health and Human Services; National Institutes of Health; National Heart, Lung and Blood Institute

CFC chlorofluorocarbon; *DPI* dry powder inhaler; *HFA* hydroxyfluoroalkane; *MDI* metered-dose inhaler; *NA* no data available

[a] Children ≤12 years old

The safety of inhaled corticosteroids has been studied extensively. Systemic effects have been identified, particularly at high doses, but their clinical significance is unclear. There may be interindividual variations in dose–response effects. In general, the potential for adverse effects must be weighed against the risk of uncontrolled asthma; to date, the evidence supports the use of inhaled corticosteroids.

The most common side effects from inhaled corticosteroids are local adverse effects: oral candidiasis (thrush) and dysphonia. Oral candidiasis is more frequent in adults than children. It typically is seen when high doses of inhaled corticosteroids are used. To significantly decrease the risk of oral candidiasis developing, a spacer device should be used with the MDI formulations and, with all methods of inhalation, the mouth should be rinsed after inhaler use. Dysphonia is seen primarily with high doses of inhaled corticosteroids. This can be prevented and treated by rinsing the mouth after inhalation, using a spacer device, reducing the dosage, and resting the voice.

The most studied systemic side effects of inhaled corticosteroids include linear growth, bone metabolism and osteoporosis, hypothalamic-pituitary axis function, and cataracts. The effect of inhaled corticosteroids on growth in children is difficult to study because of multiple confounding factors on growth, including the concomitant use of systemic corticosteroids, concomitant atopy, and asthma itself. A few studies of children with asthma treated with inhaled corticosteroids have identified some growth delay, but others have not shown a difference. Even with growth delay, it appears that the expected height is still attained or decreased by 1 cm. Low-to-medium doses of inhaled corticosteroids appear to have no serious adverse effects on bone mineral density in children. A small, dose-dependent decrease in bone mineral density may be found in adults, but the clinical significance is not clear. In children, low-to-medium dose of inhaled corticosteroid therapy has no significant effect on the incidence of subcapsular cataracts or glaucoma. In adults, high lifetime exposure to inhaled corticosteroids may increase the prevalence of cataracts. An association between glaucoma and long-term high-dose inhaled corticosteroids may be seen in those with a family history of glaucoma.

6.7.2.3 Leukotriene-Modifying Agents

Leukotrienes are inflammatory mediators that are released from mast cells, eosinophils, and basophils. They are products of arachadonic acid metabolism. Leukotrienes cause the contraction of airway smooth muscle, increase vascular permeability, increase mucus secretions, and recruit inflammatory cells into the airways. Leukotriene-modifying agents are divided into two groups: the 5-lipoxygenase inhibitor (zileuton) and the leukotriene-receptor antagonists (zafirlukast and montelukast). Zileuton inhibits the formation of leukotrienes B_4, C_4, D_4, and E_4. Zafirlukast and montelukast inhibit the binding of the cysteinyl leukotrienes C_4, D_4, and E_4 to the leukotriene receptor. The leukotriene modifiers are indicated as monotherapy for the treatment of mild persistent asthma. They should be considered for these patients who prefer an oral agent or who are unable or unwilling to use inhaled corticosteroids. When comparing the overall effectiveness of leukotriene modifiers with inhaled corticosteroids, most outcome measures significantly favor inhaled corticosteroids. Leukotriene modifiers can be used in combination with an inhaled corticosteroid for moderate or severe persistent asthma. The leukotriene modifiers can help reduce symptoms of allergic rhinitis. This may be a consideration for patients with coexisting asthma and allergic rhinitis.

Zileuton may increase liver transaminases, and follow-up with liver transaminase testing is recommended monthly for 3 months, then every 2–3 months for the rest of the first year and periodically thereafter for long-term therapy. No specific recommendation has been made for monitoring liver transaminases in conjunction with zafirlukast or montelukast therapy. Leukotriene modifiers have been linked to cases of Churg–Strauss vasculitis. Some observers have suggested that these cases were primary eosinophilic disorders that were unmasked as systemic corticosteroids were tapered with leukotriene-modifier therapy. However, eosinophilic disorders have been associated with leukotriene modifier treatment even in the absence of previous corticosteroid therapy. If this association is true, it appears to be very rare.

Zileuton is approved for children older than 12 years and for adults. The dosage is 600 mg four times daily. Montelukast, 4 mg daily, is administered in granules or chewable tablet form to children 12 months to 5 years old. The dosage for ages 6–14 years is 5 mg daily and for those 15 years and older, 10 mg daily. For zafirlukast, the dosage is 10 mg twice daily for ages 5–11 years and 20 mg twice daily for those 12 years and older. Concomitant use of warfarin results in higher warfarin levels and subsequently higher prothrombin time levels; thus, close monitoring and adjustment are advised.

6.7.2.4 Chromones

Nedocromil and cromolyn are mild anti-inflammatory agents that inhibit the release of mast cell mediators. They inhibit the early and late phase responses to allergen challenge and are bronchoprotective for exercise. They are second-line agents that may be used to treat mild persistent asthma or as prophylaxis for exercise-induced asthma and allergen-induced asthma. The effectiveness of nedocromil and cromolyn are similar to that of leukotriene antagonists and theophylline. They are less effective than inhaled corticosteroids. Cromolyn is available as an MDI or DPI or in solution for nebulization. Nedocromil is available as an MDI. The usual dosing is two puffs four times daily, although nedocromil may be given twice daily. Both have very few significant adverse effects. About 20% of patients find the taste of nedocromil unpleasant. Nedocromil and cromolyn are not recommended for moderate or severe persistent asthma.

6.7.2.5 Methylxanthines

Theophylline functions as a nonselective inhibitor of cyclic adenosine monophosphate phosphodiesterases in airway smooth muscle, resulting in bronchodilatation.

Theophylline inhibits the activation of inflammatory cells in vitro; however, the clinical importance of the anti-inflammatory effect appears to be small. Theophylline is a second- or third-line agent for the daily treatment of persistent asthma. Sustained-release theophylline is effective for nocturnal asthma. For moderate or severe persistent asthma, theophylline can be given in combination with an inhaled corticosteroid.

Theophylline use is limited by its side effect profile. Adverse effects include nausea, headache, insomnia, diarrhea, irritability, and tremors. The recommended therapeutic range is 5–15 µg mL^{-1}. Lower doses, providing a serum level of 5–10 µg mL^{-1}, usually are tolerated better than higher doses. Because theophylline is metabolized through cytochrome P-450, it has significant drug interactions. Medicines that decrease the clearance of theophylline and, thus, increase theophylline levels include macrolide antibiotics, fluoroquinolone antibiotics, propranolol, diltiazem, verapamil, disulfiram, and oral contraceptives. Medications that increase theophylline clearance and decrease theophylline levels include phenytoin, phenobarbital, and cimetidine. If patients have been treated for several years with theophylline, care must be taken when discontinuing the medication. The abrupt withdrawal of theophylline can cause an exacerabation of asthma. If theophylline treatment is being discontinued, it is recommended that the theophylline be tapered slowly and the patient be aware of the possibility of asthma being exacerbated.

6.7.2.6 Long-Acting β$_2$-Agonists

In November 2005, the FDA issued an advisory on the use of long-acting β-agonists for asthma, requesting manufacturers to include warnings on the labels that these agents may worsen asthma exacerbations and increase the risk of death. This was based primarily on the Salmeterol Multicenter Asthma Research Trial (SMART). In this 28-week, randomized, double-blind placebo-controlled observational study, there was a small but statistically significant increase in respiratory-related and asthma-related deaths and combined asthma-related deaths or life-threatening experiences in the total population that received salmeterol. The risk appeared to be greater in African Americans than in Caucasians. The effect of concomitant inhaled corticosteroid use was not able to be interpreted in this study because of the design and lack of control of multiple variables. The interpretation of the results of this study and the subsequent FDA warning have engendered significant controversy, with some experts favoring the warning and others thinking it is overreaching. There is general agreement that in mild-to-moderate persistent asthma, inhaled corticosteroids should be administered in sufficient amounts to control symptoms, whereas for patients with more severe disease and who still require daily administration of albuterol in addition to adequate doses of inhaled corticosteroids, long-acting β-agonists may be added to relieve symptoms.

Long-acting β-agonists have extended hydrophobic side chains that interact with the lipid bilayer of the cell membrane, leading to a prolonged duration of action. Bronchodilatation begins approximately 10 min after inhalation of salmeterol, and the peak response is reached after several hours. Bronchodilatation begins in only 3 min after inhalation of formoterol, with peak bronchodilatation in about 1 hours. The duration of action of both salmeterol and formoterol is approximately 12 hours. Salmeterol is available in both MDI and DPI forms and formoterol is available in a DPI form.

The primary adverse effects of long-acting β-agonists are similar to those of short-acting β-agonists, namely, tremor and increased heart rate. Continuous use of salmeterol can decrease the bronchoprotective effect of salmeterol against exercise or bronchial challenge. Inhaled long-acting β-agonists should not be used for rescue or quick relief of asthma symptoms. As a controller agent, long-acting β-agonists should not be used as a single agent because they lack an anti-inflammatory effect.

Long-acting β-agonists are most effective as an adjunct to inhaled corticosteroids in the treatment of moderate-to-severe persistent asthma. They are particularly effective in the treatment of nocturnal asthma. The recommended dose of an inhaled long-acting β-agonist is two puffs twice daily for salmeterol MDI and one puff twice daily for salmeterol or formoterol DPI.

6.7.2.7   Short-Acting β_2-Agonists

Inhaled short-acting β_2-agonists are indicated for the immediate, as-needed control of asthma symptoms. This is often described as a "rescue" therapy. Also, short-acting β_2-agonists are used for prophylaxis of exercise-induced asthma and asthma provoked by allergic triggers. Short-acting β_2-agonists are selective β_2-agonists that act on bronchodilators through the relaxation of bronchial smooth muscle. Because β_2 receptors are also found in the heart, β_2-agonists can cause sympathomimetic side effects such as tachycardia, palpitations, and tremor.

Short-acting β_2-agonists can be given in nebulized, MDI, or oral forms. The primary β-agonists used are albuterol, pirbuterol, and levalbuterol. Levalbuterol is the R-isomer of racemic albuterol. Because it only contains the R-isomer, less albuterol can be used to achieve the same amount of bronchodilation. For short-acting β-agonists, the onset of bronchodilation occurs within minutes, peaks at about 15 min, and has a duration of action of about 4–6 hours.

Overuse of β-agonists has been linked to increased asthma morbidity and mortality. Most authors believe that β-agonists themselves are not the cause of the morbidity or mortality but rather their overuse is a marker for severe undertreated asthma. If a patient is using a canister of short-acting β_2-agonist monthly, the entire treatment program should be reviewed because this amount represents a warning for overall poorly controlled asthma. Short-acting β_2-agonists should be taken on an as-needed basis. Regular, daily treatment with short-acting β_2-agonists has no advantage.

6.7.2.8   Oral Corticosteroids

Systemic oral corticosteroids are indicated for the treatment of acute asthma and for severe persistent asthma of patients whose asthma is not well controlled by high-dose inhaled corticosteroids and long-acting β-agonists. Many oral corticosteroid products are available. Prednisone is the best studied and least expensive oral corticosteroid commonly used to treat asthma. The adverse effects of prolonged use of oral corticosteroids include hyperglycemia, growth suppression, osteoporosis, posterior subcapsular cataracts, fat redistribution, skin thinning and bruising, mood changes, and suppression of the hypothalamic-pituitary axis. In hospitalized patients without risk for impending ventilatory failure, oral prednisone appears to be as effective as intravenous corticosteroids. Prednisone, 40–80 mg per day or 1–2 mg kg^{-1} daily for children, may be given in divided doses. For patients with mild asthma that is typically well controlled, an exacerbation of asthma generally resolves with a 3- to 10-day course of prednisone. For patients who require long-term prednisone treatment, the dose should be titrated to the lowest effective dose. Prednisone can be administered daily or on alternate days. The alternate-day regimen may help reduce systemic adverse effects. Control of asthma should be assessed periodically by the evaluation of symptoms, supplemental bronchodilator use, exacerbations, peak flow, and spirometry to adjust the dose to the lowest effective dose. For patients receiving continuous dosing, blood pressure, height, weight, glucose, bone density, and cataracts should be assessed periodically. Adults may benefit from a preventive approach with calcium (1,200–1,500 mg per day) and vitamin D (age 51–70 years, 400 IU per day and >70 years, 800 IU per day) supplementation.

6.7.2.9   Anticholinergic Agents

Anticholinergic medications do not carry an approved indication for use in asthma, although they may be a useful alternative for people who are intolerant to the side effects of β-agonists. Anticholinergic medications are a first-line bronchodilator in patients with COPD. Patients with a combination of asthma and COPD are most likely to benefit from this medication. Anticholinergic agents block muscarinic receptors that regulate airway tone and mucus production, resulting in bronchodilation.

Anticholinergic agents are available in a short-acting form, ipratropium bromide (Atrovent), and a long-acting form, tiotropium bromide (Spiriva). Ipratropium can be given in nebulized form or by MDI. The bronchodilation peaks approximately 1 hours after inhalation and lasts for 4 hours. Ipratropium is also available in a combination form with albuterol (Combivent) that is available in both MDI and nebulized forms. Tiotropium is available as a DPI through a HandiHaler device. It is dosed as one inhalation once daily, with bronchodilation occurring over a 24-hours period. The main side effects from anticholinergic agents are dry mouth and occasional cough. They may potentially worsen symptoms associated with narrow-angle glaucoma, prostatic hyperplasia, or bladder neck obstruction and should be pre-scribed with caution in patients with these conditions.

6.7.2.10   Anti-Immunoglobulin E Antibody

Omalizumab is a humanized anti-IgE monoclonal antibody. This drug binds to the Fc portion of IgE, preventing the IgE from binding to the IgE receptor on mast cells. Omalizumab decreases the serum levels of IgE by at least 95% and disrupts type I IgE-mediated hypersensitivity reactions. Therefore, omalizumab is used in the treat-ment of allergic asthma. The current FDA-approved indication for omalizumab is for moderate-to-severe persistent allergic asthma. The medication is given subcutane-ously either every 2 weeks or every 4 weeks, depending on the dosage required. Dosing is based on the patient's weight and total IgE level. Allergen testing is required to establish allergic sensitivity. This can be performed with allergen skin prick testing or in vitro studies of IgE binding to the pertinent aeroallergens. In clini-cal studies, omalizumab, in both children older than 12 years and adults, resulted in improved symptoms, fewer disease exacerbations, and decreased use of other asthma medications such as corticosteroids. However, only minimal changes in measured airflow and airway hyperreactivity have been shown with omalizumab. No published clinical studies have compared the safety and effectiveness of omalizumab with cor-ticosteroids. Currently, omalizumab appears to be an effective anti-inflammatory agent, primarily in severe allergic asthma; its precise role in the management of allergic asthma has not been defined fully. In 2007, a boxed warning was added to the product label of omalizumab (Xolair). This addresses the risk of anaphylaxis, which is estimated to be at least 0.2% in postmarketing studies. Because of the risk of anaphylaxis, it is recommended that omalizumab be administered under medical supervision by providers who are able to treat anaphylaxis. Anaphylaxis can occur after any dose of the drug, and its onset can be delayed after administration.

6.7.2.11   Allergen Immunotherapy

Allergen immunotherapy consists of injections of allergen extracts to which the patient is allergic to induce an immunologic tolerance. In asthma, the airborne allergens, that is, animal dander, dust mites, mold, and tree, grass, and weed pollens, are injected to neutralize the allergic triggers of asthma in sensitive patients. There appear to be multiple mechanisms by which allergen immunotherapy is able to induce tolerance, including an increase in IgG blocking antibodies, the generation of suppressor T-cells, deviation from a Th2 to a Th1 cytokine release profile, and the production of T-cell tolerance.

  Several studies have documented improvement of asthma symptoms of patients receiving immunotherapy; however, not all controlled studies have been consist-ently positive. A 1995 meta-analysis found an odds ratio of symptomatic improve-ment with immunotherapy of 3.2 (95% CI, 2.2–4.9). A revision of this meta-analysis by the same authors in 2003 incorporated 20 new studies and again showed highly significant improvement in symptoms, nonspecific bronchial hyperreactivity, and risk of symptom deterioration in the immunotherapy groups.

Patients who have persistent or seasonal allergic nasal symptoms as well as asthma appear to benefit the most. The National Asthma Education and Prevention Program Expert Panel Report recommends that allergen immunotherapy be considered if there is clear evidence of a relation between symptoms and exposure to an unavoidable allergen, symptoms occur during a major portion of or through the entire year, or symptoms are difficult to control with pharmacologic management. An evaluation of the airborne allergens is required to establish allergic sensitivity. This can be performed with allergen skin prick testing or in vitro studies of IgE binding.

In the United States, standard practice of allergen immunotherapy starts with dilutions of 1:1,000 or 1:10,000 of the maintenance concentrate. Various protocols can be used, but the dose is typically increased at intervals of every 3–10 days during the "build-up" phase until the maintenance dose is achieved. Once the maintenance dose is achieved, the injections are given every 2 or 4 weeks. The length of treatment with immunotherapy is not well defined, although 3–5 years is considered a normal course of treatment. The initial response to treatment requires approximately 3–12 months. Among the patients who improve with immunotherapy, the majority continue to have improvement after a 3- to 5-year course of treatment ends. Approximately 25% have a return of symptoms soon after treatment. No method predicts which patients will have prolonged improvement or recurrence of their allergies.

The main risk of allergen immunotherapy is the development of a severe allergic reaction or asthma exacerbation to the immunotherapy injection. Severe reactions to immunotherapy are rare, with fatalities occurring in fewer than one per million injections. To reduce the risk of reactions, patients should be selected appropriately and educated about warning symptoms. Patients who have brittle or unstable asthma or a baseline $FEV_1 < 70\%$ are at increased risk for a reaction and should be excluded from immunotherapy. For asthma patients, peak flow rates should be measured before the injections and injections should be postponed if there is clinical or peak flow evidence of an exacerbation. Patients should be observed for 30 min after an immunotherapy injection, and the injections should only be given by personnel who are trained and equipped to use epinephrine, parental glucocorticoids, intravenous fluids, intubation equipment, and nebulizers.

6.7.3 Treatment of an Acute Asthmatic Attack

Physical findings in patients with exacerbations do not always correlate well with the degree of airflow obstruction. Although diffuse expiratory wheezing is a common finding, patients with the most severe impairment may have decreased breath sounds that limit auscultatory wheezing. Once treatment is initiated, the wheezing may become manifest. Symptoms of an acute asthma attack include a sensation of air hunger, chest tightness, cough, fatigue, or inability to lie flat. Signs of an acute exacerbation include the use of accessory muscles during respiration, wheezing, diaphoresis, and inability to complete sentences. Altered mental status is an ominous sign and necessitates immediate emergency care or hospitalization. Physical examination should include close monitoring of vital signs: blood pressure, pulse, and respiratory rate and a detailed examination of the nose, throat, and chest. Patients with a severe exacerbation usually have increased pulse and respiratory rates and abnormal pulsus paradoxus. Pulsus paradoxus is the difference in systolic blood pressure taken between inspiration and expiration. Pulsus paradoxus of 10–20 mmHg occurs with moderate obstruction and one more than 25 mmHg, with severe obstruction. Peak expiratory flow readings and spirometry can further quantify the obstruction. Spirometry may be difficult to perform in the setting of a severe exacerbation. A peak flow reading <50% of predicted or personal best is consistent with a severe exacerbation; 50–80% is consistent with a moderate exacerbation and >80%, with a mild exacerbation.

Treatment is based on clinical findings, both subjective and objective, peak flow readings, and previous underlying disease and treatment. The approach is different for a patient with mild asthma who has a seasonal pollen-induced exacerbation than for one who has moderate-to-severe persistent asthma and a respiratory infection who has already been using nebulized albuterol at home. The latter patient usually requires more aggressive management. β-Agonists and corticosteroids form the cornerstone of initial treatment. Oxygen is also recommended for all except mild acute exacerbations. An overview of the management of acute asthma is given in Fig. 6.3.

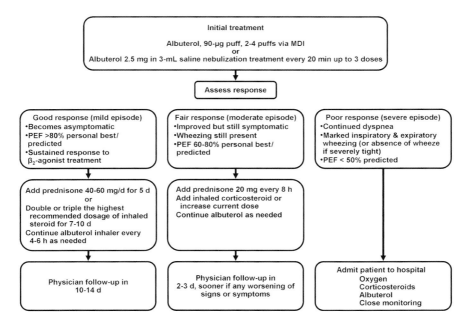

Fig. 6.3 Management of acute asthma. *PEF* peak expiratory flow

Approximately 50% of patients achieve maximal bronchodilation after one unit dose, or 2.5 mg of albuterol nebulized in 2.5–3.0 mL of normal saline. This therapy can be repeated every 15–20 min until the patient's condition is stable or the decision has been made to hospitalize the patient. Approximately 90% of patients achieve this response after three doses or 7.5 mg of inhaled albuterol. Therefore, the patient's clinical status after 3–4 doses of albuterol is often a better indicator rather than the initial presentation of whether inpatient care is required. Levalbuterol, a third-generation β-agonist, consists of the *R*-enantiomer of albuterol, which is responsible for the bronchodilatory effect. It is approved for ages 12 years and older. The usual starting dose is 0.63 mg in 3-mL unit dosages and, thus, has fewer systemic β-agonist side effects than albuterol 2.5 mg. The highest levalbuterol dose recommended is 1.25 mg in a 3-mL solution. It is approved for use every 6–8 hours, but likely can be given repeatedly, like albuterol. Because of conflicting study results, there is no clear-cut benefit when levalbuterol is compared with albuterol.

Corticosteroids are helpful in the treatment of acute asthma. Even though they do not have a rapid onset of action that immediately reverses the process, the anti-inflammatory properties can help prevent the exacerbation from escalating further and can shorten the time of the exacerbation. In addition to treatment with β-agonists, many patients with a mild exacerbation of asthma can be treated successfully with a higher-than-recommended dose of inhaled corticosteroid. For example, the dose of inhaled fluticasone may be increased to 220 μg, two puffs four times daily, instead of the usual top dose of 220 μg, two puffs twice daily for a 10-day period. Other inhaled corticosteroids can be used similarly by doubling or tripling the highest recommended dose. However, this strategy is less likely to work in patients who have a moderate or severe exacerbation, who overuse a β-agonist, or who have a severe upper respiratory infection exacerbating their asthma. Short courses of prednisone or other systemic corticosteroid are usually effective for establishing control of an exacerbation of asthma. These medications are most effective when given early in the exacerbation. For children, a common "steroid burst" is 1–2 mg kg^{-1} daily for 5 days, and for adults, prednisone 45–60 mg daily for 5 days. Most patients have considerable improvement in 5 days. Tapering the dose of systemic corticosteroids is not required after a short course (<1 week). When systemic corticosteroid treatment is longer than 10 days, it is advisable to taper the medication to help lessen the side effects of steroid withdrawal, including fatigue, depression, myalgias, and arthralgias. In essentially all exacerbations of asthma, corticosteroid treatment should be implemented or increased and continued for 5–10 days after the exacerbation to ensure stabilization. For example, a mild or moderate exacerbation that improves considerably with two treatments of nebulized albuterol is often followed by a relapse if corticosteroids, either inhaled or systemic, are not also started or increased. Corticosteroids can also be given intravenously or intramuscularly. There is no evidence that intravenous or intramuscular corticosteroids have a faster onset of action than oral corticosteroids. In hospitalized patients, a common approach is to administer intravenous methylprednisolone at 60 mg three times daily for the first 48 hours, with further dosage adjustment depending on the patient's response. Intravenous corticosteroids are advisable in the setting of severe dyspnea or nausea and vomiting associated with the asthma exacerbation. For asthma patients who present at the emergency department, the early use of corticosteroids results in fewer hospitalizations.

6.7.4 Status Asthmaticus Treatment

Status asthmaticus is defined as a severe exacerbation of asthma that does not respond to aggressive bronchodilator therapy. Patients in status asthmaticus are on the verge of acute respiratory failure and are at risk for intubation and mechanical ventilatory support. Common signs are tachypnea, tachycardia, and the use of the accessory muscles of respiration despite aggressive bronchodilator treatment. Status asthmaticus is treated with oxygen, intravenous corticosteroids, and nebulized β-agonist on a frequent (every 1–2 hours) or continuous basis. Patients are weaned from the β-agonist as their condition improves. Treatment includes close observation in an intensive care unit, especially during the first 6–12 hours, to monitor for progression to respiratory failure. Correction of acid-base imbalances helps in therapy. If respiratory failure occurs despite intensive medical management, artificial mechanical ventilation is indicated.

6.7.5 General Approach

6.7.5.1 Initial Therapy Based on Level of Severity and Subsequent Step-Wise Management

Previously, guidelines for asthma management outlined treatment recommendations on the basis of the assessment of asthma severity. These guidelines provided algorithms for increasing the dosages of medications and for adding other treatments. The practical application of these recommendations can be challenging because of the variable nature of asthma, the minimization of symptoms by patients, and poor compliance with the medications and home-based measurements. For patients who are already taking control medications, asthma severity can be assessed by their response, or lack of it, to treatment. Asthma severity and therapeutic response, however, are not always strictly correlated. To help circumvent these issues, the 2007 NAEPP guidelines recommend evaluating asthma severity to guide the choice of appropriate medication and other therapeutic interventions in only patients with newly diagnosed, untreated asthma. Once therapy is initiated, the evaluation of patients with asthma should shift to assessing the level of asthma control to guide decisions to adjust therapy.

Asthma control is assessed by several parameters, including symptoms, nighttime awakenings, interference with normal activity, β-agonist use, spirometry, validated questionnaires, and exacerbations. After asthma is controlled, the goal is to reduce the anti-inflammatory medication to the lowest effective dose. Currently, the level and duration of control required before a downward titration is undertaken and the strategy by which such adjustments should be accomplished are not known. A general rule is to consider stepping down treatment if the asthma has been well controlled for at least 3 months. Biologic markers of inflammation, such as eosinophil sputum counts and exhaled nitric oxide levels, may help in this process after they have been refined for application to the clinical setting.

6.7.5.2   Initial Therapy: Pediatric Asthma

The classification of asthma severity, which takes into account both the impairment and the risk, provides a guide for initiating asthma therapy. Initial therapy based on severity is outlined in Tables 6.7 and 6.14 for ages 0–4 years and in Tables 6.8 and 6.15 for ages 5–12 years. Once therapy is selected, the patient's response to treatment guides decisions about adjusting the therapy based on control of the impairment and risk factors. Although each asthma patient requires individualized care, some general rules are helpful in guiding therapy decisions.

For children with persistent asthma, whether mild, moderate, or severe, a daily long-term controller medication is indicated. Inhaled corticosteroids are the preferred therapy for initiating long-term control therapy. For children with mild asthma, recognition of the appropriate long-term controller therapy can be difficult, because children are often asymptomatic between episodes. Indications for the use or consideration of a long-term controller medication for the 0–4-year-old age group also includes the following:

- More than three episodes of wheezing that lasted longer than 1 day within the past year and risk factors for developing asthma, including (1) atopic dermatitis, (2) sensitization to aeroallergens, or (3) parental history of asthma or two of the following: food allergy, more than 4% blood eosinophilia, or wheezing in the absence of a viral respiratory infection
- Requires symptomatic treatment 3 days or more weekly for more than 4 weeks
- Required systemic corticosteroids for severe exacerbation of asthma two or more times within the last 6 months

In these situations, treatment with a daily low-dose inhaled corticosteroid can help reduce exacerbations and decrease symptoms but does not appear to alter the future course of asthma severity. Another option to consider is the use of daily controller therapy only during periods of higher risk, such as the fall and winter months, when the incidence of viral upper respiratory tract infections is higher. This approach has not been evaluated systematically; however, theoretically, it should help reduce symptoms and exacerbations in patients with mild asthma whose symptoms are confined to these times.

Alternative anti-inflammatory long-term controller options include leukotriene receptor antagonists or cromolyn. These are less potent than inhaled corticosteroids.

Table 6.14 Stepwise approach for managing asthma in children ages 0–4 years

	Step 1	Step 2	Step 3	Step 4	Step 5	Step 6	
Inhaled short-acting β$_2$-agonists PRN		Low-dose ICS[a] *or* (in order of preference) montelukast or cromolyn	Medium-dose ICS[a]	Medium-dose ICS[a] *and* Either montelukast or LABA	High-dose ICS[a] *and* Either montelukast or LABA	High-dose ICS[a] *and* Either montelukast or LABA *and* Oral cortico-steroids	Step up if needed (first, check adherence and environmental control) ↑ *Assess control* Step down if possible →
Intermittent asthma		Persistent asthma: daily medication					
		Consult with asthma specialist if step 3 care or higher is required Consider consultation at step 2					

Patient education and environmental control at each step

Quick-relief medication for all patients

• β$_2$-Agonist as needed for symptoms. Intensity of treatment depends on severity of symptoms
• With viral respiratory infection: β$_2$-agonist q4–6h up to 24h (longer with physician consult). If treatment needs to be repeated more than once every 6 weeks, consider starting daily long-term-control therapy (step 2). Consider short course of systemic oral corticosteroids if exacerbation is severe or patient has history of previous severe exacerbations
• *Caution*: Increasing use of β$_2$-agonist or use of >2 days per week for symptom control (not prevention of exercise-induced bronchoconstriction) indicates inadequate control and the need to step up treatment

From the National Asthma Education and Prevention Program: Expert Panel Report 3. (2007) Guidelines for the diagnosis and management of asthma. NIH publication No. 07–4051. Bethesda, MD: U.S. Department of Health and Human Services; National Institutes of Health: National Heart, Lung and Blood Institute

ICS inhaled corticosteroid; *LABA* inhaled long-acting β$_2$-agonist

[a]Preferred treatment

Note: If alternative treatment is used and response is inadequate, discontinue it and use the preferred treatment before stepping up

Table 6.15 Stepwise approach for managing asthma in children ages 5–11 years

Intermittent asthma	Persistent asthma: daily medication				
	Consult with asthma specialist if step 4 care or higher is required				
	Consider allergen immunotherapy in steps 2–4 for patients who have persistent, allergic asthma				
		Consider consultation at step 3			
					Step 6
				Step 5	
			Step 4		
		Step 3			
	Step 2				
Step 1					
Preferred: SABA prn	*Preferred:* Low-dose ICS *Alternative:* LTRA, cromolyn, nedocromil, or theophylline	*Preferred:* Medium-dose ICS *or* Low-dose ICS+either LABA, LTRA, or theophylline	*Preferred:* Medium-dose ICS+LABA *Alternative:* Medium-dose ICS+either LTRA or theophylline	*Preferred:* High-dose ICS+LABA *Alternative:* High-dose ICS+either LTRA or theophylline	*Preferred:* High-dose ICS+LABA+oral corticosteroid *Alternative:* High-dose ICS+either LTRA or theophylline+oral corticosteroid

Step up if needed (first, check adherence, environmental control, and comorbid conditions)

Assess control

Step down if possible (and asthma is well controlled for at least 3 months)

Patient education and environmental control at each step

Quick-relief medication for all patients:

- SABA as needed for symptoms. Intensity of treatment depends on severity of symptoms: up to three treatments at 20-min intervals, as needed. Short course of systemic oral corticosteroids may be needed
- *Caution:* increasing use of β_2-agonist or use >2 times per week for symptoms control (not prevention of exercise-induced bronchoconstriction) indicates inadequate control and the need to step up treatment

From the National Asthma Education and Prevention Program: Expert Panel Report 3. (2007) Guidelines for the diagnosis and management of asthma. NIH publication No. 07-4051. Bethesda, MD: U.S. Department of Health and Human Services; National Institutes of Health; National Heart, Lung and Blood Institute

ICS inhaled corticosteroid; *LABA* inhaled long-acting β_2-agonist; *LTRA* leukotriene receptor antagonist; *prn* as needed; *SABA* inhaled short-acting β_2-agonist

Considerations for the initial treatment in addition to treatment effectiveness include mode of delivery of the medication, history of previous response to therapy, and anticipated compliance with the treatment regimen. The following are the FDA-approved age indications for the controller medications:

1. Inhaled corticosteroids

   - Budesonide nebulizer solution (children >1 year)
   - Fluticasone DPI (children ≥4 years)

2. Leukotriene antagonist

   - Montelukast (children >1 year)

3. Chromones

   - Cromolyn nebulizer solution (children ≥2 years)

6.7.5.3   Initial Therapy: Adult Asthma

As for the initial therapy of pediatric asthma, the classification of asthma based on impairment and risk provides a guide for initiating therapy for adults (Tables 6.9 and 6.16). For adults, spirometry helps to clarify further the current impairment. Inhaled corticosteroids are the preferred treatment for persistent asthma that requires a long-term controller medication. Alternatives include cromolyn, leukotriene receptor antagonists, and sustained-release theophylline. The effectiveness of these alternatives is less than that of inhaled corticosteroids.

6.7.5.4   Stepwise Management of Therapy Based on Severity and Control

The aim of asthma therapy is to maintain long-term control of asthma with the least amount of medication. To achieve this, a stepwise approach to therapy has been implemented in which the number of medications and the amount of the medications are increased as necessary and decreased when possible to maintain control. The emphasis on control is a new key concept of the 2007 NAEPP report. An overview of the critical components of control and recommended actions to maintain control are shown in Tables 6.17–6.19 for the respective age groups of 0–4, 5–12 and ≥12 years.

Key issues in the stepwise approach include what to add when. Specific therapy should be tailored to the needs and circumstances of the individual patient. Short-acting inhaled β-agonists taken as needed are the primary treatment for intermittent asthma. If a β-agonist is required for quick-relief treatment more than twice weekly, then therapy should be increased to the persistent asthma regimen. Patients with persistent asthma should receive daily long-term control medication that has anti-inflammatory effects. Overall, inhaled corticosteroids are the most effective single agents. In addition, quick-relief medication should be made available to all patients

Table 6.16 Stepwise approach for managing asthma in adults and youths ages ≥12 years

Persistent asthma: daily medication

Consult with asthma specialist if step 4 care or higher is required

Consider allergen immunotherapy in steps 2–4 for patients who have persistent, allergic asthma

Intermittent asthma		Consider consultation at step 3				Step up if
Step 1	Step 2	Step 3	Step 4	Step 5	Step 6	needed (first, check adherence, environmental control, and comorbid conditions) *Assess control* Step down if possible (and asthma is well controlled for at least 3 months)
Preferred: SABA prn	*Preferred*: Low-dose ICS *Alternative*: Cromolyn, nedocromil, LTRA, or theophylline	*Preferred*: Medium-dose ICS *or* Low-dose ICS+LABA *Alternative*: Low-dose ICS+either LTRA, theophylline, or zileuton	*Preferred*: Medium-dose ICS+LABA *Alternative*: Medium-dose ICS+either LTRA, theophylline, or zileuton	*Preferred*: High-dose ICS+LABA *and* Consider omalizumab for patients who have allergies	*Preferred*: High-dose ICS+LABA+oral corticosteroid *and* Consider omalizumab for patients who have allergies	

Patient education and environmental control at each step

Quick-relief medication for all patients:

• SABA as needed for symptoms. Intensity of treatment depends on severity of symptoms: up to three treatments at 20-min intervals, as needed. Short course of systemic oral corticosteroids may be needed
• Use of a β_2-agonist >2 days per week for symptom control (not prevention of exercise-induced bronchoconstriction) indicates inadequate control and the need to step up treatment

From the National Asthma Education and Prevention Program: Expert Panel Report 3. (2007) Guidelines for the diagnosis and management of asthma. NIH publication No. 07-4051. Bethesda, MD: U.S. Department of Health and Human Services; National Institutes of Health; National Heart, Lung and Blood Institute
ICS inhaled corticosteroid; *LABA* inhaled long-acting β_2-agonist; *LTRA* leukotriene receptor antagonist; *prn* as needed; *SABA* inhaled short-acting β_2-agonist.

Table 6.17 Assessing asthma control and adjusting therapy in children ages 0–4 years

Components of control	Classification of asthma control (ages 0–4 years)[a]		
	Well controlled	Not well controlled	Very poorly controlled
Impairment			
Symptoms	≤2 days per week	>2 days per week	Throughout the day
Nighttime awakenings	≤1 per month	>1 time per month	>1 time per week
Interference with normal activity	None	Some limitation	Extremely limited
Short-acting β_2-agonist use for symptom control (not prevention of exercise-induced bronchoconstriction)	≤2 days per week	>2 days per week	Several times per day
Risk			
Exacerbations (requiring oral corticosteroids)	0–1 per year	2–3 per year	>3 per year
Recommended action for treatment	• Maintain current treatment • Attempt step down if well controlled for at least 3 months	• Step up 1 step and • Reevaluate in 2–4 week • For side effects, consider alternative treatment options	• Consider short course of systemic oral corticosteroids • Step up 1–2 steps, and • Reevaluate in 2 weeks • For side effects, consider alternative treatment options

From the National Asthma Education and Prevention Program: Expert Panel Report 3. (2007) Guidelines for the diagnosis and management of asthma. NIH publication No. 07-4051. Bethesda, MD: U.S. Department of Health and Human Services; National Institutes of Health; National Heart, Lung and Blood Institute

[a]The level of control or impairment is based on the most severe impairment category

who have persistent asthma. If the asthma is not controlled with a low-dose inhaled corticosteroid despite excellent compliance, inhaler technique, and lack of triggers or coexisting conditions, then the therapeutic options include increasing the inhaled corticosteroid dose to the medium-dose range or adding a long-acting β-agonist to a low dose of inhaled corticosteroid. These are considered essentially equal options based on risk and benefit. Alternative options include adding a leukotriene antagonist or theophylline to the low-dose inhaled corticosteroid. The next step in treatment combines a medium-dose inhaled corticosteroid and long-acting β-agonist. Alternatives to this include a leukotriene antagonist or theophylline in addition to the medium-dose inhaled corticosteroid. If further control is required, then high-dose inhaled corticosteroids and a long-acting β-agonist are recommended. No

Table 6.18 Assessing asthma control and adjusting therapy in children ages 5–11 years

	Classification of asthma control (ages 5–11 years)[a]		
Components of control	Well controlled	Not well controlled	Very poorly controlled
Impairment			
Symptoms	≤2 days per week but not more than once on each day	>2 days per week or multiple times on ≤2 days per week	Throughout the day
Nighttime awakenings	≤1 time per month	≥2 times per month	≥2 times per week
Interference with normal activity	None	Some limitation	Extremely limited
Short-acting β_2-agonist use for symptom control (not prevention of exercise-induced bronchoconstriction)	≤2 days per week	>2 days per week	Several times per day
Lung function	FEV_1 or peak flow >80% predicted $FEV_1/FVC > 80\%$	FEV_1 or peak flow = 60–80% predicted $FEV_1/FVC = 75–80\%$	FEV_1 or peak flow <60% predicted $FEV_1/FVC < 75\%$
Risk			
Exacerbations (requiring oral corticosteroids)	0–1 per year	2–3 per year	>3 per year
Recommended action for treatment	• Maintain current step • Attempt step down if well controlled for at least 3 months	• Step up at least 1 step and • Reevaluate in 2–4 weeks • For side effects: consider alternative treatment options	• Consider short course of systemic oral corticosteroids • Step up 1–2 steps, and • Reevaluate in 2 weeks • For side effects: consider alternative treatment options

From the National Asthma Education and Prevention Program: Expert Panel Report 3. (2007) Guidelines for the diagnosis and management of asthma. NIH publication No. 07-4051. Bethesda, MD: U.S. Department of Health and Human Services; National Institutes of Health; National Heart, Lung and Blood Institute

FEV$_1$ forced expiratory volume in 1s; *FVC* forced vital capacity

[a]The level of control or impairment is based on the most severe impairment category

long-term studies have assessed the efficacy of adding a leukotriene antagonist to this regimen. Omalizumab could be considered at this juncture for patients who have IgE-mediated asthma and sensitization to the pertinent perennial allergens. Allergen immunotherapy should be considered for patients with persistent asthma

Table 6.19 Assessing asthma control in adults and youths ages ≥12 years

Components of control	Classification of asthma control in patients ages ≥12 years[a]		
	Well controlled	Not well controlled	Very poorly controlled
Impairment			
Symptoms	≤2 days per week	>2 days per week	Throughout the day
Nighttime awakenings	≤2 per month	1–3 per week	≥4 per week
Interference with normal activity	None	Some limitation	Extremely limited
Short-acting β_2-agonist use for symptom control (not prevention of exercise-induced bronchoconstriction)	≤2 days per week	>2 days per week	Several times daily
FEV_1 or peak flow	>80% predicted/personal best	60–80% predicted/personal best	<60% predicted/personal best
Validated questionnaires			
ATAQ	0	1–2	3–4
ACQ	≤0.75	≥1.5	Not applicable
ACT	≥20	16–19	≤15
Risk			
Exacerbations	0–1 per year	2–3 per year	>3 per year
Progressive loss of lung function	Evaluation requires long-term follow-up care		
Treatment-related adverse effects	Medication side effects can vary in intensity from none to very troublesome and worrisome. The level of intensity does not correlate with specific levels of control but should be considered in the overall assessment of risk		
Recommended action for treatment	• Maintain current step • Consider step down if well controlled for at least 3 months	• Step up 1 step • Reevaluate in 2–6 weeks • For side effects, consider alternative treatment options	• Consider short course of systemic oral corticosteroids • Step up 1–2 steps • Reevaluate in 2 weeks • For side effects, consider alternative treatment options

From the National Asthma Education and Prevention Program: Expert Panel Report 3. (2007) Guidelines for the diagnosis and management of asthma. NIH publication No. 07-4051. Bethesda, MD: U.S. Department of Health and Human Services; National Institutes of Health; National Heart, Lung and Blood Institute

ACQ asthma control questionnaire; *ACT* asthma control test; *ATAQ* asthma therapy assessment questionnaire; *FEV₁* forced expiratory volume in 1s

[a]The level of control or impairment is based on the most severe impairment category

when there is a relationship between symptoms and exposure to an allergen to which the patient is sensitive.

Asthma can be highly variable over time, and the treatment should be adjusted accordingly. Reassessment is critical in determining asthma control. Key areas that should be monitored include the following:

1. Impairment

- Symptoms
- Nighttime awakenings
- Interference with normal activity
- Short-acting β-agonist use
- Spirometry or peak flow
- Validated questionnaires

2. Risk

- Exacerbations
- Loss of lung function
- Treatment-related adverse effects

These factors help in determining the level of treatment required to maintain control and in preventing exacerbations. Once well-controlled asthma is achieved and maintained for at least 3 months, a reduction in pharmacologic therapy should be considered. This will allow for using the minimal therapy for well-controlled asthma. If well-controlled asthma is not achieved and maintained, secondary causes should be assessed. These include patient compliance and technique in using the medications and the presence of a coexisting condition or a provocateur.

An asthma action plan should be reviewed for essentially all patients who have asthma. Even patients with mild intermittent asthma may experience sudden, severe exacerbations of asthma. It is essential that the exacerbations be recognized early so treatment can be implemented. The action plan should include symptoms of worsening asthma, peak flow meter reading guidelines, and recommendations for using β-agonist rescue therapy, increasing the use of controller medications, administration of systemic corticosteroids, and seeking medical care. An example of an asthma action plan is shown in Table 6.4.

6.7.6   Treatment of Persistent Severe or Intractable Asthma

Severe asthma represents <10% of all cases of asthma, but these patients account for a disproportionate share of the health costs and morbidity associated with the disease. Several severe asthma phenotypes have been described on the basis of the age of the patients, age at disease onset, corticosteroid resistance, chronic airflow obstruction, and evidence for eosinophilic airway inflammation on biopsy. In this group of patients, it is particularly important that the diagnosis of asthma is confirmed, that correct use and compliance with medications are confirmed, and that all possible exacerbating factors (airsmog) are optimally managed. The mainstay of pharmaco-therapy are high-dose inhaled corticosteroids and long-acting β-agonists. Possible adjunctive long-acting controller medications include leukotriene antagonists, theo-phylline, omalizumab, and anticholinergic agents. Systemic corticosteroids are used for exacerbations and may be required for maintenance therapy. The goal is to use as little systemic corticosteroid as possible to maintain stable airway function. For some patients, the asthma can be controlled with an every-other-day corticosteroid regimen. Patients who require systemic corticosteroids need monitoring and treatment for side effects, particularly increased glucose levels in those with diabetes mellitus, posterior subcapsular cataracts, and osteopenia or osteoporosis. Monitoring and corticosteroid dosage based on inflammatory markers such as sputum eosinophils and nitric oxide hold promise for the future as a way to prescribe as little systemic corticosteroid as possible. Various immunomodulating steroid-sparing agents have been attempted over the years, but generally the experience with methotrexate, troleandomycin, gold, and intravenous gamma globulin have been disappointing. Patients with severe asthma require specialist management of their condition.

6.7.7 Special Groups

6.7.7.1 Occupational Asthma

Occupational asthma is a disease characterized by variable outflow obstruction and hyperresponsiveness due to causes and conditions attributable to a particular occupational environment and not due to stimuli encountered outside the workplace. It has been estimated that 5–10% of all cases of asthma in industrialized nations are occupationally related. Occupational asthma can be separated into two main subtypes: immunologic and nonimmunologic. The immunologic subtype can be subdivided further into immunologically mediated asthma and hypersensitivity pneumonitis. The nonimmunologic subtype is due to an irritant type of reaction, usually with large exposure to the offending substance, and is termed *reactive airways dysfunction syndrome* (RADS). RADS is characterized by a high level of exposure to the offending agent, acute onset of asthma symptoms, persistence of asthma symptoms for 3 months, and development of airway hyperreactivity with subsequent irritant exposure (exercise, cold air, fumes, etc.). These subtypes can overlap. Many reactive chemicals can cause disease by inducing immunologic asthma or RADS. With other substances, for example, Western red cedar, the pulmonary response is not well delineated as being either immunologically mediated or an irritant response.

Most agents that cause occupational asthma are high-molecular-weight proteins of plant, animal, or bacteria origin. Low-molecular-weight chemicals act as irritants and can aggravate underlying asthma or produce RADS. Low-molecular-weight chemicals can also form an immunologically mediated reaction by haptenizing proteins in the respiratory tract, enabling binding by IgE. Common causes of occupational asthma are listed in Table 6.20.

Table 6.20 Major causes of occupational asthma

High-molecular-weight agents	Workers at risk
Plant proteins (wheat, grains, coffee beans, cotton, etc.)	Farmers, bakers, textile workers, food processors, millers
Animal proteins (domestic animals, birds, mice, etc.)	Farmers, veterinarians, laboratory workers, animal handlers
Latex	Healthcare workers, laboratory workers, rubber manufacturers
Enzymes (Bacillus subtilis, trypsin, papain, etc.)	Detergent manufacturers, pharmaceutical workers
Seafood	Seafood processors
Gums	Carpet makers, pharmaceutical workers

Low-molecular-weight agents	Workers at risk
Isocyanates (toluene diisocyanate, diphenylmethane diisocyanate, naphthalene diisocyanate)	Spray painters; insulation installers; polyurethane workers; plastics, rubber, and foam workers
Anhydrides (trimellitic anhydrate, phthalic anhydride)	Paint, plastic, and epoxy resin manufacturers
Metals (nickel, platinum, etc.)	Platers, welders, metal and chemical workers
Wood dusts (Western red cedar)	Forest workers, carpenters, woodworkers
Fluxes (colophony, etc.)	Solderers, electrical workers
Dyes (carmine, henna extract, etc.)	Textile workers, fur dyers, beauticians
Acrylate (methacrylate, cyanoacrylate)	Health professionals, body shop workers
Drugs (psyllium, antibiotics, etc.)	Pharmaceutical workers, health professionals

All asthma subjects should be questioned not only about their occupation, but also about their work environment. The work environment history should include details about the building they work in, the agents or chemicals they work with directly, and the other processes ongoing in their work area. Typically, the symptoms of occupational asthma occur only at work and improve when a person is away from the work environment. With progression of the disease, however, the relation between the work environment and the symptoms become less clear-cut. This is particularly true for workers with underlying asthma whose symptoms are made worse by nonspecific irritants at work or those with poorly controlled asthma. Also, workers may not be exposed to the offending agent every day, and intermittent exposures can be hard to identify. The latency period between the onset of exposure and the onset of symptoms is highly variable. Generally, the latency period is shorter with exposure to low-molecular-weight agents than to high-molecular-weight agents.

The initial evaluation of the patient should first confirm whether the patient indeed has asthma. Pulmonary function testing is indicated to obtain baseline pulmonary function and to determine the presence of asthma. Asthma can be confirmed by an increase of 12% or more in FEV_1 after administration of a bronchodilator or a decrease of 20% or more in FEV_1 after bronchoprovocation, for example, as with methacholine. Establishing that asthma is occupational can be difficult. The underlying principle is to identify the offending substance and show sensitivity with skin or in vitro testing or to detect an objective change in pulmonary function with work exposure. Skin and in vitro testing to substances present in the work environment, when positive, suggest a causal relation. In many instances, however, reagents for skin or in vitro testing are not available. Also, in RADS, skin and in vitro testing will be negative. Often, it is necessary to reproduce the symptoms by challenge. The challenge may be conducted by natural exposure of the patient to the work environment or by controlled bronchoprovocation to the suspected substance in the laboratory. When the challenge consists of normal work environment exposure, serial measurement of the PEFRs is helpful. With one method of monitoring, the patient records the PEFR four times daily for 2 weeks at work and for a similar period away from work. This approach has several potential problems, including reproducibility of the readings, compliance and honesty of the patients, and interpretation of the results. Similarly, spirometry can be performed, with measurements of FEV_1 in the workplace compared with measurements made on a nonwork day. This may need to be done repeatedly, because measurement of a single FEV_1 when the patient is at work instead of at home does not have sufficient sensitivity to detect a relation between work and asthma. Another method to determine the effect of the work environment is induced sputum measurement for eosinophils. An increase of 1% or more of sputum eosinophils obtained after 2 weeks of work exposure compared with a sample obtained after 2 weeks with no work exposure increases the sensitivity and specificity of occupational asthma diagnosis compared with PEFR monitoring alone.

Many workers with occupational asthma do not recover completely, even after they leave the work environment. Early diagnosis and removal from the work environment are critical for the goal of complete recovery. Sometimes, changes can be made in the work environment to eliminate or significantly decrease exposure. However, levels of exposure below the legal limit that are based on toxicity may still precipitate an IgE-mediated reaction. Consultation with an industrial hygienist may be helpful in measuring the exposure. Although no preemployment screening test has been effective in predicting the development of occupational asthma, effort should be made to educate workers and managers in high-risk industries so that affected workers can be recognized early.

6.7.7.2   Asthma in Pregnancy

The prevalence of asthma in pregnancy is approximately 7%. Managing asthma during pregnancy is unique because of the effect of pregnancy on asthma and the effect of asthma and the treatment of asthma on the developing fetus and mother. The primary goal is to optimize both fetal and maternal health.

During pregnancy, about one-third of patients with asthma experience improvement in symptoms, one-third experience worsening of symptoms, and one-third remain the same. The first trimester is generally well tolerated by asthma patients. An increase in symptoms and exacerbations have been reported to occur most commonly between weeks 17 and 36 of gestation, but there are fewer symptoms and exacerbations during weeks 37–40. Asthma generally remains controlled during labor and delivery. Overall, the first trimester and last month of pregnancy appear to be relatively free of asthma exacerbations, and the second and early third trimester have more potential for an increase in symptoms. The course of the asthma is often consistent in a woman during successive pregnancies. The mechanisms responsible for the changes in the course of asthma during pregnancy are not known; however, the changes do not appear to be due to random fluctuations in the disease. Possibilities include the physiologic changes during pregnancy, stress, underuse of medication, infection, immunologic response to the fetus, and atopic changes.

The general principles of asthma management during pregnancy do not differ substantially from those of nonpregnant asthma patients. The primary concern is the control of asthma, not the avoidance of asthma medications. The patient needs to be educated about the potential adverse effects of uncontrolled asthma on the well-being of the fetus and needs to understand that treating asthma with medications is safer than an increase in asthma symptoms that may lead to maternal and fetal hypoxia. The goal is to have no limitation of activity, no exacerbations, normal pulmonary function, minimal chronic symptoms, and minimal adverse effects of medications.

Objective assessments and monitoring should be performed on pregnant asthma patients. Patients with an $FEV_1 < 80\%$ of predicted are at increased risk for asthma morbidity and pregnancy complications. Because asthma has been associated with decreased fetal growth and preterm birth, accurate dating is helpful. There should be open lines of communication with the patient's obstetrician, and the obstetrician should be involved in the management of the patient's asthma and obtain information about the asthma status during prenatal visits.

Avoidance of asthma triggers, such as fumes, tobacco smoke, pollutants, and allergens, should be reviewed. Allergen immunotherapy can be continued during pregnancy in patients who tolerate the immunotherapy well without systemic reactions and are at a maintenance dose and do not require escalation of the dose. Immunotherapy should not be started during pregnancy because of the risk of a systemic reaction during the build-up phase and the latency of the immunotherapy effect.

Pharmacologic management of pregnant women with asthma has been updated recently in the document "NAEPP Working Group Report on Managing Asthma during Pregnancy: Recommendations of Pharmacologic Treatment – Update 2004." This update supercedes the initial report from 1993 and the 2002 update. The primary recommendations include the use of inhaled corticosteroids as the preferred controller therapy for mild, moderate, or persistent asthma. In addition, for moderate persistent asthma, the combination of a low-dose inhaled corticosteroid plus a long-acting β-agonist or medium-dose inhaled corticosteroid were considered equal treatment options. In 1979, the FDA established five categories to describe a drug's potential for causing adverse effects during pregnancy (Table 6.21). These categories are based on human data, animal studies, and consideration of whether the benefit of the drug's use during pregnancy outweighs the risk. No asthma or allergy medication meets the requirements for category A.

There do not appear to be clear-cut recommendations for the choice of specific medications in each medication category. In 1993, the Working Group on Asthma and Pregnancy recognized as treatment options during pregnancy the inhaled

Table 6.21 U.S. Food and Drug classification scheme for medications in pregnancy[a]

Category	Animal studies	Human studies
A	Negative	Negative
B	Negative	Not done
B	Positive	Negative
C	Positive	Not done
C	Not done	Not done
D	Positive or negative	Positive
X[b]	Positive	Positive

[a]Negative = no teratogenicity demonstrated; positive = teratogenicity demonstrated
[b]Drug contraindicated in pregnancy

corticosteroids used at that time, namely, beclomethasone dipropionate, triamcinolone, and flunisolide. Because most of the experience was with beclomethasone, it was considered the inhaled corticosteroid of choice. Since then, reports have supported the overall safety of inhaled corticosteroids in pregnancy. Currently, most of the available safety data are for budesonide, which is considered the preferred inhaled corticosteroid in pregnancy. There have not been data to suggest that other corticosteroids are less safe in pregnancy; therefore, if a pregnant woman with asthma is using an alternative inhaled corticosteroid and doing well, then it is reasonable to continue with the medication. Data about the use of systemic corticosteroids during pregnancy have raised some concern. Although there is no definite increased risk of total congenital malformations, a statistically significant increased risk of oral clefts in infants of mothers treated with oral corticosteroids during the first trimester has been shown. Other adverse outcomes associated with systemic corticosteroid use include preeclampsia, low birth weight, and preterm delivery. However, it is difficult to determine if these outcomes are due to the corticosteroids or the underlying asthma. The current recommendations support the use of oral corticosteroids when indicated for long-term management of severe asthma or for severe exacerbations during pregnancy.

The initial guidelines did not make a recommendation about a specific short- or long-acting β-agonist. On the basis of current data, albuterol is recommended as the inhaled short-acting β-agonist of choice. Few data have been published about the safety of salmeterol and formoterol. Because salmeterol has been available for a longer time, it is considered the long-acting β-agonist of choice. Other medications recommended during pregnancy as alternative choices for mild persistent asthma include cromolyn, theophylline, zafirlukast, and montelukast. Theophylline, zafirlukast, and montelukast can also be used as add-on therapy to inhaled corticosteroids. Serum theophylline levels need to be monitored closely, with maintenance serum levels targeted at $5–12$ μg mL^{-1}.

Practitioners should be aware of the potential side effects that commonly used labor medications may have on asthma. Prostaglandin $F_{2\alpha}$, ergonovine, and methylergonovine, which are used for postpartum hemorrhage, can induce bronchospasm.

Transcervical or intra-amniotic prostaglandin E_2 used for cervical ripening can also induce bronchospasm. Intravaginal or intracervical prostaglandin E_2 gel, prostaglandin E_2 suppositories, magnesium sulfate, and calcium channel blockers can be safely administered to asthma patients. For patients receiving regular systemic corticosteroid therapy or who have received frequent bursts during pregnancy, supplemental corticosteroids are recommended for the stress of labor and delivery. A typical stress dose is 100 mg hydrocortisone intravenously at admission and repeated every 8 hours for 24 hours.

6.7.7.3 Exercise-Induced Asthma

Exercise-induced asthma is the term often used to describe bronchoconstriction that follows exercise in asthma patients and produces the symptoms of cough, wheeze, dyspnea, or chest tightness (or some combination of these). This has also been termed, more accurately, *exercise-induced bronchoconstriction*, because exercise does not induce asthma, but rather exacerbates underlying asthma. Exercise-induced asthma occurs in 80–90% of patients with asthma and occurs with equal frequency in children and adults. The prevalence of exercise-induced asthma in the general population is approximately 6–13%, and approximately 10% of patients with this condition have no history of asthma or allergic disease. The magnitude of exercise-induced asthma is correlated with the underlying degree of airway hyper-responsiveness; therefore, in many patients with mild, episodic asthma, even strenuous exercise does not cause clinically significant bronchoconstriction.

The underlying pathophysiologic mechanism of exercise-induced asthma is not entirely clear. Under normal breathing conditions, the majority of the warming and humidification of inspired air is done by the nasal mucosa. During vigorous exercise, the large airways are recruited to provide the extra heat and humidity to condition the inspired air. As a person exercises, minute ventilation increases and, thus, respiratory water and heat loss increase. There is disagreement about the relative contributions of airway water loss versus airway cooling versus airway rewarming (after exercise). It is difficult to separate the roles of these potential triggers of exercise-induced asthma, but it has been shown that experimental inhalation of hot dry air can produce this condition but that it is attenuated when the inspired gas is humified and closer to body temperature, implying that water loss is the principal trigger. An interesting observation is that approximately 50% of patients who have exercise-induced asthma are refractory to exercise-induced symptoms if they exercise again within 60 min after the first exercise session. However, if the second exercise challenge is more than 3 hours after the first, the refractory period is lost and the symptoms are similar to those after the first exercise session. The refractory period does not occur if the patient is pretreated with indomethacin, suggesting that prostaglandins help provide protection during the refractory period. Other observations in exercise-induced asthma include an increase in inflammatory mediators, including histamine and leukotrienes C_4 and D_4, activation of peripheral Th2-type lymphocytes, and eosinophil influx and activation. In contrast, exhaled nitric oxide levels do not appear to correlate well with the development or severity of exercise-induced asthma.

The primary symptoms associated with exercise-induced asthma include any combination of cough, dyspnea, chest tightness, chest discomfort, and wheeze. The symptoms may occur during exercise, usually 10–15 min into the exercise or 5–15 min after the completion of the exercise. The symptoms typically clear within 60 min after the exercise is completed. As noted above, there is a refractory period of up to 3 hours after the initial exercise. If the exercise is resumed within this time, little or no bronchoconstriction occurs. Symptoms are usually more pronounced with aerobic exercise such as with bicycling, running, and cross-country skiing, which involve a significant increase in the ventilatory rate. Activities that are less aerobic, such as weight lifting, diving, or yoga, are less likely to trigger exercise-induced asthma. Patients usually note that symptoms are increased when exercising in cold dry air compared with warm moist air.

Conventionally, exercise-induced asthma testing is performed in the laboratory, with 6–8 min of treadmill exercise sufficient to increase the heart rate to 85% of the predicted maximum. Spirometry is performed before the exercise and should be at least 75% of the patient's predicted value. Spirometry is then repeated immediately upon completion of the exercise and repeated 5–10 min after exercise stops. The lowest postexercise value is obtained and compared with the preexercise level. A decrease in the FEV_1 of 15% or more is considered a positive test. If spirometry is not available, peak expiratory flow rates can also be used. These should also be obtained before exercise and repeated upon completion of the exercise and at 3, 5, and 10 min after exercise. The initial peak flow reading should be 75% or more of the personal best. A decrease of 15% is considered a positive test.

If the diagnosis is unclear despite attempts to measure pulmonary function, further evaluation is required. The primary differential diagnosis for exercise-induced respiratory symptoms includes normal physiologic exercise limitation, upper airway obstruction, vocal cord dysfunction, parenchymal pulmonary disease, and cardiac disorders. Further evaluation may require formal exercise testing in a referral center that uses pulmonary function testing with lung volumes, diffusion capacity, and oxygen saturation.

Several nonpharmacologic therapeutic modalities are available to aid in the treatment of exercise-induced asthma. Patients should be advised to have a warm-up period before more strenuous exercise. This should consist of 5–10 min of stretching and mild exercise. This warm-up may help decrease the severity of exercise-induced asthma. The patient should be encouraged to increase cardiovascular fitness. Improvement in overall fitness lowers the minute ventilation required for a given level of exercise, thereby decreasing one of the primary stimuli for bronchoconstriction. Because breathing warm and humidified air is helpful, nasal breathing should be recommended. Similarly, patients should be instructed to breathe through a loosely fitting scarf or mask when exercising in cold, dry conditions to further humidify the air.

The pharmacotherapy of exercise-induced asthma varies with the clinical setting. Generally, if exercise-induced asthma occurs in poorly controlled asthma, the most important strategy is to improve the overall control of the underlying asthma. Once the underlying asthma is well controlled, the treatment strategy is the same as for those in whom the exercised-induced symptoms are the only provocateur of airway hyperreactivity. The inhaled short-acting β-agonists are the primary prophylactic treatment for exercise-induced asthma. They significantly reduce or eliminate the condition in 85–90% of patients. A typical dose is two puffs of albuterol taken 15–45 min before exercise. This protects from exercise-induced asthma for approximately 2 hours, although the duration of bronchodilation is nearly 4 hours.

Another approach is the use of chromones. Inhaled cromolyn or nedocromil may be considered for patients in whom short-acting β-agonists are not fully effective. The dosage can range from 2 to 6 puffs 20 min before exercise. In addition, they may have a synergistic effect when used in combination with β-agonists. Long-acting β-agonists have also been shown to be effective in prophylaxis of exercise-induced asthma. The advantage of these medications is that they may be taken hours before exercise. There has been concern about the development of tolerance to the drug over time. Leukotriene receptor antagonists have also shown benefit in exercise-induced asthma. The long half-life of these agents allows for protection from exercise-induced asthma for up to 12 hours after ingestion. Inhaled corticosteroids do not prevent exercise-induced asthma in the short term. With long-term use, however, they improve airway hyperresponsiveness and decrease the bronchoconstriction associated with exertion.

If patients experience acute breakthrough symptoms despite prophylactic treatment or in the absence of prophylactic treatment, the primary treatment is a short-acting β-agonist. Other prophylactic measures, such as chromones and leukotriene antagonists, are not effective for acute treatment of exercise-induced asthma.

6.7.7.4 Allergic Bronchopulmonary Aspergillosis

Allergic bronchopulmonary aspergillosis (ABPA) is a complex hypersensitivity reaction to the antigens of *Aspergillus fumigatus*, a ubiquitous airborne fungus. This reaction occurs primarily in patients with asthma or cystic fibrosis. The aspergillus spores within the bronchial tree activate the immune system to cause tissue inflammation that results in proximal bronchiectasis and bronchiolitis obliterans. ABPA occurs in 1–2% of patients with persistent asthma and in 2–15% of those with cystic fibrosis. ABPA can occur in asthma of any severity, but it is more common in patients with moderate or severe persistent asthma.

The pathogenesis of ABPA is incompletely understood. T-cells likely have an important role by generating cytokines such as IL-4, IL-5, and IL-13 that contribute to the eosinophilia and elevated IgE seen in ABPA. In addition to the Th-2-mediated eosinophilic inflammation, enzymes and toxins released from the fungi and neutrophilic-mediated inflammation likely contribute to airway damage and central bronchiectasis. Besides the histologic features of asthma, ABPA is characterized by mucoid impaction of the bronchi and bronchocentric granulomatosis. The fungi do not invade the mucosa, but instead serve as the instigator of the immune response.

The clinical presentation of ABPA is characterized by persistent asthma complicated by recurrent episodes of bronchial obstruction, expectoration of brownish mucous plugs, and difficult-to-control asthma. No single test confirms the diagnosis of ABPA. Because of the marked inflammatory response, several laboratory abnormalities are typically noted. The diagnostic criteria for ABPA include the following:

1. History of asthma
2. Positive skin prick test or in vitro test to *A. fumigatus*
3. Elevated serum levels of IgG and IgE to *A. fumigatus*
4. Elevated total serum IgE ($>1,000$ ng mL^{-1})
5. Eosinophilia (>500 μL^{-1})
6. Pulmonary infiltrates on chest X-ray or chest CT
7. Central bronchiectasis

To make the diagnosis of ABPA, both a history of asthma (or cystic fibrosis) and a positive skin prick test or in vitro test to *A. fumigatus* should be documented (criteria 1 and 2 above). However, asthma patients can have IgE sensitivity to *A. fumigatus* without having ABPA. Approximately 20–30% of asthma patients have positive immediate skin prick testing to *A. fumigatus*. The diagnosis of ABPA-S (seropositive) is made when the first four criteria are met. The diagnosis of ABPA-CB (central bronchiectasis) is made when criteria 1–4 and 7 are met. A staging system has also been devised for ABPA.

- Stage 1 (acute): patient first appears with ABPA-S
- Stage 2 (remission): IgE level has decreased to 50–75% of the peak IgE
- Stage 3 (exacerbation): new radiographic infiltrates; IgE doubles
- Stage 4 (corticosteroid dependent): prednisone cannot be tapered without worsening asthma symptoms; increase in IgE level or development of radiographic infiltrates
- Stage 5 (fibrosis): lungs are fibrotic; pulmonary function testing shows restrictive defect with irreversible obstruction

The treatment of ABPA is designed to control the episodes of acute inflammation and to prevent the development of progressive lung injury and fibrosis. An acute flare of ABPA (stage 1 or 3) is treated with 0.5–1.0 mg kg^{-1} of prednisone for 14 days, followed by reduction to every-other-day dosing and tapering over 2–4 months. The total serum IgE is an excellent marker of disease and should be monitored at 4 weeks and then monthly or bimonthly for 1 year. Clinical improvement is generally accompanied by a 35% decrease in serum IgE. If serum IgE does not decrease, one should consider medicine noncompliance, a continuing ABPA exacerbation, or another diagnosis. If patients are treated early and aggressively, few will have the disease progress to stage 5. Corticosteroids do not appear to benefit stage 5 disease. Itraconazole has also been studied in ABPA, and it should not be administered in place of corticosteroids for ABPA. Itraconazole may provide additional benefit to corticosteroid treatment. It should be considered for patients with a slow or poor response to corticosteroids or stage 4 disease. The daily dose should

not exceed 400 mg. Typical duration of therapy is 3–6 months. With itraconazole therapy, liver function tests should be monitored monthly.

6.7.5 Churg–Strauss Syndrome

Churg–Strauss syndrome is a systemic small-vessel vasculitis that occurs in patients with severe asthma and sinusitis. Four different definitions of the diagnosis of Churg–Strauss syndrome have been developed: the pathologic criteria of Churg and Strauss, the clinical criteria of Lanham and colleagues, the clinical criteria from the American College of Rheumatology, and the criteria from the Chapel Hill Concensus Conference (Table 6.22). This syndrome is a systemic disease that develops in patients with a history of upper airway disease and sinusitis. Involvement of other organs varies but typically includes the heart, gastrointestinal tract, cerebral vessels, joints, muscles, skin, and nerves. There is no single confirmatory laboratory test for Churg–Strauss syndrome. The diagnosis depends on the clinical presentation of the disease, with its histologic hallmarks. Tissue eosinophilia is essential, and blood eosinophilia in an untreated patient is almost always present. Although perinuclear anti-neutrophilic cytoplasmic antibody (p-ANCA) is usually detectable, its absence does not rule out the syndrome.

Churg–Strauss syndrome should be considered in a patient with moderate to severe asthma who has any of the following features: new-onset footdrop (mononeuritis

Table 6.22 Definitions of Churg–Strauss syndrome

Churg and Strauss 1951 (autopsy pathologic material)
History of asthma
Tissue eosinophilia
Systemic vasculitis
Extravascular granulomas
Fibrinoid necrosis of connective tissue

Lanham et al. (1984) (clinical with or without pathologic condition)
Asthma
Eosinophilia, $>1.5 \times 10^9 \ L^{-1}$
Evidence of vasculitis that involves at least two organs

American College of Rheumatology 1990 (Masi, A. T. et al.) (clinical with or without pathologic condition; diagnosis likely when four of the six criteria are present)
Asthma
Eosinophilia, $>10\%$
Neuropathy, mononeuropathy, or polyneuropathy
Pulmonary infiltrates
Paranasal sinus abnormality
Extravascular eosinophil infiltration on biopsy

Chapel Hill Consensus Conference 1994 (Jennette, J. C. et al.) (pathologic/clinical)
"Eosinophil-rich and granulomatous inflammation involving the respiratory tract and necrotizing vasculitis affecting small- to medium-sized vessels and associated with asthma and eosinophilia"

From Lilly, C. M., Churg, A., Lazarovich, M., et al. (2002) Asthma therapies and Churg–Strauss syndrome. J. Allergy Clin. Immunol. 109, S1–S19. Used with permission

multiplex); palpable purpura, bruising, or chronic urticarial-type lesions (small-vessel vasculitis of dermal blood vessels); migratory pulmonary infiltrates (eosinophilic infiltration of the lung); or cardiac enlargement with or without failure. Other associated symptoms include decreased appetite, paresthesias, headache, arthralgias, abdominal pain, proteinuria or hematuria, or worsening sinusitis. The differential diagnosis includes hypereosinophilic syndrome, the vasculitides, ABPA, hyperplastic rhinosinusitis with nasal polyposis, eosinophilic pneumonia, parasitic disease, and drug allergy.

Laboratory evaluation includes a complete blood count with differential cell count, ANCA studies, erythrocyte sedimentation rate, urinalysis, chest radiography, aspergillus skin testing, total IgE, stool examination for ova and parasites, and biopsy. Diagnostic biopsy should be performed on the most accessible affected tissue. Biopsy of sites that are not affected clinically is of limited value and therefore discouraged. Helpful biopsy sites include the sural nerve or affected muscle of patients with footdrop, skin biopsy of those with purpura, and lung biopsy of those with migratory pulmonary infiltrates.

The clinical course of Churg–Strauss syndrome varies, and there are no proven markers of disease activity. Nevertheless, monitoring of blood eosinophil counts and acute phase reactants are generally recommended for monitoring disease activity. Elevations in these may presage clinical exacerbation and help the physician in guiding medical management. For most patients with evidence of active vasculitis, corticosteroids and immunosuppressive agents are considered first-line therapy. Treatment for Churg–Strauss syndrome requires high doses of corticosteroids, with adjustment of the dose based on disease response. When corticosteroid therapy does not induce remission, the primary immunosuppressive agents used are cyclophosphamide and α-interferon.

6.8 Clinical Vignettes

6.8.1 Vignette 1

A 70-year-old man presented with continued cough, dyspnea, and wheeze. He had no previous history of respiratory problems until 1 year ago when concomitant sinusitis and cough, dyspnea, and wheeze developed. At that time, evaluation showed the following: normal chest radiograph; pulmonary function testing with a markedly decreased FEV_1/FVC ratio and an FEV_1 of 0.91 L, 28% predicted, and normal D_Lco; coronal sinus CT with chronic pansinusitis and nasal polyps; negative ANCA studies; normal IgE; and negative allergen skin prick testing to common aeroallergens, including *Aspergillus*. He subsequently had functional endoscopic sinus surgery, after which his sinus symptoms improved significantly. However, over the course of the year, he continued to have cough, dyspnea, and wheeze essentially daily. He states that he does not have nighttime symptoms. He states that he has no other health problems, specifically no skin rash, weakness, or kidney problems.

Currently, he reports taking a combination of fluticasone and salmeterol (Advair) 250/50 one puff twice daily, prednisone 20 mg per day, montelukast (Singulair) 10 mg per day, pantoprazole (Protonix) 20 mg per day, and albuterol inhaler approximately once daily. Physical examination showed normal vital signs and normal skin. Ears, nose, and throat examination was normal. The cardiac examination was unremarkable. Lung examination was notable for scattered mild expiratory wheeze. There were no increased breath sounds over the sternal notch or inspiratory breath sounds. Currently, spirometry showed a decreased FEV_1/FVC ratio with an FEV_1 of 1.64 L, 51% predicted. Inspiratory loop was normal. Peripheral blood eosinophils were undetectable. Chest radiographic findings were unremarkable.

Comment: This situation represents a difficult process. The patient is currently symptomatic despite prednisone therapy and an intensive asthma management program. Always in severe asthma or steroid-dependent asthma, one must ensure that asthma is the correct diagnosis. In this case, the patient's clinical symptoms and pulmonary function testing are compatible with asthma. Other considerations that have been assessed include special subsets of asthma: ABPA (unlikely given the negative *Aspergillus* skin test and normal IgE) and Churg–Strauss syndrome (unlikely given the lack of peripheral eosinophilia, negative ANCA studies, and lack of skin or neurologic symptoms). Other conditions, including cardiac conditions, upper airway disorders, and other pulmonary conditions should also be assessed. On the basis of the above studies and thorough physical examination, these other conditions do not appear to be involved at this point. The next step is to consider all the factors that can contribute to asthma. The main issues to address are compliance, technique, and evaluation of exacerbators, using the mnemonic "air-smog," which includes *a*llergens, *i*rritants, *r*hinosinusitis, *s*moking, *m*edications, *o*ccupational history, and *g*astroesophageal reflux.

These issues were reviewed with the patient. Compliance did not appear to be an issue. Both he and his wife were quite clear in confirming his medication schedule. Technique was an issue. It was noted he was using the fluticasone/salmeterol inhaler incorrectly. He was given instruction and observed using the medication until it was mastered. Possible exacerbators of his asthma were reviewed. Allergens were thought not likely to be a factor based on negative skin prick testing to the common aeroallergens. He did not have exposure to irritants at his home. The rhinosinusitis had been stable since his surgery. He received maintenance treatment with intranasal corticosteroid and saline irrigations. He was a nonsmoker. He was not taking any β-blocker medication, in either pill or eye drop form. He was retired but continued to haul fertilizer by truck (occupation) and would occasionally note increased symptoms when loading and unloading the truck. He often forgot to wear a mask when loading and unloading. Although he had a history of gastroesophageal reflux, it was well controlled with pantoprazole.

Comment: Further review uncovered areas for improvement. The main areas were improved inhaler technique and the use of a mask when loading and unloading the fertilizer. Also, to maximize his inhaler regimen, fluticasone/salmeterol was increased to a high dose 500/50 one puff twice daily, with plans for a slow prednisone taper.

At follow-up 2 months later, the patient noted significant improvement, although he still required prednisone 5 mg per day to maintain good symptom control. He did not develop any other symptoms. He continued his inhaler regimen and his rhinosinusitis treatment. Further evaluation showed peripheral eosinophils 200 μL^{-1} (normal, <500), sputum eosinophils of 8% (normal, <3%), and exhaled nitric oxide 50 parts per billion (normal, <30). His FEV_1 increased to 70% predicted.

Comment: This patient would be considered to have severe asthma on the basis of the medications required to keep his symptoms controlled. He appears to have the late-onset, eosinophilic inflammation phenotype. In this phenotype, it is not uncommon to have concomitant sinus disease. This phenotype is typically difficult to treat. The patient will require close follow-up and should have preventive measures placed and close monitoring for corticosteroid adverse effects, particularly for posterior subcapsular cataracts and osteoporosis. Compliance, technique, and exacerbating factors (airsmog) need to be assessed routinely. The development of Churg–Strauss syndrome should be kept in mind. The goal is to decrease the corticosteroid dose whenever possible based on symptoms, pulmonary function, and inflammatory parameters.

6.8.2 Vignette 2

A 26-year-old female nurse with a history of anxiety presents for evaluation of asthma symptoms that have developed over the past 8 months. Despite the use of daily high-dose inhaled corticosteroids, long-acting β-agonist, and frequent use of albuterol, she continues to have symptoms of dyspnea. No cough is associated with this, but at times she feels that she wheezes. She states that she has no symptoms of rhinitis or gastroesophageal reflux. Her respiratory symptoms occur either randomly or sometimes with exposures to strong odors. There is not a strong association with exercise. She does feel it is worse when she is under increased stress. She has been treated with oral corticosteroids three times over the past 8 months. Currently, she is asymptomatic, and physical examination findings, with close attention paid to the ears, nose, and throat; heart; and lung examinations, are completely normal. Previous evaluations have included chest radiography, spirometry, electrocardiography, and echocardiography, and the results were normal.

Comment: She already has had many tests performed that have been nonrevealing. It is extremely important to obtain a good description of her dyspnea and wheeze.

The patient describes the dyspnea as typically occurring suddenly. Within minutes, she will quickly go from feeling fine to feeling that she is short of breath or cannot get a deep breath. Sometimes, the symptoms last up to 30 min and other times for days. In between episodes, she is asymptomatic. The albuterol does not seem to help when she uses it. She is not sure if the prednisone made any difference in her symptoms. She describes the wheeze as "loud breathing," typically more pronounced during inspiration.

Comment: The details of her symptoms are helpful. The sudden onset of symptoms can be seen in asthma, but asthma is generally slower in onset. The lack of benefit from albuterol and prednisone is highly suggestive of a process other than asthma. The noisy breathing during inspiration may be more consistent with stridor than with wheeze. Stridor can be a sign of an upper airway obstruction. In fixed upper airway obstruction, symptoms typically are precipitated initially by exertion and may progress to the point of occurring at rest. Currently, she is asymptomatic; it would be most helpful to evaluate her at a time she is symptomatic.

The patient returns when she is symptomatic. She appears dyspneic, with a respiratory rate of 24 breaths per minute and has audible stridor. Pulse oximetry is normal at 98% oxygen saturation. The lung examination shows increased breath sounds over the sternal notch with inspiration. The chest is clear.

Comment: The physical examination findings are not typical for asthma. An upper airway process is suggested by stridor and increased breath sounds over the sternal notch. Evaluation of the upper airway is needed.

While the patient was symptomatic, rhinolaryngoscopy was performed and showed paradoxical vocal cord adduction during inspiration.

Comment: This finding is diagnostic of vocal cord dysfunction. Unfortunately, it is often difficult to perform rhinolaryngoscopy when the patient is symptomatic. An inspiratory loop performed when the patient is symptomatic can be helpful, because it would show a flattened inspiratory loop and normal expiratory loop. Management of vocal cord dysfunction includes speech therapy and treatment of possible exacerbating factors, such as anxiety, depression, gastroesophageal reflux, and rhinitis.

6.8.3 Vignette 3

A 27-year-old woman presents during her first trimester of pregnancy for evaluation of her asthma. She describes a history of mild asthma dating back to childhood. She has never been hospitalized for asthma but did require an emergency department visit 7 months ago. She believed her asthma worsened with her previous pregnancy 3 years ago. Currently, she describes daily symptoms of wheeze and shortness of breath and nighttime symptoms once or twice weekly. She is using her albuterol inhaler three times daily. She was prescribed an inhaled corticosteroid 7 months ago, but discontinued it 3 months ago when she discovered she was pregnant. She has intermittent rhinitis symptoms but says she has no gastroesophageal reflux. She thinks her asthma is worse when cleaning the house. She has had a cat in the home for the last year. She does not smoke cigarettes. Physical examination showed scattered end-expiratory wheezes. Spirometry showed a decreased FEV_1/FVC ratio and an FEV_1 of 75% predicted. This improved to 85% predicted after two puffs of inhaled albuterol.

Comment: This patient has mild-to-moderate persistent asthma that is not optimally controlled. In an effort to improve her asthma, education should be undertaken to explain the management of asthma in pregnancy. It should be emphasized that the main risk to her and her baby is not the common medications used to treat asthma, but rather poorly controlled asthma. Allergy testing, particularly to dust mite and cat, would be helpful to assess possible exacerbators of her asthma. She is at risk for worsening asthma during this pregnancy because it occurred with her last pregnancy.

Allergy skin testing was strongly positive to dust mite, but negative to cat.

Comment: A comprehensive asthma management plan should be outlined that includes the following: (1) education about asthma and pregnancy, (2) environmental measures to decrease dust mite exposure, primarily by encasing the mattress and pillows with allergen-impermeable covers and washing the bedding in hot water weekly, (3) institution of low-dose inhaled corticosteroid, with instruction on inhaler technique, (4) peak flow rate instruction and development of a peak flow-based asthma action plan, and (5) follow-up in 2–4 weeks and scheduled visits thereafter, with easy availability for any problems between scheduled visits.

6.8.4 *Vignette 4*

A 42-year-old woman presents for evaluation of a 6-month history of chest tightness, nonproductive cough, and dyspnea. The patient reports a long-standing history of mild allergic rhinitis, with symptoms primarily in the spring and fall; however, these symptoms have been rather constant over the past year. She does not recall respiratory problems or asthma being diagnosed when she was a child. The patient has never smoked, and there have not been any changes in the home environment over the past decade. She says she does not take any prescription or over-the-counter medications or have symptoms of gastroesophageal reflux. Overall, she was in good general health. Her vital signs were normal. Nasal examination was notable for boggy edema of the inferior turbinates, with a small amount of clearish discharge. The heart examination was normal. The lung examination showed scattered expiratory wheezes. Spirometry showed a slightly decreased FEV_1/FVC ratio and an FEV_1 of 80% of predicted. This improved to 94% of predicted after two puffs of albuterol.

Comment: The patient's history, physical examination findings, and spirometry are consistent with rhinitis and asthma. Although she has a history of seasonal allergies, it is not clear why persistent rhinitis and asthma have developed. More information is required about her home and work environment to search for clues to why this may have progressed.

The patient relates she has lived in the same home for the past 12 years. No major remodeling has been done, and there has not been any dampness or water damage. She does not have any pets. However, she reports that she changed jobs approximately 1 year ago. She previously had worked as a cashier and now works in a bakery for a local supermarket. Her primary jobs are cake decoration and baking. On further questioning, she thought her symptoms were worse on days she baked cakes and better on days when she was not at work. She did not have a history of food allergies.

Comment: Possibilities for her increasing symptoms include a new sensitivity to dust mite or occupational exposure. The patient's report of increased symptoms at work raises the question of occupational asthma. In a bakery, wheat flour is the most common allergen, followed by soy flour. The role of an occupational exposure can be measured by having the patient stay off work for 1 week, then remeasuring the FEV_1, or performing serial peak flows before and after work exposure.

The patient stayed home from work for 1 week, treating her respiratory symptoms with inhaled albuterol. Her symptoms were well controlled with albuterol. Albuterol was discontinued 24 hours before her follow-up visit at the end of the week. On the follow-up visit, her lungs were clear to auscultation. Spirometry showed a baseline FEV_1 of 95% predicted and a normal FEV_1/FVC ratio. Allergen skin prick testing was markedly positive to wheat flour and was negative to soy flour and dust mite.

Comment: The findings are consistent with allergy to inhaled wheat flour, or "bakers' asthma," resulting in allergic rhinitis and asthma. Ideally, she should be moved to an area with limited exposure to wheat flour. Continued exposure to wheat flour would result in persistent rhinitis and asthma symptoms. It is important to treat the rhinitis as part of the asthma management. Masking and aggressive pharmacologic measures, including intranasal corticosteroid, H_1-blocker, inhaled corticosteroid, and inhaled β-agonist (as needed), should be used if the patient remains on the job. However, this would not be ideal.

6.8.5 Vignette 5

A 36-year-old female day care worker has a history of mild persistent asthma. She developed a persistent cough, maxillary discomfort, and purulent nasal secretions 7 days after contracting an upper respiratory tract infection. Her asthma had worsened, and she reported only partial relief with the use of inhaled albuterol. The physical examination was notable for a low-grade temperature of 100.4°F, right maxillary tenderness, purulent nasal secretions, and scattered end-expiratory wheezes. The peak expiratory flow was 330 L min^{-1}, 70% of predicted. Initial treatment included amoxicillin-clavulanate (Augmentin), 875 mg twice daily; increasing the daily inhaled steroid budesonide 200 μg from one puff twice daily to two puffs twice daily, and albuterol MDI, two puffs as needed every 4 hours.

Comment: The patient has had an upper respiratory tract infection, and now she has sinusitis and worsening asthma. Upper respiratory tract infections are the most common trigger for acute worsening of asthma. Increasing the inhaled corticosteroid may help improve the asthma exacerbation. This is likely most effective when done earlier in the course. The sinusitis is being treated appropriately with amoxicillin-clavulanate.

The patient returns 2 days later with increasing shortness of breath, chest tightness, and cough. She has been using her albuterol inhaler 4 times daily with only mild improvement in symptoms. On physical examination, she is afebrile with frequent coughing and a respiratory rate of 20 breaths per minute. The lung examination shows scattered expiratory wheezes throughout all lung fields. There are no crackles. Peak flow is 220 L min^{-1}, 50% of predicted. She was given albuterol, 0.5 mg in 3 mL of saline by nebulization × 3 and prednisone 40 mg by mouth. Following the nebulizations, the lung examination showed a decrease in the expiratory wheezes, with good air movement. The peak flow rate improved to 360 L min^{-1}, and, subjectively, the patient felt better. She was prescribed prednisone 40 mg per day for 5 days and albuterol inhaler two puffs every 4 hours, with continuation of budesonide 200 µg, two puffs twice daily. Plans were made for follow-up in 5 days, or sooner if her symptoms worsened.

Comment: Patients, even with mild asthma, can have severe exacerbations in conjunction with respiratory infections. These require aggressive treatment. The earlier use of high-dose inhaled corticosteroid or oral prednisone may have prevented the severe exacerbation.

At follow-up 5 days later, the lung examination showed only rare expiratory wheeze, and peak flow increased to 410 L min^{-1}. She was asked to continue the budesonide at two puffs twice daily for 6 weeks, with probable resumption to one puff twice daily at that time.

Comment: The patient had significant improvement with the use of oral prednisone. Even though her condition was clinically improved, the asthma, particularly from an inflammatory viewpoint, has not returned to baseline. To help prevent relapse and to hasten recovery to preexacerbation levels, she will continue the higher dose of inhaled corticosteroid for 6 weeks. At that time, she should have a follow-up examination and a review of her peak flow measurements to aid in reestablishing her management program.

Suggested Reading

Abramson, M. J., Puy, R. M., and Weiner, J. M. (1995) Is allergen immunotherapy effective in asthma? A meta-analysis of randomized controlled trials. Am. J. Respir. Crit. Care Med. 151, 969–974.

Abramson, M. J., Puy, R. M., and Weiner, J. M. (2003) Allergen immunotherapy for asthma. Cochrane Database Syst. Rev. (4), CD001186.

Agertoft, L. and Pedersen, S. (1994) Effects of long-term treatment with an inhaled corticosteroid on growth and pulmonary function in asthmatic children. Respir. Med. 88, 373–381.

Bakker, D. A., Berger, R. M., Witsenburg, M., and Bogers, A. J. (1999) Vascular rings: a rare cause of common respiratory symptoms. Acta Paediatr. 88, 947–952.

Bousquet, J., Van Cauwenberge, P., and Khaltaev, N. (2001) Allergic rhinitis and its impact on asthma. J. Allergy Clin. Immunol. 108, S147–S334.

Churg, J. and Strauss, L. (1951) Allergic granulomatosis, allergic angiitis, and periarteritis nodosa. Am. J. Pathol. 27, 277–301.

Ciftci, T. U., Ciftci, B., Guven, S. F., Kokturk, O., and Turktas, H. (2005) Effect of nasal continuous positive airway pressure in uncontrolled nocturnal asthmatic patients with obstructive sleep apnea syndrome. Respir. Med. 99, 529–534.

Froudarakis, M., Fournel, P., Burgard, G., et al. (1996) Bronchial carcinoids: a review of 22 cases. Oncology 53, 153–158.

Gilmour, M. I., Jaakkola, M. S., London, S. J., Nel, A. E., and Rogers, C. A. (2006) How exposure to environmental tobacco smoke, outdoor air pollutants, and increased pollen burdens influences the incidence of asthma. Environ. Health Perspect. 114, 627–633.

Girard, F., Chaboillez, S., Cartier, A., et al. (2004) An effective strategy for diagnosing occupational asthma: use of induced sputum. Am. J. Respir. Crit. Care Med. 170, 845–850.

Green, R. H., Brightling, C. E., McKenna, S., et al. (2002) Asthma exacerbations and sputum eosinophil counts: a randomised controlled trial. Lancet 360, 1715–1721.

Haahtela, T., Jarvinen, M., Kava, T., et al. (1994) Effects of reducing or discontinuing inhaled budesonide in patients with mild asthma. N. Engl. J. Med. 331, 700–705.

Hoffman, G. S., Kerr, G. S., Leavitt, R. Y., et al. (1992) Wegener granulomatosis: an analysis of 158 patients. Ann. Intern. Med. 116, 488–498.

Jennette, J. C., Falk, R. J., Andrassy, K., et al. (1994) Nomenclature of systemic vasculitides: proposal of an international consensus conference. Arthritis Rheum. 37, 187–192.

Lange, P., Parner, J., Vestbo, J., Schnohr, P., and Jensen, G. (1998) A 15-year follow-up study of ventilatory function in adults with asthma. N. Engl. J. Med. 339, 1194–1200.

Lanham, J. G., Elkon, K. B., Pusey, C. D., and Hughes, G. R. (1984) Systemic vasculitis with asthma and eosinophilia: a clinical approach to the Churg–Strauss syndrome. Medicine (Baltimore) 63, 65–81.

Lilly, C. M., Churg, A., Lazarovich, M., et al. (2002) Asthma therapies and Churg–Strauss syndrome. J. Allergy Clin. Immunol. 109, S1–S19.

Masi, A. T., Hunder, G. G., Lie, J. T., et al. (1990) The American College of Rheumatology 1990 criteria for the classification of Churg–Strauss syndrome (allergic granulomatosis and angiitis). Arthritis Rheum. 33, 1094–1100.

Napierkowski, J. and Wong, R. K. (2003) Extraesophageal manifestations of GERD. Am. J. Med. Sci. 326, 285–299.

National Asthma Education and Prevention Program: Expert Panel Report 2 (1997) Guidelines for the diagnosis and management of asthma. NIH publication No. 97-4051. Bethesda, MD: U.S. Department of Health and Human Services; National Institutes of Health; National Heart, Lung and Blood Institute.

National Asthma Education and Prevention Program: Expert Panel Report (2002) Guidelines for the diagnosis and management of asthma update on selected topics. J. Allergy Clin. Immunol. 110, S141–S219.

National Asthma Education and Prevention Program (2005) Working group report on managing asthma during pregnancy: recommendations for pharmacologic treatment: update 2004. NIH publication No. 05-3279. Bethesda, MD: U.S. Department of Health and Human Services; National Institutes of Health; National Heart, Lung, and Blood Institute.

National Asthma Education and Prevention Program: Expert Panel Report 3 (2007) Guidelines for the diagnosis and management of asthma. NIH publication No. 07-4051. Bethesda, MD: U.S. Department of Health and Human Services; National Institutes of Health; National Heart, Lung and Blood Institute.

Nelson, H. S., Weiss, S. T., Bleecker, E. R., Yancey, S. W., and Dorinsky, P. M (2006) The Salmeterol Multicenter Asthma Research Trial: a comparison of usual pharmacotherapy for asthma or usual pharmacotherapy plus salmeterol. Chest 129, 15–26.

O'Byrne, P. M., Pedersen, S., Busse, W. W., et al. (2006) Effects of early intervention with inhaled budesonide on lung function in newly diagnosed asthma. Chest 129, 1478–1485.

Park-Wyllie, L., Mazzotta, P., Pastuszak, A., et al. (2000) Birth defects after maternal exposure to corticosteroids: prospective cohort study and meta-analysis of epidemiological studies. Teratology 62, 385–392.

Salpeter, S., Ormiston, T., and Salpeter, E. (2002) Cardioselective beta-blockers for reversible airway disease. Cochrane Database Syst. Rev. (1), CD002992.

Smith, A. D., Cowan, J. O., Brassett, K. P., Herbison, G. P., and Taylor, D. R. (2005) Use of exhaled nitric oxide measurements to guide treatment in chronic asthma. N. Engl. J. Med. 352, 2163–2173.

Chapter 7
Urticaria and Angioedema

Abbreviations AAE: acquired C1 esterase inhibitor deficiency; ACE: angiotensin-converting enzyme; ANCA: antineutrophil cytoplasmic antibodies; CCP: cyclic citrullinated peptide; HAE: hereditary C1 esterase inhibitor deficiency; MPO: myeloperoxidase; NSAID: nonsteroidal anti-inflammatory drug; PR3: proteinase 3; PUPPP: pruritic urticarial papules and plaques of pregnancy; SPEP: serum protein electrophoresis.

7.1   Description and Epidemiology

Urticarial skin lesions are commonly known as hives or wheals. Urticaria represents transient localized areas of edema within skin tissue that appear as pruritic, raised erythematous, skin-colored or white, nonpitting, blanching plaques of variable size. Urticaria can be found anywhere on the body but is most common on the trunk and extremities. Angioedema is an edematous area that involves inflammation in the dermis and deeper subcutaneous tissue. It presents as nonpitting swelling without any color change. The size of the angioedema varies, and although it can appear anywhere on the body, it is most common in the periorbital and perioral regions. Because the deeper skin layers contain few mast cells, angioedema usually produces little or no pruritus. In contrast to other forms of edema, angioedema is distributed asymmetrically and does not characteristically occur in dependent regions.

It has been estimated that 20% of the population may have urticaria sometime during their lifetime. Angioedema accompanies urticaria in approximately 40% of patients, another 40% have hives alone, and about 20% have angioedema but not urticaria. Urticaria and angioedema are manifestations of the same underlying process, and in this chapter, discussion of urticaria also implies the possible presence of angioedema, except where specified. Urticaria is broadly divided into acute and chronic urticaria. *Acute urticaria* is defined as urticaria lasting less than 6 weeks and *chronic urticaria*, as lasting more than 6 weeks. This distinction can be helpful in the initial evaluation, although clearly, this is somewhat arbitrary because acute urticaria can "progress" into chronic

G.W. Volcheck, *Clinical Allergy: Diagnosis and Management*   279
DOI: 10.1007/978-1-59745-315-8_7, © 2009 Mayo Foundation for Medical
Education and Research

urticaria. Acute urticaria is a self-limited disorder typically caused by an allergic reaction to food or a drug and found more commonly in children and young adults. In contrast, chronic urticaria is typically nonallergic and is more common in middle-aged persons. Typical causes of acute urticaria include food products, medications, infections, and insect bites and stings. Chronic urticaria may occur in up to 25% of all patients with urticaria. However, in chronic urticaria, a specific cause is seldom identified. Although rarely life threatening, chronic urticaria causes significant discomfort and has an impact on an individual's quality of life comparable with that of severe coronary artery disease.

7.2 Pathophysiology

No unifying mechanism has been identified that accounts for all the mechanisms and clinical presentations of urticaria and angioedema. Urticaria can be IgE mediated, complement mediated, autoantibody mediated, and physically mediated. Although these mechanisms have been described, there are likely additional mechanisms because of the high frequency of idiopathic chronic urticaria. The end point for these mechanisms in most types of urticaria is the release of histamine and other inflammatory mediators by mast cells in the skin.

In acute urticaria, the most common mechanism is IgE-mediated mast cell activation. In this situation, food allergens or medication allergens cross-link membrane-bound IgE on mast cells, triggering mast cell degranulation. Mast cell products, primarily histamine, induce the wheal by increasing capillary permeability, the erythema by vasodilatation, and the itch through stimulation of the irritant receptors. The mechanism for infection-mediated hives, another primary cause of acute urticaria, is not clearly defined but likely includes complement activation.

In chronic urticaria, the known mechanisms consist primarily of an autoimmune process or a relationship to another underlying disease process. It appears that a significant percentage, approximately 40–50%, of chronic urticaria is autoimmune. Autoimmune urticaria is caused primarily by IgG antibody directed against the α subunit of the IgE receptor or possibly against IgE. The cause of the IgG formation is not known. This IgG–IgE receptor or IgG–IgE interaction activates basophils and mast cells, producing hive formation.

Complement activation leads to the production of the anaphylatoxins C3a, C4a, and C5a, causing the non-IgE-mediated release of mast cell mediators. Anaphylatoxins are produced in infections (hepatitis), connective tissue disorders (lupus erythematosus), medication reactions (serum sickness), and malignancies.

A variety of compounds are capable of releasing mediators from cutaneous mast cells through unknown mechanisms. Substance P, endorphins, enkephalins, and endogenous peptides, including gastrin, vasoactive intestinal peptide, and somatostatin, have been shown to release histamine from cutaneous mast cells at concentrations slightly above physiologic levels. These compounds may have a significant role in mast cell mediator release, particularly when there is a decrease in the threshold of mast cell activation.

Skin biopsy has been only minimally helpful in elucidating the specific pathogenic mechanisms in urticaria. Acute and physical urticarias show only dermal edema without cellular infiltrate. Chronic urticaria shows a perivascular mononuclear infiltrate with mast cells without evidence of vasculitis. The mononuclear infiltrate is composed predominantly of T-lymphocytes, specifically CD4+ helper cells. Biopsy specimens of hives induced by intradermal injection of autologous serum showed a mixed Th1/Th2 lymphocyte response, neutrophil infiltration, and increased chemokine activity. Skin biopsy is helpful to confirm vasculitis. The examination of skin biopsy specimens with immunofluorescence helps identify specific forms of connective tissue disease-induced vasculitis and urticarial vasculitis.

Despite current understanding of the autoimmune etiology of chronic urticaria, 40–50% of cases still remain idiopathic. Currently, it is thought that autoimmune and other yet unknown processes lower the threshold for mast cell activation, rendering the mast cell susceptible to mediator release by endogenous substances.

7.3   Acute Urticaria: Etiologies

Acute urticaria is self-limited urticaria that resolves in 6 weeks. The most common causes are drug reactions, foods, insect bite and stings, and infections. Occasionally, urticaria can be caused by inhalant allergens. In these situations, the inhalant allergen, primarily tree, grass, and weed pollens and pet allergens, also produce significant upper and lower respiratory tract symptoms, which aid in the diagnosis.

7.3.1   Medications

Antibiotics, in particular β-lactam antibiotics, are the most common medications associated with acute urticaria. However, all medications have the potential for eliciting an urticarial reaction; thus, it is extremely important that the entire medication list be reviewed upon evaluation for acute urticaria, with special attention paid to start and stop dates of the medications. This medication list should also include nonprescription medications, particularly nonsteroidal anti-inflammatory medications (NSAIDs) and health supplements. Hives may occur anywhere from minutes after administration of the drug to days or weeks later. In an IgE-mediated reaction, bronchospasm, gastrointestinal symptoms, and hypotension may be present in addition to the hives. The time from the administration of a medication to the development of symptoms is usually less than 1 hour. Direct mast cell release can occur with radiocontrast material, codeine, aspirin, and other NSAIDs with or without other symptoms of histamine release. Urticaria that occurs 1–3 weeks after antibiotic administration may be due to a serum sickness or serum sickness-like reaction. Antibiotics are the most frequent cause of this type of reaction. Therefore, when assessing acute urticaria, it is important to review all medications the patient has taken over the preceding month.

7.3.2 Foods

Foods are an important cause of acute urticaria. For children, the most commonly implicated foods include milk, soy, wheat, egg, peanut, tree nuts, and fish. For adults, the most common foods are peanuts, tree nuts, and fish. However, all foods have the potential to cause an urticarial reaction. The key point in the history is that the hives almost always occur within an hour after the food is ingested and typically within minutes. If the hives occur more than 2 hours after ingestion of the food, it is difficult to implicate the food as the cause of the hives. Also, it would be unusual for the food to cause hives in one instance, then be eaten without causing hives at a later time. Allergen skin prick testing or in vitro testing to foods can be performed to identify a food allergen. Testing should only be performed on foods suspected from the clinical history. If it appears that the hives are closely related to food ingestion, a food diary can be helpful in identifying the causative food.

7.3.3 Insect Stings and Bites

The bites of fleas, mites, mosquitoes, or lice can cause papular urticaria. The lesions present as pruritic tiny hives primarily on the extremities and represent a delayed hypersensitivity response to the bites. Hymenoptera stings can cause urticaria at the site of the sting or throughout the body. The urticaria may be seen alone or in conjunction with other IgE-mediated symptoms, including angioedema, bronchospasm, gastrointestinal symptoms, or hypotension. The presence of a sting is usually obvious from the history.

7.3.4 Infection

Common viruses, particularly *Rhinovirus* and *Rotavirus*, frequently cause acute urticaria, especially in children. It is important to ask specifically about viral symptoms (fever, nasal congestion, sore throat, cough, diarrhea, myalgia, arthralgia). The viral symptoms may occur before or concomitant with the urticaria, and they may have resolved by the time of the evaluation. Therefore, it is important to include questions about the presence or absence of previous viral symptoms as part of the history. The usual time course for viral-induced hives to resolve without other complicating factors is 1–3 weeks.

Urticaria has also been associated with specific infection syndromes. Hepatitis B, mononucleosis, herpes infection, mycoplasma infection, and group A streptococcal pharyngitis have been reported as causes of acute urticaria.

7.4 Chronic Urticaria

Chronic urticaria is defined by the presence of hives for more than 6 weeks, differentiating it from acute urticaria. Chronic urticaria is a very difficult condition to evaluate and manage (Fig. 7.1). It can divided into three groups: (1) idiopathic and

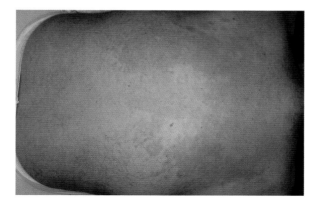

Fig. 7.1 Chronic urticaria. Widespread urticaria with coalescence of hives and erythema

autoimmune chronic urticaria (70% of cases), (2) physical urticaria (20% of cases), and (3) chronic urticaria secondary to underlying or associated disease (10% of cases). There can be overlap between these groups, particularly with the physical urticarias, because there can be a significant physical trigger in chronic urticaria of any cause. In addition, thyroid disease can be classified in the autoimmune or secondary disease category.

In approximately 70% of cases, chronic urticaria is autoimmune or idiopathic (Table 7.1). It is extremely important to educate the patient about this fact. Often, patients make drastic lifestyle changes and pursue a myriad of unconventional means in an effort to find a cause and treatment. Although chronic urticaria has been considered to be a manifestation of a reaction to foods, food preservatives, or food dyes or an anxiety disorder, these suppositions have not been substantiated on a large scale. Adherence to specialized diets has not had an effect on chronic urticaria. Anxiety, although sometimes associated with worsening of hives, is not the underlying cause. Approximately half of the patients in this category have chronic autoimmune urticaria secondary to an IgG antibody directed primarily against the IgE receptor or possibly IgE, and the other half have true idiopathic disease. Clinically, there is little distinction between the two entities, and they often are referred to together as *idiopathic urticaria* or simply *chronic urticaria*. Typically, the urticaria arises spontaneously and leaves a particular skin area in 4–6 hours. When the urticaria stays in one place for more than 24–36 hours or leaves bruises, then vasculitis or another underlying cause should be strongly considered.

In approximately 10% of patients, a secondary cause is found for chronic urticaria. A large number of disorders either have hives as part of their symptom complex or initiate changes resulting in hives. In some instances, the urticaria is present before or overshadows the signs and symptoms of the underlying disorder. The most common underlying disorders are infection, thyroid disease, connective tissue disease, and malignancy. Food allergy or environmental allergy is rarely associated with chronic urticaria. If food is the cause, it is usually obvious from the history from the temporal profile (development of hives within 1 hour after ingestion, with

Table 7.1 Etiology of chronic urticaria[a]

Idiopathic or autoimmune chronic urticaria (~70%)
    Autoimmune (~35%)
        IgG against α-subunit IgE receptor (25–30%)
        IgG against α-subunit of IgE (5–10%)
    Idiopathic (~35%)
Physical urticarias (20%)
    Dermatographism
    Cholinergic urticaria
    Cold urticaria
    Exercise-induced urticaria
    Delayed pressure urticaria
    Solar urticaria
    Vibratory urticaria
    Aquagenic urticaria
Associated underlying disorder (~10%)
    Infection
    Thyroid disease
    Connective tissue disease
    Malignancy
    Allergy

[a]Percentage values are percent of cases

subsequent resolution until the food is eaten again), and the patient often suspects the diagnosis. In other instances, hives are part of several other signs and symptoms, as in vasculitis, mastocytosis, and pruritic urticarial papules and plaques of pregnancy (PUPPP).

When the primary presenting symptom is chronic, recurrent angioedema in the absence of urticaria, C1 esterase inhibitor deficiency and medications are the primary causes, in addition to the above conditions (Fig. 7.2). Angiotensin-converting enzyme (ACE) inhibitors, in particular, are associated with recurrent angioedema in the absence of urticaria. This class of medication can cause recurrent angioedema at any time. ACE inhibitor-induced angioedema has been reported in patients who have taken the medication without symptoms for more than 5 years. Any patient with angioedema should stop taking ACE inhibitors.

A thorough review of systems and complete physical examination are helpful in assessing for these possible underlying disorders. An exhaustive array of tests usually is not indicated in the evaluation of chronic urticaria. Specialized testing can be performed on the basis of the findings of the history and physical examination.

7.4.1 Autoimmune and Idiopathic Urticaria

Abnormal immunologic findings in a significant number of patients with chronic urticaria have led to the term *autoimmune urticaria*. About half of the patients who have chronic urticaria without a secondary cause are positive on autologous serum

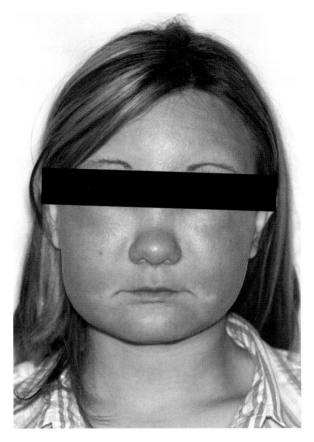

Fig. 7.2 Angioedema

skin testing and have antibodies to the alpha unit of the IgE receptor or to IgE. The other half are considered to have idiopathic chronic urticaria. Ongoing studies are investigating whether patients with autoimmune urticaria have a more prolonged and severe course or have a better response to immunomodulatory agents than those with idiopathic urticaria. Evaluation has been difficult because the sensitivity and specificity of the autologous serum skin test has varied from 50–80%, making identification of a specific autoimmune group difficult. Testing to antibodies against the IgE receptor or IgE are performed primarily in research centers, although some commercial assays are becoming available. The commercial assays have been plagued by poor specificity.

Clinically, in patients with autoimmune or idiopathic chronic urticaria, the urticaria arises spontaneously and leaves a particular skin area in 4–6 hours. When the urticaria stays in one place for more than 24–36 hours or leaves bruises, then vasculitis or another underlying cause should be strongly considered.

Angioedema accompanies the urticaria in approximately 40% of patients. The urticaria typically occurs on a daily basis and has the potential to last for years. Chronic urticaria lasts more than 1 year in 50% of patients and more than 5 years in 15%. Occasionally, the urticaria can disappear and then recur years later.

7.4.2 *Physical Urticaria*

Physical urticarias are a unique group of chronic urticaria caused by physical stimuli to the skin. They have a significant role in approximately 20% of all cases of chronic urticarias, either as the sole cause or as an exacerbator of an underlying chronic urticaria. In the evaluation of the chronic urticaria, it is important to inquire about the effect of these physical stimuli. These types of urticaria are not IgE mediated, and the exact pathophysiology is unknown. Physical urticarias include dermatographism, delayed pressure urticaria, solar urticaria, cholinergic urticaria, cold urticaria, aquagenic urticaria, and vibratory urticaria.

7.4.2.1 Dermatographism

Dermatographism means "write on the skin" and appears in varying degrees in approximately 5% of the population. Patients note linear hives that develop within minutes after the skin surface is scratched (Fig. 7.3). This can easily be reproduced in the office by stroking the skin with a pointed instrument. Within minutes, erythema, pruritus, and linear streaks of edema or wheal formation develop. Note that erythema formation alone does not constitute true dermatographism; a wheal also needs to be raised. Severe dermatographism can be the sole cause of hives when it is clear that the hive formation occurs only after skin contact.

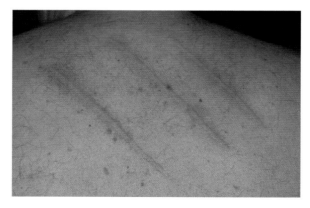

Fig. 7.3 Dermatographism. A wheal and flare reaction is elicited after stroking the skin

Usually, however, dermatographism is seen in patients with chronic urticaria from other causes. In this situation, the dermatographism worsens the underlying urticaria. Dermatographism has been passively transferred with plasma, but no antigen has been shown to initiate the response. Antihistamines are usually effective if treatment is required.

7.4.2.2 Delayed Pressure Urticaria

Delayed pressure urticaria is characterized by the gradual development of urticaria or angioedema (or both) at the site where pressure has been applied to the skin. The onset of symptoms is at least 4–6 hours after the pressure was applied and can occur up to 24 hours later. The symptoms commonly occur around tight clothing. Foot swelling is common after walking or standing for long periods, and buttock swelling may be prominent after sitting for a few hours. The mechanism of these reactions is not known. Treatment is based primarily on avoidance of pressure situations, for example, loosening a tight belt, adjusting a brassiere strap or purse strap, and avoiding prolonged stationary pressure positions. This condition is difficult to treat, and antihistamines are generally ineffective. In severe cases, low-dose, alternate-day corticosteroid treatment is an option. NSAIDs and H_2 blockers have been helpful occasionally. Immediate pressure urticaria, in contrast, is rare and associated with hypereosinophilic syndrome.

7.4.2.3 Solar Urticaria

Solar urticaria is a rare disorder characterized by the development of pruritus, erythema, and edema within minutes after exposure to light. Typically, the lesions occur only in the light-exposed areas and last 1–3 hours. The different types of solar urticaria have been classified on the basis of the wavelength of light that causes the urticaria. The diagnosis can be established by challenging with light of various wavelengths. Treatment consists primarily of avoidance through the use of protective clothing and topical preparations to absorb and reflect light. Antihistamines taken before exposure to sunlight can help in some instances.

7.4.2.4 Cholinergic Urticaria

Cholinergic urticaria is small, punctate urticaria 1–3 mm in diameter produced by heat. The most common provocateurs are exercise, sweating, a hot shower, fever, and anxiety. The small size of the hives and intense pruritus are characteristic and help to differentiate this condition from the other types of urticaria. This condition is most commonly seen in teenagers and young adults. The hives occur most commonly on the upper trunk and arms. Antihistamines, particularly hydroxyzine, are usually helpful in treating this condition.

7.4.2.5   Cold Urticaria

Cold urticaria is characterized by rapid onset of urticaria or angioedema (or both) after exposure to cold. The hives are generally confined to the cold-exposed areas, such as the face and hands. In extreme cases, total body exposure, such as jumping into cold water, can result in hypotension and subsequent drowning. This condition is usually idiopathic, but it also has been associated with cryoglobulinemia, cryofibrinogenemia, cold agglutinin disease, and paroxysmal cold hemoglobinuria. The diagnosis of cold urticaria can be confirmed by placing an ice cube on the forearm for 4 min and observing the immediate development of a large wheal at the site of the ice cube. Prevention consists of limiting exposed skin to the cold. The patient should be advised to enter swimming areas cautiously. Antihistamines are the usual treatment of choice. When an abnormal protein is present, treatment and monitoring of the underlying disease are indicated.

7.4.2.6   Aquagenic Urticaria

Aquagenic urticaria is a rare form of physical urticaria. Patients develop small wheals after contact with water, regardless of water temperature. The wheals can be reproduced by applying a water compress to the skin.

7.4.2.7   Vibratory Urticaria

Vibratory urticaria is a rare form of physical urticaria characterized by localized urticaria and angioedema in areas exposed to vibratory stimuli. The mechanism is not known, although histamine release is evident. Treatment consists of avoidance and antihistamines.

7.4.2.8   Exercise-Induced Urticaria

Exercise-induced urticaria is an uncommon form of urticaria. It may appear as a spectrum of urticaria ranging from small, 1–3 mm, punctate urticaria resembling cholinergic urticaria alone, to large, widespread welts with associated systemic anaphylaxis. The urticaria typically begins within the first 10 min after exercise and progresses if the exercise is continued. These patients have hives only with exercise. There are subgroups of exercise-induced hives/anaphylaxis based on food ingestion. In food-associated urticaria/anaphylaxis, a specific food eaten within 4 hours before the exercise triggers the urticaria/anaphylaxis reaction, although the patient can tolerate the food in the absence of exercise and can exercise without symptoms if the food is not ingested. The majority of patients with exercise-induced urticaria/anaphylaxis have increased symptoms with the ingestion of any food before exercise. The underlying pathophysiology is unknown. Treatment depends on the severity of the symptoms. The medications primarily used are H_1 blockers for mild urticaria and epinephrine for anaphylaxis. Prophylactic treatment with H_1 and H_2 blockers before exercise has been only minimally helpful in preventing symptoms. Patients should be instructed to refrain from eating for 4 hours before exercise, to exercise with a partner, to stop exercising at the first sign of symptoms, and to carry an epinephrine injection kit.

7.4.3   Underlying Causes of Chronic Urticaria

7.4.3.1   Infection

Generally, infections that contribute to chronic urticaria are low-grade, subclinical infections. In the history, clues to an infectious cause include intermittent or persistent fever, sinus symptoms, chronic pharyngitis, cough, nausea, and diarrhea. Parasitic infections are probably the most commonly identified infectious cause of chronic urticaria. For this reason, it is important to obtain an environmental, occupational, travel, and immigration history. Environmentally, it is important to note if the patient has close contact with animals or lake water (or both). *Giardia* is a parasite associated with chronic urticaria that can be obtained by exposure to lake water. Occupationally, exposures are more likely to occur if patients have close contact with animals. Travel, particularly outside the United States, can be a clue to a parasitic infection. Often, with a parasitic infection, the eosinophil count is increased. Other infections that have been associated with chronic urticaria include chronic sinusitis, tooth abscess, hepatitis, and endocarditis. Typically, the patient has some clinical signs or symptoms that point to these conditions. If the patient is completely asymptomatic, an extensive search for occult infection is not recommended.

7.4.3.2   Thyroid Disease

Thyroid disease, most frequently Hashimoto disease, has been implicated in chronic urticaria. Less common is an association with Graves disease. In these situations, the hives resolve with treatment of the disease. Patients with chronic urticaria have a higher prevalence of thyroid antibodies than the general population, even if euthyroid. The thyroid abnormality appears to be a parallel abnormality and may reflect the presence of an underlying autoimmune process. Although treatment with low-dose thyroid replacement in these patients (thyroid antibody positive, euthyroid [normal sensitive thyrotropin-stimulating hormone test]) has been associated with improvement in hives, the results overall have been inconsistent.

7.4.3.3   Connective Tissue Disease

Connective tissue disease can present with chronic urticaria. In this case, the patient usually has significant symptoms associated with the connective tissue disease. Disorders associated with chronic urticaria include rheumatoid arthritis, lupus erythematosus, mixed connective tissue disease, and scleroderma. Evaluation for these processes is not regularly indicated unless the patient exhibits signs or symptoms consistent with these diseases.

7.4.3.4   Malignancy

In young people, urticaria is rarely associated with malignancy. Malignancy and chronic urticaria are associated most often in the elderly. Urticaria and angioedema have been reported in association with lymphoma, leukemia, myeloma, and colon, rectum, liver, lung, ovarian, and testicular cancer. In some patients in whom malignancy and urticaria are clearly associated, a recurrence of urticaria can be associated with recurrence of the malignancy. Generally, the evaluation of chronic urticaria should include routinely recommended cancer screenings based on the age and risk factors of the patient.

7.4.3.5   Allergy

Chronic urticaria is not usually caused by sensitivity to foods, food preservatives, medications, or environmental allergens, even though most patients believe such sensitivities must be causative. In food allergy, symptoms usually occur reproducibly within 60 min after food ingestion. Unless there is a time relation between food ingestion and hive formation, IgE-mediated food allergy can usually be excluded. If the history is suggestive of food sensitivity, further evaluation such as skin testing or in vitro testing to the suspected foods can be helpful. Without a corroborating history, random skin testing to numerous foods is not indicated. The relation of food preservatives and additives to chronic urticaria has been a matter of controversy. Despite occasional reports, no significant relation has been shown. A 2-week preservative and additive elimination trial could be instituted to assess their relevance.

Medications have the potential to cause chronic urticaria, but they are not considered a common cause. The main clue historically is the onset of urticaria within 1 month after the patient starts taking a medication. Testing to medications is very limited and evaluation requires careful medication withdrawal, with substitution for those medications integral to health. If medications are suspected, they should be withdrawn one at a time for a 2–4-week period. Perhaps more importantly, over-the-counter medications, supplements, vitamins, and alternative medical preparations should be considered. These substances also can potentially cause chronic urticaria and may be easier to eliminate.

7.5 Urticaria-Angioedema-Associated Disorders

A few systemic disorders have urticaria or angioedema (or skin changes resembling urticaria or angioedema) as primary symptoms in association with other findings typical of the disorder. These conditions include urticarial vasculitis, C1 esterase inhibitor deficiency (hereditary and acquired), mastocytosis, and PUPPP.

7.5.1 Urticarial Vasculitis

Urticarial vasculitis presents as recurrent episodes of urticaria that have the histopathologic features of leukocytoclastic vasculitis. The clinical signs and symptoms that help differentiate this from chronic idiopathic or autoimmune urticaria are (1) a painful or burning sensation to the pruritic hives, (2) persistence of individual lesions for more than 24 hours, and (3) palpable purpura, bruising, or residual hyperpigmentation after the hives resolve (Fig. 7.4). Confirmation of urticarial vasculitis requires skin biopsy. Urticarial vasculitis generally has a more severe course than idiopathic or autoimmune chronic urticaria. It typically is idiopathic but can be associated with cryoglobulinemia, IgA myeloma, connective tissue disorders (particularly lupus erythematosus and Sjögren syndrome), infections (particularly hepatitis B, hepatitis C, infectious mononucleosis, coxsackievirus infections, and Lyme disease), and paraneoplastic syndromes. Normocomplementemic patients usually have minimal or no systemic involvement, whereas hypocomplementemic patients have a propensity for more severe multiorgan involvement. Response to treatment varies. Recommendations for treatment of urticarial vasculitis manifested only by nonnecrotizing skin lesions include antihistamines, dapsone, colchicine, hydroxychloroquine, or indomethacin, but corticosteroids are often required. With visceral involvement, corticosteroids are regularly indicated.

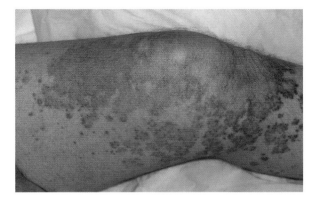

Fig. 7.4 Urticarial vasculitis

7.5.2 C1 Esterase Inhibitor Deficiency

C1 esterase inhibitor deficiency can be divided broadly into two categories: hereditary and acquired (Table 7.2). The clinical manifestations of C1 esterase inhibitor deficiency consist of localized angioedema that can occur spontaneously or be triggered by trauma, menstruation, infections, emotional stress, medications, or medical, surgical, or dental procedures. The angioedema is nonpitting, swollen, and asymmetric. It usually lasts for 3–5 days before spontaneously resolving. Urticaria or pruritus (or both) is only rarely associated with C1 esterase inhibitor deficiency, and the presence of either one essentially rules out C1 esterase inhibitor deficiency. The areas most commonly affected include the lips, eyelids, tongue, extremities, and genitalia. Visceral edema may cause intestinal obstruction, with anorexia, vomiting, and abdominal pain. The most serious symptoms are related to the airway, because angioedema of the oropharynx can result in life-threatening airway obstruction.

7.5.2.1 Hereditary C1 Esterase Inhibitor Deficiency

Hereditary C1 esterase inhibitor deficiency (HAE) is an autosomal dominant disorder defined by a deficiency of functional C1 esterase inhibitor. All HAE patients are heterozygotes and possess one normal *C1-INH* gene, which is encoded on chromosome 11. There are two types of HAE. Type 1 HAE accounts for 85% of cases and results in decreased production of C1 esterase inhibitor; thus, both the detectable level of C1 esterase inhibitor and C1 esterase inhibitor function are decreased. Type 2 HAE is caused by mutations in the C1 esterase inhibitor reactive site, and even though the circulating level of C1 esterase inhibitor is normal, the enzyme is not functional.

The age at symptom onset helps to clinically differentiate hereditary angioedema from acquired angioedema. Patients with hereditary angioedema typically have onset of episodic angioedema during childhood, but the symptoms may not be severe until the teenage years or early adulthood. In contrast, acquired angioedema occurs at a much older age, rarely before age 50 years.

The C4 level should be determined when evaluating for C1 esterase inhibitor deficiency. It is decreased in both conditions at all times and not dependent on

Table 7.2 C1 esterase inhibitor deficiency

| | | C1 esterase inhibitor | | |
	C4	Level	Function	C1q
Hereditary				
Type 1	↓	↓	↓	Normal
Type 2	↓	Normal	↓	Normal
Acquired				
Type 1	↓	↓	↓	↓
Type 2	↓	Normal	↓	↓

whether the patient is symptomatic at the time of the testing. The C1 esterase inhibitor level should be determined and a function assay should be performed if the C4 level is decreased.

The primary treatment of acute attacks is the rapid administration of anabolic steroids, such as danazol (200 mg four times daily) or stanozolol (4 mg four times daily). Intubation or tracheostomy to secure the airway can be potentially lifesaving. Antihistamines, glucocorticoids, and epinephrine have not proven efficacious. Intravenous purified C1 esterase inhibitor concentrate has been used successfully in Europe but is not currently available in the United States. The use of fresh frozen plasma that contains C1 esterase inhibitor is debated because the C4 component may contribute to further complement activation and angioedema.

Chronic prophylactic therapy with attenuated androgens such as danazol or stanozolol should be considered for patients who have frequent attacks (one or more monthly). These agents stimulate the synthesis of C1 esterase inhibitor from the one normal gene. Dosing ranges for danazol vary from 200 to 800 mg per day and for stanozolol 2–12 mg per day. Some studies suggest a role for every-other-day treatment. Because of adverse effects, the lowest effective dose should be used, and it often needs to be individualized for patients. Short-term prophylaxis for surgical and dental procedures may be achieved with 1 week of androgen therapy. Adverse effects include weight gain, altered libido, hirsutism, and liver enzyme abnormalities. These medications are contraindicated in pregnancy, during lactation, and for children. Antifibrinolytic agents such as E-aminocaproic acid may be used for prophylaxis in children as well as adults in whom androgens have failed. The dosing range varies from 2 to 10 g d^{-1}. The mechanism of action is unclear, and they generally are less effective than androgens. Adverse effects include myalgias, muscle weakness, fatigue, and increased serum level of creatine kinase.

Because the angioedema occurs intermittently and patients can have subclinical disease for years before symptoms are apparent, it is recommended that all family members of patients with HAE have screening.

7.5.2.2 Acquired C1 Esterase Inhibitor Deficiency

Acquired C1 esterase inhibitor deficiency (AAE) results from increased destruction or metabolism of C1 esterase inhibitor. The onset is usually after age 50. Two forms have been described. Type 1 AAE occurs predominantly in patients with malignancy, lymphoproliferative or hematologic disorders, or rheumatologic disease. In these patients, immune complexes form that activate C1 and consume C1 esterase inhibitor. In type 2 AAE, an autoantibody is produced that inactivates C1 esterase inhibitor, but it remains detectable as "normal" C1 esterase inhibitor. Therefore, as in type 2 HAE, the circulating level of C1 esterase inhibitor is normal but the functional activity is decreased. As in both hereditary forms, the C4 level is low during both active and quiescent periods in AAE and serves as an excellent screening tool. Unlike HAE, C1q is decreased in both types of AAE. This helps in differentiating HAE from AAE.

The critical issue in acquired C1 esterase inhibitor deficiency is the evaluation for an underlying malignancy. Patients should have a detailed physical examination, with special attention to lymph nodes, liver and spleen. Further evaluation with a complete blood count, with differential; T-cell and B-cell markers; computed tomography of the chest, abdomen, and pelvis; and bone marrow biopsy may be indicated, depending on the clinical presentation.

The primary treatment is treatment of the underlying disorder. Androgen therapy, as in HAE, may also benefit some patients.

7.5.3 Mastocytosis

Mastocytosis is characterized by mast cell hyperplasia in the skin and other organs such as the gastrointestinal tract, bone marrow, lymph nodes, liver, and spleen. The primary clinical symptoms include varying combinations of pruritus, urticaria, nausea, vomiting, abdominal pain, diarrhea, flushing, and vascular instability. Several classes of mastocytosis reflect the extent of mast cell involvement. The primary classes are cutaneous mastocytosis, systemic mastocytosis with or without skin involvement, mastocytosis in association with hematologic disorders, and mast cell leukemia.

Cutaneous mastocytosis can present as a solitary mastocytoma, urticaria pigmentosa, or diffuse cutaneous mastocytosis without urticaria pigmentosa. Urticaria pigmentosa is the most common skin manifestation of mastocytosis in children and adults. It is characterized by persistent, small, yellow-tan or red-brown maculopapular lesions. Mild trauma, such as stroking or scratching the lesions, provokes wheal and erythema formation at the site of the macule. This reaction is termed the *Darier sign*. Because of the wheal and erythema formation, these lesions may be confused with typical urticaria. It is important to differentiate these lesions from typical hives so that further evaluation of the extent of the mastocytosis can be undertaken.

Evaluation of mastocytosis should be individualized depending on suspected organ involvement. Mast cell mediators that are increased in systemic mastocytosis include serum tryptase and 11-β-prostaglandin $F_{2\alpha}$ and *N*-methylhistamine, as determined with 24-hours urine studies. These levels may be normal in cutaneous mastocytosis without systemic involvement. Skin biopsy can be performed to confirm urticaria pigmentosa.

7.5.4 Pruritic Urticarial Papules and Plaques of Pregnancy

PUPPP is an extremely pruritic condition that occurs most commonly during a woman's first pregnancy. It begins in the third trimester and persists until 1 week after delivery. The papules and plaques typically begin in the abdominal striae and spread to involve the thigh, buttocks, and arms. The eruption remains fixed and increases in intensity over time.

7.6 Patient Evaluation

An algorithm for the evaluation of patients with urticaria or angioedema (or both) is given in Fig. 7.5.

7.6.1 Acute Urticaria

Laboratory evaluation of acute urticaria focuses primarily on possible triggers elicited from the history. The history should specifically address the possible role of food, medication, and infection. Allergy skin testing to specific foods can be helpful if the clinical history shows a time association between food ingestion and hive development. If the clinical history does not point to specific triggers, random skin testing to airborne allergens or foods is not indicated. Blood tests such as a complete blood count, chemistry panel, thyroid function tests, or autoimmune studies or urinalysis are not usually indicated in acute urticaria unless other signs or symptoms suggest a systemic process.

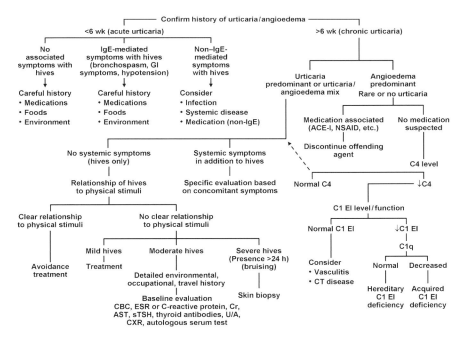

Fig. 7.5 Algorithm for the evaluation of urticaria or angioedema (or both). ACE-I, angiotensin-converting enzyme inhibitor; AST, aspartate aminotransferase; Cr, creatinine; CT, connective tissue; CXR, chest radiography; EI, esterase inhibitor; ESR, erythrocyte sedimentation rate; GI, gastrointestinal; NSAID, nonsteroidal anti-inflammatory drug; sTSH, sensitive thyrotropin-stimulating hormone; U/A, urinalysis

7.6.2 *Chronic Urticaria*

Evaluation for systemic disease is often indicated in chronic urticaria. There is no set laboratory evaluation for this condition, and it cannot be emphasized enough that the key to the evaluation is a thorough history, with a complete review of systems and a complete physical examination.

The history provides important clues to the cause of urticaria and angioedema, and an organized approach is essential. Initially, the diagnosis of urticaria and angioedema should be confirmed by the history, especially if hives are not present on the day of examination. The presence of other similar entities such as erythema multiforme or vesicular skin diseases should be excluded by the history. Once this has been established, important details about the hives should be assessed:

1. Start date of the hives
2. Situation at the onset of hives (illness, medication change, etc.)
3. Occurrence of the hives (continuously, daily, weekly, etc.)
4. Character of the hives (itchy, burning, painful)
5. Size range of the hives
6. Presence or absence of angioedema with the hives
7. Suspicions for cause of the hives
8. Treatments used for the hives
9. Complete medication (prescription and nonprescription) and health supplement list, with start and stop dates for the medications

After this baseline information about the hives has been obtained, an urticaria and angioedema review of systems (Table 7.3) should be performed to probe for possible secondary causes of the hives.

A complete physical examination should be performed on all patients who have chronic urticaria and angioedema. The purpose of the physical examination is to identify typical urticarial lesions and to evaluate for the presence of an underlying or associated disorder. Key components of the physical examination are full skin examination, lymph node examination, and liver and spleen evaluation.

Depending on the findings in the history and physical examination, laboratory evaluation needs to be tailored to each patient. When discussing the laboratory evaluation with the patient, it is important to inform him or her that most of the time chronic urticaria is autoimmune or idiopathic. Tests to consider in the evaluation of chronic urticaria are grouped in Table 7.4 on the basis of possible causes. These should be considered primarily in those patients with a positive review of systems for the etiology or positive physical examination findings. The evaluation of the patient with significant chronic urticaria in the absence of a positive review of systems and/or physical examination findings is a matter of controversy. Generally, unless there is a clue from the history, review of systems, and physical examination, an extensive laboratory investigation does not contribute substantially to the detection of underlying disorders. In a prospective study of 220 patients, Kozel et al. compared the

Table 7.3 Urticaria and angioedema review of systems[a]

Autoimmune disease
   Is there a history of thyroid disease?
   Is there a history of vitiligo, diabetes mellitus, or pernicious anemia?
Physical urticaria
   Do hives or swelling occur with lightly scratching the skin, minor trauma, or tight clothing?
   Do hives occur from vibration (pushing a lawn mower or snow blower or other activity)?
   Do hives occur with exposure to heat or cold?
   Do hives occur with exercise, hot showers or bath, or stress?
   Do hives occur with exposure to sunlight?
   Do hives occur with exposure to water?
   Do hives occur with exercise?

Vasculitis
   Do individual hives last longer than 24 hours before they disappear?
   Do hives leave bruises or other marks as they resolve?
   Is there a history of fatigue, fever, weight loss, or malaise?

Infection
   Is there a history of fever or malaise?
   Is there a history of international travel or living abroad?
   Is there any history of hepatitis?
   Is there a history of diarrhea?
   Is there a history of recurrent or chronic sinusitis?

Connective tissue disease
   Is there a history of any abnormal redness, warmth, swelling, or pain of the joints?
   Is there a history of eye or mouth ulcerations?

Malignancy
   Is there unexplained fever, night sweats, or weight loss?
   Is there a family history of early-onset cancer?
   Is age-appropriate cancer screening up to date?
   Is there significant unexplained fatigue?

Allergy
   Is there a temporal relation between food ingestion and hive formation?
   Is there a relation between the start of a medication, over-the-counter medication, supplement, or other ingestant and hive formation?
Positive answers to these questions help guide considerations for further evaluation

[a] Based on most common causes

combination of detailed history taking and limited laboratory investigations with detailed history taking and extensive laboratory screening and found only one parasitic infection that was missed in the limited laboratory investigations group. Retrospective studies have obtained similar results. Although there is no consensus, consideration could be given to performing a complete blood count with differential, erythrocyte sedimentation rate of C-reactive protein, creatinine, aspartate aminotransferase, sensitive thyrotropin-releasing hormone, and thyroid antibody, urinalysis and chest radiography in the patients with moderate chronic urticaria who are otherwise asymptomatic.

Table 7.4 Urticaria and angioedema evaluation based on review of systems

Autoimmune urticaria
  sTSH, thyroid antibodies
  Autologous serum skin test
Physical urticaria
  Physical challenge tests
  Cryoglobulins (cold-induced)
Vasculitis
  Skin biopsy
  CH50, C3, C4
  ANCA studies
  Cryoglobulins
  Hepatitis serologies
  Urinalysis
  Creatinine
  AST, ALT, AP, bilirubin
  ANA
  SPEP
  Sedimentation rate
  C-reactive protein
Connective tissue disease
  ANA, RF, CCP
  SPEP
  Sedimentation rate
  C-reactive protein
Infection
  Stool ova and parasites
  Parasite serologic testing
  Hepatitis serologic testing
  Coronal sinus computed tomography
Malignancy
  Age-appropriate cancer screening
  Computed tomography of chest, abdomen, and pelvis
  SPEP
Allergy
  Skin test or in vitro testing to suspected foods
  Trial elimination of medication, supplement
  Trial elimination of food preservatives, additives

ALT alanine aminotransferase; *ANA* antinuclear antibody; *ANCA* antineutrophil cytoplasmic antibody; *AP* alkaline phosphatase; *AST* aspartate aminotransferase; *CCP* cyclic citrullinated peptide; *RF* rheumatoid factor; *SPEP* serum protein electrophoresis

Tests used in the evaluation of chronic urticaria are outlined below:

1. A complete blood count with differential count – this should be measured if hematologic disease is suspected and to assess for eosinophilia, which can be associated with various underlying disorders ranging from parasitic disease to lymphoproliferative disorders.

2. Erythrocyte sedimentation rate or C-reactive protein – these are often elevated in urticarial vasculitis or connective tissue diseases. A significantly increased

rate or increased level can be a sign of an underlying systemic disorder and prompts further evaluation. In autoimmune idiopathic chronic urticaria, the erythrocyte sedimentation rate and C-reactive protein should be normal.

3. Thyroid function testing with thyroid antibodies – even in a euthyroid patient (normal thyroid-stimulating hormone), thyroid antibodies can be associated with chronic urticaria.

4. Antinuclear antibody – this should be determined if the history or physical examination suggests lupus erythematosus or other connective tissue disorder, but in the absence of any signs or symptoms, it usually is not helpful.

5. Hepatitis B and C serologic tests – these should be performed in patients in high-risk groups or in those with a history of jaundice, or with elevated liver enzymes, or if the findings suggest urticarial vasculitis.

6. Specific complement studies – C4 should be determined when angioedema is the primary symptom; C4 is decreased in both types of HAE and AAE, and C3 and C4 can also be decreased in urticarial vasculitis.

7. Urinalysis – if urinary tract infection or connective tissue disease is suspected, this should be performed to evaluate for proteinuria or active sediment (or both).

8. Stool examination for ova and parasites – this should be performed (usually three samples) if there are associated gastrointestinal symptoms, eosinophilia, or a travel, social, or immigration history suggestive of parasitic disease.

9. Skin biopsy – this should be performed to examine for primarily urticarial vasculitis and to characterize the urticarial inflammation. In urticarial vasculitis, the history usually includes bruising, purpura, and persistent hives (lasting longer than 24 hours) in one location. Skin biopsy is not helpful in nonaffected skin and findings are nonspecific in mild idiopathic chronic urticaria.

10. Chest radiography – this should be performed if systemic disease is suspected.

11. C1 esterase inhibitor level and function – this should be determined only if the C4 level is decreased and only when angioedema alone is the major complaint. C1 esterase inhibitor level and function should not be determined in urticaria-predominant conditions.

12. Autologous serum skin testing – this test can be performed by an intradermal injection of 20 μL of the patient's serum into the skin and checking for a significant wheal and flare reaction. Currently, no sensitive and specific test is available for IgG antibody directed at the IgE receptor or at IgE itself. This test has a variable sensitivity of 70% and specificity of 80% for functional IgG antibodies of chronic autoimmune urticaria. The autologous serum skin test has been used primarily to select patients for trials in the study of chronic autoimmune urticaria.

13. Cryoglobulins, cryofibrinogens, cold agglutinins – these should only be measured in cold-induced urticaria.

14. Anticyclic citrillinated peptide (CCP) antibodies – this test should be performed when rheumatoid arthritis is suspected. It has approximately 60% sensitivity and 90% specificity for rheumatoid arthritis.

15. Serum protein electrophoresis (SPEP) – this test is a screening procedure for the detection of a monoclonal protein. SPEP should be performed in patients who have unexplained signs and symptoms suggestive of a plasma cell disorder. These include an increased erythrocyte sedimentation rate, unexplained anemia, weakness or fatigue, renal insufficiency, hypercalcemia, and hypergammaglobulinemia.

16. Antineutrophil cytoplasmic antibodies (ANCA) – ANCA testing has a critical role in the diagnosis and classification of the vasculitidies. A c-ANCA pattern, in most cases, indicates antibodies directed against proteinase 3 (PR3), but occasionally myeloperoxidase (MPO) is responsible. The p-ANCA pattern is usually directed against MPO and only occasionally against PR3. Both c- and p-ANCA immunofluorescence results should be confirmed by antigen-specific enzyme-linked immunosorbent assays for PR3 and MPO-ANCA. The predictive value of ANCA testing depends heavily on the clinical presentation of the patient. This test should be reserved for patients in whom vasculitis is strongly suspected.

7.7 Medications Used in the Treatment of Acute and Chronic Urticaria

There is no set single treatment regimen for urticaria. Triggers for urticaria as outlined above should be avoided. The first choice of medication for chronic idiopathic or autoimmune urticaria should be a second-generation nonsedating antihistamine. These medications have been shown to reduce the intensity and frequency of urticaria episodes. If the urticaria does not resolve with these agents, the addition of first-generation antihistamines, H_2-receptor antagonists, tricyclic antidepressants, or leukotriene antagonists can be used in various combinations. Severe disease may not respond to these treatments; if not, then anti-inflammatory agents such as corticosteroids, colchicine, stanozolol, sulfasalazine, cyclosporine, dapsone, methotrexate, and hydroxychloroquine can be considered (Table 7.5). Studies of these medications are limited and the risk-benefit ratio should be reviewed thoroughly before use.

7.7.1 Antihistamines (H₁ Blockers)

Antihistamines are the mainstay of treatment in urticaria. They are competitive inhibitors of histamine and reduce the effect of histamine even during continued histamine release. Antihistamines can be divided into the older, or first-generation, agents and newer, or second-generation, agents.

Older (first-generation) antihistamines were first produced and made available in the late 1930s and 1940s. The most commonly used first-generation antihistamines are chlorpheniramine, brompheniramine, hydroxyzine, and diphenhydramine. Although effective in the treatment of urticaria and allergic rhinitis, these agents are

Table 7.5 Medication approach to chronic urticaria or angioedema

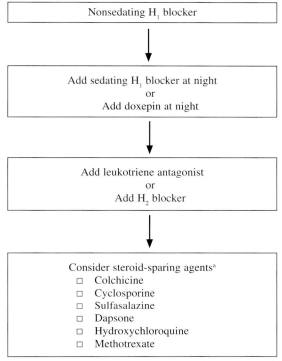

```
┌─────────────────────────────────────┐
│      Nonsedating H₁ blocker          │
└─────────────────────────────────────┘
                  │
                  ▼
┌─────────────────────────────────────┐
│    Add sedating H₁ blocker at night  │
│                 or                   │
│         Add doxepin at night         │
└─────────────────────────────────────┘
                  │
                  ▼
┌─────────────────────────────────────┐
│      Add leukotriene antagonist      │
│                 or                   │
│           Add H₂ blocker             │
└─────────────────────────────────────┘
                  │
                  ▼
┌─────────────────────────────────────┐
│   Consider steroid-sparing agentsᵃ   │
│      □  Colchicine                   │
│      □  Cyclosporine                 │
│      □  Sulfasalazine                │
│      □  Dapsone                      │
│      □  Hydroxychloroquine           │
│      □  Methotrexate                 │
└─────────────────────────────────────┘
```

[a] Should be used only by physicians familiar with the medications

limited by their adverse effects, lack of selectivity for the H_1 receptor, and a propensity to cross the blood-brain barrier, thus affecting the central nervous system. Because of the lack of selectivity, first-generation antihistamines cause anticholinergic effects such as dry mouth, headache, and urinary retention. By crossing the blood-brain barrier, they bind to H_1 receptors in the brain, resulting in sedation and cognitive impairment. Recent studies have shown first-generation antihistamines can have a significant effect on sensorimotor coordination, attention span, memory function, ability to process information, and psychomotor performance. These changes can occur without drowsiness and may not be perceived by the patient. Therefore, special counseling needs to be given with the use of these medications and the potential for decreased performance, particularly with driving or performing a job requiring considerable physical coordination. In addition to the adverse effects noted above, high doses of first-generation agents have effects beyond the H_1-receptor blockade that likely contributes to the effectiveness in the treatment of urticaria. For example, hydroxyzine has anticholinergic and antiserotoninergic effects and is considered the drug of choice for cholinergic urticaria, and it is also effective for other forms of chronic urticaria. The lack of specificity for H_1 blockade, therefore, has both pros and cons in the management of chronic urticaria. When compared with second-generation antihistamines, the first-generation agents offer similar improvement in urticaria.

Second-generation antihistamines were developed in the 1980s with the aim of being more specific for the H_1 receptor and overcoming the adverse effects associated with first-generation antihistamines. Second-generation antihistamines available in the United States include fexofenadine, desloratadine, loratadine, and cetirizine. All these medications have been shown to be effective in relieving the symptoms in chronic urticaria. A few controlled studies have directly compared second-generation antihistamines, and no evidence-based data show the superiority of one of these agents over another in the treatment of chronic urticaria. Second-generation antihistamines have better sedative profiles than first-generation agents; however, at higher-than-recommended doses, sedation and impairment can become evident. From several studies, it appears that fexofenadine has the least sedative and impairment properties, followed by loratadine and desloratadine, with cetirizine having the most. Although cetirizine is less sedating than first-generation antihistamines, the US Food and Drug Administration has classified cetirizine as sedating rather than nonsedating, and the product carries the full sedation precaution.

No clinical trials have assessed the use of two second-generation antihistamines in combination for the treatment of refractory urticaria, but this practice has been noted. Also, other off-label practices such as increased dosage of the medication have been implemented. Currently, whether these practices are superior to the regular use of antihistamines requires confirmation by randomized clinical trials. Currently, a combination of a second-generation antihistamine given in the morning and a first-generation antihistamine given at night is likely a more effective approach for refractory urticaria.

Ketotifen, a benzocycloheptathiophene, is an "antiallergic" medication that is widely used in Europe, Canada, and Mexico but has not been approved by the US Food and Drug Administration. Ketotifen has strong antihistaminic properties and has been shown to inhibit mast cell degranulation. It has been proven effective in the treatment of chronic urticaria when compared with other H_1 blockers. Small series and case reports have also shown effectiveness in severe, refractory chronic urticaria.

7.7.2 H_2 Blockers

Approximately 85% of histamine receptors in the skin are the H_1 subtype, and the other 15% are the H_2 subtype. Therefore, theoretically, the addition of an H_2-receptor antagonist, ranitidine, famotidine, or cimetidine, may yield additional benefit after H_1 blockade has been achieved. Clinical studies with a combination of H_1 and H_2 antihistamines generally have shown improvement compared with the effect of an H_1 blocker alone, but the benefit appears to be small. Because H_2 antagonists are safe and inexpensive and individual patients may exhibit a significant response, a trial of an H_2 antagonist with an H_1 antagonist is reasonable for patients who have not had a response to an H_1 antagonist alone.

7.7.3 Leukotriene Modifiers

In patients with chronic urticaria, mast cells are activated and release histamine and leukotrienes. The leukotrienes have a potent effect on the local cutaneous vasculature. Because of this effect, leukotriene modifiers have been studied in chronic urticaria. Most of the studies are anecdotal or uncontrolled. In the few placebo-controlled studies, the majority, but not all, showed therapeutic benefit compared with placebo and benefit when added to an H_1 blocker as opposed to an H_1 blocker alone. Given these data and the relative safety of the leukotriene receptor antagonists, montelukast and zafirlukast, the addition of one of these agents can be considered if the urticaria is not controlled with an H_1 blocker alone. Typically, if a therapeutic response occurs, it does so within 4 weeks.

7.7.4 Tricyclic Antidepressants (Doxepin)

Doxepin, a dibenzoxepin tricyclic antidepressant, has been used in the treatment of chronic urticaria. It is a potent inhibitor of H_1 and H_2 receptors and is a much more potent inhibitor of H_1 receptors than either diphenhydramine or hydroxyzine. It is also known to have anticholinergic and antiserotoninergic effects. It is approved for the treatment of depression in doses up to 300 mg per day, but it is highly sedating and often produces anticholinergic side effects. To help circumvent this, the dosage should begin at a low dose, 10–20 mg at night, and gradually be increased as needed, up to 75 mg at night. This should be used in conjunction with an H_1 blocker. The patient needs to be warned about sedative side effects, which often decrease with continued use and gradual increase in the medication. The patient should also be counseled that doxepin has been used to treat depression but that in this case it is being used for its antihistaminic effects and not as a treatment for depression. Other tricyclic antidepressants such as amitriptyline and nortriptyline are not used in the treatment of chronic urticaria.

7.7.5 Corticosteroids

Corticosteroids are clearly effective for the treatment of nearly all forms of chronic urticaria. However, they are not considered an option for chronic treatment because of their side effect profile. Corticosteroids should be considered mainly for the treatment of "crisis" urticaria to achieve control of severe disease. To obtain control of severe urticaria, high doses of corticosteroids (40–60 mg d^{-1}) are used in adults. This burst treatment (40–60 mg per day for 5 days, then taper by 5–10 mg per day each day) often will control the hives, so that a combination of antihistamines and other anti-inflammatory medications can help control the hives. In rare instances for which corticosteroids are required for chronic treatment, they should be given in the lowest possible doses and, if possible, on an every-other-day treatment program. Frequent attempts should be made to gradually taper the dose. Also, regular assessments for predictable adverse effects should be made. Adverse effects associated with chronic corticosteroid use include diabetes mellitus, obesity, hypertension, osteoporosis, glaucoma, and cataracts.

7.7.6 Thyroxine

Thyroxine therapy has been reported to suppress chronic urticaria in euthyroid patients with positive thyroid antibodies. Overall, the clinical results have been inconsistent. Patients treated with thyroxine should start at low doses (25–50 μg), and thyroid function tests should be performed every 6–8 weeks to assess whether hyperthyroidism is being induced by the treatment. Thyroxine is not indicated for patients with chronic urticaria who have normal thyroid function and the absence of thyroid antibodies.

7.7.7 Immunomodulatory Agents

Several immunomodulatory agents have been used in the treatment of severe refractory chronic urticaria, including sulfasalazine, dapsone, hydroxychloroquine, colchicine, methotrexate, cyclosporine, and intravenous immunoglobulin. None of these medications has been studied in large randomized controlled trials. Of these, cyclosporine has been studied most. It has been found to be effective in approximately two-thirds of patients at a dosage of 2.5–4.5 mg kg^{-1} daily in divided doses. The drug should be discontinued if a response is not obtained in 2–3 months. Because of the potential for renal toxicity, blood pressure, serum creatinine level, blood urea nitrogen, and urinalysis should be performed every 6 weeks.

Sulfasalazine may be helpful primarily when delayed pressure urticaria symptoms predominate. However, it should be avoided in patients with aspirin sensitivity or glucose-6-phosphate dehydrogenase deficiency. A complete blood count and liver enzymes should be monitored monthly for the first 3 months. Dapsone, because of its adverse effects, should be used predominately in cutaneous vasculitis. Colchicine may be beneficial for chronic urticaria with predominately neutrophilic infiltrates found on skin biopsy. In an open study, intravenous immunoglobulin (2 g kg^{-1} over 5 days) was helpful to the majority of a small group of patients with chronic urticaria. However, expense and potential morbidity pose problems, especially because it has not been studied in a controlled trial.

7.8 Therapy Recommendations

If an underlying disorder is found in the evaluation of chronic urticaria, treatment is directed at the disorder. For chronic idiopathic and autoimmune urticaria, there is no clearly established treatment program that fits every patient. Often, a stepwise approach needs to be undertaken in an effort to control the urticaria. There is general agreement that daily, nonsedating antihistamines are the first choice for treatment. If the hives are not controlled, then a first-generation antihistamine or doxepin can be added at night. The next step in treatment would be the addition of a leukotriene modifier or an H_2 blocker. Although H_2 blockers have been helpful for a small subset of patients, leukotriene modifiers appear to be of more benefit when added to H_1 blockers. In the majority of patients, chronic urticaria will be controlled with these regimens, but a small group will still have troublesome hives. At this point, the main medications used are the steroid-sparing, immunomodulating agents. There are no clear stepwise choices in this group; however, one strategy would be to start with a trial of colchicine because of the paucity of its adverse effects. If this is not effective, then cyclosporine can be used, with careful monitoring. If these medications cannot be used because of comorbid conditions, the other options include sulfasalazine, dapsone, methotrexate, hydroxychloroquine, and intravenous immunoglobulin, depending on the clinical situation. These medications should be dispensed only by physicians familiar with their use.

Corticosteroids generally should be reserved for short-term rescue during severe flares. It is very important to counsel the patient about the expectations of treatment for chronic urticaria. Most patients with chronic idiopathic or autoimmune urticaria can expect to benefit from treatment, but the expectation of becoming completely hive-free is unrealistic. For approximately half of the patients, the hives will resolve in 6 months to 1 year, and approximately 20% will have them at 20 years. The goal of treatment is to make the hives manageable until they go into remission. Chronic urticaria does not cause progressive or irreversible damage to tissues unless there is another underlying process; therefore, the use of the corticosteroids and immunomodifying agents should always be approached from a risk-benefit standpoint.

7.9 Clinical Vignettes

7.9.1 Vignette 1

A 35-year-old woman presents with a 6-month history of daily occurring hives. Her description of the hives is classic for urticaria. There is no suggestion of blistering, erythema multiforme, or other skin condition. The hives occur throughout the body, typically last for 4–5 hours rather randomly, and then disappear, only to recur the following day. There are no clear physical provocateurs. There is no bruising with the hives. She occasionally notes angioedema of the lips and extremities with this. Other than the hives, she is well. A complete review of systems is unremarkable. The hives are quite troublesome and have significantly affected her quality of life. She reports difficulty at work in her role as a bank teller because customers and coworkers ask her continually about her "disease." Socially, she has limited her activities because of the hives. She took a 2-week leave of absence from work to see if the hives were work related, but there was no difference in the hives. There is no significant travel history or home, recreational, or other environmental exposure.

The findings of a complete physical examination, with special attention paid to the lymph nodes, are unremarkable except for the skin examination, which shows urticaria ranging in size from 2–6 cm scattered throughout the body. There is no purpura, bruising, or hyperpigmentation.

She has been prescribed loratadine and cetirizine at different times but with only minimal benefit. She has never had any laboratory evaluation for the hives.

Comment: This clinical scenario is suggestive of chronic idiopathic or autoimmune urticaria. The hives have been present for more than 6 weeks and, thus, are classified as chronic. The majority of cases of chronic urticaria end up in the idiopathic or autoimmune category, and for this patient, there does not seem to be any clues to an underlying cause. Environmental review, an extensive review of systems, and complete physical examination have been performed without indicating an underlying cause. Thus far, she has not had a laboratory evaluation. On the basis of her current clinical presentation, and even though the hives are quite troubling, an extensive laboratory evaluation is not indicated. Because the hives have been ongoing for 6 months, further evaluation should screen for possible treatable disease. Without clinical clues to an underlying process, a reasonable evaluation would include a complete blood count, erythrocyte sedimentation rate or C-reactive protein, thyroid studies, creatinine, aspartate aminotransferase, urinalysis, chest radiography, and autologous serum test. The complete blood count would be performed primarily to check the hemoglobin level to screen for an anemia of chronic disease, a white cell count to screen for subclinical infection, and an eosinophil count to screen for possible parasitic infection. The erythrocyte sedimentation rate could be performed as a nonspecific screen for underlying inflammation. Thyroid studies can be performed to check thyroid function and thyroid antibodies. If the thyroid antibodies are significantly elevated, even if the patient is euthyroid, treatment with levothyroxine should be considered. Although the autologous serum test is often cumbersome to perform, it may provide evidence of autoimmune urticaria. The result of this test would not change medical management, but it provides a diagnosis for the patient.

The evaluation was performed and documented a normal complete blood count, aspartate aminotransferase, creatinine, urinalysis, chest radiograph, erythrocyte sedimentation rate, and thyroid function test without elevation of thyroid antibodies. An autologous serum skin test was not performed.

Comment: This brief evaluation did not provide any further clue to an underlying cause. At this point, additional testing is unlikely to be helpful. Management should be focused on symptomatic treatment. She already has tried second-generation H_1 blockers, loratadine and cetirizine, with only small success. Management options now would include an H_1 blocker with a sedating H_1 blocker added at night, an H_1 blocker with an H_2 blocker, or an H_1 blocker with a leukotriene antagonist. The H_1 blockers recommended are the second-generation nonsedating antihistamines: loratadine, cetirizine, desloratadine, or fexofenadine. There is no "best" H_1 blocker, although individual patients may respond more favorably to one medication than another. Because fexofenadine has not been tried, it would be a reasonable option for this patient.

Treatment was started with fexofenadine in the AM and doxepin in the PM, and the patient noticed approximately 50% improvement in the hives after 3 weeks. She was pleased there was improvement but wondered if anything else could be done.

Comment: Her improvement is encouraging. At this point, additional options include addition of an H_2 blocker or leukotriene antagonist. These two medications have not been compared head to head, but a subset of patients appears to respond well to a leukotriene antagonist.

The patient received a regimen of fexofenadine and zafirlukast in the AM and doxepin in the PM. After 2 weeks, the hives were markedly improved; she was having hives only occasionally.

Comment: She has responded well to this regimen. Once the hives are controlled, the goal is to taper the medications. A reasonable rule of thumb is to remove a medication after 3 weeks of rare or absent hives. For this patient, once she is free of hives for 3 weeks, doxepin could be discontinued, followed by zafirlukast, then fexofenadine.

7.9.2   Vignette 2

A 53-year-old woman presents with a 4-month history of progressive hives. The hives occur daily throughout the body and range in size from 5 mm–3 cm in diameter. The hives are present in one location at times for more than 48 hours and have left bruises and hyperpigmentation at the site of the hives. There is minimal to no angioedema associated with this. A review of systems is positive for generalized fatigue and occasional arthralgias and myalgias. There have been no joint effusions. A detailed travel, social, and environmental history is noncontributory. The patient is not taking any medications long term and states that she does not take over-the-counter medications or health supplements. Treatment had been attempted with both sedating and nonsedating H_1 blockers but without any significant clinical improvement.

On physical examination, the patient had hives of varying size, with small areas of ecchymoses and bruising in the lower extremities. The rest of the examination, including a detailed lymph node and joint examination, was unremarkable.

Comment: In this case, the hives remain in one location for more than 24 hours and are associated with bruising and skin hyperpigmentation. In addition, the patient notes fatigue, myalgias, and arthralgias, but these are nonspecific. Compared with idiopathic or autoimmune chronic urticaria, findings are suggestive of an underlying systemic disease, particularly vasculitis. Skin biopsy can be used to assess for vasculitis.

Skin biopsy was performed, with findings of leukocytoclastic vasculitis, an inflammatory infiltrate of predominantly neutrophils within the walls of the capillaries and postcapillary venules. Direct immunofluorescence showed IgM conjugates localized to the blood vessels.

Comment: The patient has biopsy-proven urticarial vasculitis. This can be idiopathic or occur in association with connective tissue disorders, infections, drug reactions, or paraneoplastic syndrome. Further evaluation is recommended to examine for an underlying disorder. Evaluation for urticarial vasculitis would typically include a complete blood count, erythrocyte sedimentation rate, C3, C4, serum protein electrophoresis, ANCA studies, antinuclear antibody, hepatitis B and C serologic tests, cryoglobulins, liver enzymes, creatinine, and urinalysis. Treatment is tailored on the basis of the presence of underlying disease and the extent of systemic involvement.

7.9.3 Vignette 3

A 72-year-old man presents with a 9-month history of angioedema. He describes episodic swelling of the upper and lower lips and, occasionally, the eye. Each episode lasts approximately 2 days. The episodes occur every 2–4 weeks. He has not had any respiratory distress with these episodes, nor is there any associated urticaria. Over the past 9 months, he has had a 5-lb intentional weight loss and perhaps mild fatigue. He occasionally has had crampy abdominal pain but has not noted any relationship between these episodes and the eating of certain foods.

Comment: When assessing chronic urticaria or angioedema, it is imperative to know the medication history.

The patient's current medications include hydrochlorothiazide, trazodone, baby aspirin, and vitamin E. He takes ibuprofen occasionally and has not noted any correlation between the use of the ibuprofen and the episodes of swelling.

Comment: His current medications are not typically associated with episodic angioedema. He is not taking ACE inhibitors. His symptoms are predominately angioedema. In idiopathic urticaria/angioedema, approximately 20% of patients have angioedema alone. With the angioedema predominance, the other main concern is C1 esterase inhibitor deficiency, hereditary or acquired. A family history would be helpful, as would knowledge of whether he has a past history of these events.

The patient states there is not any family history of angioedema. He does not recall any swelling episodes before the last 9 months.

Comment: The patient's age and lack of family history make hereditary C1 esterase inhibitor deficiency unlikely, although the acquired form is still a possibility. As in the evaluation of chronic urticaria, a complete review of symptoms and a physical examination should be performed.

A review of symptoms is essentially negative except for some mild fatigue and crampy abdominal pain, as previously reported. Physical examination findings are significant for a palpable spleen tip.

Comment: The physical examination finding is worrisome for acquired C1 esterase inhibitor deficiency. To evaluate further, determining the C4 level would be helpful.

The C4 level was significantly decreased at 4 mg dL^{-1} (normal, 14–40 mg dL^{-1}).

Comment: A decreased C4 level is found in both hereditary and acquired C1 esterase deficiency. To evaluate further, the C1 esterase level should be determined and a functional assay should be performed. A C1q level can help distinguish between hereditary C1 esterase inhibitor deficiency and acquired C1 esterase inhibitor deficiency.

The C1 esterase inhibitor level was decreased at 4 mg dL^{-1} (normal, 19–37 mg dL^{-1}). The C1 esterase inhibitor functional study was decreased at 24% (normal, 67–100%). The C1q was decreased at 7 mg dL^{-1} (normal, 12–22 mg dL^{-1}).

Comment: These findings are consistent with acquired C1 esterase inhibitor deficiency. In these situations, an underlying hematologic or lymphoproliferative malignancy is common. In this patient, the enlarged spleen is particularly worrisome. The patient should be evaluated further for the presence of an underlying malignancy.

Further evaluation showed the presence of non-Hodgkin lymphoma. Treatment of the underlying lymphoma resulted in improvement of the episodic angioedema.

Suggested Reading

Agostoni, A. and Cicardi, M. (1992) Hereditary and acquired C1-inhibitor deficiency: biological and clinical characteristics in 235 patients. Medicine (Baltimore) 71, 206–215

Casale, T. B., Blaiss, M. S., Gelfand, E., et al. (2003) First do no harm: managing antihistamine impairment in patients with allergic rhinitis. J. Allergy Clin. Immunol. 111, S835–S842

Hide, M., Francis, D. M., Grattan, C. E., Hakimi, J., Kochan, J. P., and Greaves, M. W. (1993) Autoantibodies against the high-affinity IgE receptor as a cause of histamine release in chronic urticaria. N. Engl. J. Med. 328, 1599–1604

Kaplan, A. P. (2002) Clinical practice: chronic urticaria and angioedema. N. Engl. J. Med. 346, 175–179

Kozel, M. M., Mekkes, J. R., Bossuyt, P. M., and Bos, J. D. (1998) The effectiveness of a history-based diagnostic approach in chronic urticaria and angioedema. Arch Dermatol. 134, 1575–1580

O'Donnell, B. F., Barr, R. M., Black, A. K., et al. (1998) Intravenous immunoglobulin in autoimmune chronic urticaria. Br. J. Dermatol. 138, 101–106

Powell, R. J., Du Toit, G. L., Siddique, N., et al., and British Society for Allergy and Clinical Immunology (BSACI). (2007) BSACI guidelines for the management of chronic urticaria and angio-oedema. Clin. Exp. Allergy. 37, 631–650

Sheikh, J. (2004) Advances in the treatment of chronic urticaria. Immunol. Allergy Clin. North Am. 24, 317–334, vii–viii

Tedeschi, A., Airaghi, L., Lorini, M., and Asero, R. (2003) Chronic urticaria: a role for newer immunomodulatory drugs? Am. J. Clin. Dermatol. 4, 297–305

Tilles, S. A. (2005) Approach to therapy in chronic urticaria: when benadryl is not enough. Allergy Asthma Proc. 26, 9–12

Toubi, E., Blant, A., Kessel, A., and Golan, T. D. (1997) Low-dose cyclosporin A in the treatment of severe chronic idiopathic urticaria. Allergy 52, 312–316

Venzor, J., Lee, W. L., and Huston, D. P. (2002) Urticarial vasculitis. Clin. Rev. Allergy Immunol. 23, 201–216

Volcheck, G. W. and Li, J. T. (1997) Exercise-induced urticaria and anaphylaxis. Mayo Clin. Proc. 72, 140–147

Wanderer A. A., Bernstein I. L., Goodman D. L., et al., Joint Task Force on Practice Parameters, American Academy of Allergy, Asthma and Immunology; American College of Allergy, Asthma and Immunology; Joint Council of Allergy, Asthma and Immunology. (2000) The diagnosis and management of urticaria: a practice parameter; part I: acute urticaria/angioedema; part II: chronic urticaria/angioedema. Ann. Allergy Asthma Immunol. 85, 521–544

Chapter 8
Atopic and Contact Dermatitis

Abbreviations AMP: antimicrobial peptide; FDA: U.S. Food and Drug Administration; GM-CSF: granulocyte-macrophage colony-stimulating factor; HBD: human B defensin; IFN: interferon; IL: interleukin; LPS: lipopolysaccaride; MCI-MI: methylchloroisothiazolinone-methylisothiazolinone; MDBGN-PE: methyldibromoglutaronitrile-phenoxyethanol; MHC: major histocompatibility complex; NK: natural killer (cell); NKT: natural killer T-cell; PAMP: pathogen-associated molecular pattern; PMN: polymorphonuclear cell; PPDA: *p*-phenylenediamine; PRR: pattern recognition receptor; SCCE: stratum corneum chymotryptic enzyme; TLR: Toll-like receptor; TNF: tumor necrosis factor; TSLP: thymic stromal lymphopoietin; VCAM: vascular cell adhesion molecule.

8.1   Atopic Dermatitis

Atopic dermatitis is a chronic, inflammatory, pruritic skin disease that affects both children and adults, primarily in industrialized countries. Both genetic mutations and cutaneous hyperreactivity to environmental stimuli are important in the pathogenesis of the disease. It is characterized by poorly defined erythema with edema, vesicles, and weeping in the acute stage and skin lichenification in the chronic stage. Although termed *atopic dermatitis*, up to 60% of children with the clinical phenotype do not have IgE positivity to allergens. Two types of atopic dermatitis have been identified: an extrinsic type associated with IgE sensitization and an intrinsic type without IgE-mediated sensitization. Asthma develops in approximately 30% of children with atopic dermatitis, and allergic rhinitis develops in 35%.

8.1.1   *Epidemiology*

Atopic dermatitis is a major public health problem worldwide. During a 1-year period, the prevalence of symptoms of atopic dermatitis among children 6 or 7 years old varied from less than 2% in China to 20% in Australia, England,

G.W. Volcheck, *Clinical Allergy: Diagnosis and Management*   311
DOI: 10.1007/978-1-59745-315-8_8, © 2009 Mayo Foundation for Medical
Education and Research

and Scandinavia. Prevalence of the disease has increased by two- to threefold during the past three decades in industrialized countries. In 45% of children, the onset of the disease occurs during the first 6 months of life, during the first year of life in 60%, and before the age of 5 years in at least 85% of those affected. Of children with onset before the age of 2 years, 20% will have persistent manifestations of the disease. Of adults with atopic dermatitis, approximately 17% have onset after adolescence.

8.1.2   Pathogenesis

Interactions between susceptibility genes, the host's environment, the skin barrier, infectious agents, allergens, and immunologic factors contribute to the development of atopic dermatitis. The clinical interplay of all these factors result in the syndrome of atopic dermatitis. These factors are summarized in Fig. 8.1.

8.1.2.1   Barrier Dysfunction

Two perspectives of the pathophysiology of atopic dermatitis are the "inside–outside" and "outside–inside" hypotheses. The "inside–outside" hypothesis suggests that barrier breakdown in atopic dermatitis is due to the inflammatory response to irritants and allergens. The "outside–inside" hypothesis suggests that xerosis, the permeability barrier abnormality, drives the activity of atopic dermatitis. It is likely that these hypotheses are not exclusive and components of both contribute to the pathophysiology of atopic dermatitis. It has been shown that barrier function fluctuates in relation to disease activity. The skin barrier is known to be damaged in patients with atopic dermatitis, both in acute eczematous lesions and in clinically unaffected skin. Many barrier factors contribute to the areas of predisposition to the disease, including the thickness of the stratum corneum, exposure to irritants and allergens at the site, and exposure to exogenous proteases from *Staphylococcus aureus* and dust mites.

The epithelium serves as the first line of defense between the body and the environment. Disturbance of this barrier predisposes to penetration by microbes and allergens. This penetration can induce sensitization and subsequently trigger the onset of inflammation. The primary barrier to penetration of irritants and allergens is located in the lower part of the stratum corneum. The structural integrity is maintained by corneodesmosomes that lock the corneocytes together. During the formation of corneocytes, the granular cells form the lipid lamellae matrix that encases the corneocytes. The lipid lamellae prevent internal water loss and penetration by water-soluble materials. This matrix is composed of ceramides, cholesterol, fatty acids, and cholesterol esters. The ceramides are the major water-retaining molecules in the extracellular space of the cornified envelope. Abnormal lamellar bodies, lipid components, and decreased ceramide production have been demonstrated in both lesional and nonlesional skin of patients with atopic dermatitis.

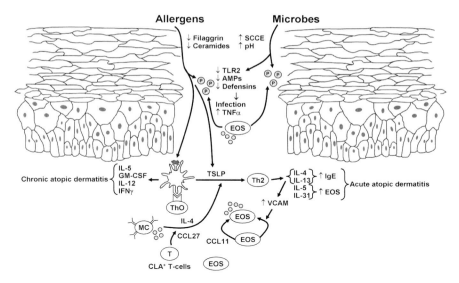

Fig. 8.1 Pathogenesis of atopic dermatitis. A decrease in filaggrin production and ceramides and an increase in protease activity and skin pH result in barrier dysfunction. This allows entry of allergens and microbes. Allergens activate Langerhans cells to prime naïve T-cells to differentiate into Th2 cells, resulting in the production of interleukin (IL)-4, IL-13, IL-5, and IL-31, which causes acute inflammation. In chronic atopic dermatitis, Langerhans cells and inflammatory dendritic epidermal cells express granulocyte-macrophage colony-stimulating factor (GM-CSF), IL-12, IL-5, and interferon (IFN)-γ, which contribute to the Th1 response characteristic of chronic atopic dermatitis. Microbial colonization occurs secondary to decreased Toll-like receptor (TLR)-2 activity, decreased antimicrobial peptide production, and decreased defensin production, resulting in infection and inflammation. Keratinocytes, endothelial cells, Langerhans cells, and monocyte/macrophages all contribute to the inflammation. Chemokines recruit inflammatory cells from the circulation
AMP antimicrobial peptide; *CLA* cutaneous lymphocyte-associated antigen; *EOS* eosinophil; *MC* mast cell; *SCCE* stratum corneum chymotryptic enzyme; *TNF* tumor necrosis factor; *TSLP* human thymic stromal lymphopoietin; *VCAM* vascular cell adhesion molecule

Corneocytes are desquamated when the corneodesmosomes are broken down by skin-specific proteases. The proteases are controlled by specific protease inhibitors to prevent overdesquamation. This regulatory pathway allows for normal sloughing and regeneration of the epidermis. The skin barrier function can be impaired by a genetic predisposition to produce increased amounts of proteolytic enzymes, causing premature breakdown of the epithelial barrier. Stratum corneum chymotryptic enzyme (SCCE), an endogenous protease involved in the process of desquamation, is overexpressed in intrinsic atopic dermatitis. The corneodesmosomes, however, are not broken down only by the skin-specific endogenous proteases. The stratum corneum is exposed to many exogenous proteases from the environment, such as products from *S aureus* and house dust mites. *S aureus* is not a part of the normal microflora of the skin, but a large number of these organisms are present in eczematous lesions of atopic dermatitis. Staphylococci produce proteases that may break down corneodesmosomes through a mechanism similar to that of endogenous skin-specific proteases. House dust mites contain cysteine and serine proteases. Apart from IgE activation, these proteases likely cause skin irritation or immune activation through direct proteolytic activity. Also, once a flare of atopic dermatitis has been triggered, cells within the inflammatory infiltrate also produce proteases that can further damage the skin barrier. Overall, when unchecked, these proteases lead to premature desquamation of the corneocytes and a damaged skin barrier.

Skin pH is important in barrier function. Normal skin pH is acidic, ranging from 5.4–5.9. The acidic pH has a strong antimicrobial effect, preserves the lipid lamellae, and decreases the endogenous protease effect. Exposure to soap and detergents has been recognized for years as an exacerbating environmental factor in atopic dermatitis. These agents are the most common environmental exposures that increase skin pH. The use of soap and detergent on skin, particularly by persons with atopic dermatitis, enhances the skin proteases, thus thinning the skin and decreasing the skin barrier. Ensuring that the washing regimen of persons with atopic dermatitis is completely free from soap or detergent is an important part of the treatment.

Genetic variants in the skin barrier protein filaggrin have been identified as a major risk factor for allergic disease, especially eczema. Filaggrin proteins are essential components of the outer skin; they serve to aggregate keratin filaments, often derived from dead keratinocytes in the stratum corneum, into bundles that promote a physical barrier against the external environment. Genetic variants that result in the loss of function of the filaggrin gene have been implicated as the cause of icthyosis vulgaris. Carriers of filaggrin mutations show a high rate of asthma and eczema. These findings support the importance of the epidermal barrier in preventing sensitization to allergens, and they identify new areas of exploration for genetic causes of atopy.

In general, barrier dysfunction and immunologic inflammation appear to feed each other. At one end of the spectrum, a single change in one skin barrier gene might predispose to atopic dermatitis but require exposure to an environmental agent for the disease to be expressed. At the other end of the spectrum, a combination of changes in several skin barrier genes could, on their own, lead to severe breakdown of the skin barrier and the development of more severe atopic dermatitis. A defective barrier enhances the penetration of irritants and allergens, which activate the immune response. The immune response results in inflammatory changes that can further escalate atopic dermatitis.

Genetic studies have shown a far greater degree of overlap between atopic dermatitis and psoriasis than between atopic dermatitis and other atopic phenotypes such as asthma. This challenges the historical view that atopic dermatitis is mediated primarily by an IgE response to allergens and the Th2 phenotype. It appears that a substantial portion of the predisposition toward atopic dermatitis is within the skin itself. A barrier dysfunction helps explain why most of the increased serum IgE is not directed against specific allergens, why intrinsic forms of atopic dermatitis exist, and why anti-IgE therapies are not uniformly successful. Therefore, atopic dermatitis may represent a primary defect of epidermal dysfunction compounded by the presence of inflammation-induced skin damage.

The awareness of the importance of barrier dysfunction in atopic dermatitis necessitates monitoring everything that comes into contact with the skin, especially soaps, detergents, microbes, and dust mites.

8.1.2.2 Immune Dysfunction and Microbial Colonization and Infection

Subjects with atopic dermatitis have an unusual propensity for colonization with certain microbes such as *S aureus* and *Candida* and aggravated infections with others such as herpes simplex and vaccinia viruses. The best characterized is *S aureus*. Approximately 90% of patients with atopic dermatitis are colonized with *S aureus*, whereas only 5–30% of controls are colonized. The colonization can advance rapidly to superinfection with 10^7 organisms per square centimeter. Eczema herpeticum is a disseminated cutaneous form of herpes simplex virus infection that requires prompt systemic antiviral therapy. Patients with atopic dermatitis who have higher IgE levels and more clinically severe disease appear to be the most at risk. Eczema vaccinatum is the severe disseminated vaccinia infection that develops in patients with atopic dermatitis exposed to individuals who were vaccinated recently with smallpox or who received the smallpox vaccination themselves. These conditions are discussed below in the section on microorganisms (1.4.3.). Although the immune dysfunction in atopic dermatitis has not been fully characterized, some deficiencies have been noted.

The immune dysfunction in patients with atopic dermatitis is likely related to the innate immune system. In contrast to the adaptive immune system that consists of antigen-presenting cells presenting antigen to T- and B-cells, the innate immune system consists of receptors and antimicrobial proteins that provide an immediate, critical response to pathogens. Components of the innate immune system include pattern recognition receptors (PRRs), pathogen-associated molecular patterns (PAMPs), and antimicrobial peptides (AMPs). When PRRs, such as Toll-like receptors (TLRs) bind PAMPs, such as bacterial cell-wall lipopolysaccaride (LPS), they initiate an immediate cellular response to the challenge. This response includes the release of AMPs, cytokines, and chemokines that have direct antimicrobial effects and recruit effector leukocytes. Abnormalities have been identified in the innate immune system of patients with atopic dermatitis.

Possible defects in patients with atopic dermatitis include abnormalities in TLR2 and the interleukin (IL)-1 pathway, which has a role in the response and containment of *S aureus* at the skin surface. AMPs, which include LL-37 and human B defensins (HBDs), have been shown to have antistaphyloccocal activity. Human keratinocytes produce LL-37 and HBDs in response to inflammatory stimuli. Patients with atopic dermatitis have been shown to have decreased levels of HBD2 and HBD3 compared with patients with psoriasis. In addition, AMP LL-37, which is necessary for an adequate response to both herpes simplex and vaccinia viruses, has been found to be significantly reduced in patients with atopic dermatitis compared with that of patients with psoriasis. Decreased production of LL-37 may predispose patients with atopic dermatitis to eczema herpeticum and vaccinatum.

An unusual finding in skin biopsy specimens from patients with atopic dermatitis is the lack of polymorphonuclear cells (PMNs), especially in light of the trauma of intense scratching and colonization and infection with *S aureus*. Various PMN defects have been reported in patients with atopic dermatitis, including impaired phagocytic function and decreased PMN chemotactic activity that correlate with disease severity and infection. Because systemic PMN dysfunction is rare in atopic dermatitis, the defect in cutaneous PMN recruitment likely emanates from defective tissue signaling from the skin. Because PMNs are critical in the initial response to pathogens, it is not unexpected that patients with atopic dermatitis are susceptible to microbes.

8.1.2.3 Inflammatory Immune Response

Skin represents the body's largest immune organ. Although the immunopathology of atopic dermatitis is not understood completely, the importance of various components of the skin's immune system, including dendritic cells, mast cells, and lymphocytes, are well established. Acute atopic skin lesions in atopic dermatitis are characterized by marked epidermal intercellular edema (spongiosis). This is associated with an increased number of CD4+ T-cells that infiltrate the epithelium. In animal models of atopic dermatitis, the eczematous rash does not occur in the absence of T-cells. Antigen-presenting cells such as Langerhans cells, inflammatory dendritic epidermal cells, and macrophages in the lesional skin bear IgE molecules. Langerhans cells have a predominant role in the initiation of the allergic immune response, and they prime naïve T-cells to differentiate into T-cells of the Th2 type with high IL-4-producing capacity. Mast cell degranulation is also observed. The number of Th2 cells that express mRNA for IL-4 and IL-13 is increased. These are the only cytokines that promote isotype switching to IgE. These cytokines also induce expression of vascular cell adhesion molecules (VCAMs) such as VCAM-1, which are involved in eosinophil infiltration. Once activated, the eosinophil is capable of releasing several cytotoxic granule proteins and chemical mediators that contribute to tissue inflammation. A subset of Th2 cells are memory cells that also express cutaneous lymphocyte-associated antigen, a homing receptor to direct inflammatory cells to the skin.

In contrast, chronic, lichenified skin lesions of atopic dermatitis have undergone tissue remodeling caused by chronic inflammation. This lesion is characterized by an acanthotic epidermis with elongation of the rete ridges, parakeratosis, and only minimal spongiosis. Fewer IL-4 and IL-13 mRNA-expressing cells are present. Macrophages, Langerhans cells, and inflammatory dendritic epidermal cells dominate the dermal mononuclear cell infiltrate. These cells are characterized by IL-5, granulocyte-macrophage colony-stimulating factor (GM-CSF), IL-12, and interferon (IFN)-γ mRNA-expressing cells. These cytokines support eosinophil and macrophage growth and promote Th1 type of inflammation. IgE-bearing FcεRI+ inflammatory dendritic epidermal cells also become more prominent in chronic disease and are thought to be involved in cell recruitment and

IgE-mediated antigen presentation to T-cells and to promote Th1 cytokine production from T-cells. Also present are eosinophils, which are thought to contribute to inflammation and tissue injury through production of reactive oxygen intermediates and release of toxic granule proteins. Increased collagen deposition is seen in the dermis.

Many chemokines are upregulated in atopic dermatitis and help recruit cells to sites of irritation. CCL5 (RANTES), CCL13 (monocyte chemoattractant protein 4), and CCL11 (eotaxin) are increased in atopic dermatitis lesions. These chemokines help in the recruitment of T-cells, macrophages, and eosinophils into the skin, in both acute and chronic lesions of atopic dermatitis. Other chemokines are being identified in atopic dermatitis. Cutaneous T-cell-attracting chemokine (CCL27) is highly upregulated in atopic dermatitis and attracts lymphocyte antigen-positive T-cells into the skin. Chemokines such as fractalkine, IFN-γ–inducible protein 10, and IFN-γ–inducible chemoattractants are upregulated in keratinocytes and contribute to Th1 cell migration toward the epidermis. Further characterization of the primary chemokines will help in better understanding the inflammatory process and timing of events.

Mechanical trauma induces the release of TNF-α and other proinflammatory cytokines from the epidermal keratinocytes in patients with atopic dermatitis. These epidermal keratinocytes produce higher amounts of RANTES after TNF-α and INF-γ stimulation. In atopic dermatitis, keratinocytes are also an important source of thymic stromal lymphopoietin (TSLP), which activates dendritic cells to prime Th-cells to produce IL-4 and IL-13. Apoptosis of keratinocytes induced by T-cells is a critical event in the formation of eczema/spongiosis in atopic dermatitis. Suppression of keratinocyte activation and induction of keratinocyte apoptosis remain potential targets for the treatment of atopic dermatitis.

The link between atopic dermatitis and allergen-specific IgE is intensely debated. The association with increased IgE levels is much less in children with mild to moderate atopic dermatitis than in those with severe disease. It has been suggested that nonallergic intrinsic dermatitis could be a transitional form of atopic dermatitis. In about 80% of adults with atopic dermatitis, the disease is associated with increased serum levels of IgE, sensitization against aeroallergens and food allergens, or concomitant allergic rhinitis and asthma (or a combination of these). However, there is a paucity of longitudinal studies on IgE measurements in atopic dermatitis. These studies could help determine whether in some subjects the increase in total serum IgE levels and allergen-specific IgE levels occurs transiently or linearly over time. An intriguing question is whether intrinsic atopic dermatitis is represented by genetic variants that predispose to a defective epidermal barrier, paving the way for the subsequent development of allergic sensitization by increased exposure through the defective epidermal barrier.

Clinically unaffected skin of patients with atopic dermatitis is not normal. It is often dry and has a greater irritant response than normal healthy skin. This skin is characterized by a sparse perivascular T-cell infiltrate and an increased number of Th2-cells expressing mRNA of IL-4 and IL-13, likely explaining the predisposition for a Th2-type response.

8.1.2.4 Genetics

Two forms of genetic studies have been performed in the study of atopic dermatitis: (1) genome-wide screens that identify broad regions of the genome linked with the disease and (2) candidate gene studies that examine a presumed contribution of genetic variants of disease-process genes in case-control association studies.

Genome screens of families with atopic dermatitis have implicated chromosomal regions that overlap with those of other skin diseases. The findings suggest an underlying abnormality of generalized epidermal dysfunction that is manifested as a compromised skin barrier and failure to protect against microbial insults and allergen exposure. These studies have identified a group of genes that are distinct from "asthma" genes. The dysfunctional skin barrier genes, which include a loss of functional filaggrin, increased protease activity, and a lack of protease inhibitors, complement the involvement of IL-4, IL-13, IL-18, and TIM-1 genes that support the role of CD4+ cells and dysregulation of Th1 and Th2 genes in atopic dermatitis. The association of atopic dermatitis with polymorphisms of the *NOD1* gene that encodes cytosolic pathogen recognition receptor and TLRs suggests an important role for microbes in the disease.

8.1.3 Clinical Manifestations and Diagnosis

The clinical pattern of atopic dermatitis varies with age. Infants typically present with a more acute atopic dermatitis manifested by poorly demarcated erythematous papules and vesicles on the cheeks, forehead, scalp, and extensor surfaces. The lesions in this phase are less defined than those that occur later. As the infant begins to crawl, lesions may localize to areas of friction on the knees and elbows. The diaper area is typically spared. During the childhood phase from age 2 years to puberty, the exudative lesions of infancy are less common; instead, lichenified papules and plaques that represent more chronic disease are present on the hands, feet, wrists, ankles, and flexural antecubital and popliteal regions. The lesional sites become more focal, but the margins of the lesions remain indistinct. The predominant areas of involvement in the adult phase include the flexural folds, the face and neck, the upper arms and back, and the dorsa of the hands, feet, fingers, and toes. Chronic hand dermatitis can be the primary manifestation in many adults. The skin lesions are characterized by dry, scaling, erythematous papules and plaques and the formation of large lichenified plaques from lesional chronicity. Photosensitivity may occur in a small number of adults, but it is not seen in the infant or childhood phases. At all stages of this disease, patients usually have dry skin. Examples of atopic dermatitis are shown in Figs. 8.2 and 8.3a, b.

Pruritus can occur throughout the day, but typically is worse at night. It results in scratching, lichenification, and prurigo papules. Patients with atopic dermatitis have a reduced threshold for pruritus. Allergens, irritants, reduced humidity, and excessive sweating can exacerbate pruritus and scratching. Clinical features of atopic dermatitis are listed in Table 8.1.

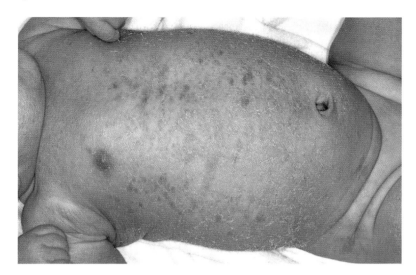

Fig. 8.2 Severe atopic dermatitis in an infant

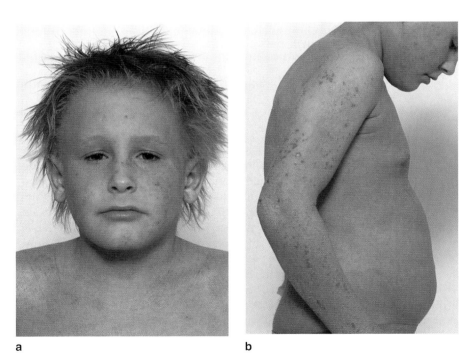

a   b

Fig. 8.3 (**a**) and (**b**), Atopic dermatitis in a child. Note the widespread underlying dry characteristic of the skin

Table 8.1 Clinical features of atopic dermatitis

Atopic dermatitis (AD) is best viewed as a syndrome. Clinical findings that define this syndrome and clinical criteria of AD include[a]:

A. Essential features (must be present)
  1. Pruritus
  2. Eczema (acute, subacute, chronic)
     a. Typical morphology and age-specific patterns[b]
     b. Chronic or relapsing history
B. Important features (seen in most cases, adding support to the diagnosis)
  1. Early age at onset
  2. Atopy
     a. Personal and/or family history
     b. IgE reactivity
  3. Xerosis
C. Associated features (these clinical associations help to suggest the diagnosis of AD but are too nonspecific to be used for defining or detecting AD for research or epidemiologic studies)
  1. Atypical vascular responses (e.g., facial pallor, white dermographism, delayed blanch response)
  2. Keratosis pilaris/hyperlinear palms/ichthyosis
  3. Ocular/periorbital changes
  4. Other regional findings (e.g., perioral changes/periauricular lesions)
  5. Perifollicular accentuation/lichenification/prurigo lesions

From Eichenfeld, L.F., Hanifin, J. M., Luger, T. A., Stevens, S. R., Pride, H. B. (2003) Consensus conference on pediatric atopic dermatitis. J. Am. Acad. Dermatol. 49, 1088–1095
[a]Exclusionary conditions: It should be noted that a diagnosis of AD depends on excluding conditions such as scabies, seborrheic dermatitis, allergic contact dermatitis, ichthyoses, cutaneous lymphoma, psoriasis, and immune deficiency diseases
[b]Patterns include (a) facial, neck, and extensor involvement in infants and children; (b) current or prior flexural lesions in any age group; (c) sparing of groin and axillary regions

8.1.3.1 Differential Diagnosis

The most important differential diagnoses are other forms of eczema. Especially in adulthood, coexisting dermatoses include allergic contact and irritant dermatitis. Hand and foot dermatitis can include psoriasis and tinea. Discoid (nummular) eczema can present as circular areas of erythema 1–5 cm in diameter found initially on the limbs, often with secondary infection. Adult-type seborrheic dermatitis presents with erythema in seborrheic areas such as the sides of the nose, eyebrows, external ear canal, scalp, front of chest, axillae, and groin creases. Seborrheic dermatitis of infancy consists of red, shiny, well-demarcated eruptions typically involving the diaper area. The lower abdomen and armpits may also be involved, and scalp scaling (cradle cap) may be present. The condition is nonpruritic and typically clears within a few months. The differential diagnosis of acute atopic dermatitis with intense erythema of the skin in combination with exudation and blistering differs from the differential diagnoses of the chronic lichenified forms. Dermatitis herpetiformis and pemphigus foliaceus may present with blisters. Scabies may produce nonspecific eczematous changes on the entire body. Burrows and pustules on the palms, soles, and genitalia and between the fingers help establish the diagnosis. In recalcitrant

Table 8.2 Differential diagnosis of atopic dermatitis

Seborrheic dermatitis of infancy
Adult-type seborrheic dermatitis
Discoid (nummular) eczema
Irritant contact dermatitis
Allergic contact dermatitis
Frictional lichenoid dermatitis
Scabies
Insect bites
Lymphoma (cutaneous T-cell)
Dermatitis herpetiformis
Pemphigus foliaceus
Psoriasis

cases, in both children and adults, vitamin deficiencies and malignancies, especially cutaneous T-cell lymphoma/mycosis fungoides, should be suspected. An abbreviated differential diagnosis of atopic dermatitis is listed in Table 8.2.

8.1.4 Triggers of Atopic Dermatitis

8.1.4.1 Stress

The response of patients with atopic dermatitis to stressful events can be increased pruritus and scratching. Stress-induced immunomodulation is altered in patients with atopic dermatitis, but the exact mechanisms have not been well defined. Possible contributors include neuropeptides, which can be found in the blood and within epidermal nerve fibers in close association with epidermal Langerhans cells. Nerve growth factor and substance P have been shown to be increased in the plasma of patients with atopic dermatitis, and this increase correlates with disease activity. The level of brain-derived growth factor, which decreases eosinophil apoptosis and increases eosinophil chemotaxis, is also increased in these patients.

8.1.4.2 Allergens

Patients with atopic dermatitis can have very high serum levels of IgE. This likely explains multiple positive results to specific allergen testing in these patients. Three patterns of skin reaction occur in patients with atopic dermatitis with food challenge. The first pattern is an immediate IgE-mediated response such as urticaria, angioedema, and erythema within minutes after ingestion of the food, but without an exacerbation of the atopic dermatitis. This is a typical IgE-mediated response and can also include respiratory, gastrointestinal, and cardiovascular symptoms. In the second pattern, pruritus occurs soon after the ingestion of the food, with subsequent scratching and worsening of the underlying atopic dermatitis. In the third pattern, exacerbations of atopic dermatitis alone occur 6–48 hours after the food is ingested. Food allergens can induce skin changes, either IgE-mediated changes or worsening of atopic dermatitis, in approximately 30% of children with moderate to severe atopic dermatitis. Food sensitivity is less common in patients with mild disease.

The foods most commonly implicated in infants and young children who have atopic dermatitis and food sensitivities are egg, milk, wheat, soy, and peanut. It is important to note that specific IgE allergen food positivity, whether measured by skin prick testing or by in vitro testing, in patients with atopic dermatitis does not establish the presence of clinical allergy or define clinical relevance in a given patient. Properly performed skin prick tests to food allergens generally have a high negative predictive value, but the positive predictive value is only approximately 50% because of nonspecific false positivity due to the increase in total IgE. Patients with multiple positive food test results may need to undergo formal food challenges or elimination diets to delineate the role of food in the disease. Consultation with a dietician may be necessary to ensure that the elimination of various foods from the diet does not cause malnutrition. Although foods that are negative on skin prick testing and in vitro testing typically do not cause an IgE-mediated reaction or worsening of the dermatitis, there are instances in which these foods do worsen the atopic dermatitis, presumably through a cell-mediated response. For this reason, food atopy patch testing over a 4-day period is being investigated as a way of identifying foods that may worsen atopic dermatitis but produce a negative result on skin prick or in vitro tests.

Airborne allergens can also be important in atopic dermatitis. Exposure to aeroallergens has been shown to increase the risk factors for the disease and its severity. Pruritus and skin manifestations can develop after intranasal or bronchial challenge with aeroallergens. Aeroallergens are also a trigger for exacerbations of the disease in adults. The application of aeroallergens such as house dust mite and animal danders by atopy patch test on unaffected atopic skin has been shown to elicit eczematoid skin reactions in patients with atopic dermatitis. In healthy volunteers or those with only respiratory allergy, the atopy patch tests are usually negative. In dust mite-sensitive patients with atopic dermatitis, measures to reduce house dust mites have been associated with improvement in the disease.

8.1.4.3 Microorganisms

Flares of atopic dermatitis are often associated with bacterial infection by *S aureus* that leads to skin inflammation. An increased number of *S aureus* organisms are found in more than 90% of atopic dermatitis skin lesions. *S aureus* exacerbates skin inflammation by several mechanisms. One way is by the secretion of superantigens that stimulate marked activation of T-cells and macrophages. Analysis of these patients has shown that they have undergone a T-cell receptor expansion consistent with superantigenic stimulation. In addition, patients make specific IgE antibodies directed against the superantigens that correlate with disease severity. Treatment of *S aureus* infection depends on the extent of the disease. Short courses of systemic antistaphylococcal antibiotics can be administered for moderate to severe flares. Topical therapy can be applied for localized, milder impetiginized skin. It is critical not to start prolonged antimicrobial therapy because of the possible development of resistant organisms. Of interest, treatment with topical immunomodulators such as steroids and calcineurin inhibitors has been shown to decrease *S aureus* colonization. Therefore, the increased binding of *S aureus* to the skin is likely related to the underlying barrier dysfunction and inflammation. Methicillin-resistant *S aureus*, which is increasingly reported, does not appear to cause increased toxicity and does not require parenteral treatment. Repair of the epidermal barrier and the use of anti-inflammatory agents are critical components of therapy.

Patients with atopic dermatitis are also susceptible to herpes simplex virus infections. After an incubation period of 5–12 days, many itchy vesiculopustular lesions erupt in a disseminated pattern. Close examination is required to detect the punched-out lesions with an erythematous base with or without a vesicle. The presence of these punched-out erosions and vesicles that do not respond to treatment with oral antibiotics should raise the suspicion of herpes simplex virus infection. Diagnosis can be made by obtaining viral polymerase chain reaction, Tzanck smear, or culture from the base of the lesion. Patients should receive treatment with oral antiviral agents such as acyclovir or valcyclovir. After antiviral treatment has been started, topical immunomodulators should be continued to allow repair of the skin barrier. Disseminated infection with herpes simplex virus or eczema herpeticum is a possible life-threatening emergency and requires systemic antiviral treatment.

Fungal colonization is common in atopic dermatitis. Recently, *Malassezia* spp. have been demonstrated in patients with atopic dermatitis. *Malassezia* sensitivity can be diagnosed with skin prick tests or in vitro specific IgE testing. Antifungal therapy has been shown to be helpful in those with sensitivity to *Malassezia*. The minimal effective dose for adults is itraconazole 100 mg per day for 1 week, followed by 200 mg weekly. It is unclear if the antifungal or anti-inflammatory activity of antifungal agents has a major role in the improvement in atopic dermatitis.

8.1.5 Evaluation

The evaluation for exacerbating factors in atopic dermatitis involves a thorough patient history, history-dependent allergen skin or in vitro tests (or both), and history and physical examination–driven patch testing. The presence of other similar skin processes needs to be considered (see above, Sect. 1.3.1).

8.1.5.1 Allergy Testing

Both skin prick tests and in vitro food specific IgE testing can be used to assess for sensitization to food at any age. The positive and negative predictive values of these tests vary considerably according to the history and total IgE of the patient. Generally, food allergy testing is helpful when the results are negative. Negative testing results usually imply that the food is not involved in the disease process. Positive tests, however, are not absolutely indicative of the specific food involvement because the false-positive rate is high. Depending on the clinical situation, positive findings can be assessed further with a detailed diet history, trial diet elimination, or a controlled food challenge. Care must be taken with diet elimination to ensure that a nutritionally adequate diet is maintained. The need for challenges should be decided on an individual basis.

Airborne allergens such as dust mite, animal dander, and pollens can exacerbate atopic dermatitis by inhalation, direct contact with the skin, or ingestion. Sensitization can be detected with skin prick tests or in vitro specific IgE antibodies. The positive and negative predictive values for these allergens are not well delineated; however, improvement in the disease has been shown with dust mite avoidance measures in those sensitized.

8.1.5.2 Contact Allergy

Contact dermatitis, whether irritant or allergic, can either mimic atopic dermatitis or occur concomitantly with it. The specific areas of involved skin need to be scrutinized carefully to assess for possible contact dermatitis (see below, 2.0. Contact Dermatitis). In particular, if eczema worsens despite topical treatment, the development of sensitization to the topical treatment should be assessed. Patch testing is the gold standard for identifying the cause of contact dermatitis.

8.1.6 Management

Successful management of atopic dermatitis requires a multipronged approach involving skin care, avoidance of flare factors, and anti-inflammatory treatment.

8.1.6.1 Basic Treatment

Basic therapy of atopic dermatitis should comprise optimal skin care with regular use of emollients and skin hydration in combination with the identification and avoidance of specific and nonspecific trigger factors.

Nonspecific irritants include contactants, such as clothing made from occluding or irritating synthetic or wool material. Clothing should consist of soft fabrics such as cotton. Fabric softeners added to clothing during the drying cycle may irritate patients with atopic dermatitis. Fabric softeners added to the wash cycle do not appear to cause a problem. Soap or detergent wash products should be avoided. These products can be replaced with emollient wash products. Patients should try to be as active as possible. Some sports such as swimming may be better tolerated than other sports involving intense perspiration and irritating clothing. Chlorine should be rinsed off immediately after swimming and the skin lubricated.

Specific allergen triggers should be addressed. Potential allergens can be identified with a careful history and selective allergy testing. Negative skin prick tests or in vitro specific IgE tests have a high predictive value for ruling out suspected allergens. Positive allergy tests, especially to foods, do not always correlate with clinical symptoms and should be confirmed with controlled food challenges, elimination diets, or, if available, atopy patch tests. Extensive elimination diets have not been found to be helpful and pose the risk of malnutrition. Food allergy is a more common factor for those younger than 4 years. Most children outgrow the food sensitivity unless the allergen is peanut, a tree nut, or seafood.

Avoidance of house dust mites by sensitized patients improves the skin disease. However, even for patients without IgE sensitivity to dust mites, exposure to dust mites means exposure to their proteases, which can break down corneodesmosomes, further compromising barrier function. Therefore, measures to reduce exposure to house dust mites might be important for all patients with atopic dermatitis. Avoidance measures include using dust-mite impermeable encasings on the pillow and mattress and washing the bedding weekly in hot water.

Dry skin contributes to the development of epithelial microfissures, which allow entry of skin pathogens, irritants, and allergens. Emollient bath, shower, and wash products should be used in combination with emollient creams and ointments to improve barrier function. The regular use of emollients and skin hydration is the mainstay of the general management of atopic dermatitis. Emollients should be applied continuously, even if no actual inflammatory skin lesions are obvious. Although general bathing can deplete the moisture of the epidermis, it does not have to be avoided. A shower, which is preferable to a tub bath, should be taken in moderately heated water, not hot water. Cleansing should be performed with a nonalkaline bar, superfatted soap, or a lipid-free cleanser. Several emollient wash products are available for the shower and bath and hand washing, including Aveeno cream and wash; Balneum plus cream and wash; E45 cream, bath, and wash; Hydromol cream and bath; Lipobase cream; and Oilatum cream and bath. After the shower or bath, the skin should be patted dry gently and any topical medication and hydrating lotion applied within 3 minutes. The proper use of emollients is critical for improving appearance, controlling itch, and reducing the need for topical corticosteroids. Two commercial emollient products often used are Eucerin cream and Cetaphil Moisturizing Cream. Patients should start with a more lubricating cream and, once hydrated, use a lighter cream. These should be applied over steroid creams and liberally over the skin after a shower and once or twice more during the day. Not all patients are comfortable with each type of emollient; patients should select which emollient they find most suitable for their skin.

8.1.6.2 Topical Treatments

Topical Corticosteroids

Topical corticosteroids are an important medication for the treatment of acute flares of atopic dermatitis. In addition, for children and adults, applying corticosteroids to unaffected skin twice weekly prevents further flare-ups of atopic dermatitis in those with frequent flares. Topical corticosteroids also reduce skin colonization with *S aureus*, contributing to the management of *S aureus* in those with infectious flares.

The adverse effects of uncontrolled topical corticosteroid use are well documented. Atrophy of the skin and damage to the stratum corneum are related to the potency of the corticosteroid and the length of therapy. Prolonged treatment with topical corticosteroids might damage the skin barrier at delicate skin sites sufficiently to enhance the penetration of irritants and allergens. Topical corticosteroids should be applied no more than twice daily as short-term therapy for acute lesions. Only mild-to-moderate strength preparations should be applied to genital, facial, or intertriginous skin areas. Studies of the percutaneous penetration of hydrocortisone into the skin found the greatest penetration in the face, eyelid, and scrotum and the lowest penetration in the plantar skin. The penetration of hydrocortisone through the eyelid is 300-fold that of the plantar skin. For infants, 1 or 2% hydrocortisone in a base of emollient may be used. Because infants are more susceptible to absorption, the weakest corticosteroid that is effective should be used. It is important to emphasize to the parent that the corticosteroid cream is not used simply as a skin lubricant. For children, only mild-to-moderate strength preparations should be used, groups IV–VII. Teens are more susceptible to topical corticosteroid complications such as striae. Most adults can be treated with a group IV preparation. For limited areas of thick, resistant eczema, higher potency corticosteroids can be used short term. Newer corticosteroid preparations, such as prednicarbate, mometasone furoate, fluticasone, and methylprednisolone aceponate, appear to have lower risk:benefit ratios and lower atrophogenic potential. The potencies of topical corticosteroids from most potent (group I) to least potent (group VII) are listed in Table 8.3.

Table 8.3 Topical corticosteroids classified by relative potency

Brand name	Generic name	Vehicle
Group I: superpotent		
Clobex	0.05% Clobetasol	Lotion, spray, shampoo
Cormax	0.05% Clobetasol	Cream, ointment, solution
Diprolene	0.05% Augmented betamethasone diproprionate	Ointment
Olux	0.05% Clobetasol	Foam
Psorcon	0.05% Diflorasone diacetate	Cream, ointment
Temovate	0.05% Clobetasol	Cream, ointment, solution
Ultravate	0.05% Halobetasol	Cream, ointment
Vanos	Fluocinonide	Cream
Group II: high potency		
Cyclocort	0.1% Amcinonide	Ointment
Diprolene AF	0.05% Augmented betamethasone dipropionate	Cream
Diprosone	0.05% Betamethasone dipropionate	Ointment
Florone	0.05% Diflorasone diacetate	Ointment
Halog	0.1% Halcinonide	Cream, ointment
Lidex	0.05% Fluocinonide	Cream, ointment, gel
Topicort	0.05–0.25% Desoximetasone	Cream, gel, ointment
Group III: mid to high potency		
Aristocort	0.5% Triamcinolone acetonide	Cream, ointment
Cutivate	0.005% Fluticasone propionate	Ointment
Cyclocort	0.1% Amcinonide	Cream, ointment, lotion

(continued)

Table 8.3 (continued)

Brand name	Generic name	Vehicle
Diprosone	0.05% Betamethasone dipropionate	Cream, lotion
Elocon	0.1% Mometasone furoate	Ointment
Group IV: mid potency		
Cloderm	0.1% Clocortolone pivalate	Cream
Elocon	0.1% Mometasone furoate	Cream, lotion
Kenalog	0.1% Triamcinolone	Ointment
Luxiq	0.12% Betamethasone valerate	Foam
Pandel	0.1% Hydrocortisone probutate	Cream
Synalar	0.025% Fluocinolone	Ointment
Valisone	0.1% Betamethasone valerate	Ointment, cream, lotion
Westcort	0.2% Hydrocortisone valerate	Ointment
Dermatop-E	0.1% Prednicarbate	Ointment
Group V: mid to low potency		
Cordran	0.05% Flurandrenolide	Cream, lotion
Cutivate	0.05% Fluticasone propionate	Cream
Locoid	0.1% Hydrocortisone butyrate	Cream
Westcort	0.2% Hydrocortisone valerate	Cream
Westcort	0.1% Hydrocortisone butyrate	Cream
Dermatop-E	0.1% Prednicarbate	Cream
Group VI: low potency		
Aclovate	0.05% Alclometasone dipropionate	Cream, ointment
DesOwen	0.05% Desonide	Cream, ointment
Tridesilon	0.05% Desonide	Cream
Valisone	0.01% Betamethasone valerate	Cream
Aristocort A	0.025% Triamcinolone acetonide	Cream
Group VII: low potency		
Hydrocortisone	1 and 2.5%	Cream, ointment, solution, lotion

From Beltrani, V. S., Bernstein, I. L., Cohen, D. E., and Ponacier, L., Joint Task Force on Practice Parameters, American Academy of Allergy, Asthma and Immunology, American College of Allergy, Asthma and Immunology. (2006) Contact dermatitis: a practice parameter. Ann. Allergy Asthma Immunol. 97 (Suppl 2), S1–S38. Used with permission. And also from Habif, T. P. (2004) Clinical dermatology: a color guide to diagnosis and therapy, 4th ed. Edinburgh: Mosby; p. 958–959. Used with permission

Topical Tacrolimus and Pimecrolimus

Tacrolimus is a topically applied calcineurin inhibitor that inhibits activation of T-cells, dendritic cells, mast cells, and keratinocytes. Tacrolimus has been shown to be effective for mild, moderate, and severe atopic dermatitis in adults and children. A local burning sensation that decreases over time is the most common adverse event, and most patients have greatly reduced pruritus within 3 days after treatment. Tacrolimus is available in 0.03 and 0.1% ointment forms. Tacrolimus 0.03% is approved for children as young as 2 years, and tacrolimus 0.1% is approved for adults. Unlike topical corticosteroids, tacrolimus ointment does not thin the skin and has been used safely for facial and eyelid eczema.

Pimecrolimus has the same mechanism of action as tacrolimus and has been shown to be effective for children and adults with various degrees of atopic dermatitis. Pimecrolimus is available as a 1% cream ointment. In the United States, it is approved for children as young as 2 years and, in several countries, for patients younger than 2 years. Like tacrolimus, pimecrolimus is not atrophogenic to the skin and is not associated with an increased number of skin infections. Compared with tacrolimus pimecrolimus has less local burning sensation associated with its use.

On 15 February 2005, the Pediatric Advisory Committee of the US Food and Drug Administration (FDA) recommended "black box" warnings for pimecrolimus (Elidel) and tacrolimus (Protopic) because of a potential risk for cancer. A postmarketing nonhuman primate study with an oral formulation of pimecrolimus demonstrated an occurrence of lymphoma in monkeys at a dosage 30 times the maximal recommended human dose. In humans, there is no evidence of an increased risk for malignancy. A comprehensive review by the Topical Calcineurin Inhibitor Task Force of the American College of Allergy, Asthma, and Immunology and the American Academy of Allergy, Asthma, and Immunology concluded that the current data do not support the use of the black box warning on topical pimecrolimus and tacrolimus and that the risk:benefit ratios of topical pimecrolimus and tacrolimus are similar to those of most conventional treatments for chronic relapsing eczema. They noted that the reported cases of lymphoma from topical pimecrolimus and tacrolimus are not consistent with lymphomas observed with systemic immunomodulator therapy, and the actual rate of lymphoma formation reported in patients taking topical calcineurin inhibitors is lower than that predicted for the general population.

The recommendations from the Topical Calcineurin Inhibitor Task Force include the following:

- Topical pimecrolimus and tacrolimus are indicated for the short-term or intermittent long-term treatment of atopic dermatitis in patients 2 years or older who are unresponsive to or intolerant of other conventional therapies or in whom these therapies are inadvisable because of potential risks.
- Children and adults with a compromised immune system should not use pimecrolimus or tacrolimus.
- In children younger than 2 years with poorly controlled persistent atopic dermatitis who require more than hydration and use of emollients to control the skin lesions, use of off-label therapy might be necessary because most topical corticosteroids or other immunomodulators have not been studied or approved for this age group.

No consensus guidelines are available for the use of topical corticosteroids versus topical calcineurin inhibitors. Topical calcineurin inhibitors can have an advantage over topical corticosteroids in some circumstances, including treatment for patients with a poor topical corticosteroid response and treatment of the face, particularly periocular and perioral areas and other "thin skin" areas where corticosteroid-induced skin atrophy could be a problem. In the longest comparative study of a topical corticosteroid versus a topical calcineurin inhibitor, tacrolimus 0.1% was significantly more efficacious than 0.1% hydrocortisone butyrate ointment for adults with moderate to severe atopic dermatitis. Long-term surveillance studies of pimecrolimus and tacrolimus are in progress. It is reassuring that in a recent study over a 2-year period of children aged 3–23 months, those treated intermittently with pimecrolimus cream 1% had normal responses to vaccinations and did not have an increased number of skin infections.

8.1.6.3 Anti-Infectious Management

Baths and gentle cleansers reduce *S aureus* colonization, and antibacterial cleansers can reduce them even further if these cleansers can be tolerated. Most patients with atopic dermatitis do not tolerate harsh antibacterial products such as chlorhexidine or bleach baths, although these can be considered for patients prone to bacterial infections when their skin is in adequate repair. Triclosan and chlorhexidine offer the advantage of a low sensitizing potential and low resistance rate. They can be used in emollients or as part of a wet wrap dressing therapy. Antistaphylococcal antibiotics can be helpful in treating poorly controlled disease of patients who are heavily colonized or infected with *S aureus*. Topical mupirocin or fusidic acid is useful in the treatment of localized impetiginized lesions. These agents should be used for only short periods (about 2 weeks). For patients with extensive superinfection, a course of systemic antibiotics is usually beneficial. First-generation cephalosporins, amoxicillin-clavulanic acid, or macrolide antibiotics can be used. It is important not to start prolonged antimicrobial therapy because patients can become colonized with resistant organisms.

8.1.6.4 Systemic Treatment

Antihistamines

There is little evidence to support the use of antihistamines for the treatment of atopic dermatitis, although they sometimes are recommended for their sedative effects. Because pruritus is usually worse at night, sedating antihistamines such as hydroxyzine or diphenhydramine may help at bedtime. Doxepin has both tricyclic antidepressant and H_1 and H_2 blocking effects and also causes sedation. Reports on nonsedating antihistamines are conflicting, although they may be useful for atopic dermatitis with concomitant urticaria. Topical antihistamines usually are not recommended and can induce cutaneous sensitization.

Systemic Corticosteroids

Systemic corticosteroids are rarely indicated for atopic dermatitis except as a short course for a severe flare. They should not be used for long-term management. When they are used, it is imperative to maximize anti-inflammatory topical treatment and intensify skin care with the application of emollients to help prevent rebound flares. The systemic corticosteroid should also be tapered to prevent rebound.

Phototherapy

Broad-band UV-B, broad-band UV-A, narrow-band UV-B, UV-A-1, and combined UV-A and UV-B phototherapy can be useful adjuncts in the treatment of atopic dermatitis. This is a standard second-line treatment for adults. UV treatment should be administered under the guidance of a dermatologist. Also, it should be restricted to patients older than 12 years. Short-term adverse effects include erythema, skin pain, pruritus, and pigmentation. Potential long-term adverse effects include premature aging of the skin and skin cancer.

Cyclosporine

Cyclosporine is a potent immunosuppressive drug. Like tacrolimus and pimecrolimus, it inhibits calcineurin-dependent T-cell pathways that result in decreased levels of proinflammatory cytokines such as IL-2 and INF-γ. Although cyclosporine has been found to be effective treatment for adult and childhood atopic dermatitis, relapse is often observed after therapy is discontinued. Because of possible adverse effects, namely renal toxicity, cyclosporine should be reserved for treating severe refractory disease. Blood pressure and serum creatinine levels need to be monitored closely.

Immunosuppressants

Various immunosuppressants such as azathioprine, mycophenolate mofetil, and methotrexate have been used to treat severe recalcitrant atopic dermatitis. Because these agents have several adverse effects, including myelosuppression and cytopenias, patients require close monitoring. These medications should be administered only by physicians familiar with their use.

8.1.6.5   Other Treatment Modalities

Allergen-Specific Immunotherapy

Although several anecdotal and case reports suggest clinical benefit from allergen-specific immunotherapy, very few blinded, placebo-controlled studies have been performed. One double-blind controlled study in children failed to show efficacy after 8 months of immunotherapy compared with placebo, but did show improvement at 14 months. However, the number of children was too small to generate definitive conclusions. In adults, a multicenter, randomized, blinded dose-response trial with three different doses of weekly subcutaneous dust mite immunotherapy over 1 year reported a dose-dependent decrease in SCORAD scores and a significant reduction in topical corticosteroid and antihistamine use in the high-dose immunotherapy group. The results of this study suggested that specific immuno-therapy may be useful for patients with atopic dermatitis who are sensitized to dust mites. Additional trials are needed for a definitive answer about this treatment.

Anti-IgE Therapy

The role of omalizumab remains to be defined. It may be of limited usefulness in atopic dermatitis because of its limitations in patients with markedly elevated IgE levels. Controlled studies are needed, particularly in those whose IgE levels are above the limits typically used in defining the dosage.

8.1.6.6   Future Possibilities

Traditional therapeutic strategies for atopic dermatitis have focused on skin hydra-tion, topical and systemic corticosteroids, and immunosuppressive agents. With the advent of new technologies such as gene expression microarrays and whole genome association, our understanding of the pathogenesis of atopic dermatitis will improve. Identification of candidate genes and contributory disease pathways will help with disease recognition and classification and culminate in the development of novel efficacious treatment options. Intrinsic immune keratinocyte immune defi-ciencies, abnormal stratum corneum barrier function, and protease regulators may represent viable therapeutic targets for the future. Inhibitors of allergic inflamma-tory response may include cytokine modulation such as TNF inhibitors, blockade of inflammatory cell recruitment by chemokine receptor antagonists, and inhibition of T-cell activation.

8.1.7   Guidelines for Management

Consensus-driven guidelines have not been available for atopic dermatitis. Although scoring systems are available for assessing acute disease severity, they do not emphasize the differences in disease burden over time. There is no distinction between persistent disease versus frequently recurrent disease versus disease with long remissions. Knowledge of the disease time pattern is crucial in outlining a preventive treatment plan. When outlining the treatment plan, consideration needs to be made regarding the following: (1) extent of the disease (acute), (2) persistence or recurrence pattern of the disease (long-term), and (3) quality of life and emo-tional impact.

Eichenfield has proposed an algorithm for the treatment of atopic dermatitis (Table 8.4). Good skin care and avoidance of irritants and allergens are part of the base therapy preceding step 1. The severity can be based on the amount of medication needed to keep the disease under control or on the extent and persistence

Table 8.4 Treatment Algorithm for Atopic Dermatitis[a,b]

A. Mild dermatitis (defined by disease extent or persistence)

Step 1	Step 2	Step 3
Emollient bid	Emollient bid	Emollient bid
	Intermittent low-potency TS for flare control	Mid-potency TS for flare control
	(? TCI alternative)	TCI alternative
	± Antihistamines	± Antihistamines

Step forward if necessary, back to step 1 if controlled
Maintenance therapy beyond step 1 if frequent recurrence or persistence of disease

B. Moderate dermatitis (defined by disease extent or persistence)

Step 2	Step 3	Step 4
Emollient bid	Emollient bid	Emollient bid
Intermittent low-potency TS for flare control	**Mid to higher potency TS for flare control (may be used instead of or in addition to TCI)**	**Higher potency TS for flare control**
TCI alternative	**TCI long-term intermittent**	TCI long-term intermittent
± Antihistamines	± Antihistamines	± Antihistamines
	Antibiotic if clinical infection	Antibiotic if clinical infection

Step forward if necessary, back one step if controlled
Maintenance therapy as Step 2 if frequent recurrence or persistence of disease
Consider Step 5 if uncontrolled: phototherapy, other systemic therapy

C. Severe dermatitis (defined by disease extent or persistence)

Step 3	Step 4	Step 5
Emollient bid	Emollient bid	Emollient bid
		Phototherapy or systemic therapy
Mid to higher potency TS for flare control (may be used instead of or in addition to TCI	**Higher potency TS for flare control**	
TCI long-term intermittent	TCI long-term intermittent	TCI long-term intermittent
(? Intermittent low to mid-potency TS as alternative)		
± Antihistamines	± Antihistamines	± Antihistamines
	Antibiotic if clinical infection	Antibiotic if clinical infection

Step forward if necessary, back one step if controlled
Maintenance therapy standard; Step 4 if uncontrolled; Step 5 as needed

From Eichenfield, L.F. (2004) Consensus guidelines in diagnosis and treatment of atopic dermatitis. J. Allergy Clin. Immunol. 118, 287–290. Used with permission
bid twice daily; *TCI* topical calcineurin inhibitor; *TS* topical steroid
[a] Proposed algorithm for severity-based step therapy of atopic dermatitis. Note: good skin care and avoidance of irritants and allergens are part of base therapy preceding step 1
[b] Changes in steps are in bold

of disease. Because of the complex scoring systems, the most commonly reported and validated scales such as SCORAD and EASI are difficult to use in everyday clinical practice. This management plan includes a plan for acute care, transition to maintenance regimen, and then further transition to the lowest possible maintenance dose.

8.2 Contact Dermatitis

8.2.1 Overview

Contact dermatitis is a common inflammatory dermatosis affecting primarily adults. Whether due to an allergic or irritant cause, contact dermatitis is the most common cause of occupational disease in the United States and accounts for 90% of workplace-acquired skin disorders. It accounts for nearly 6 million physician visits annually. Nearly 3,000 chemicals have been shown to cause allergic contact dermatitis. Contact dermatitis can be divided into irritant contact dermatitis and allergic contact dermatitis. Distinguishing between irritant and allergic triggers of contact dermatitis by clinical and histologic examinations can be challenging. Irritant contact dermatitis, which reflects an antigen-nonspecific (nonimmunologic) reaction, is responsible for approximately 80% of all cases of contact dermatitis. The reaction results from direct damage of epidermal keratinocytes after contact with a material. Allergic contact dermatitis, an antigen-specific, lymphocyte-mediated hypersensitivity reaction, occurs after previous sensitization to the allergen material. Despite the differences in mechanisms, both irritant contact dermatitis and allergic contact dermatitis involve skin inflammatory pathways. The two types of contact dermatitis are compared in Table 8.5.

Table 8.5 Characteristics of Irritant Contact Dermatitis (ICD) and Allergic Contact Dermatitis (ACD)

Characteristic	ICD	ACD
% of all cases of contact dermatitis	70–80%	20–30%
Mechanism	Direct tissue damage, nonimmunologic	Immunologic, delayed-type hypersensitivity
Histologic feature	Spongiosis	Spongiosis
Symptoms	Burning, stinging, pain	Pruritus
Signs	Erythema, edema, fissures, desquamation	Erythema, edema, vesicles, lichenification
Onset after exposure	Minutes to hours	Hours to days
Causative agents	Soaps, detergents, acids, bases, solvents	Urushiol (poison ivy), metals, cosmetics, fragrances, adhesives, preservatives
Diagnostic test	None	Patch test

8.2.2   *Pathogenesis*

Contact dermatitis results from nonallergic, irritant (irritant contact dermatitis), or allergic (allergic contact dermatitis) mechanisms. The primary factors that affect a response to a specific contact agent include the properties of the agent, the patient, the type and degree of exposure, and the state of the underlying skin. Thinner skin sites such as the eyelids, ear lobes, and genital areas are the most vulnerable areas, whereas thicker skin sites such as the palms and soles are more resistant to irritant or allergic contact dermatitis. Most contact dermatitis reactions occur directly at the site of exposure to the offending agent. Any previous damage to the skin compromises the integrity of the epidermal barrier, leaving it more vulnerable to irritants.

Irritant contact dermatitis is a multifactorial response involving contact with a substance that chemically abrades or physically damages the skin. This irritation can be produced by a wide variety of agents, including chemicals, detergents, solvents, alcohol, lotions, and powders. The irritant effect is augmented by physical factors such as scrubbing, washing, excessive hydration or drying, perspiration, and temperature extremes. This nonimmunologic, direct tissue reaction is usually a direct cytotoxic reaction. Inflammatory cytokines TNF-α, IL-1, IL-8, and GM-CSF are released by T-cells, resulting in cellular damage. In addition, host-innate immune cells such as macrophages, neutrophils, natural killer (NK), or natural killer T (NKT) cells likely contribute to the inflammatory response. The inflammatory reaction is dose dependent and typically limited only to the skin site in contact with the offending agent. Although this is a direct nonallergic tissue reaction, it can be difficult to differentiate from allergic contact dermatitis.

In contrast, allergic contact dermatitis results from a T-cell–mediated, delayed hypersensitivity immune response against haptens that come into contact with skin. Most of the contact sensitizers are small-molecular-weight molecules (haptens) that become immunogenic by coupling to the peptides loaded on the major histocompatibility complex (MHC) molecules of antigen-presenting cells in the skin. The most chemically reactive haptens are lipid-soluble, low-molecular-weight molecules that can easily penetrate the stratum corneum and strongly bind carrier proteins. Less commonly, large-molecular-weight peptides or proteins such as latex may induce the classic T-cell immune-mediated response.

Allergic contact dermatitis develops in two sequential phases: sensitization and activation. Sensitization is initiated when the offending substance comes into contact with the epidermis, activating keratinocytes that release proinflammatory cytokines, GM-CSF, and chemokines. In this environment, the hapten-protein conjugate or the protein alone is endocytosed by Langerhans or other dendritic cells and taken to draining regional lymph nodes for T-cell recognition. There, naïve CD4$^+$ T-cells are activated and sensitized. Once activated, the CD4$^+$ T-cells generate CD4$^+$CD25$^+$ regulatory and CD8$^+$ effector cells that become either memory or effector cells. When this cascade follows a patient's initial contact with the allergen, the number of responding T-cells is not sufficient to elicit a clinically visible response. These cells then "home" to the original induction skin site and circulate in the cutaneous environment. The cells contain homing and chemokine receptors that are maintained during their lifespan. This differentiation process enables the cells to be ready for the activation phase.

The activation phase, or efferent phase, of allergic contact dermatitis is provoked by hapten reexposure and requires several events, including recruitment of specific T-cells into the skin, in situ activation, and the expression of effector mechanisms responsible for tissue damage. The immune response is boosted by the existing supply of circulating memory T-cells. When activation occurs, the sensitized effector cells release proinflammatory cytokines or cytoxins, leading to an intense perivascular infiltrate and spongiosis. The latency period from allergen contact to clinical dermatitis corresponds to the travel time for Langerhans cells to present the allergen to the T-cells plus the time for the T-cells to proliferate, to secrete cytokines, and to home with the other inflammatory cells to the site of contact (18–96 hours). Haptens can be retained in the skin for a long time; however, without further contact with the substance, the inflammatory response ends in days or weeks. Subsequent exposure to sensitizing agents shortens the latency period. The reaction occurs more rapidly because T-cells are retained for long periods in the original allergic contact dermatitis skin sites.

Spongiosis, intercellular edema in the epidermis, is the predominant histologic feature of contact dermatitis. This edema stretches and eventually ruptures the intercellular attachments, resulting in vesicle formation. There generally is more spongiosis in allergic contact dermatitis than in irritant contact dermatitis. Irritant reactions tend to result in necrosis, acantholysis, and pustulosis. Despite these differences, there is significant overlap between the two types, and no distinct dermatopathologic feature is diagnostic of either irritant or allergic contact dermatitis.

Several genetic polymorphisms have been described, but the overall functional significance is not clear. Gene polymorphisms of TNF-α and IL-16 are more common in patients with multiple contact sensitivities. A TNF-α polymorphism has also been associated with increased irritant susceptibility in healthy persons. A keratinocyte CD80 gene up-regulation has been found useful in predicting allergic contact dermatitis for specific sensitizers.

8.2.3 Clinical Manifestations and Diagnosis

The approach to patients with contact dermatitis should consist of a thorough history and skin examination; patch tests with trays of allergens based on history, physical examination, and environmental exposure; education on materials that contain the allergen; and acute therapy and prevention.

8.2.3.1 History

To diagnose contact dermatitis, physicians should take a complete medical history that includes questions about sun or water exposure, hobbies, contact with pets and pet products, new exposures, and skin care and personal hygiene products and an occupational history that details the nature of the work, duration of activities, chemical exposures, protective wear and compliance with its use, dermatitis in coworkers, and remissions or exacerbations related to the work schedule. Industries in which workers are at highest risk for occupational skin diseases include food production, construction, printing, metal plating, machine tool operation, engine service, leather work, health care, cosmetology, and forestry. Although recent exposures are studied most often, long-term exposures are frequently the cause of allergic contact dermatitis. Unlike strong allergens such as poison ivy that may elicit a reaction after only one exposure, many occupational allergens are weak sensitizers and may require repeated exposures over months or years to cause skin sensitivity. Household exposures to items such as jewelry, clothing, cosmetics, fragrances, soaps, detergents, household cleaning agents, paints, and topical medicines should also be thoroughly reviewed. Of interest, it has been estimated that physicians accurately predict a sensitizer for only 10–20% of patients when relying solely on history and physical examination findings.

The prevalence of contact dermatitis is slightly higher among women than men, likely because of exposure to specific contactants, particularly cosmetics. There is age variability, with peaks during the teen years and at ages 40–60 years. The one uniformly present feature of allergic contact dermatitis is pruritus, without which the diagnosis of allergic contact dermatitis is essentially excluded. In addition, the site of irritation must have come in contact with the causative agent.

8.2.3.2 Physical Examination

The appearance of contact dermatitis can vary depending on which stage is present when the patient is examined. The acute stage is characterized by marked erythema, edema, and vesicle formation. The vesicles of allergic contact dermatitis are filled with a clear, transudative fluid that ruptures during the subacute phase. The fluid does not contain an appreciable amount of allergen and does not spread the dermatitis to other areas of the body. This is followed by oozing and erosion of the skin, with an eczematous appearance. The vesicles are replaced by papules, which are followed by crusting and scaling with lessening of the erythema and edema. As allergic contact dermatitis enters the chronic phase, lichenification and scaling predominate. The eruptions often have sharp, linear edges with geometric outlines, providing a helpful clue of contactant reactivity. The appearance, however, may be nonspecific.

The site of skin involvement is critical in the diagnosis of contact dermatitis because the area of involvement reflects the area of contact with the agent. The areas most commonly involved are the eyelids, face, neck, scalp, hands, axillae, and lower extremities (Fig. 8.4a–c). These exposed areas of the skin are more likely to have contact with an agent. The area of involvement can provide clues to the underlying causative agent.

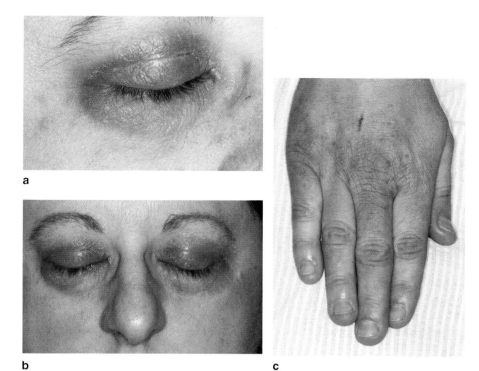

a

b

c

Fig. 8.4 Contact dermatitis involving the eyes (**a** and **b**) and hand (**c**) in classic distribution

Eyelids

The eyelids are particularly susceptible to allergic contact dermatitis because of minimal barrier protection, frequent touch, and constant aerogenic exposure to irritants. Of note, eyelid dermatitis is due more often to materials applied to the fingernails, face, or hair than to agents applied directly to the eyelids. Because the eyelid skin is not thick, materials in shampoos, conditioners, hair sprays, facial cosmetics, and gels may cause eyelid dermatitis without the scalp, face, or forehead being involved, despite exposure. Also, the methods of application and removal of cosmetics should be recognized.

Face

As with eyelid dermatitis, facial dermatitis occurs when substances are brought into contact with the face from other regions of the body. Cosmetics and fragrances are the most common cause of facial dermatitis. A partner's fragrance or cosmetics (or both) can cause facial dermatitis.

Scalp

Because of its thickness and covering, scalp skin is relatively resistant to allergic contact dermatitis. Hair dyes are the most common cause of scalp contact dermatitis. Irritant reactions may occur to hair straighteners and relaxers, particularly if they are not used correctly.

Neck

Similar to the eyelids, the skin of the neck is highly reactive, making it susceptible to allergic contact dermatitis. Hair products, cosmetics, jewelry, and clothing are common causes of allergic contact dermatitis on the neck.

Hands

More than half of all cases of contact dermatitis involve the hands (10% of women and 4% of men 30–40 years old). Contact dermatitis occurs primarily on the dorsal surface of the hands where the skin is thinner and the density of Langerhans cells greater than on the palmar surface. Both the irritant and allergic types occur in high frequency on the hands and are difficult to differentiate. Irritant contact dermatitis tends to have fewer vesicles than allergic contact dermatitis but occurs more often on the fingertips. When hand dermatitis continues into the forearms and is associated with facial dermatitis, a photosensitive process may be occurring.

Axilla

The primary agents that come into contact with the entire axillary vault include antiperspirants, deodorants, and dyes that leach out of the clothing in sweat. Contact with topically applied agents typically involves the apex of the axillary vault, whereas clothing agents usually spare this area. Aluminum hydroxide in antiperspirants is a common cause of irritant contact dermatitis of the axilla. Other causes of dermatitis in the axillary area include fragrances, formaldehyde-based resin systems, and shaving and depilatory agents.

Lower Extremities

Allergic contact dermatitis over the dorsal aspect of the feet may be caused by various shoe components, including chrome-tanned leather, glues, and rubber. Stasis dermatitis substantially increases the risk of allergic contact dermatitis due to an impaired skin barrier. Increased absorption of a topical medication through this area may cause a systemic sensitization and a generalized eruption termed an id reaction. The diagnosis of an id reaction should not be made unless there is an acute inflammatory reaction at a site distant from the contact sensitivity.

8.2.3.3 Differential Diagnosis

The differential diagnosis of contact dermatitis is broad and includes other papulo-squamous dermatoses. Endogenous forms of dermatitis, such as atopic, nummular, dyshidrotic, and seborrheic dermatitis, may mimic contact dermatitis, particularly in the more chronic forms. Both atopic dermatitis and contact dermatitis may appear eczematous; however, the onset of atopic dermatitis is typically in infancy or early childhood, whereas contact dermatitis is rare in childhood. Atopic dermatitis tends to be symmetrically distributed, primarily on the extensor surfaces in infancy and on flexural surfaces in childhood. Seborrheic dermatitis appears as a mild pruritus and a yellow, greasy coating with scaly irregularly shaped erythema on the eyebrows, nasal folds, and scalp. Nummular dermatitis consists of coin-shaped eczematous patches 2–10 cm in diameter on the torso or extremities. Dyshidrotic eczema appears as multiple, small vesicles 1–2 mm in diameter on the palms, soles, and lateral aspects of the fingers and toes. Other diseases of the skin, including psoriasis, fungal infections, cutaneous T-cell lymphoma, lupus, and pityriasis rosea, can also have an appearance similar to that of contact dermatitis.

8.2.4   Evaluation

8.2.4.1 Patch Testing

Patch testing is the gold standard for identifying a contact allergen. Patch testing attempts to artificially reproduce the circumstances that caused the initial reaction. The allergens are applied by a "patch" to a hairless region of the upper back between the spine and scapula that has been washed with plain water and gently dried. If shaving is required, an electric razor is preferable. A nonallergic adhesive tape is used to keep the allergens secured. The patch is left in place for 48 hours. Patients are instructed not to shower or exercise to the point of perspiring. The patients return to the physician's office 48 hours after the initial application for patch removal. The reaction is graded 30 minutes after the patch is removed. The 30-minutes wait allows time for nonspecific mechanical irritation to resolve. The patient is instructed to keep the skin dry and additional gradings are made 3, 4, or 7 days after the initial application of the test. It is essential that a second, delayed reading be made. The second reading assists in differentiating irritant from allergic responses and in identifying more delayed positive responses to allergens. Because elderly patients tend to take longer to mount an allergic response, 96-hours readings are preferred for these patients. Approximately 30% of relevant allergens that are negative at the 48-hours reading become positive in 96 hours. Conversely, some irritant reactions at 48 hours can disappear by 96 hours.

Table 8.6 Interpretation of patch testing as recommended by the International Contact Dermatitis Research Group

No.	Grade	Meaning/appearance	Clinical relevance[a]
1	–	Negative reaction	Excludes ACD; if ACD is still suspected, recheck technique or do ROAT
2	R	Irritant reaction	Controls show similar response or there was an excited skin response
3	±, +, or ?	Doubtful reaction	Negative test results; repeat readings at 3, 4, and 7 days after patch removed; if ACD still suspected, recheck technique or do ROAT
4	1+	Light erythema, nonvesicular	Equivocal test result; could either be negative or indicative of waning prior sensitization; false-positive test result or excited skin syndrome must be ruled out by test in control subject. Repeat steps in number 3
5	2+	Edema, erythema, discrete vesicles	Positive test result; indicative of prior or current sensitization; should correlate with history and physical findings. False-positive test result or excited skin syndrome must be ruled out by test in control subject
6	3+	Coalescing vesiculo-bullous papules	Strongly positive result; same conditions in number 5 apply

From Beltrani, V. S., Bernstein, I. L., Cohen, D. E., and Ponacier, L., Joint Task Force on Practice Parameters, American Academy of Allergy, Asthma and Immunology, American College of Allergy, Asthma and Immunology. (2006) Contact dermatitis: a practice parameter. Ann. Allergy Asthma Immunol. 97 (Suppl 2), S1–S38. Used with permission
ACD allergic contact dermatitis; *R* reaction; *ROAT* repeat open application test
[a] Clinical relevance is based on the Joint Task Force's appraisal of current literature

If no detectable changes are noted in the skin, the test is graded 0, signifying a negative test. Areas of erythema with edema covering at least half of the test area are graded 1+ and indicate a positive test. If papules are also present, the test is graded 2+. Coalescing vesicles or bullae indicate an extremely strong reaction, and the test is graded 3+. The scoring system and interpretation of patch test results are summarized in Table 8.6. A patch test tray, application of the patch tests, and patch test results are shown in Fig. 8.5a–d.

Patients receiving systemic corticosteroid therapy of more than 20 mg per day of prednisone or its equivalent or those undergoing cancer chemotherapy may have a diminished response or absence of response to patch tests. Corticosteroid therapy of less than 20 mg per day of prednisone is not likely to suppress strong positive responses to patch tests, but it can suppress mild responses. The skin site where the patch tests are to be applied should not have topical corticosteroid or calcineurin inhibitor for 5–7 days before testing. Systemic antihistamines do not affect the interpretation of patch tests. Patch testing should not be performed if the patient has acute contact dermatitis because a positive patch test reaction may induce a flare-up of existing allergic contact dermatitis. Also, the increased reactivity of the skin during

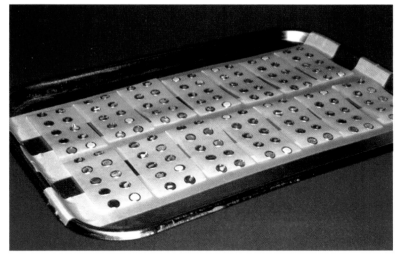

a

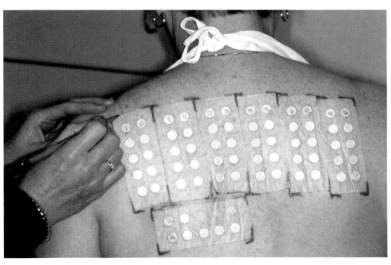

b

Fig. 8.5 Contact allergen patch testing. (**a**), A patch test tray containing various contact allergens in vehicle ready for application. (**b**), Patch tests applied to the upper back. (**c**), At 48 hours, the patches are removed from the back and results recorded. (**d**), Close-up view of a positive response to black rubber mix manifested by erythema, edema, papule, and vesicle formation

acute allergic contact dermatitis may lead to false-positive patch test results. Because patch testing does not completely reproduce the clinical scenario, local factors such as sweating, friction, and pressure that contributed to the dermatitis may not be present, leading to a false-negative result.

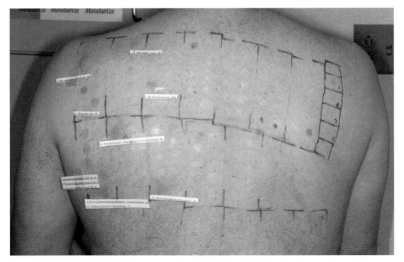

c

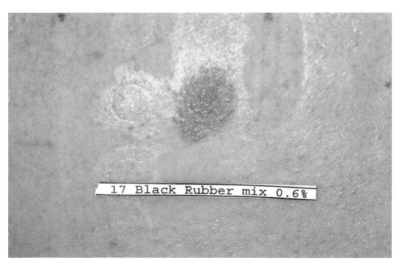

d

Fig. 8.5 (continued)

Types of Patch Testing

Although patch testing is relatively simple to perform, the selection of allergens for the test and the interpretation of the results can be difficult. Because it is impractical to test an unlimited number of contactants, standardized sets have been designed and validated by dermatologic societies. The standard tray or screening series allergens should be viewed as the starting point for patch testing all patients because the patient's history may not provide enough clues about the causative agent or can be misleading. Frequently, unexpected positive patch test reactions occur and lead to correct diagnosis. For example, patients with a suspected cosmetic allergy benefit from having the primary preservative or fragrance specifically identified to prevent further exposures. Although individual series contain different materials, the application is similar for them. Aluminum is the major carrier for current patch tests. Standardized samples of allergens are manufactured within or placed on small delivery vehicles before application on the skin. One popular system is the Finn chamber, which uses small 8-mm aluminum chambers that are occlusive and allow for quantification of the dose of allergen per unit area of skin. The chosen allergens are applied to the disk in combination with a 5-mm ribbon of petrolatum for allergen dispersion and then applied to the skin. Another method of application uses liquid antigens (one drop) that are placed on a filter paper disk and applied to the skin. Petrolatum patches can be made a few hours in advance; liquid patches should be made at the last minute. The number of allergens applied on a patient depends on the number and type of suspected allergens. Routine, ready-to-apply screening panels are often used because of the simplicity of application.

The TRUE (thin layer rapid use epicutaneous) test is an FDA-approved method for screening contact allergens. The TRUE test is preloaded with 23 common contactants and a vehicle control. These substances have been previously incorporated into a dried gel delivery system and are ready for application. The components of the TRUE test are listed in Table 8.7. When the patch is applied to the skin, the allergens are released as the gel becomes moisturized by transepidermal water. Each of the 12 panels per column is only 1 cm^2, and the panels are adequately spaced apart from each other. The standardized TRUE test identifies about 70% of clinically relevant allergens when compared with the more extensive screening series of the North American Contact Dermatitis Group. The TRUE test does not include bacitracin, gold, or poison ivy. Poison ivy should not be included in patch testing because the strong sensitizing properties of urshiol may cause severe reactions. The North American Contact Dermatitis Group currently uses 65 allergens or allergen mixes for the standard panel.

The standard tray is sometimes not sufficient for discovering the allergen responsible for the contact dermatitis. When a suspected agent is not included in the standard set, kits for specific occupations and exposures can be used. These include, for example, beautician and machinist kits and shoes, plants, and photosensitivity kits. Patch tests can be customized at times on the basis of the patient's exposure history. Cosmetics that are worn, such as nail polish and lipstick, or other contactants such as clothing, gloves, and food can be applied directly to the skin, constituting an open test.

There are variations to open testing. In the open test, the substance, as is or after being dissolved in water or other solvent, is dropped on the skin without the use of an occlusion device. The usual site is the volar forearm, and the surface is usually limited to 5 × 5 cm. This is recommended as the first step when testing poorly defined or unknown substances, such as those brought to the office by the patient.

Table 8.7 The standard true test series

Allergens	μg cm^{-2}
Panel 1	
1 Nickel sulphate	200
2 Wool alcohols	1,000
3 Neomycin sulphate	230
4 Potassium dichromate	23
5 Caine mix	630
6 Fragrance mix	430
7 Colophony	850
8 Epoxy resin	50
9 Quinolone mix	190
10 Balsam of Peru	800
11 Ethylene diamine dihydrochloride	50
12 Cobalt chloride	20
Panel 2	
13 *p-tert*-Butylphenol formaldehyde resin	50
14 Paraben mix	1,000
15 Carba mix	250
16 Black rubber mix	75
17 Methylchloroisothiazolinone/methylisothiazolinone (Kathon CG)	4
18 Quaternium 15	100
19 Mercaptobenzothiazole	75
20 *p*-Phenylenediamine	90
21 Formaldehyde (*N*-hydroxymethyl succinimide)	180
22 Mercapto mix	75
23 Thimerosal (thiomersal)	8
24 Thiuram mix	25

Modified from Frosch, P. J., Menné, T. and Lepoittevin, J.-P. (eds). (2006) Contact Dermatitis, 4th ed. Springer, Berlin Heidelberg New York, p. 454

Readings are similar to those adopted for conventional patch testing. A negative test does not preclude that allergy is not present, because a false-negative result may be due to insufficient exposure. With unknown substances, a negative open patch test indicates that one may proceed with an occlusive patch test. Care must be taken with this type of testing, because patch testing with a high concentration of caustic material may cause skin necrosis.

The semiopen test is like the open test except the substances applied to the skin are covered with nonocclusive tape after they have dried. This is particularly useful with industrial or domestic products. Various skin sites can be used, including the upper back, the extensor aspect of the arm, and the volar aspect of the forearm. The main advantage over conventional patch testing is the avoidance or reduction of skin irritation. However, false-negative results are common because of inadequate penetration.

The repeated open application test (ROAT) involves application of the substance twice daily for 7 days to the outer aspect of the skin of the upper arm, antecubital fossa, or back. A positive response usually appears on days 2–4, but, if no response occurs, it is recommended that the applications be extended beyond 7 days so late-appearing reactions are not missed. It occasionally is helpful to test at three sites simultaneously. The patient should stop the test at the first sign of a reaction. When symptoms appear after the first application, irritation cannot be ruled out and similar applications in control subjects are needed. Lack of a reaction constitutes a negative test. Cosmetics that are washed off, such as shampoos, conditioners, and cleanser, should be diluted 100- or 1,000-fold before application. Customized contactants should be incorporated into a petroleum base to allow for better absorption.

Common Materials Tested

Although hundreds of contact allergens have been identified, most cases of allergic contact dermatitis are due to only several dozen substances. The ten most frequent reactions are to nickel, balsam of Peru, neomycin, cobalt, fragrance mix, potassium dichromate, bacitracin, thimerosol, formaldehyde, and *p*-phenylenediamine (PPDA).

Nickel

Nickel is the metal that most commonly causes allergic contact dermatitis. Sensitization often occurs through ear or body piercing. Although the principal exposure is through jewelry, nickel is ubiquitous in the environment and found in numerous objects, including buttons, zippers, watchbands, glasses, bobby pins, safety pins, and shoelace eyelets. All alloys of steel, except most stainless steel, can also cause nickel allergy.

Balsam of Peru

Balsam of Peru is obtained from an extract of a tree (*Myroxylon pereirae*) that grows in Central America. It contains many constituents used commonly in fragrances. Patients who react to balsam of Peru should avoid all scented products, including perfumes, colognes, and scented toiletry products. If perfume sensitivity is suspected, the fragrance mix or the specific perfume needs to be tested, because testing with only balsam of Peru misses approximately half of fragrance-sensitive patients. Balsam of Peru is also used in the artificial flavoring industry and can be found in condiments, mouthwashes, toothpaste, and liquors.

Neomycin

Neomycin is one of the most common sensitizers in topical antibacterial preparations. It can cause contact allergy primarily because it is used topically on skin whose barrier function has been damaged. Neomycin may cross-react with gentamicin and other aminoglycosides. Patients are often sensitive to both neomycin and bacitracin, although there does not appear to be significant chemical cross-reactivity between the two substances.

Cobalt

Cobalt is a metal combined with other metals to make hard alloys. Cobalt salts are colored and used as pigments in colored glass and pottery as well as in makeup and hair dyes. It can be found in flypaper adhesives, light brown hair colors, hard metals, polyester resins, paints, cements, pottery, ceramics, and lubricating oils. Objects containing nickel and chromium also often contain cobalt, resulting in a cosensitivity. Sensitization to nickel or chromate in conjunction with active dermatitis appears to predispose to sensitization to cobalt. Occupational exposure varies and includes hard metal industries, tool and die making, paint industries, masonry, construction, cement industry, print industry, and dentistry.

Fragrance Mix

Fragrance products are found in a wide variety of cosmetics. Fragrance is not a single ingredient but a general name that includes many different fragrance ingredients. The fragrance mix has varied over the years. The TRUE test contains a blend of eight common fragrance ingredients: oak moss absolute, cinnamic aldehyde, cinnamic alcohol, alpha-amyl cinnamic alcohol, geraniol, hydroxycitronellal, isoeugenol, and eugenol. This mixture can corroborate the diagnosis in about 80% of patients allergic to fragrance. It is reasonable to test to an extended series of fragrances and the patient's own cosmetics if fragrance allergy is still suspected and the fragrance-mix patch test is negative.

Potassium Dichromate

Chromium causes both allergic and irritant reactions; however, allergic reactions are more common. Chromium is present in a wide variety of materials, including chrome-plated metals, tanned leathers, cement, plasters, glues, and paints. Although chromium is present in chrome-plated metals, reactions are typically due to the nickel in the product. Because chromium is present in cement, plasters, glues, and paints, it is a common occupational cause of contact dermatitis, particularly in workers in construction, tanning, metal, printing, and ceramics industries. People who work with wet cement are especially at risk for developing allergic contact dermatitis to chromium.

Thimerosol

Thimerosol is a preservative for liquid products used for the eyes, nose, and ears, including contact lens solutions and topical medications. It is also used as a preservative in vaccines and is found in cosmetics, primarily mascaras. For those who are sensitive, thimerosol in contact lens solutions can cause conjunctivitis and eyelid dermatitis. It is not clear whether patients with patch tests positive for thimerosol develop untoward reactions to thimerosol-containing vaccines.

Formaldehyde

Formaldehyde is produced and released in the general environment as a result of incomplete combustion found in cigarette smoke, automobile exhaust, and inciner-ation products. Formaldehyde is manufactured to make urea and phenol formalde-hyde resins; other uses include textile finishes, preservatives, and disinfectants. It is an effective cosmetic preservative against gram-negative bacteria. Substances that release formaldehyde and are used in skin care and cosmetic products include quaternium 15, imidazolidinyl urea, diazolidinyl urea, DMDM hydantoin, and Bronopol. Cross-reactivity is high among formaldehyde-releasing preservatives; therefore, it is best for patients to avoid all these substances if patch testing to one of them is positive. Formaldehyde-containing resins are used to make natural fibers such as cotton more resistant to wrinkling and shrinking. Textile dermatitis charac-teristically involves the peripheral parts of the axillae, antecubital fossa, neck, and upper part of the trunk. Allergy to free formaldehyde has become less common in recent years because manufacturers have reduced levels of free formaldehyde in fabrics. However, it is possible to have contact allergy to the formaldehyde resins used in these fabrics, but not to formaldehyde itself. The most common allergens are dimethylol dihydroxyethylene urea and melamine, which can be tested as a screening agent. Fabrics of 100% polyester knit and 100% Orlon consistently show the least amount of formaldehyde. Those of 100% cotton often have substantial amounts of formaldehyde. Patients who are allergic to formaldehyde resins should avoid natural fibers that are treated with formaldehyde resins and, instead, wear synthetic fabrics.

P-Phenylenediamine

PPDA is a pigment present in many inks and dyes. It is one of the most important dyes used for permanent hair coloring and is found in hair dye and fur dye and in black, blue, and brown clothing. In consumers, PPDA produces acute dermatitis that involves the scalp, eyelids, face, and hairline and may extend to include the neck, upper portion of the trunk, and arms. In hairdressers, the most common region affected is the hands.

Miscellaneous Contact Allergens

In addition to the above, textile coloring dyes and latex are commonly associated with allergic contact dermatitis. The most common textile dyes are disperse azo dyes. These water-soluble dyes are used to color synthetic materials such as poly-ester and nylon. In contrast to patients sensitive to formaldehyde resin dyes, patients sensitive to disperse azo dyes should wear natural fibers and avoid synthetic blends. Latex is a common occupational cause of allergic contact dermatitis. Unlike the

IgE-mediated allergy to latex, which is caused by sensitivity to the natural rubber proteins, latex allergic contact dermatitis is caused by the accelerators and antioxidants added to the latex during the vulcanization process. Thiurams, carbamates, and mercapto compounds are the accelerators most commonly associated with latex allergic contact dermatitis.

8.2.5 Special Exposures Associated with Contact Dermatitis

8.2.5.1 Occupational Contact Dermatitis (General)

The distribution of irritant contact dermatitis and allergic contact dermatitis as the cause of occupational contact dermatitis varies widely among reports. The range for irritant:allergic contact dermatitis varies from approximately 40:60 to 80:20. In approximately 80% of cases of occupational contact dermatitis, the hands are involved; the face is involved in 10% of cases.

Determination of a relation between contact dermatitis and occupation is not always easy. Mathias has proposed that "yes" answers to four of the following seven questions helps establish probable occupational causality:

1. Is the clinical appearance compatible with contact dermatitis?
2. Are there workplace exposures to potential irritants or allergens?
3. Is the anatomic distribution of the eruption compatible with job exposure?
4. Is the temporal relation between exposure and onset consistent with contact dermatitis?
5. Have nonoccupational exposures been excluded as causes?
6. Does the dermatitis improve away from work exposure to the suspected irritant or allergen?
7. Do patch or provocation tests identify a probable allergic cause?

Occupational irritant contact dermatitis can be classified as corrosion, acute irritation, chronic cumulative irritation, and phototoxicity. Chronic cumulative is the most prevalent form of occupational irritant contact dermatitis. It results from the ongoing exposure to mild irritants (waters, soaps, solvents, etc.). Over time, chronic friction can produce subclinical irritation that eventually leads to clinical irritant contact dermatitis. Phototoxicity is the least commonly reported form of occupational irritant contact dermatitis. Because the phototoxicity form requires exposure to both a photoabsorbing chemical and light, it is most commonly seen in outdoor workers such as roofers and agricultural workers. Acute irritation and corrosion result from exposure to caustic materials such as highly alkaline materials, strong acids, and powerful oxidizing or reducing agents.

A collaborative study of the North American Contact Dermatitis Group found carba mix, thiuram mix, epoxy resin, formaldehyde, and nickel to be the most common causes of allergic occupational contact dermatitis. Hand occupational allergic occupational dermatitis has been caused most frequently by chromium (leather exposure), rubber additives (gloves), and nickel (work tools and metal working). In farmers, allergic contact dermatitis has been shown to occur most frequently to metals, disinfectants, rubber, and pesticides. Unfortunately, the distinction is rarely made between irritant and allergic contact dermatitis, making it difficult to identify the specific source. Overall, the most commonly affected occupational groups are mechanics, housekeepers, metalworkers, cleaners, health care workers, construction workers, hairdressers, beauticians, bakers, and cooks.

8.2.5.2 Plant Dermatitis

Toxicodendron dermatitis (poison ivy) is the most common form of plant allergic contact dermatitis in the United States, with up to 85% of the population developing a clinical reaction when exposed. In Europe, poison ivy is not part of the natural flora and poison ivy dermatitis is virtually unknown. *Toxicodendron* plants (poison ivy, poison oak, and poison sumac) grow nearly everywhere in the continental United States. The sensitizing substances occur mainly in the oleoresin fraction. Urushiol, a catechol derivative found in the plants' sap, is an invisible oleoresin that easily spreads. It can be carried on sports equipment, animal fur, and lawn tools and can be disseminated by burning brush fires. Urushiol rapidly penetrates the skin, precipitating sensitization. Once exposed, the potential for sensitization occurs unless the substance is removed immediately. Facilities for adequate removal are limited in the outdoor environment when exposure occurs. Sensitivity typically develops after several exposures. Approximately 10–15% of the population is markedly sensitive to poison ivy and poison oak, resulting in significant swelling of the face, arms, and genitalia. The typical rash is a linear papulovesicular rash that develops 12–48 hours after exposure. Over a period of 5–7 days, the vesicles rupture, form crusts, and scale. Although the vesicular fluid is often believed to be contagious, there is no evidence that it is allergenic. However, continued unintentional exposure can occur to the urushiol on clothing, tools, and animal fur. Resolution occurs over 2 weeks to 2 months. Cross-reactions may occur in patients exposed to similar catechol derivatives found in mangoes and cashews. Patch testing is not indicated for *Toxicodendron* dermatitis because the dermatitis is self-limiting and there is danger of exacerbating allergic contact dermatitis.

Plant dermatitis also occurs in flower workers, particularly to Peruvian lily. The dermatitis affects the areas of highest contact, typically the first three fingers and exposed areas of the hands, forearms, and V-region of the neck and the face. Airborne pollen, particularly weed pollen, has been reported to cause seasonal allergic contact dermatitis. It appears this is less common with tree and grass pollen. Open patch testing with fresh plants and flowers should be done with caution because a high allergen content may cause severe bullous reactions. A positive reaction must be differentiated from an irritant reaction by testing nonsensitized controls. Because of the lack of standardized test antigens, testing for this reaction is difficult.

8.2.5.3 Cosmetics

Cosmetics include skin care products, facial makeups, personal cleanliness products, nail and hair products, perfumes, and shaving preparations. It has been estimated that adverse reactions to cosmetics occur, on average, once every 10–15 years per person. Fragrances have consistently been shown to be the most common cause of cosmetic allergic contact dermatitis. Positive reactions to fragrances on patch testing are seen in nearly 50% of patients who have suspected cosmetic dermatitis. In addition to perfumes and colognes, exposure to fragrance allergens can occur through soaps, toothpastes, household cleaning products, medications, and perfumed products worn by others. It is important to realize that products marked "unscented" may not be fragrance free and may contain a masking fragrance to make it "unscented."

Preservatives, used in cosmetics to prevent the overgrowth of microorganisms, are the second most common class of cosmetic allergens. They are divided into three categories: antimicrobials, antioxidants, and UV light absorbers. Common antimicrobials include formaldehyde, formaldehyde releasers (Bronopol, DMDM hydantoin, diazolidinyl urea, imidazolidinyl urea, and quaternium 15), and nonformaldehyde releasers (methyl-chloroisothiazolinone-methylisothiazolinone [MCI-MI], methyldibromoglutaronitrile-phenoxyethanol [MDBGN-PE], and iodopropynyl butylcarbamate). The use of formaldehyde in cosmetics has been decreasing because it is a frequent sensitizer. Exposure still occurs through other products such as cleaning agents. Complete avoidance of formaldehyde is difficult; however, patients who practice avoidance have significantly fewer eruptions. The formaldehyde-releasing preservatives are inherently antibacterial and antifungal but also act by formaldehyde release because of an easily detachable formaldehyde moiety. Despite being the most commonly used formaldehyde releaser, imidazolidinyl urea seems to be the least common sensitizer. Allergy to one formaldehyde-releasing preservative may result in sensitization to the entire class, but there are exceptions to this. Previously, MCI-MI was the most common sensitizer of the nonformaldehyde-releasing preservatives. Because of the high rates of sensitization, the concentration of MCI-MI allowed in rinse-off and leave-on products has been decreased. Although still used, it is being replaced with newer preservatives such as MDBGN-PE. Parabens are the most widely used preservatives but are rare causes of allergic contact dermatitis.

Antioxidants protect products from the development of odor and discoloration. Antioxidants that cause contact dermatitis include butylhydroxyanisole, butylated hydroxytoluene, and tertiary butylhydroquinone. UV absorbers are added to cosmetics to prevent deterioration of the product and to function as a sunscreen. Oxybenzone (benzophenone-3) is a common sensitizer.

Other cosmetic allergens include emulsifiers such as glycerin, lanolin, castor oil, and cocamidopropyl betaine. The primary noncosmetic allergens that can mimic cosmetic allergy are gold, nickel, and rubber. Rubber can produce the same distribution of lesions as cosmetics, because rubber can be found in cosmetic applicators and sponges.

8.2.5.4 Medicinal Contact Dermatitis

Contact dermatitis often develops after exposure to topical medications because of an interrupted skin barrier. The most common sensitizers are lanolin, para-amino benzoic acid, "caine" derivatives, antibiotics, antihistamines, nonsteroidal anti-inflammatory drugs, and corticosteroids. Topical antibiotics, especially neomycin and bacitracin, induce allergic contact dermatitis more often than any other class of medicines. A medicinal contact dermatitis should be suspected when an eruption worsens rather than improves after the application of the topical agent. The ester class of topical anesthetics is frequently implicated in allergic contact dermatitis, whereas the amide class of topical anesthetics is rarely implicated. Although most patients who have a reaction to topical corticosteroids are sensitive to preservatives and other vehicle components in the preparations, corticosteroid molecules themselves and their degradation products are capable of producing allergic contact dermatitis. The screening agents most commonly used for topical corticosteroid allergic contact dermatitis are budesonide and tixocortol pivalate. This does not cover the entire spectrum of topical corticosteroid sensitivity. Topical corticosteroids are divided into four groups: class A hydrocortisone, class B triamcinolone acetonide, class C betamethasone, and class D hydrocortisone butyrate. There is considerable cross-reactivity within each group, but cross-reactivity between the groups is infrequent. Class C corticosteroids are associated with the least amount of reactions. The medicinal preservative with the highest prevalence of positive patch tests is thimerosol.

8.2.6 Treatment

8.2.6.1 Prophylaxis

The primary tenet of prevention is to identify the culprit allergen and to institute avoidance measures. When the allergen is identified, the patient must be educated about all potential sources of exposure because many contact allergens are found in several different products. For example, when managing a plant sensitizer, the patient should be instructed in the proper identification of the offending plant. The patient also should be counseled about possible cross-reacting allergens and given practical suggestions for allergen avoidance. An exposure list for each allergen of significance should be provided to the patient. When the allergen cannot be avoided, the implementation of a protective barrier is the next preventive option. Protective clothing should be worn, for example, long-sleeved shirts and long pants. For hand dermatitis, appropriate gloves may be helpful. The gloves should be vinyl, waterproof, and heavy duty. They can be worn over cotton gloves for comfort. Barrier creams containing dimethicone, perfluoropolyethers, or high-lipid-content moisturizers may prevent the development of irritant contact dermatitis.

Toxicodendron dermatitis may be reduced or prevented with quaternium 18 bentonite lotion and topical skin protectant (an emulsion with perfluoroalkylpolyether), similar to Teflon.

8.2.6.2 Symptomatic Treatment

Avoidance of the contact allergen is the first step in treatment of allergic contact dermatitis. This requires identifying the offending allergen and educating the patient about avoidance measures. If the contact continues, the dermatitis may become chronic or generalized. For topical palliation, cold compresses can help both allergic and irritant contact dermatitis. Other palliative treatments include saline, aluminum subacetate (Burow's solution), or other soothing agents such as Aveeno. Oozing lesions may be dried with calamine and colloidal oatmeal baths. More chronic, dry lesions do not require compresses.

Topical corticosteroids are the first-line treatment for localized allergic contact dermatitis. Appropriate selection of a topical corticosteroid is determined by the size of the lesion, the location of the dermatitis, and the phase of evolution. Areas of thick skin, such as the palms and soles, generally require potent agents; midpotency agents can be used on the trunk and limbs. Ointments are best suited for thicker, drier lesions, whereas creams or lotions should be used on more exudative lesions or intertriginous areas. Ointments and potent corticosteroids should not be applied to areas of thinner skin such as flexural surfaces, eyelids, and face. Topical corticosteroids are most effective when applied after hydration. Localized acute lesions respond best to midpotency–high-potency topical corticosteroids. Applying the topical corticosteroid more frequently than recommended is not more effective. The relative potency of topical corticosteroids is listed in Table 8.3.

If allergic contact dermatitis involves an extensive area of skin (>20%), systemic corticosteroids are helpful. Improvement is seen in 12–24 hours. A commonly used dosage is 0.5–1 mg kg^{-1} prednisone daily for 5–7 days, and if there is clinical improvement, the dose is decreased by 50% for 5 days, with further decrease in or tapering of dosage dependent on continued clinical response and contactant avoidance. The usual treatment time is 2–4 weeks. Tapering the corticosteroid dosage too quickly may cause a rebound flare of dermatitis.

8.2.6.3 Complications and Other Contact Reactions

Contact dermatitis may become impetiginized. This typically is manifested as a sudden worsening of the contact dermatitis. If the area of involvement is limited, topical antibiotics should be used to treat the area and to prevent more serious infections. If widespread staphylococcal or β-hemolytic streptococcal bacterial infections occur, systemic antibiotics may be required.

Photocontact dermatitis occurs when a substance produces a contact dermatitis when exposed to sunlight. The clinical distribution of photocontact dermatitis includes only sun-exposed areas. The face, arms not covered by clothing, and the V of the neck are the most common areas affected. Typically, the skin under the chin and behind the ears and the upper eyelids are spared. Photocontact dermatitis produces a pruritic, papulovesicular, eczematous dermatitis similar to allergic contact dermatitis. Substances associated with photoallergic reactions include tars, dyes, psoralens, fragrances, and sunscreens. Medications associated with photocontact dermatitis include sulfonamides, tetracyclines, fluoroquinolones, oral contraceptives, thiazides, and phenothiazines.

Although much less common, contact reactions can take the form of cheilitis, dyspigmentations, acneiform eruptions, lichenoid eruptions, and urticaria.

8.3   Clinical Vignettes

8.3.1   Vignette 1

A 9-year-old boy with a history of atopic dermatitis since age 1 presents with progressively worsening atopic dermatitis. His mother reports that over the last 6 months his rash, described as red and itchy, has gotten "angrier" in his usual areas of involvement, namely, the trunk and extremities. Initially, she noted primarily increased redness, but now has also noted increased drainage. The itching, particularly at night, has interfered with his sleep. He has been reluctant to go to school because of his skin. Topical hydrocortisone has been applied once daily for the last month, but the rash has not improved.

On physical examination, the patient is found to have diffuse eczema over the trunk and extremities. There are multiple areas of excoriation, primarily on the flexural surfaces of the upper and lower extremities, with impetiginization.

Comment: This child clearly has had a significant worsening of atopic dermatitis. Impetiginization manifested as a superficial honey-colored exudate on eczematous skin is usually a sign of superficial infection. In patients with atopic dermatitis, *S aureus* is the usual microbial pathogen. *S aureus* produces proteases that can damage the skin barrier and superantigens that activate T-cells, macrophages, and eosinophils, perpetuating the inflammatory response in atopic dermatitis.

It appeared that the control of atopic dermatitis was worsening before the *S aureus* superinfection developed. At this time, it is prudent not to just treat the flare but also to outline a long-term management plan. To do this, it is important to inquire about the overall nature of the boy's atopic dermatitis. Does he have persistent atopic dermatitis, frequent flares, or infrequent flares? What is the baseline treatment regimen? What is his environment like, especially with regard to possible allergen and irritant exposure? What have been the known triggers for his atopic dermatitis in the past?

The mother reports that, overall, the atopic dermatitis is mild to moderate. The boy always has dry skin and is never completely without lesions, but he has grown accustomed to it. His current flare is the worst one he has had in years. Typically, he has mild eruptions approximately monthly that respond to topical corticosteroids. He does not have a baseline treatment regimen. He and his mother simply apply topical corticosteroids whenever his skin is bothering him. He has not been using any emollients. Their home is nearly 80 years old. They do not have any pets. He washes with regular commercial soap and hair shampoo and showers either every day or every other day. His bed was moved from the second floor in the house to the basement 4 months ago when they remodeled the house. Currently, he is sleeping on a mattress on the floor. The mother is not aware of obvious triggers for his atopic dermatitis. Foods have not been a problem for him.

Comment: Currently, this child's atopic dermatitis is not being managed optimally. The boy and mother need to be educated about the overall management strategy for the condition. First, and most important, the role of skin hydration needs to be stressed to the boy and mother. There is no substitute for this. With good, consistent skin hydration, his atopic dermatitis may be completely controlled. In this regard, proper shower technique and the use of emollients twice daily need to be emphasized. Irritants and allergens should be assessed. Clothing, fingernail status, and bedding should be discussed. His soap should be switched to a nonirritating, moisturizing soap. From the allergen perspective, the current bed situation is a set-up for dust mite exposure. He should be evaluated for dust mite allergy. At his current age, without a specific history for food sensitivity, food allergy testing is not likely to be helpful.

Specific allergen in vitro testing to dust mite was markedly positive.

Comment: Because of the potential for dust mite to worsen his disease, both by protease activity and through IgE-mediated inflammation, environmental dust mite precautions should be instituted in the overall management of his disease. Currently, for his acute flare, his treatment should consist of the following:

- Amoxicillin/clavulanic acid for 14 days for widespread *S aureus* superinfection
- Emollient use immediately after shower and twice daily
- Group V topical corticosteroid, 0.1% hydrocortisone cream twice daily
- 2-week follow-up to assess progress

  For long-term care:

- Emollient use immediately after shower and twice daily
- Dust mite precautions
- Avoidance of irritants, change of soap
- Depending on the subsequent course (day-to-day symptoms and number of flares), intermittent topical corticosteroid or topical calcineurin inhibitor may be needed

8.3.2 Vignette 2

A 42-year-old woman presents with a 3-month history of a red, pruritic rash involving primarily her hands and, to a lesser extent, the periorbital area. She does not have a past history of a similar rash. She is otherwise healthy. Physical examination shows an eczematous rash involving the dorsum of both hands characterized by erythema, papules, and few vesicles. Lichenification of the skin is also noted. The palms are spared. There is a gradual decrease in the eczema in the wrist-forearm area bilaterally. The arms, neck, trunk, and lower extremities are spared. There is mild erythema of the skin in the inferior periorbital area.

Comment: The distribution of the eczematous rash is suspicious for contact sensitivity. The presence of pruritus and involvement of both the hands and orbital area are suggestive of allergic contact dermatitis. A detailed history is required, with the focus on personal habits, including handwashing, bathing, body lotions, facial make-up, deodorant, perfume, hair products, nail cosmetics, and laundry detergent. In addition, an occupational history outlining occupation, job description, and materials should be obtained.

The salient points from the detailed history primarily involve the patient's occupation. She began working as a hairdresser 4 months ago (1 month before the onset of signs and symptoms). Her job activities include cleaning, conditioning, cutting, waving, styling, and coloring hair. She has not had more than 2 days off consecutively since starting. Currently, she is the only one at her salon who has these signs and symptoms. She becomes a bit overwhelmed when asked to describe all the materials she comes into contact with because it includes shampoos, conditioners, wave solutions, hair gels, and hair dyes. She wears nonlatex gloves for some of the styling procedures.

Comment: As a hairdresser, the number of materials the patient comes into contact with is indeed overwhelming. It is important to know common sensitizers for various occupations. Hairdressers are at risk for irritant contact dermatitis from frequent shampooing and for allergic contact dermatitis from nickel in the instruments, rubber chemicals in gloves, PPDA in permanent hair colors, glyceryl thioglycolate in permanent hair-waving solutions, and ammonium persulfate in hair bleach. Involvement of the eye area in addition to the hands suggests possible allergic contact sensitivity with transfer of the allergen from the hands to the face area. A pure irritant reaction most likely (but not exclusively) would be confined to the hands. To evaluate further, patch testing should be performed that includes nickel (scissors, clips), rubber chemicals (gloves), preservatives (cosmetics), PPDA (permanent hair dyes), fragrance mix, and balsam of Peru (fragrances) and a supplemental hairdressing tray that includes glycerol thioglycolate and ammonium persulfate.

Patch testing was performed. A 3+ response was noted to PPDA.

Comment: PPDA, an important dye for permanent hair coloring, is one of the most common allergic contact sensitivities of hairdressers. Wearing gloves appears to help prevent allergic contact dermatitis from permanent hair dyes. If

Table 8.8 Exposure list for *p*-Phenylenediamine (PPDA)

Synonyms and other names

1,4-Benzenediamine	1,4-Phenylenediamine
Orsin	PPDA
p-Aminoaniline	Rodol D
p-Phenylenediamine	Ursol D
p-Diaminobenzene	

Uses

PPDA is the parent compound for permanent hair dyes and is a component of the following products and processes:
1. Cosmetics (permanent hair colors and some dark-colored cosmetics)
2. Primary intermediate in the production of azo-type dyes
3. Rarely, fur and leather dyes
4. Photographic developers
5. Rubber and plastics industry (antioxidants and accelerators)
6. Photocopying
7. Lithography (printing inks)
8. Oils, greases, and gasoline
9. Epoxy resin hardeners
10. Milk testing
11. Temporary tattoo

Prevention

Most cases of PPDA sensitivity arise from the use of permanent hair dyes. Fully developed (oxidized), PPDA dye is no longer an allergen, so hair or fur that has already been dyed is safe. For persons who want to continue dying their hair, semipermanent (not containing PPDA) or temporary hair dyes are a good alternative. For a hairdresser, it is best to avoid dying clients' hair. Wearing of latex nitrile or 4-H gloves is helpful but interferes with manual dexterity. Besides avoiding PPDA, patients may also be sensitive to the hair dye chemicals *p*-toluenediamine, *p*-aminodiphenylamine, 2, 4-diamino-anisole, and *o*-aminophenol. Allergic individuals should be cautious about using permanent hair colors with these chemicals. Occasionally individuals with PPD sensitivity can react to other, similar chemicals, including sulfa drugs, sulfonylurea diabetes medications, *p*-aminosalicyclic acid, benzocaine and procaine anesthetics, and *p*-aminobenzoic acid sunscreens

From Marks, J. G. Jr., Elsner, P., and DeLeo, V. A. (2002) Contact & Occupational Dermatology, 3rd ed. Mosby, St. Louis, p. 118. Used with permission

possible, PPDA dyes should be avoided. The patient also needs to be aware that she should not have her hair treated with this substance. As with all patients who have contact dermatitis, an exposure sheet should be given to counsel the patient on other possible exposures. An example of an exposure sheet is given in Table 8.8.

Acute management of the dermatitis consists primarily of avoidance, moisturization, and topical corticosteroids. Topical calcineurin inhibitors generally are not very effective in contact dermatitis.

8.3.3   Vignette 3

A 35-year-old woman, an anchorwoman for television documentaries, presents with a 6-week history of eyelid dermatitis. The dermatitis is a pruritic, eczematous eruption on both right and left upper and lower eyelids. No other area of skin is involved. She has no previous history of skin problems.

Comment: An eczematous dermatitis localized just to the eyelids is suspicious for contact dermatitis. Because of its thin skin, the eyelid is highly susceptible to contact sensitivity. The initial considerations for materials causing contact sensitivity would include cosmetics, cosmetic applicators, shampoos, and hand and nail products. Materials that come into contact with the head and hands can sometimes cause eyelid dermatitis without the head and hands being affected because of the high sensitivity of the eyelids. Additional history should focus initially on the cosmetics, cosmetic applicators, shampoo, and hand and nail products the patient uses.

The patient brought in her cosmetic tray and the applicators, hand creams, nail polish, and hair care products. She has not made any change in the types of materials or products she uses.

Comment: This is important information. Unexpectedly, the patient did not report using any new products. Typically, new-onset dermatitis would be due to exposure to a new material. Because of the number of contactants in her cosmetics, cosmetic applicators, shampoo, and hand and nail products, without any one in particular being suspected, further evaluation can be performed with patch testing to a basic panel such as the TRUE panel or the North American Contact Dermatitis Group standard tray and a cosmetic tray.

Patch testing to the North American Contact Dermatitis Group standard tray and the cosmetic tray showed a positive result to nickel only.

Comment: Although the patient had a positive response to nickel, it did not appear that it was the cause of the eyelid dermatitis. Nickel in jewelry and clothes, typically causes nickel contact dermatitis, thus the ears, neck, wrist, and waist (belt buckles) are affected, not the eyelids. At this point, it would be helpful to discontinue the use of all her cosmetics and hand, nail, and hair care products.

Despite stopping the use of all cosmetic and hand, nail, and hair care products for 3 weeks, the eyelid dermatitis did not improve.

Comment: Although contact dermatitis persists after the offending agent has been removed, some improvement would have been expected after 3 weeks. At this time, it would be helpful to once again review her history in detail, focusing on all her activities throughout the day.

Upon further review of her daily routine, the patient added that she has been using an eyelash curler. Examination of the eyelash curler showed that it was made with a nickel-plated material. The patient was asked to stop using the curler, and the eyelid dermatitis markedly improved over the following weeks.

Comment: This clinical vignette demonstrates how difficult it can be to accurately list all the materials with which a patient may have contact. Evaluation of a patient with suspected contact dermatitis often requires both a detailed history and pertinent patch testing to confirm the diagnosis.

Suggested Reading

Akdis, C. A., Akdis, M., Bieber, T., et al., PRACTALL Consensus group. (2006) Diagnosis and treatment of atopic dermatitis in children and adults: European Academy of Allergology and Clinical Immunology/American Academy of Allergy, Asthma and Immunology/PRACTALL Consensus Report. J. Allergy Clin. Immunol. 118, 152–169

Belsito, D. V. (2005) Occupational contact dermatitis: etiology, prevalence, and resultant impairment/disability. J. Am. Acad. Dermatol. 53, 303–313

Beltrani, V. S., Bernstein, I. L., Cohen, D. E., and Ponacier, L., Joint Task Force on Practice Parameters, American Academy of Allergy, Asthma and Immunology, American College of Allergy, Asthma and Immunology. (2006) Contact dermatitis: a practice parameter. Ann. Allergy Asthma Immunol. 97 (Suppl 2), S1–S38

Biebl, K. A. and Warshaw, E. M. (2006) Allergic contact dermatitis to cosmetics. Dermatol. Clin. 24, 215–232

Boguniewicz, M., Schmid-Grendelmeier, P., and Leung, D. Y. (2006) Atopic dermatitis. J. Allergy Clin. Immunol. 118, 40–43

Cork, M. J., Robinson, D. A., Vasilopoulos, Y., et al. (2006) New perspectives on epidermal barrier dysfunction in atopic dermatitis: gene-environment interactions. J. Allergy Clin. Immunol. 118, 3–21

Eichenfield, L. F. (2004) Consensus guidelines in diagnosis and treatment of atopic dermatitis. Allergy 59 (Suppl 78), 86–92

Fiset, P. O., Leung, D. Y., and Hamid, Q. (2006) Immunopathology of atopic dermatitis. J. Allergy Clin. Immunol. 118, 287–290

Fonacier, L., Spergel, J., Charlesworth, E. N., et al., Task Force of the American College of Allergy, Asthma and Immunology and the American Academy of Allergy, Asthma and Immunology. (2005) Report of the topical calcineurin inhibitor Task Force of the American College of Allergy, Asthma and Immunology and the American Academy of Allergy, Asthma and Immunology. J. Allergy Clin. Immunol. 115, 1249–1253

Khumalo, N. P., Jessop, S., and Ehrlich, R. (2006) Prevalence of cutaneous adverse effects of hairdressing: a systematic review. Arch. Dermatol. 142, 377–383

Leung, D. Y. and Bieber, T. (2003) Atopic dermatitis. Lancet 361, 151–160

Mark, B. J. and Slavin, R. G. (2006) Allergic contact dermatitis. Med. Clin. North Am. 90, 169–185

Marks, J. G. Jr., Elsner, P., and DeLeo, V. A. (2002) Contact & Occupational Dermatology, 3rd ed. St. Louis: Mosby

Mathias, C. G. (1989) Contact dermatitis and workers' compensation: criteria for establishing occupational causation and aggravation. J. Am. Acad. Dermatol. 20, 842–848

Paul, C., Cork, M., Rossi, A. B., Papp, K. A., Barbier, N., and de Prost, Y. (2006) Safety and tolerability of 1% pimecrolimus cream among infants: experience with 1133 patients treated for up to 2 years. Pediatrics 117, e118–e128

Reitamo, S., Ortonne, J. P., Sand, C., et al. (2005) A multicentre, randomized, double-blind, controlled study of long-term treatment with 0.1% tacrolimus ointment in adults with moderate to severe atopic dermatitis. Br. J. Dermatol. 152, 1282–1289

Saary, J., Qureshi, R., Palda, V., et al. (2005) A systematic review of contact dermatitis treatment and prevention. J. Am. Acad. Dermatol. 53, 845

Werfel, T., Breuer, K., Rueff, F., et al. (2006) Usefulness of specific immunotherapy in patients with atopic dermatitis and allergic sensitization to house dust mites: a multi-centre, randomized, dose-response study. Allergy 61, 202–205

Williams, H. C. (2005) Clinical practice: atopic dermatitis. N. Engl. J. Med. 352, 2314–2324

Chapter 9
Drug Allergy

Abbreviations AERD: aspirin-exacerbated respiratory disease; COX: cyclooxy-genase; DRESS: drug rash with eosinophilia and systemic symptoms; HIV: human immunodeficiency virus; HSS: hypersensitivity syndrome; NSAID: nonsteroidal anti-inflammatory drug; PCP: *Pneumocystis jiroveci* (formerly *carinii*) pneumonia; TMP-SMX: trimethoprim-sulfamethoxazole.

9.1   Epidemiology

Adverse drug reactions are a major cause of morbidity and mortality worldwide. It has been estimated that 5–15% of patients develop adverse reactions to medications during treatment. This number increases to 30% for hospitalized patients. Of all hospital admissions, approximately 0.3% are due to adverse medication reactions. Fatal drug reactions occur in 0.1% of medical inpatients. Immunologic drug reactions account for 5–10% of all adverse drug reactions. The first step to properly diagnose and treat drug reactions is to identify correctly the different types of drug reaction that occur.

9.2   Definitions

Reactions to drugs can be divided into two main categories: predictable (type A) drug reactions and unpredictable (type B) drug reactions. Predictable drug reactions account for approximately 80% of all drug reactions and are due to the pharmacologic effects of the drug. These reactions are typically dose dependent and include reactions due to overdosage, adverse effects, secondary effects (indirect effects such as *Clostridium difficile* colitis with antibiotic use), and drug–drug interactions. A patient often claims an allergy to a drug on the basis of adverse effects, secondary effects, and drug–drug interactions; therefore, appreciating the distinction between type A and type B when obtaining a detailed history will help correctly categorize the drug reaction. Unpredictable reactions are typically dose independent and not

G.W. Volcheck, *Clinical Allergy: Diagnosis and Management*   361
DOI: 10.1007/978-1-59745-315-8_9, © 2009 Mayo Foundation for Medical
Education and Research

related to the pharmacologic action of the drug. Examples include drug intolerance, idiosyncratic reactions, and immune-mediated (including hypersensitivity) reactions. Drug intolerance is defined as an undesired effect produced at therapeutic or subtherapeutic dosages, whereas idiosyncratic reactions are uncharacteristic reactions that cannot be explained by the known pharmacologic reactions of the drug. With the Gell and Coombs classification, immune-mediated reactions can be characterized further according to mechanism: type 1, immediate hypersensitivity (IgE); type 2, cytotoxic; type 3, immune complex; type 4, cell mediated. Many immune-mediated reactions to drugs do not fall neatly into these categories, and, in a large number of immune-mediated drug reactions, the actual immune mechanism is unknown. These include the following: exanthematous (morbilliform) eruptions, fixed eruptions, erythema multiforme, Stevens–Johnson syndrome, toxic epidermal necrolysis, and hypersensitivity syndrome/drug rash with eosinophilia and systemic symptoms (DRESS) syndrome, among others. Clearly, the majority of immune-mediated drug reactions are not "allergic" (type 1) in the classic sense.

Categorizing the type of immune-mediated reaction is important for developing a management plan.

9.3   Pathophysiology and Clinical Manifestations

9.3.1   Type 1 Immediate Hypersensitivity (IgE Mediated)

Immediate hypersensitivity reactions are IgE mediated and constitute a true drug allergy. Nearly every drug has the potential of inducing an IgE-mediated hypersensitivity reaction. High-molecular-weight drugs can induce the production of IgE without being coupled to a carrier protein. High-molecular-weight drugs are more likely to provoke an allergic reaction than low-molecular-weight drugs. Often, low-molecular-weight drugs cannot induce an immune response alone but can act as haptens and combine with a carrier protein. The resultant hapten-carrier complexes are multivalent and capable of eliciting either a humoral or cellular response. The interaction of the complex with the T-cell starts the process for the subsequent production of specific IgE antibody to the drug. With further exposure, the drug binds and crosslinks IgE on mast cells, activating the mast cell. The mast cell releases several mediators, including preformed mediators (histamine, proteoglycans, proteases [tryptase]), newly synthesized prostaglandins and leukotrienes, and cytokines that are chemotactic for eosinophils and neutrophils. These mediators have many systemic effects such as smooth muscle spasm, bronchospasm, increased capillary leakage, and mucosal edema and inflammation. The clinical manifestations can involve any organ system but mainly affect the cutaneous, respiratory, gastrointestinal, and cardiovascular systems. Classic signs and symptoms include any combination of urticaria and angioedema, pruritus, dyspnea, wheezing, upper airway edema, dizziness, hypotension and shock, nausea, vomiting, crampy abdominal pain, and flushing. After a medication is administered orally, the reaction may occur within minutes, although there can be a delay of 1–2 hours before symptoms occur. With intravenous administration of the medication, the reaction often occurs almost immediately. These reactions can occur at any time in the course of treatment.

Several factors seem to affect the incidence and severity of anaphylaxis. The route of administration of the drug affects the frequency of occurrence and the severity. Events may occur if the drug is given by any route but are most frequent and severe with the intravenous route. If previous therapy was interrupted, thus creating gaps in administration, the risk of an anaphylactic reaction increases. Antibiotics are the most important class of drugs that cause anaphylactic reactions. Penicillin is the most common cause of anaphylaxis, accounting for nearly three-fourths of fatal anaphylactic cases in the United States each year. Other commonly used drugs associated with true allergic reactions include other antibiotics and proteins of high molecular weight, such as enzymes, insulin, protamine, tetanus toxoid, and heparin. Drugs that haptenize to cause an IgE-mediated reaction include muscle relaxants, antituberculous drugs, anticonvulsants, thiopental, and quinidine.

The clinical evaluation of an acute allergic reaction is usually straightforward, with the signs and symptoms compatible with histamine release involving the skin, respiratory, gastrointestinal, or cardiovascular system. Serum levels of tryptase, a neutral protease stored in mast cell granules, can help confirm mast cell activation. Tryptase levels peak approximately 90 minutes after an anaphylactic episode has started and remain increased for up to 4 hours after the reaction. Unless the patient has underlying mastocytosis, an increased tryptase level supports the occurrence of an anaphylactic event.

The two main methods for testing possible offending drugs in an IgE-mediated reaction are in vivo skin testing and in vitro testing of drug-specific IgE. These are discussed in Sect. 9.4.3 (Laboratory Testing of Suspected Drug Sensitivity).

9.3.2 Type 2 Hypersensitivity

Type 2 hypersensitivity reactions, or antibody-dependent cytotoxic hypersensitivity, involves IgG, IgM, and IgA antibodies to erythrocytes, leukocytes, and platelets. The antibodies interact with drug antigens bound to the cell membranes, for example, erythrocyte-bound penicillin or drug-modified cell surface antigens. Once the immune response has been elicited, complement is activated and cells with antigen and those without are removed or damaged by the reticuloendothelial system. Immunohemolytic anemias have been associated with penicillin, cephalosporins, quinidine, and α-methyldopa. Thrombocytopenia has been associated with quinine, quinidine, acetaminophen, sulfonamides, gold, and propylthiouracil. Granulocytopenia has been associated with phenothiazines, thiouracils, sulfonamides, and anticonvulsants. During evaluation, other possible causes of the cytopenias should be assessed. Knowledge of the drugs typically associated with this type of reaction is important. A thorough review of the medication list, including start and stop dates of the medications, is helpful.

9.3.3   Type 3 Hypersensitivity

Serum sickness is produced by circulating immune complexes of drug antigen and IgG or IgM antibodies that deposit in tissue. Tissue damage occurs when the complex activates complement. The first detailed descriptions of this type of reaction were given in the early 1900s; the reactions were observed in patients treated with horse serum that contained diphtheria antitoxin. Eight to 12 days after injection, the patients experienced a syndrome of fever, lymphadenopathy, skin eruptions, arthralgias, and proteinuria. These still constitute the symptom complex seen in serum sickness. The skin manifestations can vary, but typically they are primarily urticarial and morbilliform skin rashes, with a predilection for the sides of the hands, fingers, feet, and toes at the junction of the palmar or plantar skin with the skin of the dorsolateral surface.

Serum sickness generally begins 2–21 days (usually 7–10) after the medication has been given. The delay in symptoms corresponds to the time needed for antibody and the subsequent immune complexes to form. Decreased complement levels (C3, C4), from consumption, and abnormal urinalysis findings are useful in making the diagnosis. It is helpful to differentiate true serum sickness from serum sickness-like reactions. Serum sickness-like reactions include fever, rash, and arthralgias that occur 1–3 weeks after exposure to the drug. Lymphadenopathy and eosinophilia may also be present; however, immune complexes, decreased complement levels, and renal lesions are not seen. The medications most commonly associated with this type of reaction are penicillin, cephalosporins, sulfonamides, hydantoin, *P*-aminosalicylic acid, and streptomycin. Cefaclor in particular has been associated with a serum sickness-like syndrome. Management of serum sickness is primarily symptomatic because the reaction is usually self-limited. Nonsteroidal anti-inflammatory drugs (NSAIDs) and glucocorticoids may be helpful in controlling symptoms.

9.3.4   Type 4 Hypersensitivity

Type 4 hypersensitivity reactions, also known as delayed-type hypersensitivity reactions, are mediated by activated T-lymphocytes. Recent investigation has proposed that type 4 reactions be divided into four subtypes (4 A–D) on the basis of the cytokine release profile and effector cells activated after drug hapten and T-lymphocyte interaction. Contact dermatitis represents the most common medication-induced delayed-type hypersensitivity, although systemic reactions such as exanthematous (morbilliform) eruptions, fixed eruptions, Stevens–Johnson syndrome, toxic epidermal necrolysis, and bullous exanthema are also included.

For contact dermatitis, knowing the start date of the topical medication can be helpful. Typically, it takes 7–20 days for the initial sensitization to occur. With subsequent exposures, reactions may occur within 8–120 hours, depending on the patient's sensitivity and amount of exposure. In contact dermatitis, Langerhans' cells internalize the hapten-carrier complex and travel to the regional lymph nodes where clonal T-cell expansion occurs. The T-cells are redistributed in the skin, and once the antigen is reencountered, the T-cells are activated, resulting in cytokine release and inflammatory cell recruitment. The clinical manifestations of allergic contact dermatitis depend on the severity of the eruption, which is determined by the sensitivity of the patient, the exposure dose, and the potency of the dose. The clinical skin lesions range from mild erythema to edematous erythematous papules that become vesicular and weep. Pruritus is a hallmark of the disease and varies in intensity depending on the sensitivity. Initially, the dermatitis is limited to the skin area that has come in contact with the topical medication, but, over time, it may spread to other areas.

More than 3,000 different compounds have been implicated as causes of allergic contact dermatitis. The most common of these are topical formulations of penicillin, local anesthetics, antihistamines, and neomycin. Medical personnel and personnel in the pharmaceutical industry are at greatest risk for developing a medicinal contact dermatitis. In addition to the drug itself, preservatives and excipients can elicit contact dermatitis. Potent topical sensitizers include parabens, formaldehyde, ethylenediamine, lanolin, and thimerosal. Diagnosis is confirmed with patch testing (reviewed in Sect. 9.4.3 below).

9.3.5 Exanthematous (Morbilliform) Drug Eruptions

Exanthems, or morbilliform skin eruptions, resemble skin lesions caused by viruses and are the most common type of cutaneous drug eruption. These reactions are often confused with IgE-mediated drug allergy. This type of reaction can occur with a wide range of drugs, including, among others, penicillins, sulfonamides, phenytoin, and NSAIDs. The actual pathogenesis of these reactions is unclear, and they do not always occur with rechallenge. On the basis of the delay between exposure to the drug and the morbilliform reaction, a T-cell mediated process is likely. Penicillin- and sulfonamide-specific T-cell clones have been isolated from patients with morbilliform reactions due to these drugs.

Morbilliform reactions typically occur 4–10 days after therapy is initiated, but they can occur up to 2 weeks after therapy has ceased. The lesions begin as erythematous macules that can evolve into papules and coalesce into plaques (Fig. 9.1). The eruption usually begins on the upper trunk or neck and then spreads outward to the limbs in a bilateral and symmetric pattern. Typically, the face, palms, and soles are spared. The involved areas often develop regions of confluence and can be accompanied by pruritus and low-grade fever. True urticarial lesions usually are not present. When the patient is examined at the time of the reaction, it generally is clear whether the reaction is a morbilliform or urticarial reaction; however, if the reaction is remote, by history, it can be difficult to differentiate a morbilliform from an urticarial reaction. This differentiation is important because an urticarial reaction could be IgE mediated and a specific drug could be contraindicated, unless a desensitization procedure is performed. In contrast, a morbilliform reaction is not necessarily a strong contraindication to future treatment with the drug. The exanthem typically lasts 1–2 weeks and resolves without sequelae.

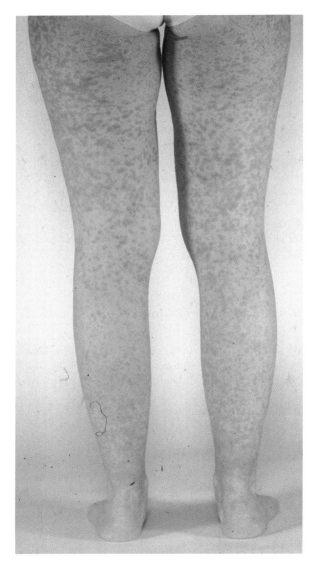

Fig. 9.1 Exanthematous, or morbilliform, drug eruption

9.3.6 Erythema Multiforme

Erythema multiforme is a hypersensitivity reaction associated with infectious agents and medications. Of all cases of erythema multiforme, 50% are thought to be drug induced. The mechanism has not been defined completely, but it is thought to be a lymphocyte cell-mediated mechanism. The development of cutaneous lesions in erythema multiforme usually begins symmetrically from the distal extremities and progresses proximally. Initially, the palms, soles, and dorsal aspects of the hands and feet are usually involved. The distinctive target lesions have a dusky center and pink-red periphery (Fig. 9.2). The size and morphology can vary; however, a single morphology is usually present in a patient. The skin manifestations typically occur 1–2 weeks after exposure to the drug. Multiple drugs have been associated with erythema multiforme. The most common ones include sulfonamides, penicillins, NSAIDs, hydantoins, phenothiazines, and barbiturates. Rechallenge with the medication usually precipitates recurrence of the erythema multiforme. The time course for erythema multiforme is typically 4 weeks if there is no progression to erythema major/Stevens–Johnson syndrome/toxic epidermal necrolysis. It is difficult to predict when and if erythema multiforme will progress to erythema major/Stevens–Johnson syndrome. The patient should be monitored carefully for progression of lesions. Treatment with systemic corticosteroids is controversial. There is no clear evidence that this treatment will prevent the progression of lesions. Also, this treatment may produce immunosuppression.

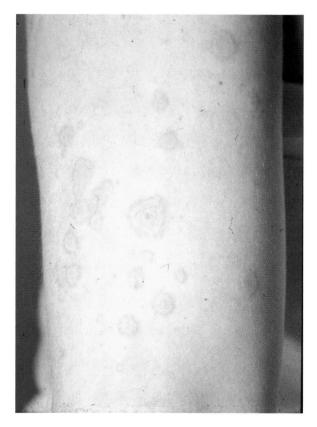

Fig. 9.2 Erythema multiforme

9.3.7 Fixed Drug Eruptions

Fixed drug eruptions appear as solitary lesions or multiple well-demarcated lesions on the skin, typically within 1–2 weeks after treatment is initiated with a new medication (Fig. 9.3). The color of the lesions, often papules or plaques, varies and includes red, red-brown, blue, and violaceous. Blisters can develop in the center of the lesions, making it difficult to distinguish between a fixed drug eruption and erythema multiforme. When the patient is rechallenged with the offending drug, the reaction occurs at the exact location previously involved. The recurrence often develops within 30 min after drug ingestion but can take up to 8 hours. After a flare-up, some patients have a refractory period of up to several months, during which time challenge with the offending drug does not activate the lesion. Lesions can occur anywhere on the body but are most common on the face, lips, hands, feet, and genitalia. Hyperpigmentation of the skin can persist for weeks to months after the eruption has resolved. The drugs that most commonly cause fixed drug reactions are sulfonamides, oral contraceptives, acetaminophen, tetracyclines, NSAIDs, barbiturates, and carbamazepine. In general, most fixed drug reactions are asymptomatic and do not require specific treatment. The mechanism of fixed drug eruptions is not known, but familial cases have been reported and genetic susceptibility may have a role.

9.3.8 Photosensitive Drug Eruptions

Photosensitive drug eruptions occur on sun-exposed skin and are classified as a phototoxic or photoallergic rash. A phototoxic drug reaction involves the absorption of ultraviolet radiation and the release of energy, damaging epithelial cells. In comparison, a photoallergic reaction occurs when ultraviolet light causes the drug to bind as a hapten to native protein on the epidermal cells, creating an antigen that

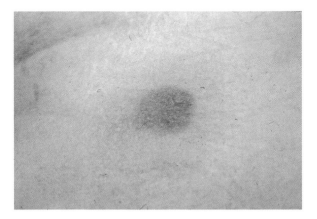

Fig. 9.3   Fixed drug eruption

sensitizes nearby lymphocytes. After cessation of treatment with the drug, reexposure to sunlight may cause recurrence of skin lesions with photoallergic reactions, but not with phototoxic reactions. Medications most frequently associated with phototoxic reactions include hydrochlorothiazide, furosemide, diltiazem, sulfonamides, psoralens, fluoroquinolones, and tetracyclines. The medications commonly associated with photoallergic reactions include dapsone, quinidine, hydrochlorothiazide, and chlorpromazine.

Phototoxic and photoallergic reactions occur most often in sun-exposed areas: the face, "V" area of the neck, dorsa of the hands, and forearms. The hair-bearing scalp, postauricular and periorbital areas, and submental portion of the chin are usually spared. Phototoxic reactions often occur within minutes or hours after exposure to light. The reaction begins with an exaggerated sunburn reaction with erythema and edema, with development of vesicles and bullae in severe reactions. The lesions can be pruritic and often heal with residual hyperpigmentation, which resolves in weeks to months. In chronic cases, lichenification can occur because of repeated rubbing and scratching of the photosensitive area. In contrast, photoallergic reactions typically develop in sensitized patients 1–2 days after exposure. The reaction usually presents as a pruritic eczematous eruption. Erythema and vesiculation are present in the acute phase. Chronic exposure results in erythema, lichenification, and scaling, but hyperpigmentation usually does not occur. The incidence of photoallergic reactions is less than that of phototoxic reactions. The amount of drug required to elicit a photoallergic reaction is less than that required for a phototoxic reaction. Distinguishing between phototoxic reactions and photoallergic reactions strictly on the basis of the physical appearance of the lesions may be difficult, but the timing of the lesions in relation to the administration of the drug can be helpful. The clinician should assess for symptoms of other diseases known to cause photosensitivity, including connective tissue diseases, primarily lupus erythematosus, which can present with only cutaneous symptoms (subacute cutaneous lupus erythematosus).

9.3.9 Erythema Multiforme Major, Stevens–Johnson Syndrome, and Toxic Epidermal Necrolysis

Erythema multiforme major, Stevens–Johnson syndrome, and toxic epidermal necrolysis are thought to be similar disorders of varying severity of erythema multiforme. Erythema multiforme major is characterized by target and bullous lesions that involve the extremities and mucous membranes. Stevens–Johnson syndrome features confluent purpuric macules on the face and trunk and severe mucosal erosions, usually at more than one mucosal site (Fig. 9.4). This appearance is accompanied by severe constitutional symptoms and high fever. There is often a prodrome of nausea, vomiting, diarrhea, malaise, headache, cough, myalgias, and arthralgias up to 14 days before the skin eruption. Toxic epidermal necrolysis is also associated with bullous lesions, mucosal involvement, and skin detachment. Toxic epidermal necrolysis and Stevens–Johnson syndrome are distinguished by the amount of skin detachment, which is less than 10% in Stevens–Johnson syndrome

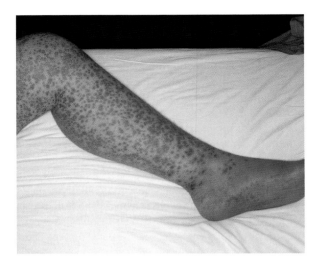

Fig. 9.4 Stevens–Johnson syndrome

and more than 30% in toxic epidermal necrolysis. Epidermal detachment between 10 and 30% is considered an overlap of the two conditions.

Drug-induced erythroderma may be confused with toxic epidermal necrolysis but is usually much less severe. Diffuse erythema with scaling and exfoliation occurs in erythroderma syndrome, but full-thickness epidermal detachment is not found. Exfoliative dermatitis can be associated with vancomycin, penicillins, and sulfonamides. Unlike toxic epidermal necrolysis, erythroderma often responds to corticosteroid treatment.

The pathophysiologic mechanism underlying Stevens–Johnson syndrome and toxic epidermal necrolysis is not known. Patients may have a genetic defect or defects in metabolic pathways that lead to the accumulation of toxic metabolites. These metabolites may have direct toxic effects or act through a hapten-mediated mechanism to activate cytotoxic T lymphocytes, with the subsequent release of inflammatory cytokines. Complications include stomatitis and mucositis, which hinder oral intake. Buccal, nasopharyngeal, pulmonary tract, esophageal, and perineal desquamation and erosion may also occur.

About 50% of cases of Stevens–Johnson syndrome and 80% of cases of toxic epidermal necrolysis are drug induced. More than 100 drugs have been associated with these two conditions. The medications with the highest relative risk are sulfonamides, β-lactam antibiotics, imidazole agents, and NSAIDs. Drugs in the moderate-risk category include quinolones, aromatic anticonvulsants, and allopurinol.

9.3.10 Anaphylactoid Drug Reactions

Anaphylactoid drug reactions are caused by the direct release of mediators from mast cells and basophils without IgE cross-linking. Clinically, the signs and symptoms resemble those of anaphylaxis, but IgE is not involved. These reactions can occur with a large number of medications and excipients, most commonly with opiates, aspirin, and radiocontrast material. Reactions may include any combination of the following: pruritus, urticaria, angioedema, bronchospasm, hypotension, syncope, nausea, emesis, and flushing. Anaphylactoid reactions may occur after first exposure to a drug. Management of these reactions is essentially the same as for anaphylaxis.

9.3.11 Hypersensitivity Syndrome/Drug Rash with Eosinophilia and Systemic Symptoms

DRESS syndrome, previously termed hypersensitivity syndrome (HSS), is a distinct drug reaction characterized by a morbilliform skin rash that may develop into exfoliative dermatitis, fever, lymph node enlargement, and differing degrees of involvement of internal organs. The more frequent and potentially serious organ involvement includes lymphadenopathy, hepatitis, nephritis, pneumonitis, and hematologic conditions. The prodrome of this syndrome includes fever, malaise, and pharyngitis, followed by skin lesions. Skin lesions range from an exanthematous eruption to erythroderma and a toxic epidermal necrolysis-like pattern. Patients often have atypical lymphocytosis and neutrophilia early in the syndrome, with eosinophilia appearing later. Symptoms usually start within 8 weeks after therapy is initiated and occur during the first prolonged course of the causative drug. The aromatic anticonvulsants (phenytoin, phenobarbital, carbamazepine) and sulfonamides are the most common causes of DRESS syndrome. Other drugs associated with this syndrome include lamotrigine, allopurinol, NSAIDs, captopril, calcium channel blockers, mexiletine, fluoxetine, dapsone, metronidazole, minocycline, and antiretroviral drugs.

Patients with DRESS syndrome are often very ill; full recovery may take months. Careful evaluation and monitoring of patients are required because new organ involvement can become manifest even after treatment with the drug has ceased.

Other systemic syndromes associated with drug hypersensitivity are systemic lupus-like syndromes and various forms of vasculitis. Hydralazine and procainamide are most commonly associated with lupus-like syndromes. The clinical symptoms resolve with discontinuation of the drug. Drug-induced vasculitis can be limited to the skin or be systemic. The skin lesions may mimic urticaria in appearance early in the course of the vasculitis. However, the lesions persist in one area for more than 48 hours and often develop a painful or burning quality. Palpable purpura can also be apparent in these conditions. Medications associated with vasculitis include amiodarone, penicillins, sulfonamides, and thiazides.

9.4   Clinical Evaluation of Suspected Drug Sensitivity

9.4.1   History

Despite the difficulties inherent in evaluating drug allergy, appropriate clinical data should be obtained to evaluate a drug reaction. Key points that should be addressed include the following:

- Complete review of all the presenting signs and symptoms
- Identification of any other causes (underlying illness) of the signs and symptoms
- List of *all* medications, with starting time, stopping time, route of administration, and dose changes
- Temporal relation between the administration of the drug and the drug reaction
- Complete history of previous drug reactions
- Knowledge about whether the medications used have been associated with similar drug reactions

The history is the primary tool in trying to discern a drug reaction. Obtaining a complete drug history can be tedious, especially for the patient who has multiple medications, but there is no substitute for the history, including a complete list of medications preceding the time of the drug reaction. A complete list can be obtained for hospitalized patients and can be confirmed with the hospital pharmacy. Obtaining a complete list for outpatients can be more difficult. It is especially important to inquire about over-the-counter medications, health supplements, or any other type of ingestant because patients often do not report these as medications. After the list is complete, the timing of the use of the medications in relation to the reaction is important, as is a history of how long the patient has been taking each medication. Often, the drug reaction is caused by the last medication added to the overall regimen. In complex situations, a flow diagram with a date and time chart of all medications can help delineate the relation between the medications and the reaction. A reaction can be immediate or delayed depending on the mechanism. For example, a type 1, IgE-mediated reaction is immediate as compared with a serum sickness-like reaction that can occur 3 weeks after drug administration. A history of a previous drug reaction, regardless of how remote or seemingly unrelated, can be helpful because different medications in the same drug class can be associated with the same drug reaction. Because the patient may have only limited or erroneous knowledge of the specific past reaction, a thorough review of the medical record can yield more information. A detailed history of the actual reaction is important to help ensure that a systemic reaction (as opposed to a skin-only reaction) is not overlooked. Alternative causes, such as infection or concomitant underlying illness, should be excluded. Knowledge of the classes of drugs most likely associated with the type of reaction can help narrow the list.

9.4.2 Physical Examination

A complete physical examination is helpful in categorizing the drug reaction because multiple organ systems potentially can be involved. The skin is the organ system most often involved, and a detailed description of the skin findings aids in diagnosis. The most frequent skin finding is an exanthematous or morbilliform eruption. This maculopapular eruption can be difficult to differentiate from a viral exanthem and consists of red or pink macules and papules distributed in a symmetric pattern throughout the body, often sparing the face. This eruption tends to be mildly pruritic. Urticaria, in contrast, is manifested by pruritic red wheals that vary in size from small papules to large plaques. These wheals can be associated with angioedema and swelling of the deep dermal and subcutaneous tissues. Erythema multiforme is a distinctive exanthem characterized by a "target" lesion that consists of a central clearing and erythematous outer ring. This lesion can progress to erythema multiforme major, with the development of blisters and involvement of mucous membranes; therefore, an examination of the mouth and throat is required for these patients. Further along this spectrum is toxic epidermal necrolysis, in which the death of epidermal cells results in sloughing of the skin and the appearance of "scalded" skin.

Localized skin changes can help determine the causative drug. Phototoxic and photoallergic reactions produce erythema and eczematous changes localized to or significantly more prominent in sun-exposed areas. Localized, well-demarcated plaques and papules in only one area of the body can represent a fixed drug eruption. This can be confirmed with recurrence of the rash in exactly the same location with subsequent administration of the offending drug. Topical medications that cause contact dermatitis leave a characteristic rash of raised erythema, papules, and vesicles over the area of application.

In addition to a detailed skin examination, a complete physical examination can provide more clues. Vital signs should be monitored. Tachycardia, tachypnea, and hypotension can occur with an anaphylactic or anaphylactoid reaction. Fever, alone or in combination with other signs and symptoms, can occur with a systemic drug reaction. Other critical components of the physical examination include assessments of the lymph nodes, lungs, liver, spleen, and joints. These examinations are critical in determining the extent, severity, and type of the drug reaction.

9.4.3 Laboratory Testing of Suspected Drug Sensitivity

There is no set battery of tests for the evaluation of all drug reactions. The selection of laboratory tests used must take into account the mechanism of the type of drug reaction suspected. Currently, the number of readily available tests specific for drug allergy is small.

9.4.3.1 Skin and In Vitro IgE-Specific Testing

The two main methods for testing for immediate IgE-mediated drug allergy are (1) in vivo skin testing and (2) in vitro testing of drug-specific IgE. It needs to be remembered that these test only for IgE-mediated sensitivity. A negative skin test does not have any meaning for type 2–4 reactions, exanthematous, morbilliform, erythema multiforme, photosensitive, fixed, Stevens–Johnson syndrome, toxic epidermal necrolysis, anaphylactoid, or DRESS syndrome reactions. When carefully performed, skin testing is safe. For penicillin, reactions to properly performed skin tests are rare, occurring in less than 1%. The reactions that occur are mild.

In prick testing, a small amount of the test solution containing a concentration of the suspected medication is placed on the skin. A sterile needle or standard skin prick test lancet is then placed through the test solution into the epidermis. The area is evaluated after 15 min for a wheal and flare reaction. If negative, an intradermal test can be performed. After intradermal placement of the test solution, the area is evaluated after 15 min, with measurement of the wheal and flare response. Prick and intradermal skin testing can be performed to test for β-lactam antimicrobial agents, latex, local anesthetics, ciprofloxacin, trimethoprim, cisplatin, neuromuscular blocking agents, thiobarbiturates, and some anticonvulsants. However, standardized skin testing has been established only for penicillin. Sensitivity and specificity and, thus, positive and negative predictive values have not been established for the other drugs.

During penicillin degradation, several metabolites are formed that potentially can cause an IgE-mediated reaction. Mainly, it is degraded to the "major" determinant, the benzylpenicilloyl determinant. The major determinant mix is available commercially as Pre-Pen. This detects approximately 80% of the patients allergic to penicillin. The other breakdown products that can cause an allergic reaction are termed the "minor" determinants. The original minor determinant mixture consisted of benzyl penicilloate and benzyl penilloate. The minor determinant mix is not available commercially in the United States. When the minor determinant mix is synthesized and used according to published protocols, patients with negative skin tests to both the major and minor determinants can receive penicillin safely. In addition, benzylpenicillin (penicillin G) has been used as a minor determinant, but it is not clear if it is as accurate as the benzyl penicilloate and penilloate mix. To achieve maximal predictive accuracy for penicillin allergy, both the major and minor determinants should be used in skin testing. For patients with a history of penicillin allergy and negative skin tests to the major and minor determinants, even though adverse reactions have occurred with administration of the drug, the incidence of IgE-mediated reactions is the same as for those with no history of previous penicillin allergy. Negative skin testing to the major and minor determinants generally allows for safe administration of penicillin to a patient with a history of suspected IgE-mediated penicillin allergy. This has been studied extensively for penicillin but not for the other drugs listed above. For other drugs, a positive skin test, in the absence of an irritant reaction, generally confirms an IgE-mediated sensitivity, although a negative test does not rule out drug allergy.

In vitro testing of allergen-specific IgE antibodies is performed most often by measuring circulating IgE antibodies with a solid phase radioimmunoassay, a RAST assay. The application of this assay is limited by insufficient knowledge of the relevant drug metabolites in the allergic drug reactions. Assays have been developed to measure IgE antibodies to the major determinant of penicillin but not to the minor determinants. Only a small number of reliable drug RAST tests are available commercially.

Other measures of a type 1 response have been used primarily in research settings. These include in vitro measurement of leukotriene synthesis, basophil activation, and basophil histamine release. Currently, their sensitivity and specificity are not well delineated, but they hold promise as a possible way in the future to assess a type 1 hypersensitivity response.

9.4.3.2   Commonly Used Tests in Drug Reaction

Because drug-specific tests are generally limited, the majority of laboratory tests performed to evaluate a drug reaction are used to categorize the type and extent of the reaction.

Tryptase is a mast cell mediator released approximately 1–2 hours after an anaphylactic reaction. An increased level is helpful in implicating a mast cell-mediated process. The tryptase level is elevated in anaphylactic and anaphylactoid reactions. A normal tryptase level in the acute setting makes a mast cell-mediated process unlikely.

The Coomb's test is a useful screening procedure for drug-induced hemolysis. If it is positive, additional testing can be performed with drug-specific antibodies, if available. A complete blood count with a differential count is helpful in outlining the cytopenias that occur with a type 2 reaction and for the presence of eosinophilia seen with several drug reactions, primarily DRESS syndrome. Complement levels, particularly C3 and C4 levels, are depressed in a true serum sickness reaction (type 3) but are normal in a serum sickness-like reaction. Liver enzymes, creatinine level, and urinalysis help define the extent of DRESS syndrome and should be determined or performed for any drug reaction with systemic symptoms.

For type 4 reactions, patch testing can confirm the diagnosis of contact dermatitis. Patch testing can be performed open or closed. During an open patch test, the suspected allergen is applied to the skin and left uncovered. The application is repeated twice daily for 2 weeks and then read. With closed patch testing, the material is applied to the skin and covered with an adhesive, which is removed in 48 hours for the initial interpretation. Additional readings are performed at 72 and 96 hours.

For other suspected type 4 reactions (exanthematous [morbilliform], erythema multiforme, and fixed), studies have been conducted with patch testing and delayed reading (>48 hours) of intradermal skin tests. Overall, patch testing has a good positive predictive value for delayed cutaneous reactions to drugs. Nevertheless, a negative result is difficult to interpret. Generally, the use of a drug that produces a positive result on a patch test or delayed intradermal skin test should be avoided when possible. It is important to note that this type of drug testing is not widely available in the United States and the majority of the studies using these tests are being performed in Europe.

9.5   Therapy and Management

After a drug reaction has been characterized, specific treatment can be instituted. In addition to immediate clinical management of the reaction, other issues that need to be addressed include the type of drugs that can be substituted for the medication that caused the reaction and consideration for future use of the medication. The general rule is that the offending medication should always be discontinued immediately. A possible exception to this is a mild morbilliform reaction. The identification and future management of the most common drug reactions are outlined in Table 9.1.

Table 9.1 Identification and future management of the most common drug reactions

Reaction type	Clinical characteristics	Laboratory testing	Future use of medication
Gell and Coombs			
Type 1	Urticaria, angioedema, wheezing, hypotension, nausea, vomiting, abdominal pain, diarrhea	Skin testing, radioallergosorbent testing, tryptase	Desensitization
Type 2	Hemolytic anemia, granulocytopenia, thrombocytopenia	Complete blood count, direct/indirect Coombs' test	Contraindicated
Type 3	Fever, urticaria, arthralgias, lymphadenopathy 2–21 days after therapy initiated	Complement levels, erythrocyte sedimentation rate, C-reactive protein	Contraindicated
Type 4	Skin erythema, skin blistering	Patch testing	Likely contraindicated
Morbilliform	Maculopapular rash becoming confluent	Possibly patch testing, intradermal skin testing (delayed reaction)	Use with caution
Erythema multiforme	Distinctive target lesions	None	Contraindicated
Stevens–Johnson/TEN	Target lesions, mucous membrane involvement, skin desquamation	None	Contraindicated
Anaphylactoid	Urticaria, wheezing, angioedema, hypotension	Tryptase	Pretreatment with prednisone and diphenhydramine for radiocontrast sensitivity
HSS/DRESS	Exfoliative dermatitis, fever, lymphadenopathy	Complete blood count, liver enzymes, creatinine, urinalysis	Contraindicated

From Volcheck, G. W. (2004) Clinical evaluation and management of drug hypersensitivity. Immunol. Allergy Clin. North Am. 24, 357–371. Used with permission

HSS/DRESS hypersensitivity syndrome/drug rash with eosinophilia and systemic symptoms; *TEN* toxic epidermal necrolysis

9.5.1 Type 1 Reactions

The treatment for a type 1 reaction is determined by the severity of the reaction. For mild urticaria, H_1 blockers are usually effective. The primary concern is anaphylaxis. The initial steps in the management of drug-induced anaphylaxis are the same as for anaphylaxis of any cause: control of the airway, breathing, and circulation. The most critical medication is epinephrine. For children or adults, intramuscular epinephrine can be used. Intramuscular administration is preferred to subcutaneous administration.

The intramuscular dosage for adults is 0.2–0.5 mL (0.3–0.5 mg) of 1:1,000 epinephrine. For children, the dose is 0.01 mg kg^{-1} (maximum, 0.5 mL [0.5 mg] per dose). If the patient's condition worsens despite repeated doses of intramuscular epinephrine, intravenous epinephrine could be given. This dose is initially titrated at 1 µg min^{-1}, which can be increased to 2–10 µg min^{-1} as needed. Of course, this would be done in conjunction with the administration of oxygen and intravenous fluid resuscitation and vasopressors, depending on the clinical scenario. Histamine receptor antagonist therapy can be used with epinephrine. In adults, diphenhydramine may be given intramuscularly or intravenously at a dose of 25–50 mg. Diphenhydramine can be administered orally, intramuscularly, or intravenously to children at a dose of 1–2 mg kg^{-1}. The role of corticosteroids in the initial management of the acute event is unclear; however, because of a possible late-phase reaction, corticosteroids may help from a preventive standpoint, although studies in this area have not been performed. After stabilization, patients with mild symptoms should be observed for at least 2 hours and those with severe anaphylaxis for 24 hours. The management of type 1 (IgE-mediated) drug allergy is summarized in Table 9.2.

For type 1 reactions (IgE-mediated), the therapeutic indication for a drug often persists despite the need for withdrawal of the medication. Structurally unrelated drugs are the preferred substitute. Closely related β-lactams and carbapenems should not be administered to patients allergic to penicillin. Patients with positive skin tests to penicillin have an estimated 4–8% risk of having a reaction to cephalosporins. First- and second-generation cephalosporins are more likely than third-generation cephalosporins to cause allergic reactions in penicillin-sensitive patients. For patients in whom skin testing is not available and who describe a remote, nonanaphylactic reaction to penicillin, the chance of a reaction to a cephalosporin is approximately 1%. Monobactams, such as aztreonam, generally do not cross-react with the penicillins, but cross-reactivity has been shown between ceftazidime and aztreonam.

Table 9.2 Management of type 1 (IgE-mediated) drug allergy

Mild (hives only)
  Discontinue medication
  H$_1$ blocker
  Observe for systemic symptoms

Moderate–severe (systemic symptoms)
  Airway, breathing, circulation
  Supplemental oxygen
  IV access, fluids
  Epinephrine
    Children 0.01 mg kg^{-1} (maximum, 0.5 mL [0.5 mg] IM)
    Adults 0.3–0.5 mL (0.3–0.5 mg) 1:1,000 IM

H$_1$ blocker: diphenhydramine
    Children 1–2 mg kg^{-1} IM
    Adults 50 mg IM

IM intramuscular; *IV* intravenous

If a clinical situation arises in which the drug must be used, a desensitization procedure can be performed. This procedure induces tolerance by the induction of a desensitized state in IgE-primed cells by low-dose antigen. Desensitization is performed by cautious incremental increases in drug dosage according to a protocol. Extremely dilute solutions (such as 1,000- to 10,000-fold dilution) are administered initially, with incremental increases every 15–30 minutes. An example of intravenous desensitization for β-lactam antibiotics is outlined in Table 9.3. After desensitization, the drug must be administered continuously until the required dose is completed. The desensitization procedure does not result in long-term desensitization. When treatment with the drug stops, sensitization can recur. If the medication is required again in the future and has not been given continuously, the patient should be desensitized again. Desensitization is recommended only for type 1 reactions. It is not recommended for reaction types 2–4, erythema multiforme, Stevens–Johnson syndrome, toxic epidermal necrolysis, or DRESS syndrome.

9.5.2   Types 2, 3, and 4 Reactions

Type 2, cytotoxic, reactions usually require only discontinuation of the offending drug. Corticosteroids may help with recovery, and transfusions may be required in

Table 9.3   Protocol for intravenous desensitization with β-lactam antibiotics

β-Lactam concentration, mg mL^{-1}	Penicillin G concentration, U mL^{-1}	Dose no[a]	Amount given, mL	Dose given, mg U^{-1}
0.1	160	1	0.10	0.01/16
		2	0.20	0.02/32
		3	0.40	0.04/64
		4	0.80	0.08/128
1	1,600	5	0.15	0.15/240
		6	0.30	0.30/480
		7	0.60	0.60/960
		8	1.00	1.0/1,600
10	16,000	9	0.20	2.0/3,200
		10	0.40	4.0/6,400
		11	0.80	8.0/12,800
100	160,000	12	0.15	15.0/24,000
		13	0.30	30.0/48,000
		14	0.60	60.0/96,000
		15	1.00	100.0/160,000
1,000	1,600,000	16	0.20	200.0/320,000
		17	0.40	400.0/640,000
		18	0.80	800.0/1,280,000

Observe patient for 30 min; administer full therapeutic dose intravenously

From Ditto, A. M., Greenberger, P. A., and Grammer, L. C. (2002) Drug allergy. In: L. C. Grammer and P. A. Greenberger, (Eds.), Patterson's Allergic Diseases, 6th ed. Philadelphia: Lippincott, Williams & Wilkins. pp. 295–386. Used with permission

[a]Dose approximately doubled every 15 min

severe cases. Completely different classes of medications should be used in substitution. Medications that cause this reaction generally are contraindicated for life.

Type 3, antigen–antibody, reactions usually respond to discontinuation of the offending medication. Symptomatic treatment with NSAIDs and corticosteroids can be used as necessary. Different classes of medications should be used in substitution.

Type 4, delayed hypersensitivity, reactions usually respond to removal of the contactant agent. Topical corticosteroids and H$_1$ blockers provide relief from symptoms. Systemic corticosteroids can be considered in cases of severe dermatitis.

For these aforementioned reactions, future use of the drug is contraindicated. In addition to avoiding the offending drug, one must make the patient and other physicians aware of the avoidance of medicines in the same class.

9.5.3 Morbilliform Reaction

The usual recommendation is that the offending drug be stopped at the time of the morbilliform reaction to help prevent the skin manifestations from progressing to a generalized erythroderma or exfoliative dermatitis. The reaction typically subsides without any significant sequelae. The primary difficulty occurs when the history of the reaction is remote. In these situations, it is difficult to differentiate a morbilliform reaction from an urticarial one that could be IgE mediated or another immunologic response. A true morbilliform reaction is not a strong contraindication to future use of the drug. It has been estimated that the chance of recurrence of the same reaction with future use is approximately 50%. The preference would be to use another medication if the option is available.

9.5.4 Erythema Multiforme

Management of erythema multiforme includes stopping the offending medication and ruling out infectious causes such as herpes simplex virus or *Mycoplasma pneumoniae* infection. It is difficult to predict when and if erythema multiforme will progress to erythema major/Stevens–Johnson syndrome. The patient should be observed closely for progression of lesions. The use of systemic corticosteroids is controversial. There is no clear evidence that such treatment will prevent progression of the lesions, and corticosteroids may immunosuppress the patient.

9.5.5 Erythema Multiforme Major, Stevens–Johnson Syndrome, Toxic Epidermal Necrolysis

The treatment of Stevens–Johnson syndrome is controversial. In some studies, the use of corticosteroids has been associated with delayed recovery, but in other studies, these agents have been of benefit. Otherwise, management is aimed at symptom relief. Pruritus can be treated with H_1 blockers, and cutaneous blisters can be treated with cool, wet Burow's solution compresses. Papules and plaques can be treated with topical corticosteroids, which should not be applied to eroded areas. Ocular involvement should be monitored by an ophthalmologist.

In contrast, most authorities recommend that corticosteroids not be used in the management of toxic epidermal necrolysis. Because the pathology of this condition is similar to that of burn injury, treatment is best provided in a multidisciplinary burn center. Intensive treatment includes temporary skin substitutes, fluid and electrolyte monitoring, internal alimentation, infection control, and pain management. In small studies, cyclophosphamide, cyclosporine, plasma exchange, and plasmapheresis have improved symptoms. Recently, intravenous immunoglobulin has been shown to produce marked clinical improvement in toxic epidermal necrolysis by inhibiting Fas-mediated keratinocyte cell death by blocking the Fas receptor.

9.5.6 Hypersensitivity Syndrome/Drug Rash with Eosinophilia and Systemic Symptoms Syndrome

The treatment of DRESS syndrome is similar to that of other severe drug reactions and consists initially of rapid removal of the offending drug. Supportive treatment includes volume replacement, nutritional support, antibiotics, and extensive skin care. The role of corticosteroid is controversial. In case reports, corticosteroids have been associated with improvement in symptoms and eosinophilia, with relapses occurring after tapering or withdrawal of the corticosteroids. Although several investigators have suggested that corticosteroids be used when internal organs are involved by the disease, the use of corticosteroid treatment cannot be recommended automatically without randomized controlled trials to support their benefit. Part of the reason for this caution is the clinically similar presentation of toxic epidermal necrolysis, for which corticosteroid treatment has shown either no benefit or increased morbidity or mortality.

9.6   Special Medication Reactions

9.6.1 Radiocontrast Media Reactions

Radiocontrast media reactions occur in approximately 5–10% of patients. There is a wide variety of reactions, ranging from mild vasomotor symptoms to severe anaphylactoid reactions. The majority of reactions are vasomotor symptoms of nausea, vomiting, flushing, or warmth. The anaphylactoid reactions range from mild to severe and consist of any combination of urticaria, angioedema, wheezing, dyspnea, nausea, vomiting, hypotension, and death. The majority of anaphylactoid reactions occur within 30 min after administration of the contrast material, with a severe reaction usually occurring within 5 min after administration. Risk factors for a reaction to contrast material include asthma or other atopic and allergic disease. Patients with a previous history of anaphylactoid reaction to contrast material have approximately a 33% (range, 17–60%) chance of having a reaction with readministration of the contrast material. The incidence of reactions decreases significantly when nonionic or low-molecular-weight radiocontrast material is used instead of high-molecular-weight material.

The cause of reactions to radiocontrast material appears to be secondary to non-IgE-mediated release of mediators from mast cells. Despite single case reports, allergy to shellfish is not associated with radiocontrast sensitivity. There is no specific test that can be performed to determine radiocontrast sensitivity.

Pretreatment strategies have been successful in decreasing the incidence of radiocontrast reactions among patients with a history of previous radiocontrast reactions. The most commonly used pretreatment regimen consists of oral prednisone (50 mg) given 13, 7, and 1 hour before the procedure and diphenhydramine (50 mg) given 1 hour before the procedure. This combination reduced reaction rates to 9% with use of high-molecular-weight contrast material. Almost all the reactions in the pretreated patients were mild. Another regimen using prednisone and diphenhydramine, as above, with ephedrine (25 mg) 1 hour before the procedure decreased the reaction rate to 3% among previous reactors. With use of low-molecular-weight radiocontrast material in addition to the pretreatment regimen, the rates of reaction among previous reactors decreased to less than 1%. The addition of H_2 blockers has been postulated to give further protection, but they appear to provide only marginal benefit.

Overall, pretreatment of patients with previous radiocontrast reactions who require radiocontrast materials consists of the following:

1. Use of nonionic or low-molecular-weight contrast material
2. Prednisone, 50 mg orally, 13, 7, and 1 hour before the procedure
3. Diphenhydramine, 50 mg orally or intramuscularly, 1 hour before the procedure
4. Ephedrine sulfate, 25 mg orally, 1 hour before the procedure; however, if the risk with the use of this medication is significant (e.g., underlying heart disease, hypertension), it can be withheld

9.6.2 Sulfa Reactions

Sulfonamides have the potential to elicit many types of adverse drug reactions. These reactions include the entire spectrum of IgE-mediated allergic reactions, including anaphylaxis, and non-IgE-mediated reactions, including morbilliform skin exanthems, serum sickness-like reactions, Stevens–Johnson syndrome, toxic epidermal necrolysis, and a special subset of primarily skin hypersensitivity reactions in patients with human immunodeficiency virus (HIV) infection.

Among the antibiotics, hypersensitivity reactions involving the penicillins and sulfonamides have been studied extensively. For the penicillins, production of the major and minor determinants has resulted in diagnostic skin testing reagents with excellent sensitivities, but the sulfonamides are not understood completely. Although IgE-mediated reactions to sulfonamides occur, other mechanisms appear responsible for the majority of hypersensitivity reactions. This may be due to sulfonamide intermediate products being directly toxic to lymphocytes and other immune cells or to activation of the immune system from an underlying infection that results in an immune response to normally tolerated intermediate products.

The most common reaction of sulfonamide hypersensitivity is a generalized maculopapular rash that develops 7–14 days after initiation of therapy. This is usually accompanied by fever and toxicity of one or more internal organs, which may be asymptomatic. Urticaria can sometimes be seen with this. This reaction typically resolves 7–14 days after discontinuation of the medication.

The other reactions are rare in non-HIV patients. Anaphylaxis is much less frequent than the aforementioned hypersensitivity reaction. Toxic epidermal necrolysis and Stevens–Johnson syndrome occur very rarely, although they account for the largest percentage of antibiotic-induced cases of these entities.

No standard in vivo or in vitro tests are available to assess for sulfonamide hypersensitivity reaction or anaphylaxis. There is some evidence that the primary IgE sensitivity is to the N4-sulfonamidoyl metabolite, but additional studies are needed because there are likely multiple haptens. Most sulfonamide reactions do not appear to be IgE mediated. Hydroxylamine metabolites have a toxic effect on lymphocytes. The lymphocyte toxicity assay involves incubating the drug with lymphocytes from the patient. In preliminary research studies of patients with sulfonamide hypersensitivity, the sensitivity and specificity of the assay were relatively high, but the negative predictive value was low. Further validation studies and improvements in the negative predictive value are still required.

Another area of clinical interest is the question of cross-reactivity between sulfonamide antibiotics with sulfonamide nonantibiotics such as diuretics, sulfonylureas, and cyclooxygenase (COX)-2 inhibitors. The N4 arylamine group is unique to sulfonamide antibiotics and is not present on sulfonamide nonantibiotics. Because the N4 arylamine group is implicated in the hypersensitivity reaction, the absence in the nonantibiotics should result in less cross-reactivity. The case reports and small studies that have addressed this topic support the notion of little or no cross-reactivity between sulfonamide antibiotics and sulfonamide nonantibiotics. In a large epidemiologic study of more than 20,000 patients, it was noted that patients with a history of penicillin reaction were more likely to react to sulfonamide nonantibiotics than patients with a history of sensitivity to sulfonamide antibiotics. The conclusion was that sulfonamide cross-reactivity is unlikely but that certain patients may have a predisposition to reactions to multiple drugs.

9.6.3 Sulfonamide and HIV

Sulfonamide antibiotics are extremely important in the HIV population because trimethoprim-sulfamethoxazole (TMP-SMX) is the antibiotic of choice for *Pneumocystis jiroveci* (formerly *carinii*) pneumonia (PCP) treatment, PCP prophylaxis, and toxoplasmosis prophylaxis. However, approximately 60% of HIV-infected patients experience TMP-SMX sensitivity during treatment. The typical TMP-SMX-induced reaction in HIV-positive patients consists of a generalized maculopapular eruption without systemic symptoms. The underlying mechanism responsible for these reactions is unknown but is not due to drug-specific IgE or IgG antibodies. Because alternative drugs for these indications pose significant risks, are more expensive, and can be difficult to administer, cautious readministration becomes an important consideration. For patients with a mild hypersensitivity reaction, desensitization has been shown to be effective, despite the mechanism of the reaction not being IgE mediated. However, for patients with severe anaphylaxis, Stevens–Johnson syndrome, or toxic epidermal necrolysis, desensitization is not an option.

Multiple protocols have been published outlining successful desensitization and continued administration of TMP-SMX to HIV patients with a history of sulfonamide sensitivity. Although most sulfa-sensitive HIV patients have been able to receive the drug safely, desensitization should be undertaken very cautiously. The protocols vary in time from desensitization in 7 hours to as long as 10 days. The longer protocols are generally favored to allow time for a delayed reaction to be recognized. Some investigators have reported that it is safe for patients with a history of a mild reaction (mild maculopapular rash only) to administer the slow protocol at home as long as safeguards are taken, including immediate access to a health facility and an understanding of the signs of a serious reaction.

TMP-SMX desensitization in non-HIV-infected patients has not been well studied; therefore, the safety of desensitization in these patients is not well known and likely requires more intensive monitoring (i.e., a hospital setting).

9.6.4 Aspirin and NSAIDs

Aspirin, the first NSAID, has been in use for more than 100 years. Within the past 30 years, several NSAIDs have been developed. Both aspirin and NSAID are generally well tolerated, but, because of the inhibition of COX-1, gastritis and peptic ulcer disease are common adverse effects. Other rare adverse effects associated with aspirin and NSAIDs include hepatitis, erythema multiforme, anemia, hepatotoxicity, interstitial nephritis, toxic epidermal necrolysis, and Stevens–Johnson syndrome. More common and challenging to the physician are the spectrum of allergic, pseudoallergic, and respiratory reactions associated with aspirin and NSAIDs. These reactions can be classified into the following groups:

1. NSAID-exacerbated asthma and rhinitis, or aspirin-exacerbated respiratory disease (AERD)
2. NSAID-exacerbated urticaria or angioedema
3. Single NSAID-induced urticaria or angioedema
4. Multiple NSAID-induced urticaria or angioedema
5. Single NSAID-induced anaphylaxis

9.6.4.1 NSAID-Exacerbated Asthma and Rhinitis, or Aspirin-Exacerbated Respiratory Disease

NSAID-induced asthma and rhinitis has also been termed aspirin-exacerbated respiratory disease (AERD). This term describes patients with underlying asthma or rhinitis who develop upper or lower respiratory tract symptoms, including rhinorrhea, nasal congestion, laryngospasm, and bronchospasm, with ingestion of aspirin or NSAIDs. These reactions tend to be dose dependent and to apply to aspirin and all NSAIDs. On the basis of history alone, approximately 3–5% of patients with asthma describe NSAID-induced asthma and rhinitis. When prospectively challenged with aspirin, a respiratory reaction occurs in 10–15% of asthma patients. In asthma patients with nasal polyps, approximately 40% develop respiratory symptoms with ingestion of aspirin or NSAIDs. For these patients, the avoidance of aspirin or NSAIDS does not change the course of their underlying respiratory inflammation, which progresses over time. This type of reaction is not IgE mediated. It is thought to be due to enhanced release of leukotrienes or greater end-target organ sensitivity to leukotrienes.

There are no skin or in vitro tests to measure aspirin or NSAID sensitivity. The only way to make the diagnosis definitively is through provocative challenge testing. In the United States, only oral provocative challenges are available. At the Scripps Clinic, the aspirin oral challenges are conducted over 3 days. The basic protocol is outlined in Table 9.4. The first day consists of placebo at 8 AM, 11 AM, and 2 PM. On day 2, the patient starts with 30 mg at 8 AM. Reactions to this dose are rare. Depending on the history, the patient may be advanced 15–30 mg at 3-hours intervals for a total of three doses during the day. The study continues on the third day, with greater escalation of the dose once 150 mg is tolerated. Most reactions occur between 45–100 mg. If the patient's FEV_1 decreases more than 15%, the challenge is stopped for the day and resumed the following day at the same dose if the goal is to desensitize the patient.

Table 9.4 Three-day oral aspirin (ASA) challenge/desensitization in aspirin-exacerbated respiratory disease[a]

Time	Day 1	Day 2	Day 3
8:00 AM	Placebo	ASA 30 mg	ASA 100–150 mg
11:00 AM	Placebo	ASA 45–60 mg	ASA 150–325 mg
2:00 PM	Placebo	ASA 75–100 mg	ASA 325–650 mg

FEV_1 forced expiratory volume in 1 min

[a]FEV_1 is measured before each dose; FEV_1 at baseline needs to be >70% predicted to proceed with challenge

Treatment of these patients with aspirin (650 mg daily or twice daily) after the challenge has been associated with reductions in clinical markers for respiratory disease and a decrease in subsequent sinus surgery and in the use of inhaled nasal and systemic corticosteroids. In one large study, 67% of patients followed for 6 years, including those who discontinued the aspirin because of side effects or other reasons, showed improvement.

9.6.4.2 NSAID-Exacerbated Urticaria or Angioedema

This type of reaction occurs in patients with a history of underlying chronic urticaria who develop an exacerbation of urticaria with or without angioedema after ingestion of aspirin or NSAIDs. This occurs in approximately 20–30% of people with chronic urticaria. The cause is thought to be due to the inhibition of COX-1. This type of reaction is not IgE mediated. No in vitro testing is available for this reaction. Avoidance of aspirin and NSAIDs may help eliminate acute flares of urticaria; however, the course of the chronic disease is unchanged. In a small group of patients who underwent aspirin challenge and desensitization, the underlying chronic urticaria worsened, unlike those with AERD. Therefore, long-term aspirin treatment does not appear to be an option for patients with NSAID-exacerbated urticaria or angioedema.

9.6.4.3 Single NSAID-Induced Urticaria or Angioedema

Ingestion of aspirin or NSAIDs can induce urticaria or angioedema in a patient who has no risk factors. These patients commonly have this reaction to only one NSAID and tolerate the others without difficulty. The likely mechanism is IgE mediated. There is no reliable skin or in vitro testing for NSAIDs. Although challenge can be done to prove the sensitivity, this poses significant risk. Use of an alternative NSAID is more practical.

9.6.4.4 Multiple NSAID-Induced Urticaria or Angioedema

This is a rare occurrence in which a patient without underlying risk factors develops urticaria or angioedema after ingestion of more than one NSAID. The mechanism is thought to be due to COX-1 inhibition. Some of these patients later develop chronic urticaria. There are no data about desensitization in these individuals. COX-2 inhibitors can be considered in this group.

9.6.4.5 Single NSAID-Induced Anaphylaxis

Similar to single NSAID-induced urticaria or angioedema, these patients react to a single NSAID. It is not clear if this is an IgE-mediated or anaphylactoid response. These patients usually can be given alternative NSAIDs without a reaction being elicited.

9.6.5   Intraoperative Anaphylaxis

The true incidence of intraoperative anaphylaxis is poorly defined because of
difficulty with reporting accuracy. The majority of the data are from France,
Australia, Norway, and New Zealand. The range of the incidence of intraoperative
anaphylaxis is 1:900–1:20,000 procedures, with 1:5,000 being quoted most often.
Neuromuscular blocking agents are the most common cause of intraoperative
anaphylaxis and account for approximately two-thirds of the episodes. The majority
of the rest of the episodes are caused by antibiotics and latex. Other less common
(<10%) causes include induction agents, narcotics, colloids, blood products, protamine,
and mannitol. Women are at highest risk for intraoperative anaphylaxis, typically
accounting for 65–70% of cases of intraoperative anaphylaxis. Atopic disease such
as allergic rhinitis or asthma does not appear to predispose patients to intraoperative
anaphylaxis, although patients with atopic disease are at higher risk for the development of latex sensitivity.

The neuromuscular blocking agents may induce IgE-mediated or non-IgE-
mediated mast cell activation. The tertiary and quaternary ammonium groups of the
neuromuscular blocking agents are considered to be the antigenic sites for IgE. The
ammonium groups are also present in cosmetics, disinfectants, and foods, explaining a possible source of sensitization in first-time anesthesia recipients and the pre-
ponderance of intraoperative anaphylaxis among females. Skin testing can be
performed to neuromuscular blocking agents to identify the source of intraoperative
anaphylaxis. There is approximately 70% cross-reactivity among neuromuscular
blocking agents with skin testing. Patients with a history of intraoperative anaphylaxis and a positive skin test to a neuromuscular blocking agent have been anesthe-
tized successfully with the use of a skin test-negative neuromuscular blocking
agent. In a French study of 518 patients with an identifiable cause of intraoperative
anaphylaxis, rocuronium and succinylcholine were the most common triggers.
Atracurium and vecuronium also were frequently involved; reactions to pancuronium, mivacurium, cisatracurium, and gallamine were less common. When examined with respect to clinical usage of the various neuromuscular blocking agents,
succinylcholine and rocuronium accounted for more than 65% of the reactions but
less than 16% of the market share usage of the neuromuscular blocking agents in
France. No comparable studies are available in North America.

The majority of intraoperative anaphylaxis episodes occur during induction,
when neuromuscular blockers, sedatives, and opiates are administered. Latex reactions often exhibit a delay, occurring during maintenance anesthesia, approximately
60 min after induction. Antibiotics usually cause a reaction within minutes after
infusion. Intraoperative anaphylaxis due to antibiotics has increased eightfold over
the last 15 years. The β-lactam antibiotics, penicillins and cephalosporins, are
involved most commonly. Treatment of intraoperative anaphylaxis is the same as
for anaphylaxis of any cause.

The patients most important to evaluate preoperatively are those with a history
of intraoperative anaphylaxis. A thorough review of the previous reaction, including the type of reaction, the time course of the reaction, and the medications

(preoperative, intraoperative, and postoperative), may provide a clue to the causative agent. Allergy testing to the previous medications and the medications planned for subsequent use helps guide management.

9.6.6 Vaccine Allergy

Allergic, IgE-mediated reactions to vaccines are rare. An allergic reaction to a vaccine consists of the same signs and symptoms as seen in allergic reactions to foods and other medications. These reactions include any combination of pruritus, urticaria, angioedema, dyspnea, wheeze, rhinitis, nausea, vomiting, diarrhea, hypotension, and tachycardia. The signs and symptoms generally develop within 30 min after the vaccine has been administered, but the reaction may be delayed up to several hours. Allergic reactions have been reported to nearly every vaccine. Minor, self-limited reactions to vaccination such as swelling or redness at the injection site are not IgE-mediated reactions and typically are not contraindications to administration of additional doses of the vaccine.

Most often, allergic reactions to vaccines are due to vaccine constituents rather than the microbial products. The vaccine constituents most commonly associated with an allergic reaction are gelatin, egg, chicken, and antimicrobial agents. Gelatin, a vaccine stabilizer, is responsible for many allergic reactions to measles, mumps, rubella (MMR), varicella, and Japanese encephalitis vaccines. Other vaccines, including influenza and diphtheria, tetanus, and pertussis (DTaP) vaccines, also contain gelatin, but in significantly smaller amounts. A history of gelatin allergy should be obtained before any gelatin-containing vaccine is administered. However, a negative history of gelatin allergy does not exclude an allergic reaction to gelatin injected with the vaccine. Patients who have a positive history of gelatin allergy should be evaluated by an allergist before the vaccine is administered. Egg is a component of influenza and yellow fever vaccines and may cause reactions in patients allergic to egg. Although influenza vaccine containing 1.2 µg egg protein per mL has been reported to be administered safely to patients with egg allergy, the egg content of commercially available influenza vaccine is not stated on the label and some vaccines contain more than this amount. The nasal influenza vaccine also contains egg protein and should not be given to patients with egg allergy. Chicken proteins may be present in yellow fever vaccine, and this needs to be considered in patients who are allergic to chicken.

Preservatives such as thimerosal, aluminum, and phenoxyethanol used in vaccines can cause delayed-type hypersensitivity reactions and contact dermatitis; however, these agents are not thought to cause immediate IgE-mediated reactions. Contact sensitivity or positive patch testing to these preservatives is not a contraindication to administering vaccines containing these agents. Antimicrobials such as neomycin, polymyxin B, and streptomycin may be added in trace amounts to vaccines. Reactions to vaccines caused by antimicrobial sensitivity appear to be very rare; however, patients who have experienced anaphylactic reactions due to these antibiotics should not receive vaccines containing them.

Evaluation of a possible vaccine allergy begins by determining if the signs, symptoms, and timing of the reaction to the vaccine are consistent with an IgE-mediated allergic reaction. If the reaction is consistent with an allergic reaction, the next step is to determine if the patient needs additional doses of the vaccine in question or, in the future, needs vaccines with the same constituents. Skin testing can be performed to the constituents of the suspect vaccine and to the vaccine itself. If the suspect vaccine contains egg (influenza and yellow fever vaccines), chicken (yellow fever vaccine), or gelatin proteins (multiple vaccines), skin testing to these constituents should be performed. Egg and chicken skin testing reagents are available commercially and the gelatin skin testing reagent can be made by dissolving one teaspoon of sugared gelatin powder of any color or flavor (e.g., Jell-O) in 5 mL of normal saline. Skin testing to vaccines is performed initially with skin prick testing to an undiluted preparation of the vaccine or a diluted preparation for patients whose reactions were severe. If the skin prick test to undiluted vaccine is negative, intradermal testing with a 1:100 dilution of the vaccine can be performed. If the vaccine or vaccine constituent component skin tests are positive, alternatives to the vaccine should be considered. However, after a risk/benefit ratio is assessed, consideration could be given to using a graded dose protocol for administering of the vaccine. For an allergic patient, the graded dose protocol would still carry the risk of an anaphylactic reaction and should be undertaken only after weighing all the options and ensuring that the knowledge and equipment required to manage an anaphylactic reaction are available. An example of a graded dose protocol for a vaccine with a usual dose of 0.5 mL would start with 0.05 mL of a 1:100 dilution, followed every 15 min by subsequent doses of 0.05 mL of a 1:10 dilution, 0.05 mL of full strength, 0.10 mL of full strength, 0.15 mL of full strength, and 0.20 mL of full strength. If skin testing with the vaccine is negative, it is recommended that the patient receive the vaccine in the usual manner. As a precaution, it is advisable for the patient to be observed for any signs or symptoms of a reaction after the vaccine has been given.

9.7 Clinical Vignettes

9.7.1 Vignette 1: Immediate Hypersensitivity Type 1 Reaction

A 35-year-old man presents with widespread urticaria beginning 1 hour after his AM dosage (second day) of amoxicillin. He reports no other symptoms. On physical examination, the vital signs are normal. Skin examination shows multiple classic urticarial lesions scattered throughout the integument. There is no angioedema. The rest of the physical examination, including ears, nose, throat, lymph nodes, heart, lungs, abdomen, and joints, is unremarkable.

Comment: This vignette is an example of a typical presentation of a mild type 1 hypersensitivity reaction. In this situation, immediate treatment would be with an H_1 blocker. The patient would also be educated about drug allergy to penicillin. His risk for another IgE-mediated reaction to penicillin would be approximately 60%, with the potential for an anaphylactic reaction.

Three years later, the patient is being treated for endocarditis. His physician would like to prescribe high-dose penicillin. Because of the patient's history, further evaluation is performed with skin prick, followed by intradermal testing to the major and minor determinants of penicillin. Intradermal testing shows a positive response to the benzyl penicilloyl determinant.

Comment: Because appropriate testing to the major and minor determinants of penicillin shows a positive response, the patient has persistent IgE-mediated sensitivity. In this situation, the use of high-dose penicillin is considered the treatment of choice. The penicillin can be administered according to a desensitization protocol.

The patient tolerates the desensitization protocol and finishes the course of penicillin for endocarditis. Two years later, he is evaluated because of a sinus infection and the physician wants to prescribe penicillin.

Comment: Because the patient has not received penicillin continuously, he must still be considered allergic to penicillin until proven otherwise. The desensitization procedure only desensitizes the patient for that initial course of treatment. The patient's current status could be assessed with skin testing to both the major and minor determinants of penicillin.

9.7.2 Vignette 2: Exanthematous (Morbilliform) Reaction

A 44-year-old woman presents with a measleslike (maculopapular) rash that started on day 7 of a 10-day course of cephalexin for sinusitis. She states that she does not have any other symptoms except for mild pruritus. She specifically says she does not have fever, joint pain, myalgias, or shortness of breath. The vital signs are normal, as is the physical examination, including the lymph nodes, heart, lungs, liver, spleen, and joints. Skin examination discloses a symmetric pink-red maculopapular exanthema, confluent in parts, over most of the skin. No target lesions, urticarial wheals, or angioedema is noted. Allergy skin prick and intradermal testing to cephalexin was performed and was negative.

Comment: This scenario is typical for an exanthematous reaction, which is thought to be T-cell mediated. Skin prick and intradermal testing is not indicated because the reaction is not IgE mediated. The skin tests would be expected to be negative. Despite the patient's rash, this is not a true allergy. The medication usually is discontinued at this time to prevent further spread of the exanthem. This type of reaction is not an absolute contraindication to future use of the medication.

9.7.3 Vignette 3: DRESS Syndrome

A 37-year-old woman is hospitalized for a constellation of flulike signs and symptoms, with no clear-cut diagnosis. Because of a sore throat, low-grade fever, and fatigue, treatment with azithromycin was started 3 days ago. Currently, she is febrile, with temperatures in the range of 101–103°F, slightly tachycardic, with a pulse rate of 104 min^{-1}, and a respiratory rate of 14 min^{-1}. The skin examination shows a widespread maculopapular rash without urticaria or angioedema. No target lesions or skin blistering is noted. Mucous membranes are intact. Examination of lymph nodes shows large anterior cervical and axillary lymph nodes bilaterally. Heart and lung examinations are normal. Abdominal examination shows a palpable liver edge and normal spleen. Examination of the joints is unremarkable. Her medications, including start dates, are listed below:

Medication	Start date	12/1 (fever, fatigue, sore throat)	12/2	12/3 (skin rash)	12/4 (examination)
Azithromycin	12/2/07		X	X	X
Omeprazole	3/15/07	X	X	X	X
Ibuprofen	1/30/07	X	X	X	X
Phenytoin	11/20/07	X	X	X	X

Laboratory tests: hemoglobin 12.4 g dL^{-1}, leukocytes 15.3 × 10^9 L^{-1}, eosinophils 1.2 × 10^9 L^{-1}, aspartate aminotransferase (AST) 105 U L^{-1}, alanine aminotransferase (ALT) 120 U L^{-1}.

Comment: This scenario is consistent with DRESS syndrome, which is characterized by fever, malaise, lymphadenopathy, eosinophilia, and liver inflammation. Although azithromycin was the most recently added medication, the most likely culprit in this case is phenytoin. Phenytoin is more commonly associated with DRESS syndrome reaction than is azithromycin. Treatment with both medications should be discontinued. Making a chart of her entire list of medications and knowing the type of reactions associated with these medications are helpful in making the diagnosis. In this type of situation, it is also important to evaluate for another underlying medical illness.

9.7.4 Vignette 4: Aspirin Sensitivity

A 58-year-old man with a long-standing history of asthma, nasal polyps, and aspirin sensitivity comes to the office to discuss his aspirin sensitivity. He is known to have coronary artery disease and several risk factors for cardiac disease, including elevated cholesterol level, strong family history of early coronary artery disease, and hypertension. His primary physician recommends that he take a daily low dose of aspirin (81 mg per day), but the patient is concerned because of his history of aspirin sensitivity.

Comment: There are different types of aspirin sensitivity, and management depends on the type. It is imperative to obtain a detailed history of the aspirin sensitivity.

The patient reports that approximately 15 year ago increased nasal congestion, rhinorrhea, and wheezing developed within 15 min after he ingested aspirin. The wheezing responded to albuterol treatment. The symptoms lasted for approximately 4 hours; he did not require any other treatment measures. There were no associated angioedema, urticaria, cardiovascular, or gastrointestinal symptoms. Since that time, he has avoided aspirin and other NSAIDs. He does not recall reactions to any other medication.

Comment: The type of reaction described is consistent with NSAID-exacerbated asthma and rhinitis or AERD. If his asthma is well controlled, he could be a candidate for aspirin challenge and desensitization, which would allow him to take the aspirin daily long term.

Suggested Reading

Berges-Gimeno, M. P., Simon, R. A., and Stevenson, D. D. (2003) Long-term treatment with aspirin desensitization in asthmatic patients with aspirin-exacerbated respiratory disease. J. Allergy Clin. Immunol. 111, 180–186.

Bernstein, I. L., Gruchalla, R. S., Lee, R. E., Nicklas, R. A., and Dykewicz, M. S., Joint Task Force on Practice Parameters; the American Academy of Allergy, Asthma and Immunology; the American College of Allergy, Asthma and Immunology; and the Joint Council of Allergy, Asthma and Immunology. (1999) Disease management of drug hypersensitivity: A practice parameter. Ann. Allergy Asthma Immunol. 83, 665–700.

Ditto, A. M., Greenberger, P. A., and Grammer, L. C. (2002) Drug allergy. In: L. C. Grammer and P. A. Greenberger (Eds.), Patterson's Allergic Diseases, 6th ed. Philadelphia: Lippincott, Williams & Wilkins. pp. 295–386.

Greenberger, P. A. and Patterson, R. (1991) The prevention of immediate generalized reactions to radiocontrast media in high-risk patients. J. Allergy Clin. Immunol. 87, 867–872.

Gruchalla, R. S. (2003) Drug allergy. J. Allergy Clin. Immunol. 111(Suppl. 2), S548–S559.

Lawley, T. J., Bielory, L., Gascon, P., Yancey, K. B., Young, N. S., and Frank, M. M. (1984) A prospective clinical and immunologic analysis of patients with serum sickness. N. Engl. J. Med. 311, 1407–1413.

Mertes, P. M., Laxenaire, M. C., and Alla, F.; Groupe d'Etudes des Reactions Anaphylactoides Peranesthesiques. (2003) Anaphylactic and anaphylactoid reactions occurring during anesthesia in France in 1999–2000. Anesthesiology 99, 536–545.

Namazy, J. A. and Simon, R. A. (2002) Sensitivity to nonsteroidal anti-inflammatory drugs. Ann. Allergy Asthma Immunol. 89, 542–550.

Primeau, M. N. and Adkinson, N. F. Jr. (2001) Recent advances in the diagnosis of drug allergy. Curr. Opin. Allergy Clin. Immunol. 1, 337–341.

Stella, M., Cassano, P., Bollero, D., Clemente, A., and Giorio, G. (2001) Toxic epidermal necrolysis treated with intravenous high-dose immunoglobulins: Our experience. Dermatology 203, 45–49.

Strom, B. L., Schinnar, R., Apter, A. J., et al. (2003) Absence of cross-reactivity between sulfonamide antibiotics and sulfonamide nonantibiotics. N. Engl. J. Med. 349, 1628–1635.

Tas, S. and Simonart, T. (2003) Management of drug rash with eosinophilia and systemic symptoms (DRESS syndrome): An update. Dermatology 206, 353–356.

Volcheck, G. W. (2004) Clinical evaluation and management of drug hypersensitivity. Immunol. Allergy Clin. North Am. 24, 357–371.

Chapter 10
Food Allergy

Abbreviations DBPCFC: double-blind: placebo-controlled food challenge: FD&C: Food Dye & Coloring; IL: interleukin; MSG: monosodium glutamate; MSG: monosodium glutamate; TNF: tumor necrosis factor.

10.1 Definitions

Approximately 20% of the population alters their diet because of a perceived adverse reaction to food. Adverse reactions to food can be grouped according to the pathophysiologic mechanism underlying the reaction. In this chapter, adverse reactions to food are classified as IgE-mediated disorders (classic food allergy), probable combination IgE-associated-cell-mediated disorders (atopic dermatitis and eosinophilic gastroenteropathies), non-IgE-associated-cell-mediated immunologic disorders (protein enteropathies, celiac disease, and dermatitis herpetiformis), and nonimmunologic disorders (food intolerances). Disorders with acute onset of symptoms after the ingestion of food are usually mediated by IgE or toxins, whereas subacute or chronic symptoms that develop after food ingestion tend to be caused by other mechanisms, particularly cell-mediated immunologic mechanisms. Some foods can result in several types of adverse reactions. For example, wheat can cause an IgE-mediated reaction (hives, anaphylaxis), an IgE-associated-cell-mediated reaction (worsening of atopic dermatitis), or a non-IgE-associated-cell-mediated immunologic disorder (celiac sprue). The age at onset of the food sensitivity, the specific signs and symptoms associated with food ingestion, and diagnostic testing can help categorize the type of adverse food reaction and aid in subsequent management.

10.2 Epidemiology

Knowledge of the epidemiology of food allergy is helpful in the diagnostic approach to patients with adverse food reactions. According to food allergy surveys of adults, without confirmatory testing, approximately 12–20% of respondents

G.W. Volcheck, *Clinical Allergy: Diagnosis and Management*
DOI: 10.1007/978-1-59745-315-8_10, © 2009 Mayo Foundation for Medical Education and Research

Table 10.1   Prevalence of food allergy in the United States

Food	Children (%)	Adults (%)
Cow's milk	2.5	0.3
Egg	1.3	0.2
Peanut	0.8	0.6
Tree nuts	0.2	0.5
Fish	0.1	0.4
Shellfish	0.1	2.0

From Sampson, H. A. (2004) Update on food allergy. J. Allergy Clin. Immunol. 113, 805–819. Used with permission

report food reactions and approximately 25% of parents believe their children have food allergies. However, further studies on these patients, such as skin prick testing and food challenge, have shown that true food allergy occurs less commonly than indicated by patient or parent self-report. Therefore, physician assessment is helpful not only in identifying or confirming suspected food allergy but also in discounting food allergy in patients with incorrect assumptions about certain foods.

Approximately 6% of young children and 3.7% of adults in the United States have food allergy. Any food can cause an allergic reaction, and in young children, the most common food allergies are to cow's milk, egg, peanut, wheat, soy, tree nuts, fish, and shellfish. These account for approximately 90% of significant reactions. In adults, the most common food allergies are to shellfish, peanut, tree nuts, and fish (Table 10.1). Early childhood allergies to milk, egg, soy, and wheat usually resolve by school age. Although peanut, tree nuts, and seafood allergies are generally considered permanent, approximately 20% of children may become tolerant to peanut. Reactions to fruits and vegetables are common but usually not severe and usually not life long. Allergy to seeds, particularly sesame, is becoming more common in children. Although few studies have been performed, approximately 20% of children appear to outgrow sesame seed allergy.

10.3   Pathophysiology

The pathophysiology of adverse food reactions are broadly divided into immunologic and nonimmunologic reactions. The immunologic reactions are divided further into IgE-dependent, IgE-associated-cell-mediated, or non-IgE-associated-cell-mediated reactions (Table 10.2). The IgE-mediated food reaction is considered the classic food allergy reaction. The main function of the gastrointestinal tract is to process ingested food for energy production and cell growth. This requires discriminating between harmful and harmless foreign proteins. The process by which the gastrointestinal immune system avoids attacking food antigens is termed oral tolerance. In food allergy, there is a disruption in the development of food tolerance. Several mechanisms are involved in oral tolerance. The primary mechanism is the gastrointestinal mucosal barrier, a complex physical and immunologic structure consisting

Table 10.2 IgE-dependent, IgE-associated–cell-mediated, and non-IgE-associated–cell-mediated food reactions

Reaction	Age	Associated foods	Clinical features	Laboratory findings	Treatment
IgE-dependent					
Classic food allergy	Any	Milk, egg, peanut, soy, wheat, fish, shellfish, tree nuts (potentially all foods)	Urticaria, angioedema, wheezing, vomiting, diarrhea, abdominal cramping (alone or in combination)	Positive food-specific skin prick or IgE in vitro testing	Avoidance Patient education
Oral allergy syndrome	Any	Fresh fruits, vegetables	History of seasonal allergic rhinitis; pruritus or mild edema of oral cavity	Positive food-specific skin prick or IgE in vitro testing	Able to eat food in cooked form
Anaphylaxis	Any	Milk, egg, peanut, tree nut, soy, fish, shellfish, wheat (potentially all foods)	Urticaria, angioedema, bronchospasm, vomiting, diarrhea, hypotension, tachycardia	Positive food-specific skin prick or IgE in vitro testing	Avoidance Patient education
IgE-associated–cell-mediated					
Atopic dermatitis	Child	Milk, egg, wheat, peanut, soy, fish (potentially all foods)	Exacerbation of atopic dermatitis	Positive food-specific skin prick or IgE in vitro testing	Avoidance
Eosinophilic esophagitis	Any	Milk, egg, grains, peanut, soy, fish, shellfish (potentially all foods)	Children: vomiting, regurgitation, abdominal pain Adults: as above, also dysphagia and heartburn	Positive food-specific skin prick or IgE in vitro testing >15 eosinophils/HPF on esophageal biopsy	Avoidance Corticosteroids
Cell-mediated–IgE-independent					
Protein enterocolitis	Infants	Milk, soy, rice, poultry, fish	Vomiting, diarrhea, hypotension, abdominal distension, failure to thrive	Neutrophilia Biopsy: patchy villous injury and colitis	Avoidance Supportive measures

(continued)

Table 10.2 (continued)

Reaction	Age	Associated foods	Clinical features	Laboratory findings	Treatment
Protein proctitis	Infants	Milk, soy	Well-appearing infant with bloody stools	Fecal neutrophils	Avoidance
Protein enteropathy	Infant, child	Milk, soy, egg, chicken, fish	Emesis, diarrhea, other signs and symptoms consistent with malabsorption	Biopsy: flattening of small intestinal villae	Avoidance
Celiac disease	Any	Gluten	Weight loss, chronic diarrhea, steatorrhea	IgA antigliadin antibody IgA antiendomysial antibody Biopsy: duodenal villous atrophy	Gluten-free diet
Dermatitis herpetiformis	Any	Gluten primarily, other foods possible	Pruritic, papulovesicular rash	Skin biopsy: deposits of IgA and C3 at dermoepidermal junction	Avoidance

HPF high-power field

of mucus, epithelial tight junctions, enzymes, acid, and secretory IgA, which protects the immune system from protein exposure overload. Breakdown of this barrier promotes food allergy through exposure of a large amount of food allergens to the immune system. For the small amount of food allergens normally absorbed (approximately 2%), the T-cell has a critical role in inducing tolerance through induction of T-cell anergy, deletion of reactive T-cells, and generation of suppressor T-cells. This neutralizes the immune response and allows foods to be tolerated.

The cytokine milieu of the gastrointestinal tract likely has an important role in the development of food allergy. When cytokines (interleukin [IL]-4, IL-5, and IL-13) of Th2, helper T-cells predominate, food hypersensitivity reactions associated with the production of food-specific IgE antibody can occur. Increased food absorption can affect the response by allowing more substrate for production of food-specific IgE antibody. Increased absorption likely explains why infants, who have leakier gut barriers than older people, have a higher prevalence of food allergies. Other factors, including alcohol, aspirin, and exercise, can contribute importantly to food allergy by increasing food absorption.

Although sensitization occurs most frequently through the gastrointestinal tract, it also can occur through the respiratory tract or the skin. Sensitization through the respiratory tract typically occurs occupationally, as in bakers' asthma. In this situation, millers and bakers develop IgE-mediated respiratory symptoms through the inhalation of cereal flour. Sensitization through the skin is likely less common and occurs primarily with skin conditions in which the epidermal barrier is impaired.

The production of food-specific IgE antibodies provides the primary background for a classic allergic response. When the specific food reaches IgE antibodies bound to mast cells or basophils, preformed mediators, including histamine and leukocyte chemotactic factors, and newly synthesized mediators, including leukotrienes, prostaglandins, and platelet-activating factor, are released, resulting in the symptoms of immediate hypersensitivity. These signs and symptoms include any combination of pruritus, urticaria, angioedema, dyspnea, wheezing, dizziness, hypotension, nausea, abdominal cramping, vomiting, and diarrhea.

Cell-mediated hypersensitivity has been implicated in food immunologic disorders in which the onset of symptoms occurs several hours or more after ingestion of the food. Of interest, some cell-mediated disorders have also been associated with specific food IgE antibody positivity. This has been found primarily in eosinophilic esophagitis and eosinophilic gastroenteritis. The role of IgE in these conditions has not been well delineated because IgE sensitivity is found in some, but not all, patients with these conditions. Eosinophilic infiltration of the mucosal, muscular, or serosal layers of the gastrointestinal tract results in the development of symptoms. The location and extent of the eosinophilic infiltration dictate the signs and symptoms that are manifested. The eosinophilic infiltration appears to result from the increased expression and secretion of IL-5 from T-cells. IL-5 has a critical role in eosinophil survival and activation.

Cell-mediated hypersensitivity without IgE association is found in protein-induced enterocolitis and enteropathy. The mechanism for these entities has not been clearly delineated, but the food antigen appears to induce a cell-mediated response without IgE involvement. In sensitive patients, there is increased release of mononuclear cell mediators such as tumor necrosis factor (TNF)-α with exposure to food-specific antigen, producing symptoms. In protein-induced enterocolitis syndrome, stools often contain occult blood, neutrophils, and eosinophils. Jejunal biopsy specimens show flattened villi, edema, and an increased number of lymphocytes, eosinophils, and mast cells. In dietary protein-induced enteropathy, patchy villous atrophy is seen on endoscopy and biopsy specimens show mononuclear cell infiltrates.

10.4   Food Allergens

Foods are composed of proteins, carbohydrates, and lipids. The major food allergens have been identified as water-soluble glycoproteins that range in molecular weight from 10,000 to 67,000 Da (Table 10.3). Food allergens have no known unique biochemical or immunochemical characteristics. They tend to be resistant to heat and acid treatment and to proteolysis and digestion. However, fruits and vegetables are often an exception to this. Food allergens soluble in water are classified as albumins, and those soluble in saline, as globulins. The amount of food allergen required to elicit a response varies. The lowest amounts are commonly in the range of 1–2 mg of natural foods, representing a few hundred micrograms of protein. These minimal doses characterize about 1% of patients allergic to milk, egg, or peanut, and 65 mg induces a response in approximately 17% of patients allergic to egg or peanut.

Table 10.3 Common food allergens

Food	Protein	Nomenclature
Cow's milk	Caseins	
	α_{s1}-Casein	Bos d 8
	α_{s2}-Casein	
	β-Casein	
	κ-Casein	
	Whey	
	β-Lactoglobulin	Bos d 5
	α-Lactalbumin	Bos d 4
	Serum albumin	Bos d 6
Chicken egg white	Ovalbumin	Gal d 1
	Ovomucoid	Gal d 2
	Ovotransferrin	Gal d 3
Peanut	Vicilin	Ara h 1
	Conglutin	Ara h 2
	Glycinin	Ara h 3
Soybean	Glycinin G1	
	Profilin	Gly m 3
Fish	Parvalbumin	Gad c 1
Shrimp	Tropomyosin	Pen a 1

10.4.1 Cow's Milk

Cow's milk allergy is a common food allergy of infancy and childhood, affecting approximately 2.5% of infants. Tolerance is often achieved (approximately 85%) by the age of 3–5 years. IgE antibodies may be directed to various potential allergenic proteins, particularly casein and whey proteins. Caseins constitute 80% of the total protein of cow's milk, and whey proteins constitute the other 20%. Caseins and β-lactoglobulin, a whey protein, are the major allergens in cow's milk. Most patients allergic to cow's milk cannot tolerate milk from other mammals except mare's milk. Approximately 10% of patients with cow's milk allergy may have a reaction to beef. Table 10.4 outlines food allergen cross-reactivity of the common food allergens. Of the infants with IgE-mediated cow's milk allergy, 85% tolerate a soy formula. However, the rate of tolerance is only about 50% for those with cell-mediated cow's milk sensitivity. More than 95% of infants with cow's milk sensitivity, either IgE mediated or cell mediated, tolerate extensively hydrolyzed cow's milk formula. For the few who continue to have a reaction, an amino acid–based formula is required.

10.4.2 Hen's Egg

Allergy to hen's eggs affects approximately 2.5% of infants and young children, and tolerance is usually achieved by the age of 5 years. Eggs are composed of egg white and egg yolk. Egg white appears to be more allergenic than egg yolk. The major allergenic proteins in egg white are ovalbumin and ovomucoid. Other allergenic proteins include ovotransferrin, ovomucin, and lysozyme. Hen's egg allergens cross-react with other avian egg allergens, but the clinical implications of this cross-reactivity are unclear. Several proteins that cross-react with allergens in hen's egg white are also detected in egg yolk, hen sera, and poultry meat. Clinically, most patients allergic to hen's eggs are able to tolerate poultry.

Table 10.4 Food allergen cross-reactivity

Allergy to	Risk of reaction to	Risk (%)
Cow's milk	Soy	15
Cow's milk	Beef	10
Egg	Chicken	5
Soy	Other legumes	5–10
Peanut	Other legumes	5–10
Peanut	Tree nuts	30–40
Fish	Other fish	50
Shellfish	Other shellfish	50–75
Tree nuts	Other tree nuts	40–50
Grains	Other grains	10–20

Egg allergy is important in immunizations. The influenza vaccine (both killed injected and live attenuated nasal) and yellow fever vaccine are grown in chick fluid. The egg protein content of these vaccines varies and is greater than 1 μg. Patients with a history of hen's egg allergy should be evaluated by an allergist before influenza or yellow fever immunization for consideration of skin testing with the vaccine before administration or graded dosage administration.

10.4.3   Soy

The prevalence of soy allergy among the population appears to be approximately 0.4% and transient. Soybean globulins are the major proteins of soybeans. The 2S or 7S fractions are thought to contain the major allergens. Gly m 1, a component of the 7S fraction, has at least 16 distinct soybean-specific IgE-binding epitopes along the amino acid sequence. Gly m 1 is the major soy allergen responsible for airborne soy allergen asthma outbreaks. This allergen, localized in soybean hulls, is different from proteins that cause food allergy to soybean. Glycinin and profilin are common soy food allergens. Although extensive cross-reactivity, as shown by in vitro testing, occurs between soy and the other legume foods (peanut, lima bean, pea, garbanzo bean, green bean), oral food challenges have shown that clinically important cross-reactivity to legumes in children is uncommon and usually transitory. Overall, clinical hypersensitivity to one legume does not routinely warrant dietary elimination of all legumes. Processed soybean oil is usually considered safe for patients with soy allergy.

10.4.4   Peanut

Peanut allergy is one of the most popularized food allergies because of the severity of the reactions associated with it. Peanut allergy affects approximately 0.6% of the general population. In case series of fatal food-induced anaphylaxis, peanut is generally the most common culprit, with the highest risk group being adolescents with asthma. Peanut is a legume, not a tree nut. Several peanut allergens have been identified and characterized. Ara h 1, a glycoprotein, has been identified as a major peanut allergen and has at least 23 specific IgE-binding epitopes along its amino acid sequence. Ara h 2 has at least ten specific IgE-binding epitopes along its amino acid sequence. Unexpectedly, the ingestion of other legumes generally does not induce an allergic reaction, and the avoidance of all legumes is generally unwarranted. Because challenge studies have shown significant cross-reactivity with lupin, lupine should be avoided by peanut-allergic individuals. A wide variety of peanut products, including peanut flour and pressed peanut oils, retain their allergenicity, although refined peanut oil appears to be safe for those with peanut allergy. Most patients with peanut allergy have the allergy for life. Of the children whose peanut allergy is diagnosed before age 2 years, approximately 20% eventually develop tolerance. This occurs primarily in those with milder peanut sensitivity.

10.4.5   Fish

Allergic reactions to fish are common in many areas of the world where fish is a major source of protein. The cross-reaction between different species of fish, including salt and freshwater fish, is significant, dispelling the notion that saltwater and freshwater fish have primarily exclusive allergens. The only clinically relevant distinction appears to be between fish, either saltwater or freshwater, and shellfish (crustaceans and mollusks), for which there does not appear to be any significant cross-reactivity. (Shellfish are reviewed in the next section.)

There is significant cross-reactivity between different types of fish, but the number of confirmatory double-blind placebo-controlled food challenges (DBPCFCs) has been small. Parvalbumin is the dominant allergen in finned fish. Gad c 1 is a parvalbumin with at least five IgE-binding sites on the allergen; the carbohydrate moiety does not appear to be important for its allergenicity. The most common signs and symptoms in fish allergy are vomiting and pruritus of the mouth and throat. Patients allergic to fish are often clinically sensitive to more than one species of fish. Skin test reactivity alone is not diagnostic; therefore, a patient with a fish allergy who has a specific IgE to any fish and a history of a severe reaction should exercise caution when eating fish of another species until a lack of reactivity to that species can be demonstrated. Negative results of testing to nonsuspected fish must be cautiously verified with appropriately designed, graded, challenge testing before the fish is considered safe to eat. Fish allergy is considered long-lived, although the allergy has been reported to resolve.

10.4.6   Shellfish

Shellfish are divided into two groups: (1) mollusks, which include mussel, oyster, scallop, clam, and squid, and (2) crustaceans, which include crab, crawfish, lobster, and shrimp. Shrimp is the most studied of the shellfish allergens. Pen a 1 has been identified as a major allergen from boiled shrimp and constitutes 20% of the soluble protein in crude cooked shrimp. Pen a 1 binds shrimp-specific IgE in more than 85% of patients with shrimp allergy. Met a 1, another shrimp allergen, and Pen a 1 are highly homologous with tropomyosin, which occurs in various species. Crustaceans are a frequent cause of adverse food reactions, including life-threatening anaphylaxis. Patients allergic to one crustacean species should be cautious about the ingestion of other crustaceans because of cross-reactivity. Cross-reactivity between mollusks and crustaceans is not well defined. Crustaceans do not cross-react with vertebrate fish.

Despite the common belief that a person with seafood allergy has a higher risk of a reaction to radiocontrast media, no convincing data support this and it has no theoretical basis. Seafood allergy is an IgE response to proteins in the seafood, not to iodide. Also, the mechanism of the anaphylactoid reaction to contrast material is not due strictly to the iodide but to the physiochemical properties of the radiocontrast material. For patients with shellfish allergy, special precautions are not required before the administration of radiocontrast media.

10.4.7 Wheat

The proteins of wheat include water-soluble albumins, saline-soluble globulins, ethanol-soluble prolamins, and glutelins. Sensitivity to wheat can be manifested in multiple forms. IgE-mediated reactions to wheat include classic food allergy ranging from urticaria to anaphylaxis, exercise-induced anaphylaxis, or occupational asthma. Cell-mediated responses to wheat include celiac disease and dermatitis herpetiformis. Patients with wheat allergy alone show extensive in vitro IgE cross-reactivity to other grains that is not reflected clinically. This extensive cross-reactivity is probably caused by nonspecific IgE binding to the lectin fraction in cereal grains. Patients with wheat allergy have specific IgE binding to wheat fractions of 20,000 and 47,000 Da. Wheat α-amylase inhibitor also appears to be a major wheat allergen. For patients with wheat allergy, the elimination of all grains such as rye, barley, oats, rice, and corn from the diet is clinically unwarranted. Wheat allergy typically affects children and is usually outgrown. An exception is wheat-dependent, exercise-induced anaphylaxis. This condition – manifested by wheat ingestion coupled with physical exercise resulting in anaphylaxis – occurs primarily in adults. This condition appears to be persistent, but extensive long-term studies have not been performed.

10.4.8 Tree Nuts

Clinical reactions to tree nuts can be severe and potentially fatal. Serologic studies have indicated a high degree of IgE binding to multiple tree nuts in patients with tree nut allergy. Because of the potential for severe reactions, no comprehensive studies have been performed to determine clinically relevant cross-reactivity to tree nuts. In view of the potential severity of allergic reactions to tree nuts and the difficulty with accurately identifying tree nuts in foods and the potential for cross-reactivity, the total elimination of tree nuts from the diet of a patient with allergy to a particular tree nut is generally recommended. However, total elimination of tree nuts from the diet may not be necessary if it can be clearly established that a patient can tolerate tree nuts other than the one responsible for the reaction and is able to obtain them without risk of cross-contamination.

10.5 Approach to Patients

The approach to patients with food allergy is similar to that for patients with other allergic disorders and focuses on all the signs and symptoms involved in the reaction and the timing of ingestion in relation to the onset of the reaction. A thorough review of symptoms and a physical examination can help categorize the disorder as likely being an IgE-mediated, IgE-associated–cell-mediated, non-IgE-associated–cell-mediated, or nonimmunologic reaction (Fig. 10.1).

IgE-mediated reactions show evidence of the release of mast cell mediators affecting one or more target organs. The primary manifestations involve the integumentary, respiratory, gastrointestinal, and cardiovascular systems. Similar to all systemic allergic reactions, the signs and symptoms can consist of any combination of pruritus, urticaria, angioedema, rhinitis, asthma, abdominal cramping, vomiting, diarrhea, tachycardia, and hypotension. The onset of symptoms typically occurs within minutes and up to approximately 2 hours after the food is ingested. Key considerations when evaluating the patient include the following:

- Could something other than food cause the signs and symptoms? Often, patients can present a convincing story for a particular food. However, it is important to keep in mind alternate diagnoses that can masquerade as food allergy, particularly gastroesophageal reflux, choking episode, gustatory flushing, mediator release syndromes, or panic disorder.
- Was something ingested besides the suspected food? A patient may focus on a particular food, but at the same time may have ingested other foods that may be the true allergen.

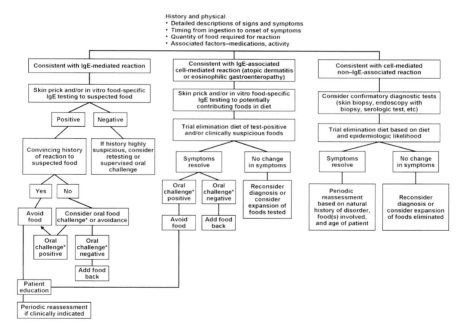

Fig. 10.1 Algorithm for the diagnosis of immunologic food reactions. *Food challenges should only be performed after careful analysis of the risks and benefits and in a supervised setting with appropriate emergency medications and equipment

- Which suspected food is the most likely culprit? Common things occur commonly. Knowledge of the most common food allergens can help narrow the possibilities, but it must be kept in mind that any food is capable of causing an allergic reaction.
- What ancillary factors may have contributed to the reaction? The most common ancillary factors that can contribute to the development of food allergy with food ingestion include exercise, alcohol, and medications, particularly nonsteroidal anti-inflammatory medications.

IgE-associated-cell-mediated reactions, unlike classic IgE-mediated reactions, do not result primarily from the release of mast cell mediators. The most common clinical manifestations are worsening of atopic dermatitis and the development of eosinophilic enteropathies. Of children who have moderate to severe atopic dermatitis, approximately 35% have food allergy. Instead of large urticaria, skin manifestations are primarily chronic pruritus dermatitis and xerosis, with worsening of atopic dermatitis. Other organ systems, such as the respiratory and cardiovascular systems, are not involved. In eosinophilic gastroenteropathies, the symptoms can vary widely with respect to the site and degree of eosinophilic inflammation. Typical symptoms include dysphagia and abdominal pain.

Cell-mediated-non-IgE-mediated disorders include protein-induced enterocolitis and enteropathy, celiac disease, and dermatitis herpetiformis. Protein-induced conditions are seen in infants and include protein proctitis, protein enteropathy, and protein enterocolitis. Protein proctitis results in mucousy, bloody stools and is usually due to milk. Protein enteropathy is manifested as malabsorption, emesis, and poor growth. Protein enterocolitis is the most serious form and is manifested as severe vomiting, diarrhea, and potentially sepsislike features, with dehydration and shock. Milk and soy are the most common causes of these syndromes, which typically resolve by age 2 years. Celiac disease and dermatitis herpetiformis can occur together or separately and at any age. Both are due to gluten sensitivity. Celiac disease results in malabsorption and signs and symptoms attributable to nutrient deficiencies. Dermatitis herpetiformis consists of pruritic papulovesicular skin lesions instead of urticaria or atopic dermatitis.

10.6 Clinical Disorders

10.6.1 IgE-Mediated Disorders

10.6.1.1 Food Allergy

Allergic reactions to a food can vary depending on the method of exposure, the condition of the food, and the sensitivity of the patient. Reactions that occur after ingestion, inhalation, or contact with foods can range from mild, gradually developing symptoms limited to the gastrointestinal tract to severe and rapidly progressive life-threatening anaphylaxis. Possible signs and symptoms include cutaneous manifestations, gastrointestinal symptoms, respiratory symptoms, hypotension, and laryngeal edema, occurring together or separately. Cutaneous and gastrointestinal symptoms are the most commonly observed acute manifestations of food allergy. In IgE-mediated reactions, the time from the ingestion of the food to the onset of symptoms is typically rapid (within minutes). It is also important to note that small amounts of food can potentially elicit severe reactions, and the reactions will continue to occur with reexposure to the food.

Cutaneous manifestations of food allergy range from acute urticaria or angioedema to a morbilliform pruritic dermatitis. Although cutaneous signs are the most common signs in an allergic food reaction, the absence of skin manifestations does not rule out food-induced anaphylaxis. The length of time that the cutaneous manifestations persist varies in IgE-mediated food allergy. With treatment, the majority of lesions subside in 24–36 hours, but this depends on the severity of the initial reaction.

Gastrointestinal symptoms can include nausea, vomiting, abdominal cramping, and diarrhea. Young children and infants with food allergy may immediately spit out food without being able to describe the sensation they experienced with the ingestion. This behavior, although nonspecific, should not be overlooked in assessing food allergy. IgE-mediated reactions to foods may be difficult to differentiate from other types of reactions such as food intolerances, especially if the symptoms are primarily or exclusively gastrointestinal. The physician should examine carefully for involvement of other organ systems.

Respiratory manifestations of food allergy include sneezing, rhinorrhea, and bronchospasm. These signs are typically part of a general anaphylactic reaction and represent a more severe disease manifestation. Isolated airway signs and symptoms without other organ system involvement are rare. Although uncommon, food allergy should be considered in those with asthma triggered after the ingestion of particular foods.

Anaphylaxis

Each year in the United States, about 150 people are believed to die because of fatal food allergic reactions. Peanut and tree nuts account for more than 90% of food anaphylaxis fatalities; however, fish, shellfish, cow's milk, and hen's egg have also caused fatality, and any food may do so. Severe bronchospasm has frequently been reported in the few case series that have examined food allergy mortality. Symptoms can initially be mild and then progress rapidly. Reactions often start immediately on contact with the food or within 1–2 min in those with severe allergy. Less commonly, the reaction may occur up to 1–2 hours later. Although the term anaphylaxis is commonly used when a systemic reaction is severe, the term applies to any systemic IgE-mediated reaction. Modifiers such as mild, moderate, or severe are often used to describe anaphylaxis, but there are no widely accepted definitions for grading anaphylaxis. The most severe manifestations of anaphylaxis are laryngoedema, bronchospasm, and hypotension with cardiovascular collapse. Other signs and symptoms that can be part of an anaphylactic reaction include any combination of pruritus, urticaria, angioedema, wheeze, dyspnea, abdominal cramping, nausea, vomiting, diarrhea, and uterine cramping.

Oral Allergy Syndrome

Oral allergy syndrome is a unique syndrome characterized by the acute onset of oropharyngeal pruritus following the ingestion of raw fruits and vegetables by patients with a history of seasonal allergies. It is a form of contact allergy to ingested fruits and vegetables that is manifested by oral pruritus and occasionally by mild edema of the lips, tongue, palate, and throat. Systemic symptoms are not part of this syndrome. Reactions progress to systemic manifestations, including anaphylaxis, in fewer than 1% of patients who initially have oral allergy syndrome.

The syndrome is attributed to initial sensitization to airborne seasonal pollens. The raw fruits and vegetables share cross-reacting proteins with particular pollens, which are the source of the initial sensitization. Of interest, it appears the allergenic protein is heat labile, because the causative foods generally can be tolerated when they are ingested in a cooked or canned form. Typical patterns of raw fruit or vegetable sensitivity are associated with certain airborne seasonal pollens. Ragweed-sensitive patients may experience oral symptoms when they eat a banana or melon, whereas birch-pollen-sensitive patients may have symptoms with the ingestion of raw carrot, celery, cherry, pear, walnut, potato, apple, or hazelnut. Mugwort allergy is associated with sensitivity to melon, apple, peach, and cherry; grass allergy is associated with sensitivity to melon, tomato, and orange. The typical clinical scenario is that of a patient with seasonal allergic rhinitis who reports an "itchy" sensation in the mouth after ingesting the raw fruit or vegetable but who tolerates it in other forms. For example, a birch-sensitive patient may note itchiness of the mouth when eating a fresh apple, yet not have any symptoms when eating a baked apple pie.

The symptoms may be more prominent after the associated pollen season. Often, the allergens are concentrated in the peels of the allergenic fruits. Patients may have oral allergy syndrome to just one fruit or vegetable, but it often occurs with more than one. It is important to distinguish this syndrome from oral symptoms caused by allergens in other foods, for example, peanut or tree nuts, in which subsequent systemic reactions may occur.

10.6.1.2   Diagnosis

Skin Testing and In Vitro Testing

Allergen skin testing remains a useful tool in the diagnosis of food allergy. As allergen extract materials have improved over the years, the proper use and interpretation of skin testing have also improved. Several techniques are used for allergy skin testing, but research studies indicate that the prick or puncture skin test is the most useful technique, with the most predictable results. Intradermal skin tests with varying concentrations of extract are widely used for venom and drug allergy skin testing but are not recommended for clinical food allergy because of the high degree of false-positive results and risk for a systemic reaction. To accurately select and interpret tests for food-specific IgE antibodies, the epidemiology, clinical history, and pathophysiology of the signs and symptoms under investigation should be considered.

Commercial extracts from foods with stable proteins are reliable for detecting specific IgE antibodies in most patients, but extracts from foods such as fruits and vegetables that contain labile proteins may be less reliable. In these situations, pricking the fresh food and then applying the testing device to the patient may be useful. The skin prick test is performed by placing a drop of the allergen extract, for example, walnut protein, on the skin. Several devices are available for pricking or puncturing the skin through the drop. The results are read in 15–20 minutes. Different scoring systems can be used to record skin test results. The initial critical piece of information is to determine whether the skin prick test is positive or negative. A wheal diameter of 3 mm or larger compared with the diluent control is considered a positive marker of food allergy in most North American and European centers. Although the sensitivity is high, the specificity is low. Conversely, a negative test, or wheal less than 3 mm in diameter, essentially rules out food allergy.

In children older than 1 year, negative skin tests for major food allergens have high negative predictive accuracies, essentially ruling out IgE-mediated food allergy if the skin test is negative. The positive predictive value is lower, approximately 50–60%, depending on the clinical history. Generally, a slightly positive skin test with a vague history often requires a food challenge to verify the allergen. Selecting which food skin test extracts to use should be based on the patient's history. The use of a large number of food skin tests applied indiscriminately often produces more questions than answers because of false-positive findings. If the history does not suggest a specific food, but the pattern of symptoms suggests a food allergy, for example, signs and symptoms of histamine release occurring within an hour after the ingestion of the food at various times, limited skin testing may be helpful. The major foods for which skin testing has been found most helpful include egg, milk, wheat, peanut, tree nuts, fish, and shellfish.

Recent studies have shown that the actual diameter of the skin test wheal helps quantify the degree of sensitivity. Sporik and colleagues calculated the likelihood ratios of a positive food challenge for a given wheal diameter to various foods in a high-risk referral population (Table 10.5). The likelihood ratio represents a measure of the odds of having a disease relative to the prior probability of the disease. This estimate is independent of the disease prevalence. For example, if a patient has a skin test wheal diameter that has a likelihood ratio of 10, he or she would have a positive challenge ten times as frequently as those with a negative test. In that situation, further evaluation such as a food challenge would not be considered. Those with lesser skin reactivity, depending on the food and the clinical history, may be candidates for food challenge. However, caution is needed in extrapolating these data broadly, because of the differences between the test setting and other care centers and patient populations. Important differences that can affect outcome include the

Table 10.5 Likelihood ratios of a positive challenge for a given wheal diameter based on skin prick testing[a]

Wheal (mm)	Cow's milk	Egg	Peanut
3	3.8	2.8	3.4
4	5.8	3.1	6.3
5	7.3	7.3	18.0
6	13.2	12.5	16.7
7	16.2	∞	∞
8	∞	∞	∞

Data from Sporik, R., Hill, D. J., and Hosking, C. S. (2000) Specificity of allergen skin testing in predicting positive open food challenges to milk, egg and peanut in children. Clin. Exp. Allergy 30, 1540–1546
[a]Likelihood ratio: compares frequency of test correctly identifying those with food allergy to the frequency of the test being positive in those without food allergy. A likelihood ratio >10 is highly predictive of a positive food challenge

use of different skin test reagents, the potency of the reagents, and the type of skin prick method.

Overall, on the basis of the high negative predictive value of the skin prick test, this is considered an excellent means of ruling out IgE-mediated food allergy. Positive tests alone are suggestive of but not diagnostic for food allergy because of the low positive predictive value. Caveats to these general statements are needed for the evaluation of fruits and vegetables in which commercially prepared extracts are used. In this situation, IgE sensitivity may not be elicited because of the lability of the allergen and the resulting false-negative test. Also, a positive skin test to a food that is suspected by history is considered diagnostic.

The major form of in vitro testing for food hypersensitivity has involved some type of immunoassay that detects the presence of circulating food-specific IgE antibody. Situations in which these tests may be valuable include patients with a history of a life-threatening reaction to the suspected food or conditions that would interfere with the interpretation of the skin test, for example, atopic dermatitis or other skin disorder or the use of medications causing a nonreactive histamine control. Modern in vitro detection systems use radioimmunoassay procedures (radioallergosorbent test) or detect serum IgE by exposing serum to allergen bound to a solid matrix and using a secondary labeled anti-IgE antibody to detect the bound IgE antibody. The in vitro tests generally have been thought to be slightly less sensitive than skin testing. Recently, however, Sampson and others have studied the quantitative CAP fluorescent enzyme immunoassay to generate positive and negative predictive values for common food allergens based on the immunoassay level (Table 10.6). With the use of these levels, decisions about the safety and need for food challenges can be determined. For example, for egg and milk, values >7 kU L^{-1} and >15 kU L^{-1}, respectively, indicate a high probability for a reaction; therefore, a challenge would be unnecessary and the food should be avoided. However, for values <0.35 kU L^{-1} for egg and milk, a reaction is unlikely, on the order of 10–25%, depending on history, and a food challenge could be performed with less risk to rule out food

Table 10.6 Predictive values of selected food allergies[a]

Food	Mean age, 5 years ~50% react	Mean age, 5 years ~95% react	Age ≤2 years ~95% react
Egg	2	7	2
Milk	2	15	5
Peanut	2/5[b]	14	–

Data from Sicherer, S. H. and Sampson, H. A. (2006) 9. Food allergy. J. Allergy Clin. Immunol. 117(Suppl. Mini-Primer), S470–S475
[a]Data are reported in kIU L^{-1} (Pharmacia CAP system FEIA)
[b]Value is 2 kIU L^{-1} for those with and 5 kIU L^{-1} for those without a clear history of peanut allergy

allergy. In vitro tests are not performed properly in every laboratory, and quality control of these tests is critical. As with any laboratory test, CAP fluorescent enzyme immunoassay must be interpreted in the context of the patient's history and physical examination and laboratory findings.

Families often inquire about other "blood tests" for allergy. There are other blood tests for food allergy that have not been validated. Several laboratories in the United States perform food-specific IgG antibody testing. These tests are often used in situations in which the problem is behavioral. Often, multiple positive findings result in highly restrictive diets that can be detrimental to the patient. Because positive IgG levels to specific foods are found frequently in the sera of normal people, there is little support for dietary recommendations based on IgG food-specific testing. It is important to remember that food-specific IgG antibody testing has no clinical validation.

Food Challenge

A food challenge is a procedure in which potentially allergenic foods are ingested by the subject in increasing increments to observe for a potential clinical reaction. Currently, food challenge is the most effective way to determine whether a person truly has a reaction to the food when the cause and effect are not clear despite a thorough history and specific testing. Challenges are most often used to eliminate incriminated foods that are highly unlikely to cause symptoms or to document whether an individual has acquired clinical tolerance to a food after experiencing food-induced anaphylaxis in the past and losing sensitization to it, as documented by skin testing and measurement of specific IgE. If an individual has a history consistent with anaphylaxis to the specific food or a skin test or an allergen-specific serum IgE level above the decision point for that food, an oral food challenge is contraindicated. Because of the potential risk to the patient, food challenges should not be undertaken casually. Challenges should not be performed in patients with active asthma or if the FEV$_1$ is <70% predicted. Anyone who performs food challenges must have the background and equipment for treating anaphylactic reactions. A food challenge is administered in the fasting state, starting with an extremely low dose (5–250 mg) of the food. The dose is then doubled every

15–60 minutes depending on the type of reaction. Most food challenges require
several hours. Other foods should not be ingested during the challenge because they
may enhance or delay absorption. Once the patient tolerates a normal serving of the
food, clinical reactivity is essentially ruled out.

Food challenges can also be performed to assess for non-IgE-mediated food
reactions. For dietary protein-induced enterocolitis, challenges may require 0.5 mg
food substrate/kg body weight and be given in one or two doses. The patient would
require observation for 8 hours after the challenge. In eosinophilic esophagitis or
eosinophilic gastroenteritis, the patient may require challenge with multiple feed-
ings over 1–3 days. Challenges to different foods for non-IgE-mediated reactions
should be at least 3–5 days apart to avoid the contamination of a delayed reaction.
Oral food challenges should be conducted in a clinic or hospital setting if an IgE-
mediated reaction or protein-induced enterocolitis is suspected. For foods suspected
of causing other non-IgE-mediated reactions, a challenge usually can be performed
on an outpatient basis. There are basically three types of food challenge: open food
challenge, single-blind food challenge, and DBPCFC.

The open food challenge is useful for ruling out suspected food allergies. It is
used most commonly in situations in which the history and testing suggest that a
reaction to the food is very unlikely, for example, a child with a remote history of
milk allergy who, despite attempted avoidance, inadvertently ingested milk occasionally without a reaction yet still has a minimally positive skin test or mildly elevated
in vitro test. Another example is an adult who describes a history of egg allergy but
ingests French toast without difficulty and has a minimally elevated in vitro test or
3 × 3-mm-response to skin prick testing. In these types of situations, an open food
challenge can be performed in which an increasing amount of the food in question
is given every 20 min while the patient is closely monitored for signs and symptoms
of an allergic reaction. An open challenge is prone to bias by both the clinician and
the patient. If an open challenge is suspected to be falsely positive, a follow-up
DBPCFC is warranted.

In the office, the single-blind food challenge is helpful in testing foods about
which the patients or parents have concern and considerable apprehension or anxiety.
In this situation, the food is hidden in another food or capsule. The physician is
aware whether placebo or actual food is being given, but the patient is not. With a
blinded study, signs and symptoms due just to anxiety, for example, feeling warm
and having a fast heart rate and increased respiratory rate, that can also be seen in
an early IgE-mediated reaction can be assessed more easily. It is important not to
telegraph which sample is the food and which is the placebo. If objective symptoms
are part of the history or if the challenge is expected to be negative, particularly if
not influenced by the beliefs of the patients or parents about the food, the single-blind
approach will often clearly implicate or rule out the food in question.

The DBPCFC is the gold standard for the diagnosis of food allergy in both clinical
and research investigations. Subjective symptoms should be challenged in this manner
to eliminate the biases of both the patient and physician. The placebo and test food
are both masked in a food vehicle that the patient tolerates. To control for potential
confounding factors, an equal number of food and placebo challenges are necessary.

A standardized scoring system should be used for the challenges. Challenges of this type are labor intensive and require a clearly delineated stepwise protocol, with the food and placebo prepared and administered by a neutral party.

10.6.1.3   Natural History

In the United States, the most common food allergens in children are egg, milk, peanut, soy, and wheat. About 80% of childhood food allergies develop in the first year of life. Sensitivity to cow's milk, egg, and wheat tends to remit during childhood. For example, most infants who are sensitive to cow's milk lose their sensitivity by age 2 years. Conversely, allergy to peanut, tree nuts, fish, and shellfish tends to persist. Children with food allergy diagnosed after age 3 years are less likely to lose their food sensitivity. Children who develop one food allergy have an increased risk of developing allergies to other foods and inhalant allergens.

Features favorable for a child outgrowing a food allergy include small-to-negative skin test results, 2 years or more without a food reaction, a history of only mild reactions, and few additional atopic diseases. It is not understood why some children outgrow food sensitivity and others do not. A positive skin test result or serum test for food-specific IgE does not necessarily mean that food allergy is persistent, because these tests can remain slightly positive even when the patient is no longer clinically sensitive. A skin test that becomes negative, however, is more likely to be associated with the loss of clinical sensitivity. An oral food challenge is sometimes necessary to prove that food allergy is no longer present. Although it is thought that strict avoidance increases the chance of outgrowing the food allergy and may hasten the process, few studies are available to confirm this.

The most common food sensitivities in adults include peanut, fish, shellfish, and tree nuts, which usually have persisted since childhood. There are no known characteristics for identifying which adults are likely to develop food allergy. The subsequent clinical course of adult-onset food allergy is not as well defined as it is for child-onset food allergy. When food allergy is discovered for the first time in adults, it often is to a food they have not been significantly exposed to previously, such as certain tree nuts or seafoods. Adults with food allergy often maintain the food allergy for life. Food challenges are performed less frequently in adults than in children.

10.6.1.4   Prevention

No specific tests are available to identify persons at risk for food allergy; however, a family history of atopic disease appears to be the best predictor. Food allergy in children born to families with a strong biparental or parental history of atopic disease is approximately fourfold higher than for an unselected patient population. The rate of allergy for a sibling of an affected person is approximately tenfold higher than the rate for the general population. Therefore, a family history of atopy is currently the best screening predictor to identify those at risk for food allergy.

Food allergy is a complex trait influenced by both genetic and environmental factors. Environmental factors that have been identified to influence atopic disease in children, primarily atopic respiratory disease, include a protective effect of breast-feeding and a detrimental effect of exposure to tobacco smoke. Specifically for food allergy, several risk factors have been studied, often with variable or controversial results. These factors have included maternal diet during pregnancy and lactation, breast-feeding in general, age at exposure to solid food, age at exposure to allergenic food, use of hypoallergenic formulas, and use of probiotics. These factors have been studied primarily in infants and children with a family history of atopic disease instead of the population in general.

Overall, the effectiveness of strategies for preventing the development of food allergies has not been established. Studies have suggested a beneficial role for exclusive breast-feeding of infants at high risk for the first 3–6 months of life and the use of hypoallergenic formulas instead of cow's milk or soy formulas if breast-feeding is not possible. Currently, no study has demonstrated conclusively that manipulation of the mother's diet during pregnancy or lactation or the restriction of allergenic foods from the infant's diet prevents the development of food allergy. The Committee on Nutrition of the American Academy of Pediatrics has taken all this into consideration and has presented recommendations for the prevention of food allergy in "at-risk" infants. The committee specified that its statements did not constitute an exclusive recommendation or an absolute standard of medical care. Highlights of the recommendations include the following:

- Breast-feeding mothers should continue breast-feeding for the first year of life or longer.
- Hypoallergenic formulas can be used to supplement breast-feeding.
- While breast-feeding, mothers should eliminate peanut and tree nuts from their diet and consider eliminating eggs, cow's milk, and fish.
- Solid foods should not be introduced into the diet of high-risk infants until 6 months of age, with dairy products delayed until 1 year of age, eggs until 2 years, and peanuts, nuts, and fish until 3 years.
- No maternal dietary restrictions are necessary during pregnancy except possibly peanut avoidance.

These recommendations apply to infants and children with a family history of atopy. There is no evidence to conclusively support the use of hypoallergenic formulas for preventive purposes in healthy infants without a family history of allergic disease.

10.6.2   IgE-Associated–Cell-Mediated Disorders

10.6.2.1   Atopic Dermatitis

Multiple clinical studies have shown that the elimination of food allergens can lead to improvement in skin symptoms and that reintroduction of the food can lead to the redevelopment of symptoms in atopic dermatitis. These studies are particularly relevant for children. The diagnosis of food allergy in atopic dermatitis is complicated by the different manifestations of food sensitivity in atopic dermatitis. The responses to food may be (1) a classic IgE-mediated reaction, (2) pruritus only, or (3) exacerbation of the atopic dermatitis alone, without any other symptoms. Unlike classic IgE-mediated food allergy, the exacerbation of the atopic deramatitis to ingestion of causal foods is delayed, making it difficult to establish an obvious cause and effect on the basis of the history. In addition, other environmental trigger factors such as other allergens, irritants, and infection may contribute to the waxing and waning of the disease, thereby masking the effect of dietary changes. From the testing standpoint, these patients, who may have high circulating IgE levels, can generate IgE to multiple allergens that may not be clinically relevant, creating a higher percentage of false-positive responses to food testing.

Despite these difficulties, identifying specific food sensitivities can significantly improve atopic dermatitis. A general approach is to begin with a complete medical history, with specific attention given to the dietary history and any acute reactions to food ingestion. On the basis of the history and the knowledge that more than 90% of reactions are caused by cow's milk, eggs, peanut, soy, wheat, tree nuts, fish, and shellfish, testing can be conducted for specific IgE antibodies. Food-specific IgE testing can be performed by skin prick testing or in vitro testing specific to IgE antibody.

Skin prick tests are most informative when the results are negative. The negative predictive value is more than 95% for an immediate IgE-mediated reaction. It is anticipated that these foods would be well tolerated. In addition, the skin test–negative foods typically do not exacerbate the atopic dermatitis. However, this is not always true. It is possible for a skin test–negative food to make the atopic dermatitis worse through a cell-mediated mechanism. Currently, atopic food patch testing is being studied as a way of assessing this type of reaction. It is not available clinically. The positive predictive value of skin prick or in vitro food-specific IgE testing is only between 30 and 50%; therefore, a positive test alone cannot be considered diagnostic of food allergy exacerbating the atopic dermatitis. Oral food challenges are helpful in the diagnosis and management in assessing whether the food is worsening the atopic dermatitis. Challenges should not be performed to a food when there is a clear recent or past history of a severe reaction in the setting of a positive IgE-specific antibody to the food. If worsening of the atopic dermatitis is suspected to only a few foods, single-blind or open challenges may be used to test for sensitivity. However, these challenges are subject to observer and patient bias and may overestimate the reactivity. The challenge may need to be performed over a period of a few days because of a delayed response to the food exacerbating the atopic dermatitis. In this situation, a food diary can be helpful. Patients are instructed to keep a record of all foods ingested over a certain period and to list any symptoms, particularly skin symptoms, during that period. This prospective information is not as dependent on the patient's memory when reviewing possible food contributors and can help identify previously unrecognized relations between certain foods and the patient's symptoms.

When a specific food sensitivity is properly diagnosed, the elimination of the offending food allergen should be part of the medical management of atopic dermatitis.

The elimination of food allergens is often difficult, and incomplete elimination of the food can lead to confusion during an open trial or dietary elimination. It is important for the patient to realize that the food protein needs to be avoided completely. This requires reading labels and not just grossly avoiding a particular food. For example, patients with milk allergy must be instructed not only to avoid all milk products but also to read labels to determine whether cow's milk protein is present in a particular product. The terms used on labels may include words that are not easily recognizable, for example, casein, whey, lactalbumin, caramel color, and nougat – all of which indicate the presence of cow's milk protein. Patients must also be made aware that the food protein, and not sugar or fat, is the reason for the allergic reaction. For example, skim milk contains the same milk protein allergens as does whole milk. Foods and ingredients that contain common food allergens are listed in Table 10.7.

Approximately one-third of children with atopic dermatitis and food allergy lose their clinical reactivity over 1–3 years with strict adherence to dietary elimination of the offending food. In this situation, the elimination appears to aid in the faster disappearance of clinical reactivity. Loss of food-specific IgE, shown either by skin prick testing or in vitro testing, lags behind the loss of clinical reactivity. Therefore, for foods to which sensitivity is usually lost over time, such as egg, milk, soy, and wheat, challenges can be considered at various intervals even though skin prick or in vitro testing still show slight positivity.

10.6.2.2 Eosinophilic Gastroenteropathies

Eosinophilic Esophagitis

Eosinophilic esophagitis occurs in children and adults. In healthy subjects, a small number of eosinophils are commonly found in almost all parts of the gastrointestinal tract except the esophagus. The clinical presentation of eosinophilic esophagitis is similar to that of gastroesophageal reflux, but pH probes record normal values and the symptoms are unresponsive to antireflux medications. In children, vomiting, regurgitation, water brash, food impaction, and abdominal pain are the most common symptoms. Older children and adults may also experience heartburn and dysphagia.

The cause of eosinophilic esophagitis is unknown. Several lines of evidence support an allergic cause in that approximately 75% of patients are atopic, the severity of the disease is reversed with the institution of an allergen-free diet, and mast cell degranulation products are found in tissue specimens. Despite the common finding of food-specific IgE in patients with eosinophilic esophagitis, actual anaphylactic responses occur in only a small fraction of patients. It appears that the sensitivity to food in these patients has properties that fall between those of pure IgE-mediated food allergy and cellular-mediated disorders. Initial research studies suggested that evaluation of food protein sensitivity with delayed skin patch testing is better for identifying food sensitivity in eosinophilic esophagitis than skin prick testing alone. Currently, food patch testing is not widely available. The diagnosis of eosinophilic

Table 10.7 Foods and ingredients containing common food allergens

Food allergy to	Avoid foods that contain these ingredients	These may indicate the presence of the food
Egg	Albumin, eggnog, lysozyme, mayonnaise, meringue, surimi	Flavoring, lecithin, macaroni, marzipan, marshmallows, nougat, pasta
Milk	Artificial butter flavor, butter, butter oil, buttermilk, casein, cheese, cream, cottage cheese, curds, custard, ghee, lactoferrin, lactalbumin, lactulose, nougat, pudding, sour cream, whey, yogurt, all forms of milk (condensed, dry, goat, half-and-half low fat, malted, skim)	Caramel candies, chocolate, high protein flour, lactose, margarine
Peanut	Artificial nuts; beer nuts; cold-pressed, expelled, or extruded peanut oil; goobers; mixed nuts; mandelonas; nut meat; peanut butter; peanut flour	African, Asian, and Mexican dishes; baked goods; candy; chili; egg rolls; enchilada sauce; marzipan; nougat
Soy	Edamame, hydrolyzed soy protein, miso, natto, soya, soybean, soy (shoyu) sauce, tamari, tempeh, textured vegetable protein, tofu	Asian cuisine, vegetable broth, vegetable gum, vegetable starch
Wheat	Bran, bread crumbs, bulgur, couscous, cracker meal, durum, farina, flour, gluten, kamut, matzo, pasta, seitan (wheat gluten), semolina, spelt, wheat germ, whole wheat berries	Hydrolyzed protein, soy sauce, starch, surimi
Shellfish	Abalone, clams, cockle, crab, crawfish, lobster, mollusks, mussels, octopus, oysters, prawns, scallops, shrimp, snails, squid	Bouillabasse, cuttlefish ink, fish stock, seafood flavoring, surimi

Data from The Food Allergy & Anaphylaxis Network, Mofidi, S., and Bock, S. A. (2004) A health professional's guide to food challenges. Fairfax (VA): The Food Allergy & Anaphylaxis Network

esophagitis is made by the identification of eosinophilic infiltration in the esophagus of patients who have refluxlike symptoms and who have normal or borderline pH studies and are refractory to acid inhibition. The number of eosinophils in the esophagus required to make the diagnosis has not been clearly established. However, most investigators have found that more than 15 eosinophils per high-power field is consistent with eosinophilic esophagitis.

Several treatment approaches have been evaluated. Investigators have demonstrated prompt clinical and histologic improvement with the use of amino acid-based formulas and strict elemental diets. Oral corticosteroids have produced both resolution of symptoms and near-complete disappearance of esophageal eosinophils. However, on discontinuation of corticosteroid therapy, the majority of patients experience relapse of symptoms within 1 year. Inhaled corticosteroids have been helpful for this condition. Instead of inhaling the corticosteroid into the lungs, the inhaler's spacer is not used and the drug is "swallowed" into the esophagus. Regimens of inhaled fluticasone metered dose inhaler (110–220 µg, four puffs twice daily) have produced clinical improvement. Relapses have been reported after the inhaled corticosteroid has been discontinued. The optimal length of treatment with inhaled corticosteroids has not been determined, and long-term treatment with inhaled corticosteroids may be necessary for some patients.

Dietary modification is the mainstay of treatment for eosinophilic esophagitis for those in whom an offending food is identified. Although corticosteroids produce clinical and histologic improvement, the improvement tends to be short-lived. In comparison, dietary restriction prevents the underlying problem after the offending antigens have been discovered and removed from the diet. Currently, allergy testing is limited primarily to the skin prick and in vitro tests, and in a variable number of patients, the allergen is identified without a strict elimination diet. A reasonable approach is to perform skin prick testing to the common food allergens and to restrict foods that show positive results. Although most patients with eosinophilic esophagitis have allergies to the typical food allergens, many can have multiple food allergies or other sensitivities that do not appear to be IgE mediated but instead represent a delayed cellular response. In these situations, the use of a strict elemental diet will allow the esophagus to heal, after which foods can be added slowly, one at a time, to identify the potential food allergens.

Eosinophilic Gastroenteritis

In contrast to the esophagus, the stomach and intestine normally have readily detectable eosinophils, making the diagnosis of eosinophilic gastroenteritis more complex. Many disorders are associated with eosinophilic infiltration of the stomach and small and large intestines, including parasitic and bacterial infections, inflammatory bowel disease, hypereosinophilic syndrome, myeloproliferative disorders, periarteritis, vasculitis, scleroderma, and drug hypersensitivity. These conditions need to be ruled out before the diagnosis of eosinophilic gastroenteritis can be made.

Eosinophilic gastroenteritis has a constellation of symptoms related to the degree and area of the gastrointestinal tract affected. The mucosal form of eosinophilic gastroenteritis, the most common variant, is characterized by vomiting, abdominal pain, diarrhea, blood loss in stools, iron deficiency anemia, malabsorption, and protein-losing enteropathy. The muscularis form is characterized by infiltration of eosinophils predominantly into the muscularis layer, leading to thickening of the bowel wall and causing symptoms of gastrointestinal obstruction. The serosal form, which occurs in a small fraction of patients, is characterized by exudative ascites, with higher peripheral eosinophil counts than in other forms of the disease.

No standards have been proposed for the diagnosis of eosinophilic gastroenteritis, but the diagnosis is supported by the presence of an increased number of eosinophils in biopsy specimens from the gastrointestinal tract wall, the lack of involvement of other organs, and the exclusion of other causes of eosinophilia. Food allergy and peripheral eosinophilia are not required for diagnosis. Approximately 25% of patients do not have peripheral eosinophilia.

Eliminating the dietary intake of the foods implicated by skin prick testing or in vitro testing has variable effects on the symptoms of eosinophilic gastroenteritis. Examples of strict elimination diets for the common food allergens are given in Table 10.8. Complete resolution is generally achieved with amino acid-based

Table 10.8 Sample meal patterns for a strict diagnostic elimination diet[a]

Pattern 1
Breakfast
  1 cup apple juice or milk substitute fortified with calcium and vitamin D
  1 cup plain, milk-free oatmeal (made with water or milk substitute)
  1–2 tsp sugar or 1 tsp 100% maple syrup
  1/2 cup canned peaches

Lunch
  2–3 ounces broiled pork or lamb chop
  1/2 cup cooked carrots
  1/2 cup canned pears
  1 cup apple juice or milk substitute fortified with calcium and vitamin D

Dinner
  2–3 ounces pan-fried chicken breast (using corn oil)
  1/2 cup milk-free mashed potatoes
  1/2 cup baked butternut squash sprinkled with brown sugar
  1/2 cup canned pears
  1 cup apple juice or milk substitute fortified with calcium and vitamin D

Pattern 2
Breakfast
  1 cup apple juice or milk substitute fortified with calcium and vitamin D
  1/2 cup canned pineapple
  1–2 corn or rice muffins with jelly

Lunch
  2–3 ounces cooked ground turkey patty (using corn oil)
  1/2 cup rice or corn noodles
  1/2 cup cooked carrots
  1/2 cup applesauce
  1 cup apple juice or milk substitute fortified with calcium and vitamin D

Dinner
  2–3 ounces pan-fried pork chop (using corn oil)
  1/2 cup steamed white rice
  1/2 cup cooked spinach
  1/2 cup canned pineapple
  1 cup apple juice or milk substitute fortified with calcium and vitamin D

Pattern 3
Breakfast
  1 cup apple juice or milk substitute fortified with calcium and vitamin D
  2 slices egg-free, milk-free, and wheat-free pan-fried bread with milk-free and soy-free margarine topped with canned fruit or 100% maple syrup
  2–3 slices bacon
  1/2 cup applesauce

(continued)

Table 10.8 (continued)

Lunch
  2–3 ounces cooked ground chicken patty (using corn oil)
  1/2 cup cooked broccoli
  1/2 cup canned pears
  1 cup apple juice or milk substitute fortified with calcium and vitamin D

Dinner
  2–3 ounces pan-fried lamb or pork chop (using corn oil)
  1 baked potato with milk-free and soy-free margarine
  1/2 cup rice or corn noodles
  1/2 cup baked sweet potato fries
  1/2 cup applesauce
  1 cup apple juice or milk substitute fortified with calcium and vitamin D

Snacks
  Trail mix of rice and corn puffs or safe cereals with raisins and dried cranberries
  Milk-free and nut-free rice cakes with grape jelly or homemade peach butter
  Fruit salad made from canned fruits
  Homemade popcorn

[a]This meal pattern eliminates major allergens such as eggs, wheat, milk, soy, fish and shellfish, peanuts, and tree nuts as well as beef. This strict elimination diet should be limited to a 2–4-week period. Modified from The Food Allergy & Anaphylaxis Network, Mofidi, S., and Bock, S. A. (2004) A health professional's guide to food challenges. Fairfax (VA): The Food Allergy & Anaphylaxis Network. Used with permission

elemental diets. Once disease remission has been obtained with dietary modification, specific food groups can be slowly introduced at approximately 3-week intervals. Endoscopy should be performed every 3 months to monitor for disease flare-up or to confirm sustained remission. Several medications used to treat atopic disorders have been used to treat eosinophilic gastroenteritis, including cromolyn, montelukast, and ketotifen, but the results have been disappointing. Systemic or topical corticosteroids are the main therapy for the patients with severe symptoms and lack of improvement despite dietary restriction. For those with disease refractory to corticosteroid therapy, azathioprine or mercaptopurine is an alternative. The overall prognosis of eosinophilic gastroenteritis has not been well documented. It is generally a chronic disorder with intermittent remissions and exacerbations. Because this disease can be a manifestation of another disease process, routine surveillance of the gastrointestinal tract and other organ systems is recommended.

10.6.3 Immunologic-Cell-Mediated (Non-IgE) Disorders

10.6.3.1 Protein-Induced Enterocolitis

Food protein enterocolitis presents in the first months of life and typically resolves by age 2 years but, in rare cases, can persist into childhood. The signs and symptoms include vomiting, diarrhea, lethargy, and dehydration and can progress into those of a severe shocklike state. Compared with IgE-mediated reactions, the onset of symptoms is delayed from 1–10 hours (median, 2 hours) after the ingestion of food. Symptoms typically start with emesis, followed by diarrhea. Cow's milk and soy are the foods most often responsible for protein enterocolitis in infants, but rice, oat, sweet potato, squash, string beans, peas, and poultry have also been reported as causes. The symptoms resolve after appropriate dietary exclusion. A distinct feature of this disease is the delayed onset of dramatic symptoms approximately 2 hours after reintroduction of the causative food.

Essentially all patients with protein enterocolitis have negative skin tests or negative specific IgE in vitro tests to the offending food. The only consistently reported laboratory finding is an increase in peripheral blood neutrophil counts during a positive challenge. Research studies have also shown an alteration in TNF-α levels in the feces. The pathophysiology of protein enterocolitis is not completely understood, but it is thought to be a T-cell mediated disease. Various in vitro studies have shown increased T-cell production of cytokines, particularly IL-5 and interferon-γ, with specific food exposure. This is suggestive of a T-cell driven process, but the exact mechanism is elusive. Jejunal biopsy specimens show patches of flattened villi, edema, and an increased number of lymphocytes, eosinophils, and mast cells.

Treatment consists of avoidance of the causative food allergen. Because of the high rate of cosensitivity to cow's milk and soy, treatment with a hydrolysated formula is recommended and usually effective. If symptoms persist, an amino acid-based formula can be used. Because resolution of the disease must be proved through oral challenges, the evaluation must be undertaken in a controlled setting, usually with intravenous access in place.

10.6.3.2   Protein-Induced Proctitis

Protein-induced proctitis typically presents from 4 days to 4 months after birth (mean age at diagnosis, 2 months). Unlike protein-induced enterocolitis, breast-fed infants may be affected. Signs and symptoms include a well-appearing infant with blood-streaked or bloody stools. The lack of systemic symptoms, vomiting, diarrhea, and growth failure help to differentiate this disorder from other food sensitivities. Cow's milk proteins and, less commonly, soy protein are the common triggers. Laboratory findings may include fecal polymorphonuclear cells or peripheral blood eosinophilia (or both). Allergy skin prick or in vitro IgE food-specific antibodies are negative. Endoscopy shows eosinophilic rectal inflammation. The treatment is avoidance of the causative protein. For breast-fed infants, maternal avoidance of cow's milk is indicated first, followed by avoidance of egg and soy. Formula-fed infants should be switched to a highly hydrolyzed hypoallergenic formula. The symptoms usually clear within several days after dietary manipulation. By 9–12 months of age, infants often tolerate the offending protein. After age 1 year, the causal food protein can be added gradually to the diet, with monitoring for visible blood. No known long-term sequelae have been reported.

10.6.3.3   Protein-Induced Enteropathy

Protein enteropathy occurs during ages 2–18 months. This is characterized by the malabsorption to protein, usually cow's milk, soy, egg, chicken, or fish. Signs and symptoms include anorexia, emesis, diarrhea, and other chronic sequelae of malabsorption (edema and anemia). No cutaneous signs are associated with this condition. Biopsy specimens show flattening of the small intestinal villae, intraepithelial lymphocytes, and few eosinophils. The immune mechanism seems to involve T-cell responses and is not associated with IgE antibodies. Treatment is avoidance of the offending protein, usually by switching to a highly hydrolyzed hypoallergenic formula. This condition usually is outgrown during childhood. No long-term sequelae have been reported.

10.6.3.4   Celiac Disease

Celiac disease is an autoimmune enteropathy induced by gliadin, the alcohol-soluble portion of gluten found in wheat, oat, rye, and barley. It occurs in genetically susceptible persons carrying the HLA-DQ2 or HLA-DQ8 haplotype. Typical symptoms include weight loss, chronic diarrhea, and steatorrhea from malabsorption caused by the extensive gastrointestinal cellular infiltration induced by gliadin. Blood tests helpful in diagnosis include IgA antigliadin and IgA antiendomysial (tissue transglutaminase) antibodies. Diagnosis is confirmed with duodenal biopsy findings that document villous atrophy and cellular infiltrate, which is reversed by the elimination of gliadin from the diet. It is important to note that typical biopsy findings are not found if the patient is following a gluten-free diet. Diagnosis of the disease is critical because removal of gluten from the diet can result in total recovery of gastrointestinal tract function and reversal of histopathologic changes. Skin prick testing to wheat, oat, rye, and barley is not of value in this condition. Life-long elimination of gluten-containing foods is necessary to prevent the recurrence of symptoms.

10.6.3.5   Dermatitis Herpetiformis

Dermatitis herpetiformis is a cutaneous non-IgE-mediated condition characterized by an intensely pruritic, papulovesicular rash distributed symmetrically over the extensor surfaces of the extremities and buttocks. Many, but not all, patients with dermatitis herpetiformis have gluten-sensitive enteropathy. With or without enteropathy, gluten-containing foods are most commonly implicated in exacerbations of dermatitis herpetiformis. Despite this, dermatitis herpetiformis can worsen when patients are taken off an elemental diet, even when gluten-containing foods are avoided. The skin is infiltrated with neutrophils and contains deposits of IgA and C3 that typically accumulate at the dermoepidermal junction. Although the histologic findings can be nonspecific, direct immunofluorescence may be helpful in making the diagnosis. The histologic features of the intestinal lesions are virtually identical to those of celiac disease.

10.6.4   Non-IgE-Nonimmunologic Food Intolerance

Food intolerance is commonly mistaken by the patient for a food allergy. A true intolerance to food occurs without IgE or other immunologic involvement. These reactions represent the most common adverse reactions to food. The mechanism typically involves a metabolic disorder or enzyme deficiency, a pharmacologic response to the food, or a toxin in the food. One of the most common enzyme deficiencies is lactase deficiency. In this condition, the patient is not able to digest lactose present in milk and other dairy products. With the ingestion of these foods, abdominal pain and bloating, excessive flatus, and watery stool develop. There is no associated urticaria or angioedema or cardiopulmonary symptoms. The diagnosis usually can be made on the basis of a careful history supported by dietary manipulation. The diagnosis can also be confirmed by a breath hydrogen or lactose tolerance test. Treatment consists primarily of avoiding lactose-containing foods. For some patients, lactase enzyme supplements may be helpful. Other disorders of this type include phenylketonuria and pancreatic insufficiency.

Patients can have a pharmacologic response to various foods that is sometimes mistaken for an allergy to the food. Foods that most frequently induce a pharmacologic sensitivity include caffeine, alcohol, and vasoactive amines such as tyramine in aged cheese. These types of foods usually cause a response consisting of flushing, headache, and tachycardia.

Toxic contaminants include histamine in scombroid fish poisoning and toxins secreted by *Salmonella*, *Shigella*, and *Campylobacter* in "spoiled" food. These toxins cause nausea, vomiting, and severe diarrhea. Food intolerances can be differentiated from a classic IgE-mediated food allergy by the lack of pruritus, urticaria, angioedema, and bronchospasm. Knowledge of the common foods that cause intolerance and the associated signs and symptoms is helpful in diagnosis.

10.7   Management

The three general approaches to the management of food allergy are avoidance, education, and pharmacotherapy.

Successful avoidance of food allergens depends on the identification of the specific food that caused the reaction, the recognition of cross-reacting allergens in other foods, education about avoidance measures, and the willingness of the patient to read labels carefully and inquire about food ingredients at restaurants and other social gatherings to prevent inadvertent exposure to known or suspected allergens. The consumption of hidden food ingredients is one of the greatest challenges and dangers facing patients with food allergy. Complete elimination of even one food may require extensive education of the patient or the patient's care provider. For example, milk may be labeled as casein, whey, caseinate, or lactalbumin, without the word "milk" being listed. Foods and ingredients that contain common food allergens are listed in Table 10.7.

High-risk environments may need to be investigated closely if the patient is highly allergic and particularly susceptible to airborne food allergens. High-risk environments include common eating places such as school cafeterias, restaurants, and other people's homes. Inquiry should be made into how various dishes are prepared. For example, at an ice cream shop, the use of chopped peanuts in various menu items can result in cross-contamination, depending on the utensils used to prepare the food.

Because elimination diets may lead to malnutrition or other adverse effects, every effort should be made to ensure that the dietary needs of the patient are met. It is important to determine the specific foods to which a patient is allergic because of the consequences of malnutrition or eating disorders if a large number of foods are eliminated from the diet for a long time. Even the elimination of a single food, for example, cow's milk, can lead to deficiencies in protein and calcium in children. Working with a local dietician can provide alternatives to obtain important dietary constituents.

Patients with food allergy, especially children younger than 7 years allergic to eggs, milk, or wheat, should be reevaluated periodically to determine if the child still has the allergy. Establishing the loss of food allergy relieves the burden of avoidance on the patients and parents.

Monitoring of skin prick testing and food-specific IgE antibody levels may be helpful in determining the time that would be appropriate for food challenge or reintroduction of the food (or both). However, because peanut, tree nuts, fish, and shellfish are more likely to persist throughout the patient's life, frequent monitoring (yearly) of specific IgE reactivity or antibody levels is not helpful. These can be tested every 3–4 years throughout childhood, depending on the clinical circumstances.

Inadvertent ingestion of a food by a person who knows that he or she is allergic to that food is not uncommon. Studies have shown that patients allergic to peanuts have a 35–50% chance of unintentional ingestion during a 3–4-year period. Patients also may experience a severe reaction after exposure to a food that previously produced only a mild reaction that caused them to think the food may have been safe. The reactions, or lack thereof, to inadvertent ingestions of the food causing allergy provides important information for determining whether a food allergy still exists.

The pharmacotherapy of food allergy consists primarily of emergency treatment of the allergic reaction. As for anaphylactic reactions in general, epinephrine is the treatment of choice for food-induced anaphylaxis. Injectable epinephrine and instructions on its use should be given to all patients who have had an immediate systemic IgE-mediated reaction to a food. Epinephrine should be administered immediately in the treatment of an anaphylactic reaction. In addition, the patient should be counseled to seek medical care immediately if he or she develops a systemic reaction to a food. The patient should not only inject the epinephrine and observe but also seek acute medical treatment.

New therapies for IgE-mediated food allergy have been studied. Subcutaneous injections of anti-IgE antibodies (TNX-901) for long-term prophylactic treatment of patients older than 12 years with peanut allergy have shown an increase in the average amount of peanut tolerated from approximately 1/2 peanut to 9 peanuts before a reaction occurred. Of the group, however, 25% showed no improvement. This treatment is not a cure for food allergy, but rather a way to increase slightly the amount of peanut a patient is able to tolerate. Clearly, this does not give a patient license to eat peanuts, but it possibly may provide more protection after the inadvertent ingestion of a small amount of peanut. The use of anti-IgE antibodies has not been studied in other food allergies. Studies have not been performed with the only anti-IgE antibody, omalizumab, currently available commercially. Future studies include the use of engineered proteins that lack IgE binding sites but can induce tolerance, either given alone or with coadministration of Th1-promoting adjuvants. Peptide immunotherapy, mutated protein immunotherapy, and DNA immunization all strive to decrease the deleterious Th2 response and subsequent IgE production and to promote the development of oral tolerance.

Various medications can provide relief for certain aspects of food-induced disorders. Antihistamines may partially relieve symptoms of oral allergy syndrome and mild IgE-mediated skin symptoms. Corticosteroids are helpful in eosinophilic esophagitis and eosinophilic gastroenteritis. It is important to note that medications taken before food is ingested will not protect patients from anaphylactic reactions to foods. Antihistamines, cromolyn, and corticosteroids are not effective in preventing the development of anaphylaxis. Currently, avoidance of the causative food is the only complete treatment. An excellent resource to help the patient in numerous aspects of practical food avoidance strategies is the Food Allergy & Anaphylaxis Network (11781 Lee Jackson Hwy., Suite 160, Fairfax, VA 22033–3309, www.foodallergy.org).

10.8 Food Additive Reactions

Despite the large number of food additives used by the food industry, only a small number have been implicated in IgE or other adverse food reactions. Food additives include antioxidants, flavoring and coloring substances, preservatives, and sweeteners, among others. The majority of reported adverse reactions to additives have been anecdotal and without well-controlled challenge procedures. Compared with the prevalence of additives, adverse reactions are exceedingly rare.

Patients with sensitivity to an additive tend to exhibit adverse reactions to foods or beverages that are inconsistent, in that on one occasion they may experience an adverse reaction to the food, yet at other times may tolerate the food without any problem. This is due to ingesting, on one occasion, the food item with the additives and then, on another occasion, ingesting the food item without the additives. An example is the ingestion of fresh fruit versus a dried fruit product.

Common Food Dye and Coloring (FD&C)–approved dyes include tartrazine (FD&C yellow #5), ponceau (FD&C red #4), brilliant blue (FD&C blue #1), erythrosine (FD&C red #3), and indigotine (FD&C blue #2). The use of FD&C–approved dyes is ubiquitous in foods and beverages. Although several dyes have been reported to cause anaphylaxis, urticaria or angioedema, or bronchospasm, the prevalence of reactions is unknown because of the lack of properly controlled studies. Of the dyes, tartrazine has been studied most, and it appears that worsening of asthma in association with tartrazine sensitivity is exceedingly rare. Also, although suspicion has been raised about tartrazine sensitivity in aspirin-sensitive patients, there does not appear to be any cross-reaction of tartrazine with cyclooxygenase-inhibiting drugs or to be any reason why tartrazine should be avoided by aspirin-sensitive patients with asthma.

Monosodium glutamate (MSG) is a dicarboxylic amino acid flavor enhancer used primarily in Asian foods. Various symptoms have been associated with MSG, including myalgia, headache, flushing, neck pain, and chest heaviness, which have been labeled the "MSG symptom complex" or "Chinese restaurant syndrome." The pathophysiology of this type of reaction is unclear. MSG has also been associated with urticaria and provocation of asthma; however, blinded, placebo-controlled challenges have not confirmed these associations.

Sulfites have been used for centuries to freshen and prevent browning of foods. Common sulfating agents include sulfur dioxide, sodium or potassium sulfite, bisulfites, and metabisulfites. High levels of sulfites are found in dried fruits, potatoes, wine, seafood, and restaurant salad bars. In double-blind, controlled studies, sulfites have clearly been shown to cause a significant and potentially life-threatening asthmatic reaction. The incidence of sulfite-sensitive asthma is unknown, but investigators have suggested that as many as 5% of the asthmatic population may experience an asthma exacerbation ranging from mild to potentially life-threatening. The mechanism of sulfite sensitivity is not fully understood. Some patients have shown positive skin test results to sulfites, implicating an IgE-mediated mechanism, but whether this is truly the case is not clear. In addition to asthmatic exacerbations, there are isolated case reports of urticaria or angioedema in nonasthmatic patients after sulfite ingestion. However, controlled studies and challenges have not been confirmatory.

The other primary artificial additives reported in the literature associated with reactions include butylated hydroxyanisole and butylated hydroxytoluene (antioxidants used in breakfast cereals and other grain products), nitrates and nitrites (preservatives used in processed meats), and aspartame (NutraSweet), an artificial sweetener. Isolated case reports have described allergic-type symptoms with these products, but confirmatory studies have not been performed.

Natural food additives, including annatto, carmine, saffron, and erythritol, have rarely been reported as causes of anaphylaxis. These natural color additives are derived from plant and animal sources, in contrast to the additives that are chemically synthesized. Annatto is a natural yellow food coloring used in cereal, cheese, ice cream, popcorn, margarine, and beverages. Carmine is the natural dark red food dye used in candy, ice cream, cookies, syrups, liqueurs, and jam. Saffron is collected from the flower *Crocus sativus*. It is used as a spice and also as coloring in soups, rice dishes, sauces, cakes, and liqueurs. Erythritol is prepared from glucose by fermentation and is used as a sweetener; it may occur naturally in wine, beer, soy, cheese, and mushrooms. Reactions to these additives appear to be exceedingly rare but occasional case reports have been published.

10.9   Summary

Adverse reactions to foods have been reported in up to 25% of the population at some point in their lives, with the highest prevalence in infancy and early childhood. Although adverse reactions to foods are common, food allergy, an IgE-mediated reaction to a food, represents only a small percentage of all adverse reactions to food. Reactions to foods can be placed into the following groups on the basis of clinical presentation and pathophysiologic mechanism: (1) IgE-mediated disorders, (2) IgE-associated-cell-mediated disorders, (3) immunologic-cell-mediated (non-IgE) disorders, and (4) non-IgE-nonimmunologic food intolerance. A detailed medical history, review of systems, and physical examination help place the reaction into one of these categories. Food-specific allergen skin prick testing and in vitro IgE food-specific allergen testing are the primary methods for confirming or ruling out the diagnosis. In situations where cause and effect are not clear, food challenges can be performed. They should be performed only after a careful risk assessment has been made and by clinicians with the knowledge and equipment to treat a severe anaphylactic reaction. After a food allergy has been confirmed, patient education is essential. Patient education should include information about foods and ingredients that may contain the food allergen, foods that may cross-react with the food allergen, and emergency treatment for a food reaction, including the use of injectable epinephrine. Currently, no specific treatment is available for preventing food allergy. Future treatments may include peptide immunotherapy and DNA immunization.

10.10   Clinical Vignettes

10.10.1   Vignette 1

A 24-year-old man presents for allergy evaluation after an "allergic reaction" that occurred 1 week earlier while he was eating at a restaurant. He reports that while eating dinner with friends he developed a sensation of itchiness of the mouth, followed by pruritus throughout his body, hives, and wheezing. He also noted abdominal cramping but no diarrhea or vomiting. He did not have syncope. He was taken to the emergency department, where he was treated immediately with epinephrine and diphenhydramine, after which his symptoms resolved in a few hours. The symptoms have not recurred since that episode. He has no previous history of food allergy or similar symptoms.

Comment: The signs and symptoms are consistent with an IgE-mediated reaction. Because the reaction occurred in a restaurant, food sensitivity seems likely. It is important, however, to remember other variables. Important questions at this time include finding out what he did before he ate at the restaurant, whether he had taken any medications that day, the contents of his meal and beverage at the restaurant, and whether anyone else at the table or the restaurant had similar symptoms.

Additional history documented that before he ate at the restaurant, he had not done anything out of the ordinary; he had been at work, where he is an accountant. He was not taking any medications and had not taken any nonprescription medications. No one else at his table or at the restaurant had become ill. His meal consisted of bread, a seafood casserole, and diet soft drink.

Comment: No other activity was suspicious for having a role in the reaction. Nonsteroidal anti-inflammatory medications can sometimes cause an allergic reaction or predispose to a food reaction. Food poisoning seems unlikely because wheezing was also part of his symptom complex and no other person at the restaurant became ill. Knowledge of the actual components of the seafood casserole would be helpful at this time. Also, it is important to inquire about how it was prepared and if there could be any contamination by other foods made similarly with the same utensils.

After discussion with the restaurant, it was discovered that the seafood casserole contained shrimp, scallops, rice, tomato sauce, cream sauce, salt, and pepper. The shrimp casserole was prepared in the same area as other seafood dishes, including lobster, crab, and clam. The patient recalled eating crab and shrimp in the past without difficulty, but was not sure whether he had ever ingested scallops, lobster, or clam.

Comment: On the basis of the general epidemiology of food allergy, seafood is the most likely culprit. Often in adults, an allergic food reaction is due to a food that has been eaten only rarely or one to which they have been cross-sensitized. In this situation, further evaluation with an allergen skin prick test to the shrimp, scallops, lobster, crab, and clam should help identify the food allergen.

Allergen skin prick testing showed an 8 × 8-mm wheal with flare to scallops. The rest of the skin test results were negative.

Comment: On the basis of his history and skin test results, scallops are the cause of his allergic reaction. Scallops should be avoided in the future. The patient was prescribed and instructed on the proper procedure for administration of injectable epinephrine. He was educated about food allergen avoidance. In this situation it would include avoidance of scallops and other shellfish, particularly mollusks.

10.10.2 Vignette 2

A 20-year-old man with a history of allergic rhinitis and mild intermittent asthma presents with worsening gastrointestinal symptoms. He reports that over the past 4 years he has had increasing dysphagia manifested by the sense of food "getting stuck" in his esophagus, causing him to vomit up the food to dislodge it. This occurs approximately every 3 weeks. The patient does not correlate this episodic dysphagia with any particular food except possibly rice. With these episodes, he has not had pruritus, hives, breathing difficulties, or diarrhea. He has had previous trials of H$_2$ blockers and proton pump inhibitors but without any significant change in his symptoms. In between these episodes, he has felt well and has not had persistent gastrointestinal symptoms.

Comment: The patient's symptoms are not typical for a classic IgE-mediated reaction because there does not seem to be a specific food involved and the symptoms are not typical of histamine release. Gastroesophageal reflux is a consideration, but the lack of response to H$_2$ blockers and proton pump inhibitors make this less likely. Because dysphagia is the primary symptom, further evaluation with imaging of the esophagus is appropriate.

The patient underwent esophagogastroduodenoscopy. The proximal and mid portions of the esophagus appeared normal. In the distal esophagus, the Z-line demonstrated a slight nodularity that was nonspecific, and biopsy was performed. The stomach, duodenal bulb, and second portion of the duodenum appeared normal. The biopsy specimen showed hyperplastic squamous esophageal mucosa with many intraepithelial eosinophils (80 cells per high-power field).

Comment: This atopic patient has findings consistent with eosinophilic esophagitis. Because specific foods appear to have a pathogenic role in a subset of patients with this condition, evaluation with skin prick testing to commonly ingested foods may provide additional information. Except possibly rice, no other specific food was suspected on the basis of the history.

Skin prick tests were performed to commonly ingested foods. A positive response was found to rice, potato, corn, and egg. On further questioning the patient reports he eats potatoes nearly every other day and egg and corn or corn products about twice a week. The patient does not recall any correlation between potato, corn, or egg ingestion and the dysphagic episodes.

Comment: Even without any clear clinical correlation between all the skin test–positive foods and the episodic dysphagia, it was recommended that the patient eliminate rice, egg, corn, and potato from his diet because of the potential for these foods to contribute to eosinophilic esophagitis. Treatment was commenced with swallowed fluticasone, 220 µg four puffs twice daily for 6 weeks.

Two months later, the patient was asymptomatic.

Comment: At this point, the foods can be reintroduced singly, with the patient monitoring for any recurrence of dysphagia. Because of the possible clinical correlation and the positive skin test, rice should be the last food to be reintroduced.

10.10.3   Vignette 3

A 6-year-old girl presents for further evaluation of food allergy. At age 8 months, she developed lip swelling and hives, primarily involving the face and neck, with the ingestion of scrambled eggs. Also, approximately 1 month later with ingestion of peanut butter, hives and cough developed immediately. Skin testing at that time was markedly positive to egg and peanut, with a 7 × 7-mm wheal with erythema and an 8 × 9-mm wheal with erythema, respectively. Since that time, the parents have been avoiding egg and peanut in the girl's diet. At age 2 years, an inadvertent exposure to egg resulted in some rash on the face. The child or parents are not aware of any further exposure to egg or peanut. The child has a history, as an infant, of mild eczema, that is currently quiescent. For the past 2 years, she has had symptoms of rhinitis in the spring. There is no history of asthma. Both parents have a history of seasonal allergic rhinitis and mild asthma.

Comment: The type of reaction described at 8 months of age is consistent with an IgE-mediated reaction to egg and peanut. The positive skin tests at that time are consistent with her reaction. She also has had an underlying eczema (atopic dermatitis) and has subsequently developed probable allergic rhinitis, which is common in atopic youth. The primary question now is whether the child has outgrown her food allergies. There have not been enough inadvertent exposures to assess this from the clinical history. Knowing that nearly all children lose egg sensitivity but approximately only 20% lose peanut sensitivity is important. To evaluate further, skin prick testing can be performed to peanut and egg.

Skin prick testing to peanut was markedly positive, with an 8 × 8-mm wheal with surrounding erythema. Skin prick testing to egg was slightly positive, with a 3 × 3-mm wheal with slight erythema.

Comment: The strongly positive skin test to peanut implies a persistent sensitivity to peanut, and strict peanut avoidance should continue to be enforced. The slightly positive response to egg is more difficult to interpret. It is known that the majority of children outgrow egg sensitivity and that positive, especially slightly positive, food skin prick tests can persist after clinical sensitivity is lost. To evaluate further, egg-specific IgE in vitro testing can be performed.

The result of egg-specific IgE in vitro testing was <0.35 kU L^{-1}.

Comment: In this setting of a low clinical likelihood of reactivity based on the type of food involved, a minimally positive skin test, and a low egg-specific IgE in vitro test, the chance of reaction with egg ingestion is low. In this situation, an open challenge under medical supervision can be performed to determine the safety of egg ingestion.

An open food challenge was performed in the clinic, with emergency resuscitation immediately available. The child tolerated initial minute doses of egg, followed by doubling the amounts of egg every 20 min until an entire egg was able to be ingested. During the challenge, no symptoms occurred.

Comment: The patient tolerated the food challenge without a reaction; therefore, egg can be added back to her diet. Peanut, however, still needs to be strictly avoided. Retesting with skin prick testing or in vitro peanut-specific IgE should be considered in 2–3 years.

10.10.4   Vignette 4

A 42-year-old African American woman presents with a concern about food allergy. She notes that after eating she has symptoms of nausea, abdominal cramping, bloating, and diarrhea. The symptoms last 30 min and then resolve. The symptoms have been present for 3 months and occur 5–6 times a week, always during or immediately after she eats. She has not had any previous history of food allergy or gastrointestinal symptoms. Otherwise, she has felt well and has not had any weight loss, hematochezia, or fatigue.

Comment: The gastrointestinal symptoms described can occur with food allergy but also with a large number of gastrointestinal disorders. In these situations, it is extremely important to check for signs of histamine release involving other organ systems (especially skin and lung) and also to carefully review her diet, inquiring about the type of food she has eaten when the symptoms occur and the type of food eaten when the symptoms do not occur.

Upon detailed questioning, the patient reports that she has not experienced pruritus, hives, angioedema, skin rash, sensation of throat closure, cough, wheeze, shortness of breath, light-headedness, or fast heart rate in association with the gastrointestinal symptoms. Her diet was reviewed in detail in relation to her symptoms. She had not made any marked changes to her diet during the previous 3 years. The symptoms have occurred both when she eats in a restaurant and when she eats at home. She reported that she never seemed to have symptoms during or after breakfast. The symptoms typically occur during or after lunch or dinner. Her breakfast typically consists of plain coffee, a donut or roll, and occasionally a piece of fruit. Lunch typically consists of either some type of sandwich, often turkey or roast beef, or a green salad with dressing. She frequently has chicken, pasta, roast beef, potatoes, green vegetables, or fish for dinner. She has not been able to correlate her symptoms with any specific foods.

Comment: Patients frequently think that any symptom associated with food ingestion must be a food allergy, but often this is not true. Her symptoms are confined to the gastrointestinal tract. The lack of other signs or symptoms of histamine release with food ingestion makes classic IgE-mediated food allergy less likely. Also, her inability to associate the symptoms with a particular food type makes IgE-mediated food allergy less likely. In a 42-year-old person without previous history of food allergy, the development of multiple food allergies would be highly unusual.

The diet history obtained is very general. Obtaining an accurate dietary history can be difficult because of the variety of foods in the diet. It is helpful to break this down by meals and to include beverages, foods, and supplements. The list needs to be comprehensive because any food has the potential to cause a reaction. Because it is often difficult to accurately detail the diet by history, patients frequently will need to start a food diary. The food diary, a comprehensive list of all foods ingested, needs to be completed after each meal, with a comment about whether any signs or symptoms occurred. In classic IgE-mediated food allergy, symptoms should occur each time the food allergen is ingested. Therefore, the process of finding foods tolerated without a reaction are as important for finding the culprit as foods ingested in association with the reaction. The food diary can be used as a tool to help find the causative food. Classically, the food is included on the list at the times the symptoms occur and not on the list of tolerated foods. At this point, because the likelihood of an actual IgE-mediated food allergy is low and no foods are suspected on the basis of the history, allergen skin prick testing or in vitro testing to foods is not indicated.

The patient kept a strict food diary for 1 week. When she reviewed the food diary, she noted that her symptoms occurred primarily with the ingestion of milk, yogurt, and ice cream. The most prominent symptoms were associated with a large consumption of dairy products.

Comment: The patient noted the association of symptoms with the consumption of dairy products. Although IgE-mediated food allergy to milk allergens is still a consideration, her gastrointestinal symptoms are more likely due to a nonimmunologic cause. Because dairy products appear to be the main problem, lactose intolerance is a consideration. If no food associations were noted, other gastrointestinal disorders, including irritable bowel syndrome and malabsorption syndromes, would need to be considered. Lactose deficiency can be assessed with the lactose tolerance test or hydrogen breath test.

The hydrogen breath test showed increased levels of hydrogen in the breath, indicating improper digestion of lactose.

Comment: The patient has lactose deficiency, which is most common among African Americans, Native Americans, and Asian Americans. It is least common among people of northern European descent. The symptoms can be controlled through diet. The extent to which the diet needs to be modified depends on how much lactose a person's body can handle. Lactose-reduced milk and other products are available at most supermarkets.

10.10.5   *Vignette 5*

A 4-year-old boy with moderate-severe atopic dermatitis continues to have prominent flares of skin disease despite intensive medical treatment. The question has been raised about whether food exacerbates the atopic dermatitis.

Comment: Details about the type of skin reactions he has been having should be sought. Three patterns of skin reactions occur in patients with atopic dermatitis with food challenge. The first pattern is an immediate IgE-mediated response, such as urticaria, angioedema, and erythema, that occurs within minutes after ingestion of the food, but without an exacerbation of the atopic dermatitis. In the second pattern, pruritus occurs soon after the food is ingested, with subsequent scratching and worsening of the underlying atopic dermatitis. In the third pattern, exacerbations of atopic dermatitis alone occur 6–48 hours after food ingestion.

Upon further questioning, the mother has not noticed skin changes suggestive of urticaria or angioedema and thinks the flares consist primarily of worsening of the underlying atopic dermatitis. She believes that the skin condition improved some-what when milk was eliminated from the diet, but because of the variability in the activity of the atopic dermatitis, it is difficult for her to know this with certainty.

Comment: The patient does not have episodes of urticaria or angioedema. If these were present, an IgE-mediated food allergy would be likely. It is estimated that

30–50% of children with atopic dermatitis have IgE-mediated food allergy. What is unclear is the percentage of children with atopic dermatitis whose atopic dermatitis is made worse with ingestion of a specific food. Estimates of food sensitivity affecting the underlying atopic dermatitis range from 25–50%. No reliable markers are available for identifying foods that contribute only to the worsening of atopic dermatitis. Because the mechanism for worsening atopic dermatitis likely is not purely IgE mediated, skin prick and in vitro IgE food testing will not identify all possible contributing foods. These tests may help identify foods that contribute to pruritus and immediate urticaria and angioedema but may not be helpful in identifying strictly those that worsen the underlying atopic dermatitis. Interestingly, skin test-negative foods are typically tolerated and do not appear to worsen atopic dermatitis. Because of the high levels of circulating IgE in patients with atopic dermatitis, multiple food tests can have false-positive results. To discover foods that worsen atopic dermatitis, additional diagnostic maneuvers are often required, including elimination diets and oral food challenges. Food patch testing is being studied for this situation. The most common contributing foods to worsening of atopic dermatitis in children are eggs, cow's milk, wheat, and soy.

The patient underwent allergen skin prick testing to a small panel of commonly ingested food allergens. Positive responses were noted to milk, egg, and wheat. Testing was negative to chicken, peanut, soy, tree nuts, and fish.

Comment: This information may be helpful as a starting point. It is difficult to know with certainty whether the foods producing positive skin tests contribute to the boy's atopic dermatitis by causing an increase in pruritus or if the test results are false positive. Considerations at this time include eliminating milk, egg, and wheat from the diet for 2–3 weeks to determine if the atopic dermatitis changes. If there is improvement, the foods can be added back singly, one food every 2 weeks, while monitoring for recurrence.

The atopic dermatitis improved notably with elimination of wheat, milk, and egg. Wheat was added back to the diet without any change in the atopic dermatitis. However, with reintroduction of the milk, the atopic dermatitis worsened. Milk was again discontinued. The same type of response was seen with egg.

Comment: It appears that milk and egg worsen the underlying atopic dermatitis. For the time being, they should be avoided. Also, foods that contain milk and egg should be avoided. Consultation with a dietician is advisable to discuss ways to maintain good nutrition without milk and egg. Because the foods have been associated only with a worsening of the atopic dermatitis, rechallenge can be performed in the future to these one at a time, initially in a controlled setting.

Suggested Reading

Agne, P. S., Bidat, E., Rance, F., and Paty, E. (2004) Sesame seed allergy in children. Allerg. Immunol. (Paris) 36, 300–305

Bischoff, S. and Crowe, S. E. (2005) Gastrointestinal food allergy: new insights into pathophysiology and clinical perspectives. Gastroenterology 128, 1089–1113

Bock, S. A., Sampson, H. A., Atkins, F. M., et al. (1988) Double-blind, placebo-controlled food challenge (DBPCFC) as an office procedure: a manual. J. Allergy Clin. Immunol. 82, 986–997

Chapman, J. A., Bernstein, I. L., Lee, R. E., et al, American Academy of Allergy, Asthma and Immunology, American College of Allergy, Asthma and Immunology. (2006) Food allergy: a practice parameter. Ann. Allergy Asthma Immunol. 96(Suppl. 2), S1–S68

Committee on Nutrition. American Academy of Pediatrics. (2000) Hypoallergenic infant formulas. Pediatrics 106, 346–349

The Food Allergy & Anaphylaxis Network, Mofidi, S., and Bock, S. A. (2004) A health professional's guide to food challenges. Fairfax (VA): The Food Allergy & Anaphylaxis Network

The Food Allergy & Anaphylaxis Network (2006) Available from http://www.foodallergy.org/. Accessed July 24, 2007

Leung, D. Y., Sampson, H. A., Yunginger, J. W., et al. (2003) Effect of anti-IgE therapy in patients with peanut allergy. N. Engl. J. Med. 348, 986–993

Perry, T. T., Matsui, E. C., Conover-Walker, M. K., and Wood, R. A. (2004) Risk of oral food challenges. J. Allergy Clin. Immunol. 114, 1164–1168

Perry, T. T., Matsui, E. C., Conover-Walker, M. K., and Wood, R. A. (2004) The relationship of allergen-specific IgE levels and oral food challenge outcome. J. Allergy Clin. Immunol. 114, 144–149

Rothenberg, M. E. (2004) Eosinophilic gastrointestinal disorders (EGID). J. Allergy Clin. Immunol. 113, 11–28

Sampson, H. A. (2001) Utility of food-specific IgE concentrations in predicting symptomatic food allergy. J. Allergy Clin. Immunol. 107, 891–896

Sampson, H. A. (2004) Update on food allergy. J. Allergy Clin. Immunol. 113, 805–819

Sicherer, S. H. (2002) Food allergy. Lancet 360, 701–710

Sicherer, S. H. (2005) Food protein-induced enterocolitis syndrome: case presentations and management lessons. J. Allergy Clin. Immunol. 115, 149–156

Sicherer, S. H., Eigenmann, P. A., and Sampson, H. A. (1998) Clinical features of food protein-induced enterocolitis syndrome. J. Pediatr. 133, 214–219

Sicherer, S. H. and Sampson, H. A. (2006) 9. Food allergy. J. Allergy Clin. Immunol. 117(Suppl. Mini-Primer), S470–S475

Simon, R. A. (1996) Adverse reactions to food and drug additives. Immunol. Allergy Clin. N. Am. 16, 137–176

Spergel, J. M., Beausoleil, J. L., Mascarenhas, M., and Liacouras, C. A. (2002) The use of skin prick tests and patch tests to identify causative foods in eosinophilic esophagitis. J. Allergy Clin. Immunol. 109, 363–368

Sporik, R., Hill, D. J., and Hosking, C. S. (2000) Specificity of allergen skin testing in predicting positive open food challenges to milk, egg and peanut in children. Clin. Exp. Allergy 30, 1540–1546

Chapter 11
Anaphylaxis and Anaphylactoid Reactions

Abbreviations 5-HIAA: 5-hydroxyindoleacetic acid; MSG: monosodium glutamate; NSAID: nonsteroidal anti-inflammatory drug.

11.1   Definition and Epidemiology

The term *anaphylaxis* was first used in 1902 by Portier and Richet to describe the reaction that occurred while they attempted to immunize dogs to a sea anemone toxin. Instead of providing prophylaxis, the injection induced a fatal hypersensitivity reaction, labeled *anaphylaxis*, the opposite of *prophylaxis*. Anaphylaxis is a systemic hypersensitivity reaction caused by IgE-mediated immunologic release of mediators from mast cells and basophils. The release of preformed mediators such as histamine and newly formed mediators such as prostaglandins and leukotrienes increases vascular permeability, mucus secretion, vascular smooth muscle relaxation, and constriction of respiratory smooth muscle, leading to the clinical manifestations of anaphylaxis. Anaphylactoid or pseudoallergic reactions are similar to anaphylaxis; however, they are not mediated by an antigen–IgE antibody interaction. This type of reaction results from antigen acting directly on mast cells and basophils, with subsequent release of mediators, or acting on other cascades such as anaphylatoxins of the complement system or prostaglandins and leukotrienes from arachidonic acid metabolism. These reactions have the same systemic manifestations as anaphylaxis.

Anaphylaxis causes approximately 500–1,000 fatalities per year in the United States. However, the true incidence is difficult to determine because of underdiagnosis and underreporting. For these same reasons, it is also difficult to determine the incidence of nonfatal anaphylaxis. In population-based studies, the overall incidence of anaphylaxis was 8.4 cases per 100,000 person-years in the United Kingdom and 21 cases per 100,000 person-years in the United States. Hospitalized patients are at increased risk for anaphylaxis compared with the general population. It has been estimated that in-hospital anaphylaxis occurs in approximately 1 of every 5,100 admissions.

Food appears to be the most frequent cause of anaphylaxis, surpassing antibiotics. In general, a cause is suspected and confirmed in two-thirds of cases of anaphylaxis and is unclear or idiopathic in the other one-third.

G.W. Volcheck, *Clinical Allergy: Diagnosis and Management*   433
DOI: 10.1007/978-1-59745-315-8_11, © 2009 Mayo Foundation for Medical
Education and Research

11.2 Pathophysiology

Classic anaphylaxis occurs when an allergen combines with a specific IgE antibody bound to the surface membranes of mast cells and basophils and activates these cells, resulting in the rapid release of preformed granular constituents and the generation of newly formed mediators. Mast cells occur in the epithelia of the upper and lower respiratory tracts and in the bronchial lumen, central nervous system, peripheral nerves, gastrointestinal tract mucosa, bone marrow, connective tissue adjacent to blood vessels, and skin. They do not circulate in the blood. Basophils, however, constitute 0.1–2.0% of the peripheral blood leukocytes and are rarely found in tissues except in disease states.

The primary preformed mediator released from mast cells and basophils is histamine. Histamine binds to H_1 and H_2 receptors in several organ systems. The primary effect of histamine on the vasculature is vasodilation, which results in flushing, decreased peripheral resistance, and, subsequently, hypotension. Histamine also increases vascular permeability, which can produce a rapid loss of intravascular volume. Fluid shifted to the extravascular space can result in a 50% loss of vascular volume within 10 minutes. Cardiac effects of histamine include increased heart rate and coronary artery vasospasm. The smooth muscle in the bronchial tree and gastrointestinal system contracts in response to histamine. These effects produce the signs and symptoms of wheeze, nausea, vomiting, abdominal cramping, and diarrhea. The release of histamine in the skin can cause pruritus, urticaria, erythema, or angioedema. In an anaphylactic reaction, histamine-induced signs and symptoms include any combination of urticaria, angioedema, flush, wheeze, dyspnea, nausea, vomiting, diarrhea, syncope, and hypotension, depending on the severity and the extent of the organ systems involved.

Other mast cell preformed mediators include neutral proteases (such as tryptase, chymase, and carboxypeptidase), acid hydroxylase, oxidative enzymes, chemotactic factors for eosinophils and neutrophils, and heparin. These mediators also contribute to the signs and symptoms of anaphylaxis. Tryptase has kallikrein activity and can activate the complement cascade and cleave fibrinogen. Heparin is an anticoagulant and a complement inhibitor and modulates tryptase activity. The mediators generated and released from mast cell membranes by arachidonic acid metabolism include prostaglandin D_2; leukotrienes B_4, C_4, and E_4; and platelet-activating factor. Prostaglandin D_2 is the predominant cyclooxygenase product generated by mast cells. It is a potent vasodilator and induces contraction of intestinal and pulmonary smooth muscle. Leukotrienes are produced by the activity of lipoxygenase on arachidonic acid. They contribute to bronchoconstriction, mucus secretion, and changes in vascular permeability.

Other inflammatory pathways are activated in anaphylaxis. The kinin system can be activated by kallikrein and tryptase. Activation of the kinin system results in the production of bradykinin at the endothelial cell level. Bradykinin causes vasodilation and increases vascular permeability. Multiple chemotactic factors are released and recruit and activate leukocytes. Among the leukocytes, eosinophils and neutrophils appear to have a significant role in prolonging and intensifying reactions through the release of toxic metabolites. They also likely have a role in the late-phase anaphylactic reaction.

The role of nitric oxide in anaphylaxis has been studied in detail. The synthesis of nitric oxide is induced by histamine, platelet-activating factor, leukotrienes, and bradykinin. Nitric oxide appears to have both deleterious and beneficial effects in anaphylaxis. It contributes to hypotension through two mechanisms: (1) relaxation of vascular smooth muscle, resulting in vasodilation, and (2) increase in vascular permeability, resulting in loss of intravascular volume. However, nitric oxide also relaxes bronchial smooth muscle, which helps prevent bronchoconstriction.

Anaphylactoid reactions are not mediated by an IgE antibody; instead, they are induced by substances that act directly on mast cells and basophils to cause the release of preformed mediators and the formation of new mediators, as in IgE-mediated anaphylaxis. Anaphylactoid reactions are due primarily to drugs, particularly radio-contrast media and opiates, and physical factors. Most cases of idiopathic anaphylaxis likely have an anaphylactoid pathogenesis.

Overall, anaphylactic and anaphylactoid events result from the release and synthesis of multiple mediators by mast cells and basophils, together with the involvement of leukocytes and their products, the complement cascade, the coagulation pathway, and the kinin system (Fig. 11.1).

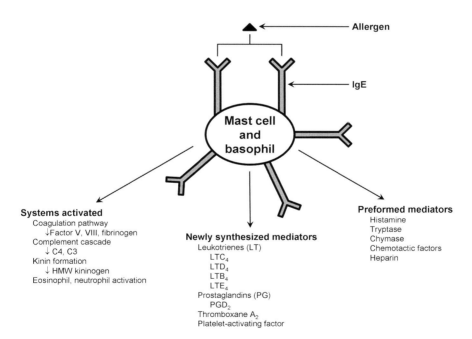

Fig. 11.1 Summary of the major systems and mediators activated in anaphylaxis. *HMW* high-molecular weight

11.3 History and Physical Examination

There is no universally accepted clinical definition of anaphylaxis. Although anaphylaxis (IgE-mediated) and anaphylactoid reactions (non-IgE-mediated) differ mechanistically, the clinical presentations are identical. The manifestations of anaphylaxis can vary depending on the severity of the reaction. The typical history contains any combination of urticaria, angioedema, flushing, pruritus, upper airway tract obstruction, lower airway tract obstruction, diarrhea, nausea, vomiting, syncope, hypotension, tachycardia, and dizziness. The primary organ systems that should be assessed for signs and symptoms of histamine release are the integumentary, cardiovascular, pulmonary, and gastrointestinal systems. Specifically, the following questions should be considered:

- Integument: Is there any history of pruritus, flush, urticaria, or angioedema?
- Pulmonary: Are there any signs or symptoms of upper or lower airway tract obstruction such as dysphonia, stridor, dyspnea, cough, or wheeze?
- Gastrointestinal: Is there any history of nausea, vomiting, abdominal cramping, or diarrhea?
- Cardiovascular: Are there any signs of tachycardia, hypotension, syncope, or presyncope?

This review of systems helps assess the likelihood of an anaphylactic event. Although no two anaphylactic events are identical, certain patterns have been noted (Table 11.1). Symptoms generally begin seconds to minutes after exposure to the inciting agent but can occur up to 2 hours later. Initial signs and symptoms often include erythema, urticaria, and pruritus, followed by signs and symptoms indicating involvement of other organ systems. The absence of cutaneous symptoms puts the diagnosis in question but does not rule it out. About 90% of anaphylactic episodes include urticaria or angioedema. However, the presence of skin findings may be delayed or absent in rapidly progressive anaphylaxis. Respiratory symptoms are the next most common, occurring in approximately 50% of anaphylactic episodes. The respiratory signs and symptoms can range from mild airway obstruction due to laryngeal edema to asphyxia. Patients with underlying asthma may have a severe exacerbation. Cardiovascular signs and symptoms occur in approximately 30–35% of patients. These are manifested primarily as syncope, hypotension, or dizziness. Respiratory compromise and cardiovascular involvement cause the most concern because they are the most frequent causes of anaphylactic fatalities. Gastrointestinal symptoms occur in 25–30% of anaphylactic episodes, primarily as nausea, vomiting, diarrhea, and cramping pain. Other signs and symptoms that have been associated with anaphylaxis include headache, feeling of impending doom, chest pain, and seizures.

A biphasic anaphylactic response can occur in up to 20% of people experiencing an anaphylactic episode. There do not seem to be any unique clinical characteristics to identify those at risk for a biphasic response. The second response can occur 1–72 hours after the initial anaphylactic episode has resolved. No definitive recommendations have been made about how long a person should be observed after an anaphylactic episode because there are no clear metrics to identify those who need longer observation.

Table 11.1 Frequency of occurrence of signs and symptoms of anaphylaxis

Signs and symptoms	Frequency (%)
Cutaneous	90
Urticaria and angioedema	85–90
Flushing	45–55
Pruritus without rash	2–5
Respiratory	40–60
Dyspnea, wheeze	45–50
Upper airway angioedema	50–60
Rhinitis	15–20
Dizziness, syncope, hypotension	30–35
Abdominal	
Nausea, vomiting, diarrhea, cramping pain	25–30
Miscellaneous	
Headache	5–8
Substernal pain	4–6
Seizure	1–2

From Lieberman, P., Kemp, S. F., Oppenheimer, J., Lang, D. M., Bernstein, I. L., and Nicklas, R. A., American Academy of Allergy, Asthma and Immunology, American College of Allergy, Asthma and Immunology, Joint Council of Allergy, Asthma and Immunology. (2005) The diagnosis and management of anaphylaxis: an updated practice parameter. J. Allergy Clin. Immunol. 115, S497. Used with permission

Generally, patients who experience severe anaphylaxis should be observed for 12–24 hours and, at the minimum, should be warned about the possibility of a biphasic response so they can immediately seek medical assistance when the symptoms recur.

If anaphylaxis is confirmed or suspected, a detailed history should be obtained to uncover the inciting agent. A checklist to help uncover the most common causes should include the following:

- Time of the event
- Location of the event
- Ingestants consumed before the event, including prescription and nonprescription medications, health supplements, and food
- Any possible stings or bites
- Any association with exercise
- Any relation with exposure to heat, cold, or sexual activity
- Any relation between the event and menstrual cycle

11.4   Risk Factors

The likelihood of an anaphylactic reaction is influenced by several factors, including age, sex, atopy, route and intensity of exposure, and history of previous anaphylactic episodes. Other factors that may provide information about the identity of the inciting antigen but are not considered predisposing factors for anaphylaxis include occupation, geographic location, season of the year, and race.

Adults are more likely than children to have an anaphylactic reaction to β-lactam antibiotics, radiocontrast media, Hymenoptera stings, anesthetic agents, and intravenous colloids. However, children have a higher incidence of food allergy. The variance between children and adults for these selected subtypes may be due to exposure patterns or maturity of the immune system. There is no exclusivity between children and adults in regard to a certain type of exposure and subsequent anaphylaxis.

Sex can have a role in the type of allergen that elicits an anaphylactic reaction. Intravenous muscle relaxants, latex, and aspirin reactions occur more frequently in females, and Hymenoptera anaphylaxis occurs more frequently in males. Exposure to cross-reacting antigens may be a factor in these differences; for example, cosmetics contain antigens that are also found in muscle relaxants and may serve as a sensitizer to these antigens. This clearly does not explain all the differences that have been found. Increased anaphylaxis to Hymenoptera stings in men is most likely related to greater outdoor exposure.

An underlying atopic state appears to predispose a patient to certain types of anaphylactic reactions. Atopic persons have an increased incidence of anaphylactic reactions to latex, exercise, food, and radiocontrast media. In addition, atopy is a risk factor for idiopathic anaphylaxis. However, atopy is not considered a risk factor for anaphylaxis from medications or insect stings. Underlying asthma is associated with greater severity of an anaphylactic reaction, particularly to foods.

Anaphylactic reactions are more common and severe when a medication is administered parenterally than when given orally. Uninterrupted administration of the medication is less likely than intermittent dosing to result in anaphylaxis. Concomitant allergen exposures theoretically increase the risk of an anaphylactic episode but are difficult to quantify.

Patients with a previous history of an anaphylactic episode are at a markedly increased risk for anaphylaxis with reexposure to the offending agent. Therefore, it is imperative to identify the causative agent so the patient can be counseled about avoidance measures for the inciting agent and any cross-reacting substances.

11.5   Common Causes of Anaphylactic and Anaphylactoid Reactions

Multiple substances can cause anaphylaxis in humans. These substances are most common in foods, medications, radiocontrast media, latex, Hymenoptera venom, blood and blood products, volume expanders, and seminal fluid (Table 11.2). Overall, foods are the most likely cause of anaphylaxis. Despite the current methods for investigation, approximately one-third of anaphylactic events appear to be idiopathic.

Table 11.2 Common causes of anaphylaxis and anaphylactoid reactions

Anaphylactic (IgE-dependent)
Foods
Food additives[a]
Medications
Insect bites and stings
Latex
Aspirin and other NSAIDs[b]
Exercise[b]
Anaphylactoid (IgE-independent)
Radiocontrast media
Medications
Opioids
Muscle relaxants
Aspirin and other NSAIDs[b]
Physical factors
Temperature
Exercise
Gamma globulin
Dialysis membranes

NSAID nonsteroidal anti-inflammatory drug
[a] Rare
[b] Can likely cause both anaphylactic and anaphylactoid reactions

11.5.1 Foods

Many foods have been reported to cause anaphylaxis. An anaphylactic reaction can occur to any food at any age. The most frequent causes of food anaphylaxis include peanuts, tree nuts, fish, shellfish, fruits, and seeds. The foods that most commonly cause anaphylaxis in children are peanuts, tree nuts, milk, and eggs, and in adults, they are shellfish, fish, and peanuts.

The time from ingestion of the food to the onset of symptoms is usually rapid, occurring within minutes, but it can take up to 2 hours. The symptoms can range from only cutaneous symptoms to full-blown anaphylaxis involving the integumentary, pulmonary, gastrointestinal, and cardiovascular organ systems. The symptoms can start slowly and progress over 1–3 hours to cardiovascular collapse. In those with exquisite sensitivity, the progression can occur over minutes. The amount of food required to elicit a response varies, but in some instances, only microgram amounts may be needed.

In some situations, a specific food cannot be easily identified. If anaphylaxis occurs repeatedly after food ingestion, a food diary should be kept to look for a common denominator. Also, a list of ingredients for the foods ingested should be compiled to search for a common constituent. Associated factors should also be reviewed, particularly exercise. Food ingestion followed by exercise can be associated with anaphylaxis as a particular food-dependent reaction or nonspecific food-dependent reaction. In the former, ingestion of a particular food before exercise evokes anaphylactic symptoms, but anaphylaxis does not occur when the food is ingested without subsequent exercise. This has been reported for various foods, including shellfish, wheat, nuts, and various fruits. In the nonspecific food-dependent reaction, eating any type of food before exercise produces anaphylactic symptoms.

The most useful diagnostic tests for food allergy are skin prick tests and in vitro specific IgE assays. Caution must be taken with skin testing because it can produce anaphylaxis. Intradermal skin testing should be avoided. When skin testing is performed, it should be done with the skin prick technique. Although many food allergens have been well characterized, uniformly standardized food extracts are not currently available, and, in certain instances, fresh food extracts, particularly for fruits and vegetables, should be used for testing. The extract for testing may require dilution, depending on the severity of the reaction. Skin testing should be performed by a physician experienced with the procedure and with appropriate rescue equipment and medications available. In certain instances, in vitro specific IgE assays can be helpful, but generally they are less sensitive than the skin prick tests. Food challenges can be performed if a causative food has not been identified but food is still suspected. The potential risk in this procedure needs to be identified. The use of a food challenge is usually limited to situations in which it is unlikely that the suspect food was responsible for the reaction (negative skin prick and in vitro specific IgE testing) and the patient needs to be assured that it is safe to ingest that particular food. The challenges can be done in various ways, including open challenges or single- or double-blind, placebo-controlled challenges. The double-blind placebo-controlled challenge is considered the gold standard. The challenges are typically performed in a graded fashion, starting with minute amounts of the food and, every 20–30 min, doubling the amount of food given. The challenge is continued until a normal serving of the food is ingested. The challenge is discontinued at the first signs of symptoms. It is important to remember that even a small amount of food can precipitate anaphylaxis, and any challenge should be conducted under physician supervision, with emergency equipment and medications available.

The role of food additives in anaphylaxis is controversial. Food additives have rarely been associated with anaphylaxis and anaphylactoid reactions. The primary food additives that have been implicated are carmine, sulfites, sodium benzoate, nitrates, and papain. Carmine is a red food colorant used in foods and beverages. For carmine, studies of small groups of patients (five in one series) and single case reports have established, with positive skin tests, in vitro specific IgE studies, and a positive transfer reaction, the likelihood of an IgE-mediated mechanism. Sulfites used as food or drug additives include sulfur dioxide and inorganic sulfate salts: sodium and potassium metabisulfite, sodium and potassium bisulfite, and sodium sulfite. These are used as food additives, but they also occur naturally in many foods, including wines. Although some patients may develop urticaria or anaphylactoid reactions to sulfites, the frequency appears to be exceedingly rare and requires confirmation by double-blind challenges. Sodium benzoate, an antimicrobial preservative in food, has been documented in several case reports to cause anaphylactic reactions that have been reproduced with oral challenge; however, the mechanism is not clear.

Nitrates are used as curing agents for meat products. Although they usually are not associated with severe reactions, a recent case report has described anaphylaxis in a young man which was confirmed with a double-blind, placebo-controlled challenge. Papain, used as a meat tenderizer, has been associated with IgE-mediated anaphylaxis. There appears to be a higher rate of sensitization among those with pollen allergies. Monosodium glutamate (MSG) is a flavor enhancer added to many foods, but it also occurs naturally. The classic symptoms reported with MSG as part of the "Chinese restaurant syndrome" include a burning sensation in the back of the neck and chest, facial pressure, headache, nausea, and upper body tingling. There does not appear to be a clear association with anaphylaxis. There are several anecdotal reports of MSG-induced asthma, but few confirmation studies. Overall, food additive-induced anaphylactic or anaphylactoid reactions appear to be very rare. Depending on the severity of the symptoms associated with the reaction, a double-blind, placebo-controlled food challenge is the best way to confirm sensitivity.

11.5.2   Medications

Multiple medications can cause anaphylaxis or anaphylactoid reactions. The relatively low molecular weight of most medications prevents them from inducing an immune response themselves. These low-molecular-weight compounds (haptens) bind with a host protein, for example, normal tissue or serum proteins, to form an immunogenic antigen. In addition, the majority of medications are degraded or metabolized to produce reactive intermediates that then bind with host proteins to elicit an IgE response. Large-molecular-weight drugs are able to elicit an IgE response without binding to a carrier protein. In most situations, the specific allergenic determinants of medications are unknown, limiting testing opportunities. The primary medications implicated in anaphylaxis are antibiotics and aspirin and other nonsteroidal anti-inflammatory drugs (NSAIDs).

Antibiotics are the most common cause of drug-induced anaphylaxis. Penicillin is the most common cause of antibiotic-induced anaphylaxis and the most studied. The allergenic determinants for specific IgE have been well characterized. Penicillin is degraded to reactive intermediates termed the *major* and *minor antigenic determinants*. Validated skin testing reagents have been developed on the basis of the immunochemistry of these determinants. Currently, only the major determinant, the penicilloyl protein, is commercially available. On the basis of studies using both the major and minor determinants, penicillin skin testing has a positive predictive value of approximately 60% and a negative predictive value of approximately 98%. Patients with a positive skin test should receive an alternate non-β-lactam antibiotic or undergo desensitization. Patients with a negative skin test to the major and minor determinants of penicillin can be treated safely with penicillin. The risk of an anaphylactic reaction is considered essentially the same as that for the general population.

This only applies to IgE-mediated reactions. Patients with a history of severe non-IgE-mediated reactions such as Stevens–Johnson syndrome or toxic epidermal necrolysis should avoid the medication and not be tested.

Cephalosporins share a β-lactam ring with penicillin but little allergenic cross-reactivity. About 2–8% of patients with penicillin allergy also have cephalosporin allergy. In patients with a history of penicillin allergy and positive skin testing to penicillin, cephalosporins should be avoided, even though the risk of a reaction is low. Patients with positive skin testing to penicillin should also avoid the carbapenem antibiotics. However, aztreonam, a β-lactam with a monobactam structure, can be given safely to those with penicillin allergy. Conversely, those with aztreonam sensitivity can receive β-lactam antibiotics except for ceftazidime, which shares a side chain with aztreonam.

Non-β-lactam antibiotics are less common causes of anaphylaxis. Diagnosis of IgE-mediated allergy to these drugs is difficult because the allergenic determinants have not been characterized and standardized testing is not available. In these situations, skin testing can be helpful if a nonirritative positive response is obtained, but a negative result is difficult to interpret because neither the positive nor negative predictive value is known.

Aspirin and NSAIDs are the second most common causes of medication-induced anaphylaxis. These medications are often overlooked in the evaluation of an anaphylactic episode because they are available over the counter and often used intermittently. Thus, they are not usually included on the patient's medication list. The anaphylactic reaction is distinguished from the other types of NSAID-induced reactions by the type of reaction, the underlying disease state of the patient, and the mechanism of the reaction. An anaphylactic reaction to NSAIDs has the same presentation as an anaphylactic reaction of any cause and is likely mediated by IgE. This is based on the fact that the reaction appears to be medication specific and the reaction does not usually occur with structurally unrelated aspirin or other NSAIDs. Other types of NSAID reactions, particularly NSAID-exacerbating respiratory disease and NSAID-exacerbating urticaria, are not IgE mediated and result in upper and lower respiratory tract symptoms in those with underlying asthma and nasal polyposis or worsening urticaria in those with underlying chronic urticaria. These types of reactions, compared with anaphylactic reactions, occur with exposure to all NSAIDs, and not just one specific NSAID. Currently, there is no accurate skin test or specific IgE in vitro test for aspirin or other NSAIDs. Although challenges can be performed, they are dangerous and should only be performed by a clinician experienced with the procedure (see Chap. 9).

Numerous other medications, especially vaccines, protamine, insulin, and chemotherapy agents, have been implicated in anaphylactic reactions.

11.5.3 Radiocontrast Media

Radiocontrast media cause an anaphylactoid reaction; IgE does not appear to be involved. The overall frequency of adverse reactions to conventional high-osmolarity radiocontrast media is 5–8%, with moderate reactions that require treatment in 1%

and life-threatening reactions in less than 0.1%. With the development of low-osmolarity radiocontrast media, the overall risk of anaphylactoid reactions is decreased to about one-fifth that of conventional radiocontrast media. The primary patients at increased risk for a reaction are those with a previous history of an anaphylactoid reaction to radiocontrast media. For these patients, the risk with subsequent reexposure ranges from 16–44%. Other risk factors for a severe reaction include underlying asthma, atopy, and use of β-adrenergic blocking agents. For high-risk patients who require radiocontrast media, a pretreatment protocol and low-osmolarity agent should be used. This strategy reduces the risk to approximately 1%. A commonly used pretreatment regimen consists of 50 mg prednisone given 13, 7, and 1 hour before the procedure and 50 mg diphenhydramine and 25 mg ephedrine, both given 1 hour before the procedure (see Chap. 9).

11.5.4 Latex

Latex or natural rubber latex is derived from the rubber tree *Hevea brasiliensis*. Over the last 20 years, life-threatening allergies to proteins in latex products have been recognized. Manufacturers, physicians, scientists, and government regulators have worked to reduce this problem. The majority of severe immediate anaphylactic reactions to latex are due to balloons, gloves, and other products manufactured by a "dipped" method. With this method, latex is not coagulated but treated with ammonia and then stored until ready for use. This method allows for retention and easier dispersion of the allergenic latex proteins in the latex product; in contrast, for products such as rubber tires and tennis balls, latex is acid coagulated and then heat vulcanized. With acid coagulation, smaller quantities of latex allergenic proteins are retained in the finished product.

An increased need for gloves throughout the health care industry occurred in the 1980s with the introduction of universal medical precautions. To meet the demand, there was increased harvesting of latex from trees by more frequent tapping of trees and use of yield-enhancing chemicals that likely produced more allergenic proteins. Also, decreased storage time for the latex and substandard manufacturing processes in which the allergenic proteins leached into the cornstarch slurry used in the production of latex gloves increased the presence of the protein allergens. With increased airborne dissemination of latex allergens, health care workers in particular became sensitized and began experiencing allergic reactions. Risk factors for latex allergy were shown to be previous contact dermatitis, atopy, multiple surgical procedures (particularly in patients with spina bifida), and regular exposure to latex gloves.

Clinical reactions to latex can be divided into irritant contact reactions, type 4 contact dermatitis, and IgE-mediated type 1 reactions. Irritant dermatitis is characterized by dry, cracked skin, with itching and erythema without vesicles or weeping of the skin. The usual presentation of contact dermatitis is intense itching, erythema, vesicle formation, and weeping of the skin in contact with the latex. There are no systemic symptoms with these entities, but both can predispose to a type 1 reaction by allowing easier allergen sensitization through the denuded skin. Type 1 IgE-mediated latex allergy may be manifested by any combination of local or generalized urticaria, angioedema, rhinitis, asthma, or severe anaphylaxis. It is not possible to predict in whom the condition may progress from a mild IgE-mediated reaction to a severe anaphylactic episode. Latex anaphylaxis can occur in various situations involving direct contact with latex. The majority of the cases occur intraoperatively, although episodes have been reported with dental procedures, obstetric or gynecologic examinations, use of latex condoms, enema preparations, and blowing into rubber balloons.

In daily medical practice, latex allergy is infrequent. In general population studies, skin test positivity has ranged from 1–6%. Because the specificity and sensitivity of the test are not optimal, it is not accurate to construe these percentages as defining true sensitivity. The prevalence rate for health care workers (a high-risk group) appears to be 5–15%, whereas for children with spina bifida, it can be as high as 70%. Other groups at risk for latex allergy include housekeepers, greenhouse workers, and workers in tire plants and toy factories.

No skin test for latex is available commercially in the United States. Other materials such as latex glove extracts can be used to produce a latex skin test reagent, but the amount of latex allergen in these extracts is highly variable and not standardized. Centers are able to make their own extracts and gauge the sensitivity and specificity of the test on the basis of clinical experience. In vitro testing for latex allergen is available, but the sensitivity and specificity are highly variable. Overall, it appears there are more than 200 polypeptides in latex, with less than 25% of the proteins reacting to IgE from patients with latex allergy. Eleven primary proteins appear to be associated with IgE sensitivity. Cross-reactivity can occur between latex and foods. The most commonly reported cross-reactive foods that produce symptoms in latex-allergic patients are banana, avocado, kiwifruit, and chestnut.

The acute management of latex anaphylaxis follows the same guidelines as for any form of anaphylaxis. It is imperative to remove exposure to latex during treatment. For prevention, avoidance is the only treatment. For health care workers, the workplace should be made safe from latex by the removal of latex-containing gloves and replacement of other latex-containing devices with nonlatex items. Over the last 5 years, more latex-free medical gloves and devices have become readily available. When a latex-sensitive patient undergoes a surgical procedure or medical, gynecologic, or dental examination, the clinical area should be free of latex devices. For surgery, a patient allergic to latex should be the first case of the day to help avoid latex contamination that can occur during the day in the operating room. Pretreatment with antihistamines or corticosteroids (or both) does not seem to attenuate the allergic reaction with subsequent exposure to latex. Strict avoidance is the only true preventive measure.

11.5.5 General Anesthesia and Intraoperative Anaphylaxis

The incidence of anaphylaxis during anesthesia has been reported to range from 1 in 4,000 to 1–25,000. The multiple physiologic changes that occur during anesthesia may limit or mask the symptoms of anaphylaxis, making it difficult to detect until significant cardiovascular or pulmonary signs and symptoms develop. The agents most commonly responsible for intraoperative anaphylaxis are muscle relaxants, latex, and antibiotics, which account for approximately 90% of anaphylactic reactions. The rest of the reactions are caused by numerous substances, including induction agents (hypnotics), colloids, opioids, blood products, protamine, isosulfan blue dye (for lymph node dissection), gelatin solution (for hemostasis), chlorhexidine, and ethylene oxide.

Muscle relaxants are responsible for 60–70% of reactions during general anesthesia. These reactions can be due to an IgE-mediated reaction or to direct activation of mast cells. The medications implicated include vecuronium, pancuronium, atracurium, and succinylcholine. The main antigenic determinants in the generation of specific IgE antibodies against muscle relaxants are substituted quaternary ammonium ions. This helps explain the cross-reactivity found between different muscle relaxants by specific IgE in vitro evaluation and skin testing in patients with a history of anaphylaxis. It has been reported that in up to 25% of cases IgE-mediated anaphylaxis may appear at first contact with a muscle relaxant. This suggests a cross-reaction with IgE antibodies from previous exposure to chemicals containing quaternary and tertiary ammonium ions, for example, cosmetics, disinfectants, foods, and medications. Skin testing to specific dilutions of muscle relaxants has been useful for determining the safest agent after a suspected reaction. The estimated sensitivity of skin tests for muscle relaxants is approximately 94–97%.

Latex is considered the second most common cause of intraoperative anaphylaxis. It has been implicated as the cause in 10–17% of cases of intraoperative anaphylaxis. With the recognition that latex is a causative factor and with the elimination of latex products from operating rooms, the incidence appears to be decreasing. During a procedure, latex anaphylaxis typically occurs later than anaphylaxis due to muscle relaxants or induction agents. Of all latex-containing operating room materials, the product most associated with latex anaphylaxis is latex gloves. High-risk groups for intraoperative latex anaphylaxis include children with spina bifida and urogenital malformations sensitized by previous surgical procedures, patients with bladder problems and long-term exposure to latex-containing catheters, and health care workers. Because no standardized skin testing reagent is available in the United States, latex glove extracts and other materials are used for testing. A Food and Drug Administration–approved in vitro test for latex-specific IgE is available, but the specificity and sensitivity have been highly variable.

Antibiotics are frequently administered before, during, or immediately after anesthesia and surgery. The antibiotics most commonly implicated in the operative setting are β-lactam antibiotics and vancomycin. Intravenous administration of these medications generally results in a more severe form of anaphylaxis than does oral administration. The reaction typically occurs during the administration of the antibiotic or within minutes after infusion is completed. The evaluation and subsequent management of β-lactam antibiotic allergy is discussed above and in Chap. 9. Vancomycin is associated with both anaphylactoid and IgE-mediated reactions. The anaphylactoid reactions are much more common and have been termed *red man syndrome*. The anaphylactoid reaction is due directly to the release of mast cell mediators and is characterized by pruritus, erythema, and flushing, particularly of the face, neck, and upper torso, and may be accompanied by hypotension. This reaction can be minimized by administering vancomycin slowly over a 2-hours period. Pretreatment with antihistamines in combination with the slow infusion rate helps to further decrease symptoms.

The other medications used in the operative setting are less common causes of anaphylaxis. Hypnotics and opioids account for approximately 3% and 1% of reactions during anesthesia, respectively. Hypersensitivity to thiopental is usually IgE mediated. Intravenous protamine used to reverse heparin anticoagulation may cause anaphylactic or anaphylactoid reactions. Acute reactions may be mild and consist of urticaria and transient increases in pulmonary artery pressure. Severe reactions include bronchospasm, hypotension, and cardiovascular collapse. Patients with diabetes mellitus who are prescribed protamine-containing insulin have a 40-fold increased risk of sensitization to protamine. Skin testing and in vitro IgE and IgG testing do not appear to predict sensitivity. Dextran and hydroxyethyl starch used for high oncotic fluid replacement during surgery are rarely associated with anaphylactoid reactions. Estimates of reaction rates are 0.008% for dextran and 0.08% for hydroxyethyl starch. Skin and serologic tests are not accurate.

11.5.6 Hymenoptera

Generalized systemic IgE-mediated hypersensitivity reactions to stinging insects are well documented. In the general population, 0.3–3.0% have had a history of a systemic reaction to a member of the Hymenoptera: honeybee, hornet, wasp, yellow jacket, and fire ant. Hymenoptera anaphylaxis accounts for approximately 40–50 deaths per year in the United States. The diagnosis and management of Hymenoptera anaphylaxis is discussed in detail in Chap. 12. Skin testing to the stinging insects is highly effective in identifying the causative insect. Venom immunotherapy decreases the risk of anaphylaxis after a subsequent sting from approximately 65 to 1% for vespids (yellow jacket, hornet, wasp) and from 65% to 5–10% for apids (honeybee).

11.5.7 Exercise Induced

Exercise-induced urticaria and anaphylaxis have become increasingly recognized as a form of physical allergy. These syndromes can be categorized as cholinergic urticaria or exercise-induced anaphylaxis. Cholinergic urticaria is characterized by punctate (1–3 mm diameter) pruritic wheals with erythematous flaring that occurs with an increase in core body temperature or stress. Classic exercise-induced cholinergic urticaria is not usually associated with vascular collapse, although in severe cases, angioedema, bronchospasm, and hypotension can be observed. Cholinergic urticaria induced by exercise manifests approximately 6 min after the onset of exercise and increases over the following 25 minutes. In contrast, exercise-induced anaphylaxis is characterized by large as opposed to punctate urticaria. The usual sequence of symptoms includes diffuse warmth, pruritus, and urticaria, with progression to angioedema (including upper airway involvement), gastrointestinal symptoms, or vascular collapse (or a combination of these). Activities that have been associated with these syndromes include jogging, brisk walking, bicycling, skiing, and aerobic exercise.

Ingestion of food in relation to exercise can have an important role in the development of symptoms. In some patients, exercise-induced anaphylaxis may occur only when a specific food is ingested before exercise; yet, the specific food is tolerated at other times. In a survey of patients with exercise-induced anaphylaxis, nearly 50% reported that ingestion of any food before exercise was associated with anaphylactic symptoms. Medications may also have a role. Patients have reported that NSAIDs taken before exercise contributed to exercise-induced anaphylaxis. Therefore, it is important to inquire specifically about the ingestion of food and use of medications before exercise, even if these foods or medications are tolerated in the absence of exercise.

The management of exercise-induced anaphylaxis is aimed primarily at prevention. Prophylactic use of H_1 and H_2 blockers has not been uniformly helpful in preventing exercise-induced anaphylaxis, but they may help decrease symptoms in certain patients. It is extremely important that exercise-induced anaphylaxis be recognized early and the exercise be discontinued at the earliest symptom. The patient should not be encouraged to "exercise through it," because the signs and symptoms worsen with further exercise. The exercise program should be modified to decrease the intensity or duration to determine if this helps prevent the onset or severity of the symptoms. Food should be avoided for 4–6 hours before exercise by patients with a history consistent with food-dependent exercise-induced anaphylaxis. The patient should always exercise with a partner and carry an injectable epinephrine device.

11.5.8   Blood and Blood Products

Blood transfusions are associated with anaphylactic reactions. The most common reaction is an IgG- or IgE-mediated reaction from the donor's IgA antibodies against the recipient's anti-IgA antibodies. The anti-IgA antibodies are found in approximately 40% of those with IgA deficiency. All patients with IgA deficiency should be counseled about the risk of an anaphylactic episode with the use of blood products and instructed to obtain an identifying necklace or bracelet. These reactions can be prevented with the use of washed red blood cells or blood from IgA-deficient donors. Other blood products capable of causing an anaphylactoid reaction include human albumin and human gamma globulin, which appear to activate complement. Cryoprecipitate and factor VIII concentrate have been reported to cause IgE-mediated anaphylaxis.

11.5.9 *Seminal Fluid-Induced Anaphylaxis*

Seminal fluid is a rare cause of anaphylaxis. The reactions occur after sexual intercourse and are due to an IgE-mediated reaction to human seminal plasma proteins. The symptoms begin seconds to minutes after ejaculation and include the following: diffuse pruritus and urticaria, uterine contractions, rhinorrhea, sneezing, wheezing, and rarely hypotension or syncope. Other possible underlying causes should be assessed, including sexually transmitted diseases, latex sensitivity, or sensitivity to other possible contactants such as lubricants or sanitary napkins. These reactions generally are not specific to one partner. The diagnosis can be confirmed by skin prick testing with whole seminal plasma prepared from the ejaculate of the male partner. Treatment consists of avoidance of coital exposure to seminal fluid. This can be achieved with the correct use of condoms. Successful pregnancies have been achieved after artificial insemination with sperm washed free of seminal fluid. In rare instances, immunotherapy with seminal plasma fractions has been administered at specialized centers.

11.6 Idiopathic Anaphylaxis

The clinical manifestations of idiopathic anaphylaxis are indistinguishable from those of other forms of anaphylaxis. This is a diagnosis of exclusion, and the diagnosis should be made only if, after appropriate evaluation, no cause can be found. It has been estimated there are 21,000–47,000 cases in the United States. The clinical manifestations include urticaria, angioedema, hypotension, tachycardia, wheezing, stridor, nausea, vomiting, flushing, diarrhea, presyncope, and syncope. Patients may experience different combinations of symptoms but generally tend to have the same manifestations on repeated episodes. The progression from hives to the life-threatening symptoms of syncope, wheezing, and laryngeal edema may vary from minutes to hours, depending on the person. In general, the first episode tends to be the worst because the patient does not understand the situation. Subsequently, after the patient learns to recognize the prodromal symptoms, he or she can initiate emergency therapy early.

Several potential mechanisms for idiopathic anaphylaxis have been studied but have not been found to be present or operative in patients with idiopathic anaphylaxis. These include an increased number of mast cells, increased releasability of mast cells or basophils, release of a greater number of mediators, increased end-organ hypersensitivity, metabisulfite sensitivity, progesterone sensitivity, presence of anti-IgE autoantibodies, and presence of histamine-releasing factors. Current promising areas of research on the pathogenesis of idiopathic anaphylaxis include the following: (1) more activated B-cells occur in the peripheral blood of patients with idiopathic anaphylaxis than in controls and (2) patients with symptomatic idiopathic anaphylaxis have a higher percentage of activated T-lymphocytes than patients with idiopathic anaphylaxis in remission. The role of these activated cells in the pathogenesis of idiopathic anaphylaxis has not been determined.

   The evaluation of patients who have idiopathic anaphylaxis should include a thorough history, physical examination, and review of medical records to document previous blood pressure readings, heart rate, lung and skin examinations, and objective findings to support the diagnosis of anaphylaxis. The common causes of anaphylaxis, such as foods, medications, stings, latex, and exercise, should be assessed. In addition, diseases that can mimic anaphylaxis should also be considered, including mastocytosis, carcinoid syndrome, pheochromocytoma, and other flushing syndromes (discussed in detail in the following section).

   Treatment for idiopathic anaphylaxis should be individualized. All patients should be educated about the disease and how to manage an acute attack. Management of an acute attack is the same as that for other causes of anaphylaxis and includes the use of antihistamines and epinephrine. Patients who experience six or more episodes in 1 year or two or more episodes in 2 months are classified as having frequent anaphylaxis. Patients in this category have been treated with prednisone, 40–60 mg daily, and an antihistamine to control the episodes. Once the symptoms are controlled, the prednisone can be slowly tapered. The antihistamines may be tapered after prednisone has been discontinued. Medications that can be used in addition to antihistamines include oral cromolyn and leukotriene antagonists. The effectiveness of these agents varies, and they should be discontinued after a 1–2-month trial if the severity or number of episodes does not decrease.

11.7   Differential Diagnosis

A large number of medical conditions can resemble anaphylaxis. These disorders should be considered, particularly in idiopathic anaphylaxis (Table 11.3). Although multiple entities have presentations similar to that of anaphylaxis and anaphylactoid episodes, the primary conditions to consider are ones that can cause the abrupt and dramatic collapse of a patient. These include vasodepressor (vasovagal) reactions, other forms of shock, myocardial dysfunction, pulmonary embolism, flushing disorders, endogenous production or exogenous intake of histamine, foreign body aspiration, hypoglycemia, seizure disorder, and anxiety and panic attacks.

   The vasodepressor (vasovagal) reaction is likely the condition most often confused with anaphylactic and anaphylactoid reactions. This reaction, which commonly can be triggered by heat, dehydration, pain, or emotional trauma, produces hypotension, pallor, weakness, nausea, vomiting, and diaphoresis, and, in severe reactions, loss of consciousness. Although the mechanism has not been clarified completely, the primary response is an increased neural response through the vagus nerve. This can be distinguished from anaphylaxis by the presence of bradycardia, as compared with tachycardia usually seen in anaphylaxis. However, occasionally bradycardia can also occur in an anaphylactic event because of the Bezold-Jarisch reflex, conduction defects, or use of sympatholytic medications. Other distinguishing factors in vasodepressor reactions are the absence of pruritus, urticaria, angioedema, or flush. The skin is typically cool and pale. Pulmonary symptoms such as dyspnea and bronchospasm are generally absent.

Table 11.3 Differential diagnosis of anaphylaxis and anaphylactoid reactions

Vasodepressor (vasovagal) reactions
Systemic mastocytosis
Urticaria pigmentosa
Basophilic leukemia
Acute promyelocytic leukemia
Other forms of shock
  Hemorrhagic
  Cardiogenic
  Endotoxic
Flushing syndromes
  Carcinoid syndrome
  Postmenopausal
  Alcohol induced
    Unrelated to drug ingestion
    Related to drug ingestion
  Medullary carcinoma of thyroid
  Vasointestinal peptide and other vasoactive peptide–secreting gastrointestinal tumors
Pheochromocytoma
Restaurant syndromes
  Scromboidosis and other fish poisoning
Monosodium glutamate
Seizure
Capillary leak syndrome
Hereditary angioedema
Pulmonary embolism
Panic attacks
Vocal cord dysfunction syndrome
Undifferentiated somatoform anaphylaxis

Other forms of shock, such as hemorrhagic, cardiogenic, or endotoxic shock, can cause the abrupt collapse of a patient. These are acute episodes, as opposed to recurrent episodes, and usually are easily differentiated from an anaphylactic event. Other single acute episodes include myocardial dysfunction and pulmonary embolism. In these situations, cutaneous signs of histamine release (pruritus, urticaria, and angioedema) will not be present.

Clinically, flushing syndromes can be difficult to differentiate from anaphylaxis and anaphylactoid episodes. Conditions and ingestants that result in flushing include carcinoid syndrome, medullary carcinoma of the thyroid, pancreatic tumors, medications, alcohol, hypoglycemia, postmenopausal state, pheochromocytoma, and mastocytosis. Carcinoid tumors have the potential to synthesize and secrete serotonin, kinins, prostaglandins, substance P, and histamine. The flush typically involves the face and upper trunk and may contain serpiginous and sharply defined borders. Diarrhea usually occurs with the flush. The first-line test is measurement of 24-hours urine excretion of 5-hydroxyindoleacetic acid (5-HIAA). The test results can be false positive with the concomitant ingestion of bananas, kiwifruit, nuts, guaifenesin, and naproxen, and they can be false negative with ingestion of aspirin and phenothiazines. Medullary carcinoma of the thyroid and pancreatic tumors can also produce prostaglandins, histamine, substance P, and serotonin, resulting in a similar presentation. Patients with medullary carcinoma of the thyroid often have telangiectasias, mucosal neuromas, and a family history of the disease.

Medications associated with flush include niacin, nicotine, catecholamines, and angiotensin-converting enzyme inhibitors. Alcohol can produce an intense erythema over the face and trunk within minutes after even a small amount is ingested. This reaction typically peaks after 30 min and subsides after 2 hours. This reaction is most common in Asians but also occurs in Occidentals. In addition, the alcohol-induced flush can occur in association with certain medications, particularly chlorpropamide, disulfiram, griseofulvin, tolbutamide, and cephalosporins. It also can be associated with nausea, vomiting, light-headedness, and anxiety.

The postmenopausal flush is a "wet" flush. This is mediated by sympathetic cholinergic nerves and is associated with perspiration. The flush lasts approximately 3–5 min and can occur several times a day. Typically, there is no accompanying pruritus or respiratory or gastrointestinal symptoms. Pheochromocytoma is a catecholamine-releasing tumor. Although flush has been seen with pheochromocytoma, it is not typical; instead, pallor is the usual skin manifestation. Numerous symptoms can be associated with pheochromocytoma, including warmth, perspiration, palpitations, tremor, anxiety, nausea, emesis, weakness, and dizziness and can sometimes be confused with anaphylaxis. Hypertension may be sustained or paroxysmal. Diagnosis is made by measuring 24-hours urine excretion of metanephrines or catecholamines.

Endogenous production and exogenous exposure to histamine can be seen in mastocytosis, leukemia, and fish poisoning. Mastocytosis is a heterogenous collection of disorders with clinical symptoms that result from an increase in mast cells in the tissues. The skin, gastrointestinal tract, lung, brain, bone, bone marrow, liver, spleen, and lymph node may be involved. Skin involvement is the most common manifestation and includes urticaria pigmentosa, violaceous macules that form a wheal when stroked (Darier's sign), and solitary mastocytomas. The symptoms vary depending on the extent of the disease. Typical symptoms are episodes of flush, pruritus, palpitations, light-headedness, dyspnea, nausea, emesis, and diarrhea, with fatigue and profound lethargy occurring after a spell. The symptoms typically last 15–30 min and can recur from daily to only a few episodes annually. Of note, bronchospasm is rarely seen in mastocytosis. The episodes can occur spontaneously or be provoked by exercise, emotional stress, aspirin, radiocontrast media, codeine, morphine, or vancomycin. Clinically, mastocytosis can be very difficult to differentiate from idiopathic anaphylaxis. In systemic mastocytosis, the baseline level of α-protryptase is markedly elevated (>20 ng mL^{-1} [mean normal, 4.5 ng mL^{-1}]). In an anaphylaxis episode, the serum β-tryptase level is elevated initially and then returns to normal over time. The half-life of tryptase is 1.5–2.5 hours, which allows it to be measured during or after the episode. The only confirmatory test diagnostic of mastocytosis is bone marrow biopsy showing an increased number of mast cells. Tryptase staining should be performed on bone marrow biopsy specimens when mastocytosis is suspected. The primary leukemias associated with histamine release are acute promyelocytic leukemia and basophilic leukemia. Tretinoin can increase symptoms in promyelocytic leukemia.

Histamine fish poisoning can resemble anaphylaxis. Scombroidosis is the most prevalent form of seafood-borne disease, but it can also result from eating non-scombroid species such as mahi mahi, anchovies, and herring, among others. The reaction is precipitated by histamine and other mediators that are increased by bacterial enzymatic activity in fish stored at elevated temperatures. Fish with increased histamine levels can appear and smell normal. Cooking does not alter the histamine content. The symptoms are similar to those of anaphylaxis (urticaria, flush, angioedema, nausea, vomiting, diarrhea, and hypotension) and occur from a few minutes to several hours after ingestion of the fish. Unlike anaphylaxis induced by a specific food allergy, many people who eat the fish will be affected.

Nonorganic disease can mimic anaphylaxis. A panic attack is characterized by a sudden onset of apprehension accompanied by palpitation, diaphoresis, flushing, gastrointestinal symptoms, and shortness of breath. The typical duration of an attack is 30 minutes. No specific diagnostic test is available, and often several episodes occur before the diagnosis is made. Psychiatric consultation can be helpful for diagnosis and management. Vocal cord dysfunction is due to an involuntary adduction of the vocal cords that occludes glottal opening. This produces obstruction primarily in inspiration. The patient presents in acute distress but usually without other organ involvement. Once confirmed, management includes speech therapy with breathing exercises. Munchausen's stridor, however, occurs in patients who intentionally adduct their vocal cords and present with self-induced symptoms of upper airway tract obstruction. This occurs in patients with underlying psychologic disease. Undifferentiated somatoform anaphylaxis describes patients with symptoms that suggest anaphylaxis but who do not have objective confirmatory signs and do not respond to therapy. They also exhibit psychologic signs of an undifferentiated somatoform disorder.

11.8   Diagnosis and Diagnostic Testing

The diagnosis of anaphylaxis depends on a thorough history and physical examination. These should corroborate the sequential exposure of an agent with the signs and symptoms typical of anaphylaxis. On the basis of the results of the history and physical examination, testing can be performed to confirm the inciting agent. If no agent is identified, the evaluation should focus on conditions that can mimic the signs and symptoms of anaphylaxis (Fig. 11.2).

The primary tests that can be performed to confirm an anaphylactic reaction due to any cause are the measurement of serum and urine levels of histamine and histamine metabolites and the serum level of tryptase. Plasma levels of histamine begin to increase within 5–10 min after the onset of symptoms in anaphylaxis and remain increased for 30–60 minutes. Histamine levels correlate with the severity and persistence of cardiopulmonary manifestations, but they do not always correlate with the development of urticaria in anaphylaxis. Because the increase in plasma levels of

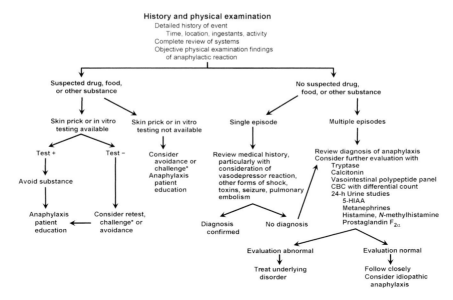

Fig. 11.2 Algorithm for the evaluation of anaphylaxis. *Challenge should be performed only after careful analysis of risks and benefits and in a supervised setting with appropriate emergency medications and equipment. *CBC* complete blood count; *5-HIAA* 5-hydroxyindoleacetic acid

histamine is transient and variable, this measurement is not usually helpful. Urinary levels of methylhistamine, a metabolite of histamine, are increased for a longer time, up to 24 hours. A 24-hours urine study is more accurate than a spot study and should be started as early as possible. Tryptase is a protease specific to mast cells. Although it is not as physiologically active as histamine, it serves as an excellent marker of mast cell activation. Serum levels of tryptase peak 1–1.5 hours after the onset of anaphylaxis and can remain elevated for as long as 5 hours. The best time to measure serum tryptase is 1–2 hours after the onset of symptoms. Tryptase has two forms: α and β. α-Tryptase is secreted continually, and β-tryptase is released only during episodes of degranulation. Patients with mastocytosis have persistently elevated levels of α-tryptase, compared with normal subjects, and patients with anaphylactic events of other causes have normal baseline levels of α-tryptase. During an anaphylactic reaction, β-tryptase is secreted in large amounts in both groups. Because the sensitivity is not 100%, a normal serum level of total tryptase does not rule out a possible anaphylactic reaction.

11.8.1 Identification of a Specific Allergen

Allergen-specific skin testing or in vitro testing can identify specific causes of anaphylaxis. Causes that can be identified include foods, medications (penicillin, insulin, and muscle relaxants), latex, and stinging insects. For most medications, standardized skin tests or in vitro tests are not available. It is important to note that for anaphylactoid reactions, for example, radiocontrast media reactions, skin testing is not helpful. In general, skin testing is more sensitive than in vitro testing and is the diagnostic procedure of choice for evaluation of potential anaphylaxis-inducing agents. If skin testing is performed, it should be performed by a physician experienced with the procedure. The timing of the skin test is important. There appears to be an autoinduced "protective phase" that occurs up to 4 weeks after an anaphylactic episode, possibly from depletion of specific IgE or mast cell mediators. Testing within that time can produce a false-negative result. If skin testing or in vitro testing or both do not identify a specific cause, challenge with the suspected agent can be considered. The risks and benefits of a challenge should always be considered because of the potential of inducing an anaphylactic reaction, even with a small amount of the substance.

11.8.2   Tests Performed in the Evaluation of Conditions That Mimic Anaphylaxis or Idiopathic Anaphylaxis

Knowledge of the differential diagnosis as outlined above is critical in the evaluation of patients who have episodes, particularly recurrent episodes, of anaphylaxis-like symptoms. Idiopathic anaphylaxis is a diagnosis of exclusion, and before this diagnosis is entertained (after an exogenous source has been ruled out), the following tests may be helpful (these apply particularly to flushing episodes):

- 24-hours Urine 5-HIAA: this is increased (normal, <6.0 mg per 24 hours) in carcinoid syndrome. Results can be false positive with ingestion of bananas, pineapple, kiwifruit, avocados, or nuts. Medications that also increase 5-HIAA levels include guaifenesin, acetaminophen, and naproxen. False-negative results can occur with aspirin, levodopa, and phenothiazines.
- 24-hours Urine metanephrines: these are increased (normal, <1.3 mg per 24 hours) in pheochromocytoma. Results can be false positive with tricyclic antidepressants, labetalol, levodopa, ethanol, sotalol, or benzodiazepines. False-negative results can occur with metyrosine and methylglucamine.
- Calcitonin: this can be increased (normal, <16 pg mL^{-1} for males and <8 pg mL^{-1} for females) in mastocytosis and medullary carcinoma of the thyroid.
- Serum vasointestinal hormonal polypeptide panel (pancreastatin, vasointestinal polypeptide, and substance P): this is useful to assess for the presence of a vasoactive polypeptide–secreting gastrointestinal tumor or medullary carcinoma of the thyroid that also can secrete vasoactive peptides.

In addition to serum tryptase, the following tests can be used to assess for mastocytosis:

- 24-hours Urine β-prostaglandin F$_{2\alpha}$ (normal, <1,000 ng per 24 hours): although the sensitivity and specificity are unknown, this mast cell product may be increased when other mast cell mediators are within the normal limits.
- 24-hours Urine N-methylhistamine (normal, 70–330 μg g^{-1} creatinine for ages 6–16, 30–200 μg g^{-1} for ages ≥ 17)

- Skin biopsy: biopsy of normal-appearing skin is not helpful. Biopsy can be performed on suspicious skin lesions that resemble urticaria pigmentosa.
- Bone marrow biopsy: this is the only test for definitively diagnosing systemic mastocytosis.

11.9   Management

11.9.1   Acute Management

The management of anaphylaxis and anaphylactoid reactions is identical and should follow established principles for emergency resuscitation (Table 11.4). The presentation can be highly variable, and treatment should be individualized for the particular symptoms and severity. Assessment and maintenance of the airway, breathing, and circulation are necessary before proceeding to other management steps. The administration of epinephrine and the maintenance of adequate oxygenation and intravascular volume have high priority. At the first sign of anaphylaxis, the patient should be given epinephrine. Mortality in anaphylaxis is associated with delayed administration of epinephrine.

11.9.1.1   Epinephrine

Epinephrine is the treatment of choice for acute anaphylaxis. Epinephrine in an aqueous solution at a 1:1,000 dilution, 0.2–0.5 mL (0.01 mg kg^{-1} in children; maximal dose, 0.3 mg) is administered intramuscularly in the lateral thigh. It is injected every

Table 11.4   Treatment of anaphylaxis

Initial assessment
Airway
Breathing
Circulation
Vital signs
Treatment
Epinephrine
Supine position, legs elevated
Oxygen
Further treatment depends on severity
Intravenous fluids
$H_1 + H_2$ antagonists
Vasopressors
Corticosteroids
Glucagon
Atropine
Nebulized albuterol

5 min as necessary to control symptoms and increase blood pressure. If the clinician deems it appropriate, injections can be given more frequently. Absorption is more rapid and plasma levels higher in children and adults who receive an intramuscular injection of epinephrine in the thigh instead of an intramuscular or subcutaneous injection in the arm (deltoid muscle). There is no absolute contraindication to the administration of epinephrine in anaphylaxis.

Epinephrine can also be administered intravenously. However, because of the risk of arrhythmias, epinephrine should be administered intravenously only during cardiac arrest or to profoundly hypotensive patients who have not responded to intravenous volume replacement and several intramuscularly injected doses of epinephrine. No established dosage or regimen is uniformly recommended for intravenous epinephrine in anaphylaxis. An epinephrine infusion may be prepared by adding 1 mg (1 mL) of a 1:1,000 dilution of epinephrine to 250 mL of 5% dextrose in water to yield a concentration of 4.0 μg mL^{-1}. This 1:250,000 solution is infused at a rate of 1–4 μg min^{-1} (15–60 drops per minute with a microdrip apparatus [60 drops per minute = 1 mL = 60 mL h^{-1}]), increasing to a maximum of 10.0 μg min^{-1} for adults and adolescents. A dosage of 0.01 mg kg^{-1} (0.1 mL kg^{-1} of a 1:10,000 solution up to 10 μg min^{-1}; maximum dose, 0.3 mg) is recommended for children. Continuous hemodynamic monitoring is essential.

11.9.1.2 H$_1$ and H$_2$ Antagonists

Antihistamines are supportive in the treatment of anaphylaxis. However, these agents have a much slower onset of action and less potency than epinephrine and should never be administered alone as treatment for anaphylaxis. They should be considered a second-line treatment after the administration of epinephrine. Antihistamines are useful in the treatment of pruritus, urticaria, and angioedema as part of the anaphylactic episode. Diphenhydramine can be administered intravenously (slowly over 20 s), intramuscularly, or, in milder cases, orally at a dose of 1–2 mg kg^{-1}, with a maximal single dose of 50 mg for children and adults. The role of H$_2$ antagonists is more controversial, but they have been shown in some studies to be helpful in clinical improvement when added to H$_1$ antagonists. Ranitidine can be given at a dose of 1 mg kg^{-1} for adults and 12.5–50 mg for children, infused over 15 minutes.

11.9.1.3 Corticosteroids

Corticosteroids are not helpful in the acute management of anaphylaxis because they have no appreciable effect for at least 4 hours, even when administered intravenously. However, on the basis of their effects in other allergic diseases, idiopathic anaphylaxis, and asthma, corticosteroids may potentially prevent protracted or biphasic anaphylaxis. When used, corticosteroids should be given early in the treatment of anaphylaxis. Aqueous hydrocortisone can be given at a dosage of 5 mg kg^{-1}, up to 200 mg, followed by 2–5 mg kg^{-1} every 4–6 hours. Oral administration of prednisone 0.5 mg kg^{-1} may be sufficient for milder attacks.

11.9.1.4   Oxygen and β-Adrenergic Agonists

Oxygen is often overlooked in the initial treatment of anaphylaxis. It should be given to patients who have dyspnea, wheezing, preexisting hypoxemia, or myocardial dysfunction or who have a prolonged reaction. Pulse oximetry should guide oxygen therapy and caution should be exercised if the patient has underlying chronic obstructive pulmonary disease. Inhaled $β_2$-agonists, such as albuterol, should be administered for bronchospasm. The medication can be given by metered dose inhaler, 2 puffs every 4 hours, or nebulization, 0.5 mL or 2.5 mg of a 5% solution.

11.9.1.5   Glucagon

Glucagon is given primarily when epinephrine is ineffective. This situation most commonly arises in patients with anaphylaxis who are receiving β-adrenergic blockers. Patients receiving these agents are more likely to experience severe anaphylactic reactions characterized by paradoxical bradycardia, profound hypotension, and severe bronchospasm due to a blunted response to epinephrine and a propensity for decreased cardiac contractility. Glucagon has been proposed to be helpful in this situation by activating adenyl cyclase directly and bypassing the β-adrenergic receptor. The recommended dosage for glucagon is 1–5 mg (20–30 μg kg^{-1} [maximal dosage, 1 mg] in children) administered intravenously over 5 min and followed by an infusion (5–15 μg min^{-1}) titrated to clinical response. Protection of the airway is important because glucagon may induce emesis.

11.9.1.6   Fluid Resuscitation

With increased vascular permeability during anaphylaxis, up to 50% of the intravascular fluid may move into the extracellular space in a short time. Because of individual variability in compensatory vasopressor mechanisms, hemodynamic stability may or may not be maintained. Patients who do not respond to epinephrine may respond to fluid replacement. Saline generally is preferred initially because it stays in the intravascular space. Intravenous fluids should be given through a large-gauge catheter at a rate necessary to maintain systolic blood pressure above 100 mm Hg in adults and 50 mm Hg in children. Large volumes are often required, and patients with underlying renal disease or congestive heart failure should be monitored for volume overload.

11.9.1.7   Vasopressors

Dopamine may be required if epinephrine and volume expansion fail to alleviate hypotension. Dopamine (400 mg in 500 mL of 5% dextrose) is administered at 2–20 μg kg^{-1} min^{-1} and titrated to maintain systolic blood pressure above 90 mm Hg.

11.9.1.8 Atropine

Atropine can be used for persistent bradycardia. Bradycardia is seen most often in patients receiving β-adrenergic antagonists. The dosage is 0.3–0.5 mg given subcutaneously, intramuscularly, or intravenously and repeated every 10 min to a maximum of 2 mg.

11.9.2 *Further Management*

Further management consists basically of detailed patient education (Table 11.5). The patient needs to be instructed about avoidance measures to prevent further exposure. The avoidance measures should not be limited to the avoidance of the substance only but also to the avoidance of possible cross-reacting substances. This is particularly important in food- and medication-induced anaphylaxis. Avoidance measures for specific foods and medications are considered in detail in Chaps. 9 and 10. The patient should also be prescribed injectable epinephrine and be instructed about its correct use. An injectable epinephrine "trainer," a sample device of injectable epinephrine that does not contain epinephrine, or a needle is valuable for demonstrating the technique and assessing the patient's ability to self-inject epinephrine. The patient should be proficient in the administration of injectable epinephrine before the need for its use arises. A commonly used commercial preparation of injectable epinephrine is EpiPen, a prefilled injection device that delivers 0.3 mg epinephrine (1:1,000 as a 0.3-mL dose) and EpiPen Jr., which delivers 0.15 mg epinephrine. Patients who weigh ≤20 kg should receive EpiPen Jr., and those weighing >20 kg, EpiPen.

In addition to patient education, the patient's sensitivity has to be made clear to the patient's health care providers. The medical records should clearly outline the patient's sensitivity and type of reaction. The patient should also carry identification of the sensitivity by a medical alert bracelet or medical card. Patients with a history of severe anaphylaxis should not be prescribed β-adrenergic antagonists, and if they currently are receiving them, these agents should be replaced with an alternative medication.

Table 11.5 Measures to reduce future anaphylactic episodes

Avoid foods and drugs that have cross-reactivity with any agent to which the patient is sensitive
Check all food ingredients and drug labels for the presence of the offending agent
Wear an alert bracelet or necklace and carry an identification card
Know the procedure for self-injection of epinephrine and carry an epinephrine kit
Avoid β-adrenergic-blocking agents

11.10   Clinical Vignettes

11.10.1   Vignette 1

A 54-year-old man presents with a 3-year history of "allergic reactions." They occur approximately every 3 weeks and have been increasing in severity over the past year. He has made meticulous notes of his activities, food ingestion, and medication use during the time before these episodes and has not found any correlations. The reactions can occur in various locations and at various times of day. He has been awakened at night with these episodes. The reactions are somewhat similar each time. The patient reports he will have some generalized itching, followed shortly by scattered small hives throughout the body and flushing, primarily in the neck and face. This is followed by nausea and abdominal cramping with diarrhea. With the more severe episodes, he also has light-headedness and, on a couple occasions, has passed out. After one of the syncopal episodes, a comprehensive cardiac evaluation was performed, including electrocardiography, Holter monitor, echocardiography, and stress echocardiography. All the findings were unremarkable. At the onset of the symptoms, he often goes to the emergency department, where he is treated with epinephrine, diphenhydramine, and corticosteroids. The symptoms start to subside within 2–3 hours after this treatment, and by the next day, he is feeling better, although very fatigued. He often feels fatigued for a couple of days and then his normal health resumes. He usually feels well between episodes. Complete blood counts, with differential counts, have been normal at the time of the episodes and in between episodes.

Comment: The symptoms described are certainly suggestive of a histamine-releasing process. The combination of pruritus, hives, flush, nausea, diarrhea, near-syncope, and syncope represents the effect of histamine and likely other mediators on multiple organ systems. All these signs and symptoms can occur with anaphylactic episodes. Because this has been long-standing, a journal or history of activities, food, and medications used in the days preceding the events is imperative for the initial evaluation. In this situation, there was no association between activities, food, and medications (prescription and nonprescription). Without any clinical clues or suspicions, random testing to airborne or food allergens is highly unlikely to uncover a cause. To further evaluate for a systemic process at this point, a complete review of symptoms and full physical examination should be undertaken.

Complete review of symptoms was negative for weight loss, night sweats, fever, chronic cough, skin changes (except with the episodes), joint pain, and bone pain. The findings of a complete physical examination were unremarkable except for possibly a palpable spleen tip, which was difficult to discern on examination.

Comment: The review of systems confirmed that in between the episodes the patient really had no other complaints. Physical examination showed the possibility of splenic enlargement but was otherwise normal. Therefore, at this point, considerations would be given to syndromes that can induce intermittent symptoms. Primary considerations would include mastocytosis, carcinoid syndrome, pheochromocytoma, and idiopathic anaphylaxis. Mediator studies should be undertaken to evaluate for these entities.

Further evaluation for mastocytosis was performed, and 24-hours urine studies documented an elevated N-methylhistamine of 300 µg g^{-1} creatinine and 11 β-prostaglandin F$_{2\alpha}$ of 1,800 ng per 24 hours. Serum tryptase was elevated at 21 ng mL^{-1}. The calcitonin level was normal. Carcinoid syndrome was evaluated with 24-hours urine 5-HIAA, which was within normal limits. Pheochromocytoma was evaluated with 24-hours urine metanephrines, which were within normal limits.

Comment: The increased 24-hours urine levels of methylhistamine and β-prostaglandin F$_{2\alpha}$ and the increased serum level of tryptase are suggestive but not entirely diagnostic of mastocytosis. For a definitive diagnosis, a tissue diagnosis must be made. This is done with tryptase staining of a bone marrow biopsy specimen. After the diagnosis has been confirmed, baseline staging studies should be performed to help quantify the accumulation of mast cells in the different organs. Hepatomegaly or splenomegaly (or both) occurs in 10–80% of patients and skeletal involvement in 10–20%.

Tryptase staining of a bone marrow biopsy specimen showed clusters of mast cells, with otherwise normal hematopoiesis. There was no suggestion of mast cell leukemia. Further evaluation included a complete blood count; liver enzyme studies; computed tomography of the chest, abdomen, and pelvis; and a skeletal bone survey. The results of these studies were all within normal limits. Anemia or thrombocytopenia due to mast cell infiltration of the bone marrow or extensive organ involvement is associated with a poor prognosis.

Comment: Treatment of mastocytosis is aimed at relieving symptoms and does not alter the course of the disease. Antihistamines are the initial primary therapy. Pruritus, urticaria, and flushing can be controlled with H$_1$ antagonists; H$_2$ antagonists are used to control oversecretion of gastric acid. Oral cromolyn sodium is used to help reduce diarrhea and abdominal pain. Systemic corticosteroids and interferon alpha can be attempted if the patient does not respond to extensive antihistamine and cromolyn regimens.

11.10.2   Vignette 2

A 53-year-old woman with invasive grade 3 transitional cell cancer of the bladder underwent cystectomy with urinary diversion. Thirty minutes into the operation, with mobilization of the lateral aspect of the bladder, severe hypotension and tachycardia suddenly developed. There was no sign of intra-abdominal bleeding. Periorbital edema and diffuse erythema and urticaria also developed. She was resuscitated with intravenous fluids, ephedrine, epinephrine, diphenhydramine, and methylprednisolone. The response to these measures was rapid, and the procedure was halted and the incision closed. Evaluation, including a complete blood count, electrolyte levels, radiography of the chest and abdomen, serial electrocardiograms, and creatine isoenzyme levels were normal. The patient's condition remained stable postoperatively, and the periorbital edema and urticaria resolved over the ensuing 24 hours.

Comment: The signs and symptoms are consistent with an anaphylactic reaction. Intraoperative anaphylaxis has many causes, and it is important to establish the timeline between the medications given and the onset of symptoms.

Three hours before the operation, the patient received intravenous ampicillin sodium and gentamicin sulfate. Anesthesia was induced with thiopental sodium, oxymorphone hydrochloride, and atracurium besylate. The procedure began 30 min after the induction of anesthesia. Thirty minutes into the operation, the symptoms began.

Comment: On the basis of the timing of the medications and onset of symptoms, it is unlikely that ampicillin sodium or gentamicin sulfate was the cause. Severe anaphylactic reactions to these antibiotics would be expected to occur during injection or within an hour after the injection. The most common cause of anaphylactic reactions during surgery is muscle relaxants. Again, the timing is critical. Typically, reactions to muscle relaxants occur as the medication is given or immediately afterward. In this patient, the reaction began approximately 1 hour after induction of anesthesia. Although this is outside the typical time frame for muscle relaxants, atracurium must still be considered. Other considerations include latex allergy or an underlying mediator-releasing process. Additional history would be helpful.

On further questioning, the patient described an episode of lip swelling and periorbital itching and edema when she blew up a balloon 4 years before the operation. She also described symptoms of itchy eyes and lips and localized vaginal irritation during her yearly pelvic examinations for the previous 4 years. She stated that she had no history of angioedema other than the above or any history of similar type reactions. She did not have a history of asthma, allergic rhinitis, or food allergies.

Comment: Her history is highly suggestive of latex sensitivity. Further evaluation can be performed with allergy skin testing or in vitro testing (or both) to latex and skin testing to the anesthetic induction agents.

Further evaluation was performed with allergen skin intradermal testing to thiopental sodium, oxymorphone hydrochloride, and atracurium besylate. The results were negative. Allergen skin prick testing to latex with a stock latex reagent prepared from latex glove extracts was positive, raising a 3 × 3-mm wheal with surrounding erythema. In vitro testing showed latex-specific IgE antibodies were elevated at 1,298% of negative control.

Comment: Allergy testing confirmed the clinical suspicion of latex allergy. It is imperative to counsel the patient on latex avoidance, particularly within the medical setting. Future surgery can be performed only in a latex-free operating room. Pretreatment with antihistamines or corticosteroids is not a substitute for strict latex avoidance.

11.10.3   Vignette 3

A 42-year-old man was stung by a yellow jacket, and signs and symptoms of anaphylaxis developed within 10 minutes. On arrival at the emergency department, his vital signs are as follows: blood pressure 84/50 mm Hg, heart rate 80 beats per minute, and respiratory rate 22 min^{-1}. Physical examination shows widespread urticaria and wheezing on lung examination. The patient reports feeling light-headed.

Comment: The reaction is consistent with a severe anaphylactic reaction. In an anaphylactic reaction, a higher heart rate would be expected. As treatment is commenced with oxygen, epinephrine, and intravenous fluids, additional medical history should be obtained.

The patient recalls a previous stinging reaction approximately 10 years earlier that resulted in widespread hives and cough. He also reports a history of hypertension and is currently being treated with metoprolol 50 mg twice daily. He is not taking any other medication.

Comment: Patients treated with β-blockers may respond poorly to treatment with epinephrine. However, epinephrine should still be given in the setting of severe anaphylaxis.

After three injections of 0.5 mL of epinephrine 1:1,000, placement of oxygen at 4 L per nasal cannula, and 50 mg of diphenhydramine, blood pressure is 86/52 mm Hg, heart rate 82 beats per minute, and respiratory rate 20 min^{-1}. Pulse oximetry shows an oxygen saturation of 97%. The urticaria is unchanged. Scattered expiratory wheezes are detected on lung examination.

Comment: The epinephrine appears to have only minimal effect. In this situation, the hypotension should be treated with vigorous intravascular volume repletion. To help increase the relative bradycardia, atropine can be administered 0.2–0.5 mg subcutaneously to a total dose of 2 mg. Nebulized albuterol should be administered for the expiratory wheezing.

The patient received 2 L of normal saline intravenously, 2 doses of 0.5 mg atropine, and nebulized albuterol. Blood pressure increased to 110/60 mm Hg, heart rate 90 beats per minute, and respiratory rate 18 min^{-1}. Although urticaria is still present, it is slightly decreased. Lung examination detected occasional expiratory wheezes.

Comment: The condition of the patient is stabilizing but will require continued close monitoring. If the patient had not started responding hemodynamically, glucagon would need to be administered 1–5 mg intravenously over 5 min, followed by a 5–15-μg min^{-1} infusion as required. If the hypotension is still refractory, vasopressors such as dopamine should be considered. Corticosteroids are not helpful acutely in treating anaphylaxis. They have not been shown definitively to prevent a late-phase systemic reaction. Generally, they are administered because of their anti-inflammatory properties in other similar clinical conditions. Although no clinical features identify which patients are most likely to experience a biphasic anaphylactic reaction, a patient with severe anaphylactic episode should be observed for at least 12 hours after the symptoms have resolved.

Suggested Reading

American Academy of Allergy and Immunology Board of Directors. (1994) The use of epinephrine in the treatment of anaphylaxis. J. Allergy Clin. Immunol. 94, 666–668

Bernstein, J. A., Sugumaran, R., Bernstein, D. I., and Bernstein, I. L. (1997) Prevalence of human seminal plasma hypersensitivity among symptomatic women. Ann. Allergy Asthma Immunol. 78, 54–58

Brown, A. F., McKinnon, D., and Chu, K. (2001) Emergency department anaphylaxis: a review of 142 patients in a single year. J. Allergy Clin. Immunol. 108, 861–866

Bush, R. K., Taylor, S. L., and Hefle, S. L. (2003) Adverse reactions to food and drug additives. In: Adkinson, N. F., Jr., Yunginger, J. W., Busse, W. W., Bochner, B. S., Holgate, S. T., Simons, F. E. R., eds. Middleton's Allergy Principles & Practice, 6th ed. Philadelphia: Mosby. pp. 1645–1663

Douglas, D. M., Sukenick, E., Andrade, W. P., and Brown, J. S. (1994) Biphasic systemic anaphylaxis: an inpatient and outpatient study. J. Allergy Clin. Immunol. 93, 977–985

Fisher, M. M. (1986) Clinical observations on the pathophysiology and treatment of anaphylactic cardiovascular collapse. Anaesth. Intensive Care 14, 17–21

Grammer, L. C., Shaughnessy, M. A., Harris, K. E., and Goolsby, C. L. (2000) Lymphocyte subsets and activation markers in patients with acute episodes of idiopathic anaphylaxis. Ann. Allergy Asthma Immunol. 85, 368–371

The International Collaborative Study of Severe Anaphylaxis. (1998) An epidemiologic study of severe anaphylactic and anaphylactoid reactions among hospital patients: methods and overall risks. Epidemiology 9, 141–146

Kemp, S. F. and Lockey, R. F. (2002) Anaphylaxis: a review of causes and mechanisms. J. Allergy Clin. Immunol. 110, 341–348

Kurek, M. and Michaelska-Krzanowsky, G. (2003) Anaphylaxis during surgical and diagnostic procedures. Allergy Clin. Immunol. Int.: J. World Allergy Org. 15, 168–174

Lieberman, P., Kemp, S. F., Oppenheimer, J., Lang, D. M., Bernstein, I. L., and Nicklas, R. A., American Academy of Allergy, Asthma and Immunology, American College of Allergy, Asthma and Immunology, Joint Council of Allergy, Asthma and Immunology. (2005) The diagnosis and management of anaphylaxis: an updated practice parameter. J. Allergy Clin. Immunol. 115, S483–S523

Lin, R. Y., Schwartz, L. B., Curry, A., et al. (2000) Histamine and tryptase levels in patients with acute allergic reactions: an emergency department–based study. J. Allergy Clin. Immunol. 106, 65–71

Sampson, H. A., Mendelson, L., and Rosen, J. P. (1992) Fatal and near-fatal anaphylactic reactions to food in children and adolescents. N. Engl. J. Med. 327, 380–384

Simons, F. E., Gu, X., and Simons, K. J. (2001) Epinephrine absorption in adults: intramuscular versus subcutaneous injection. J. Allergy Clin. Immunol. 108, 871–873

Soreide, E., Buxrud, T., and Harboe, S. (1988) Severe anaphylactic reactions outside hospital: etiology, symptoms and treatment. Acta. Anaesthesiol. Scand. 32, 339–342

Volcheck, G. W. and Li, J. T. (1994) Elevated serum tryptase level in a case of intraoperative anaphylaxis caused by latex allergy. Arch. Intern. Med. 154, 2243–2245

Volcheck, G. W. and Li, J. T. (1997) Exercise-induced urticaria and anaphylaxis. Mayo Clin. Proc. 72, 140–147

Yocum, M. W., Butterfield, J. H., Klein, J. S., Volcheck, G. W., Schroeder, D. R., and Silverstein, M. D. (1999) Epidemiology of anaphylaxis in Olmsted County: a population-based study. J. Allergy Clin. Immunol. 104, 452–456

Young, W. F., Jr. and Maddox, D. E. (1995) Spells: in search of a cause. Mayo Clin. Proc. 70, 757–765

Chapter 12
Stinging Insect Allergy

12.1   Introduction

Allergic reactions to stinging insects of the order Hymenoptera (honeybees, yellow jackets, hornets, wasps, and imported fire ants) can range from local swelling and pruritus to severe, life-threatening anaphylaxis. The prevalence of severe allergic reactions to stinging insects ranges from 0.4–0.8% in children to 3% in adults. Stinging insect anaphylaxis accounts for at least 40 deaths annually in the United States. The number is likely higher than this because of instances in which stinging insect anaphylaxis is not detected or reported. The most common type of reaction is a large local reaction, which occurs in approximately 15% of adults. Fully characterizing the extent of the allergic reaction to the stinging insect and identifying the insect by visualization and skin testing are imperative in outlining a complete management plan to decrease the risk of severe anaphylaxis from a subsequent sting. After the stinging insect is identified with skin testing, immunotherapy can be instituted to significantly decrease the risk of anaphylaxis from a subsequent sting. Difficulties arise in treating a patient who has a negative skin test but a strong clinical history of stinging insect reaction. The length of time immunotherapy is required has recently been questioned and needs to be addressed individually on the basis of risk factors. Overall, successful management requires identification of the stinging insect, careful delineation of the reaction type, management of the acute reaction, and appropriate use of venom immunotherapy.

12.2   Identification of Stinging Insects

Stinging insects belong to the order Hymenoptera of the class Insecta. Hymenoptera has three families of interest because of allergic reactions: the Apidae family, Vespidae family, and Formicidae family. The Apidae family includes honeybees and bumblebees, and the Vespidae family includes yellow jackets, wasps, and hornets. Fire ants and harvester ants are in the family Formicidae; the two imported fire ants of major importance are *Solenopsis richteri* and *S. invicta*. The similarity

G.W. Volcheck, *Clinical Allergy: Diagnosis and Management*   465
DOI: 10.1007/978-1-59745-315-8_12, © 2009 Mayo Foundation for Medical
Education and Research

between the apids, vespids, and formicidae is minimal. Among the vespids, there is a significant difference in overall venom antigenicity despite cross-reactivity between the venoms. The appearance, habitat, and aggressiveness also varies among the vespids. Thus, yellow jackets, wasps, and hornets are not interchangeable, and separate venoms are used in immunotherapy.

The apids and vespids have characteristics that can be helpful in identifying the stinging insect that causes a reaction (Fig. 12.1). However, these characteristics are not definitive and positive skin testing is required to commence specific immunotherapy. The characteristics of apids, vespids, and formicidae are listed in Table 12.1.

Honeybees are fuzzy insects with alternating black and burnt orange-tan stripes. They are generally docile and do not sting without provocation. They are often seen pollinating clover and flowering plants. Honeybee nests may be found in tree hollows or buildings. When honeybees sting a person, they leave a barbed stinger with an attached venom sac. Therefore, the presence of a stinger implies a honeybee sting, although vespids can also leave a stinger in 4–8% of cases. Most honeybee stings occur in beekeepers or in people who walk barefoot on clover-filled lawns. Bumblebees are large bees with alternating bright yellow and black stripes. They are nonaggressive and account for only a small fraction of stings.

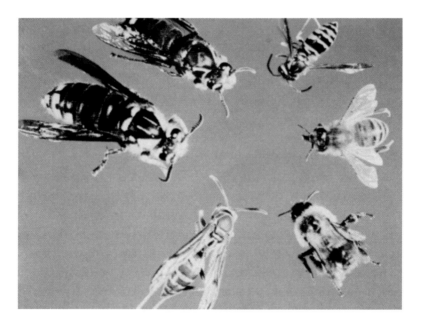

Fig. 12.1 Apids and vespids. Clockwise from top right are yellow jacket, honeybee, bumblebee, *Polistes* wasp, and two hornets From Reisman, R. E. [1994] Insect stings. N. Engl. J. Med. 331, 523. Used with permission

Table 12.1 Characteristics of Hymenoptera (apids, vespids, formicidae)

Family	Common names	Allergens[a]	Distinguishing traits
Apidae	Honeybee	Api m 1 (phospholipase A2), Api m 2 (hyaluronidase), Api m 4 (mellitin), Api m 6, acid phosphatase, allergen C	Pollinate fruit, vegetable and seed crops, and flowering plants; nonaggressive; leave stinger and sac
	Bumblebee	Phospholipase, hyaluronidase, acid phosphatase, protease	Nonaggressive; seldom responsible for stings
Vespidae	Yellow jacket	Antigen 5, phospholipases, hyaluronidases, proteases	Responsible for most human stings; aggressive; ground dweller; feed on human food
	Yellow hornet, white-faced hornet	Antigen 5, phospholipases, hyaluronidases, proteases	Build nests in tree hollows or wall cavities; paper mâché nests
	Paper wasp	Antigen 5, phospholipases, hyaluronidases, proteases	Honeycomb nests on or around buildings
Formicidae	Fire ants (red)	Sol i 1 (phospholipase), Sol i 2, Sol i 3 (similar to antigen 5 but does not exhibit immunological cross-reactivity), Sol i 4	Southeastern and south central United States; build large subterranean nests; leave sterile pustule at the site of sting
	Fire ants (black)	Sol r 2, Sol r 3 (significant cross-reactivity with corresponding Sol i allergen)	
	Harvester ants	Phospholipase, hyaluronidase, lipase	Rarely cause allergic reactions

[a]Phospholipases in bee venom are not related to phospholipases in vespid venom. There is significant cross-reactivity in the phospholipases among the vespids. There is cross-reactivity between bee venom and vespid venom hyaluronidase. Sol i 1 shows cross-reactivity with vespid phospholipase

Yellow jackets have alternating yellow and black body stripes and are ground-dwelling insects. They build their nests in concealed locations, for example, underground, in wall cavities, or in decaying logs and stumps. They are most common in the northeastern and north-central areas of the United States. They may be encountered during yard work, and because of their attraction to food, they may be found around garbage cans, soda cans, and other foodstuffs and at picnics. They tend to sting with minimal provocation and are most aggressive in the late summer and autumn months. In most areas, yellow jackets are the most common cause of allergic reactions to stings. Hornets are black or brown with white, orange, or yellow markings. They build large paperlike hives in trees or wall cavities. Wasps have slender elongated bodies and may be black, brown, or red with yellow markings. Wasp nests have a honeycomb appearance and are typically found under house eaves, outdoor furniture, or shrubbery. Wasp stings are more common in the Gulf Coast states, but wasps are found throughout the United States.

Imported fire ants are found primarily in the southeast and south-central United States. They are native to southern Brazil, Uruguay, and northeast Argentina. Imported fire ants live in dirt mounds, up to 1–2 ft high, that contain thousands of ants. These mounds are often found along the roadside. The ants attach to the skin by their mandibles and rotate circumferentially around the attachment, stinging repeatedly from their abdomen. The characteristic mark left from their sting is a sterile pustule that develops over 18–24 hours.

The raw venoms are collected in two ways: honeybee venom is collected by electrical stimulation and vespid venoms are obtained by extraction from venom sacs. A honeybee sting imparts approximately 50 μg of venom, whereas a yellow jacket sting imparts 2–20 μg. Hymenoptera venoms are assayed for protein content, moisture content, and enzyme activity. These assays are used to confirm the quality and consistency of the venom products. Imported fire ant venoms are not commercially available, and only whole body extracts are sold for diagnosis and immunotherapy.

The major allergenic components of honeybee venom are Api m 1, phospholipase A2; Api m 2, hyaluronidase; Api m 4, mellitin; Api m 6; and Api m 7. The major allergenic components of vespid venoms are phospholipase A1, hyaluronidase, serine protease, and antigen 5 (Ves v 5). Fire ant allergens have been characterized and designated Sol i 1, phospholipase A1, and Sol i 2, 3, 4 for *Solenopsis invicta*, the "red" fire ant. The "black" fire ant, *S. richteri* has allergens designated Sol r 2 and Sol r 3. Melittin is unique to honeybees, and bee venom lacks vespid antigen 5. Although honeybee venom and vespid venom contain similar enzymes, honeybee venom phospholipase A2 and hyaluronidase are different from the vespid enzymes; consequently, there is little significant cross-reactivity. Among the vespids, the yellow jackets and hornets show more cross-reactivity with each other than they do with wasps. Honeybee and fire ant venoms show limited cross-reactivity with vespid venoms. Sol i 3 shows approximately 50% homology with vespid group 5 antigens but, overall, cross-reactivity is limited. In addition to the allergens, the apid and vespid venoms contain histamine, dopamine, serotonin, toxins, kinins, acetylcholine, and vasoactive amines. These contribute to the localized pain, swelling, and erythema of the sting. Fire ant venom contains alkaloids, including solenopsin A, that contribute to the immediate burning sensation of the fire ant sting and the subsequent sterile pustules. The alkaloids are not allergenic.

12.3   Reactions to Stinging Insects

Typically, a sting reaction results in pain, erythema, and swelling at the site of the sting. The presence of pain helps to differentiate it from a nonstinging insect bite. The symptoms usually resolve in a few hours. Application of a cold compress or use of analgesics can help relieve symptoms.

12.3.1   *Large Local Reaction*

A *large local reaction* is similar to a normal sting reaction but involves more extensive erythema and edema. Approximately 15% of the population develops large local reactions. These reactions can vary in severity from a few centimeters of swelling to involvement of an entire extremity. A typical presentation is a sting on the hand that causes erythema and edema of the entire forearm, without any skin manifestations elsewhere. Contiguity is the key feature. If an extremity is stung and a noncontiguous hive or swelling occurs on the abdomen or face, this is termed a *systemic dermal reaction*; it is not simply a large local reaction. A large local reaction typically peaks at 48 hours and persists for a few days. If the swelling progresses for more than 2 days and is accompanied by fever or lymphadenitis, secondary infection should be suspected. The mechanism for large local reactions is not clear, but it appears to be IgE-mediated, because a large number of patients have positive skin tests to the stinging insect. If stung again by the same insect, the same reaction usually occurs. This type of reaction is dangerous only if the sting occurs in the oropharynx. The risk for anaphylaxis with a subsequent sting is less than 5%. Venom immunotherapy does not help to significantly reduce the risk of subsequent large local reactions to future stings. Venom immunotherapy is not recommended for patients with large local reactions only.

Most fire ant stings produce a vesicle or series of vesicles within 24 hours at the sting site(s). The vesicles fill with necrotic material, giving the appearance of a pustule. These vesicles should be left intact to help decrease the chance of secondary infection. The vesicle formation is a normal reaction to a sting; it does not represent an allergic reaction.

12.3.2   Systemic Reaction

Systemic reactions to insect stings can range from mild (dermal only) to life-threatening anaphylaxis. Dermal systemic reactions include urticaria and angioedema distant from the site of the sting in the absence of any other signs or symptoms. Signs and symptoms of anaphylaxis from stinging insects are similar to anaphylaxis of any cause and can include several organ systems, resulting in urticaria, pruritus, angioedema, bronchospasm, wheezing, tachycardia, hypotension, lightheadedness, vomiting, and diarrhea. Symptoms of anaphylaxis usually begin within 10 min after the sting, although delayed anaphylaxis has been reported. Of interest, a repeat sting by the identical species of stinging insect causes repeat anaphylaxis in only 30–65% of patients, instead of the intuitively expected 100%, with the higher percentage in those with a more severe initial reaction. In obtaining the history, it is critical to determine how many organ systems were involved in the reaction, because this is the best predictor of the likelihood of severity of systemic reaction with subsequent stings. For example, in an adult with widespread urticaria and mild nausea, the risk of a systemic reaction with a subsequent sting would be approximately 30%. However, if the patient had full-blown anaphylaxis with widespread urticaria, bronchospasm, and hypotension, the risk would be 65% with a subsequent sting. There does not seem to be a good correlation between the severity of the reaction and the size of the reaction to the skin test or titer of venom-specific

IgE. Some anaphylactic reactions may be followed by a late phase reaction, occurring 4–12 hours after the initial reaction. This occurs primarily in persons with severe reactions. The mechanism of the late reaction is poorly understood, and a patient with a severe reaction should be observed for 8–12 hours after the sting.

12.3.3 Toxic Reaction

Toxic reactions to stinging insects may occur in a person after multiple (100–500) simultaneous stings. Clinically, the reaction resembles anaphylaxis. These reactions are not IgE mediated and are likely due to the vasoactive amines, peptides, and enzymes found in the venom and are not allergic in mechanism. However, this type of reaction can cause IgE sensitization, placing these patients at a higher risk for an allergic reaction with a subsequent sting.

12.3.4 Non-IgE Reactions

Non-IgE–mediated immune reactions have rarely been reported after Hymenoptera stings. These reactions include neuritis, hemolytic anemia, glomerulonephritis, encephalitis, and vasculitis. Fever, myalgias, and chills can occur 8–24 hours after a sting. Rarely, a serum sickness-like reaction has been reported 1–2 weeks after a sting. Skin testing and in vitro testing to Hymenoptera are not helpful in these situations.

12.4 Diagnostic Testing

The clinical evaluation begins with a thorough review of the clinical presentation. The sting history is reviewed, with particular attention paid to the circumstances surrounding the sting to help identify the stinging insect. Also, the timing of the sting and all other signs and symptoms associated with the sting need to be studied closely. This is important in trying to classify the number of organ systems involved and the severity of the sting. It is important to distinguish between true IgE-mediated signs and symptoms and those from other sources. Anxiety, in particular, can complicate the clinical picture. For example, if a person experiences shaking or sweating or feels "unwell" but in the absence of any changes in vital signs, then the findings likely have a significant anxiety component.

One of the major reasons for skin testing is to determine suitability for immunotherapy, but it also is helpful in accurately identifying the stinging insect. Patients with positive skin tests who have experienced a systemic reaction to Hymenoptera are considered suitable candidates for immunotherapy. However, there is a distinction between children and adults who have urticarial reactions only. Children with urticarial reactions only have not been shown to be at significantly higher risk for a systemic reaction if stung again. This risk also decreases further over time; therefore, immunotherapy is not indicated for this group. In adults, however, a generalized urticarial reaction is considered an indication for immunotherapy. Large local reactions only are not an indication for immunotherapy. Thus, testing should be pursued only for other reasons. The indications for venom immunotherapy are summarized in Table 12.2 .

Because the stinging insect often is not easily identified by the patient, skin testing is usually performed to both the apids (honeybee) and vespids (wasp, yellow jacket, yellow hornet, and white-faced hornet). Despite these families having similar enzymes, there is little cross-reactivity. This immunochemical distinction is shown by the lack of cross-reactivity between hyaluronidase enzyme in the honeybee and hyaluronidase enzyme in the vespids. However, an enzyme (such as antigen 5) may be positive across the vespid family (yellow jacket, yellow hornet, and white-faced hornet). It is difficult to know if this represents antibody to one venom with cross-reactivity to several venoms or increased susceptibility to an allergic reaction from a number of venoms. In general, all venoms for which skin testing yields positive results should be used in treatment. Skin testing for fire ant uses a whole body extract and not strictly fire ant venom. These reagents have been shown to be highly sensitive and specific for fire ant sensitivity.

Timing is critical in skin testing. Skin tests performed within 4 weeks after the reaction can be falsely negative. The mechanism for this unknown, but it may be due to depletion of mediators from the anaphylactic event. Therefore, if the skin tests are negative when performed within this time, they should be repeated at least 4 weeks after the time of the reaction.

Evaluation involves testing for the presence of specific IgE antibodies to all the Hymenoptera. Skin testing is the primary measure because it is more sensitive than in vitro testing. Skin tests are performed initially by prick and, if negative, then intradermally. Skin prick tests use $1\ \mu g\ mL^{-1}$ concentration for the apids and vespids and 1:1,000 w/v for fire ant. In intradermal testing, the allergen is injected just under the skin. Initial intradermal tests use concentrations of 0.001–0.01 $\mu g\ mL^{-1}$ of venom for the apids and vespids and 1:1,000,000 w/v for fire ant extract. If testing at these concentrations is negative, the dose is increased in tenfold increments to a maximal test dose of $1\ \mu g\ mL^{-1}$ for the apids and vespids and 1:1,000 w/v for the fire ant. Positive responses at these concentrations are considered indicative of IgE venom-specific sensitivity. Skin tests to Hymenoptera are safe, with a severe reaction occurring to testing in only 0.25% of patients tested.

For patients who cannot be skin tested because of severe dermatitis or use of medications that blunt the histamine response, in vitro testing is an alternative. This technique, however, has a 15–20% false-negative rate compared with skin tests, is more expensive, and has not been well standardized for low-level detection of IgE

Table 12.2 Candidates for venom immunotherapy

Reaction to insect sting	Patient population[a]
Severe anaphylaxis	Children, adults
Moderate anaphylaxis	Children, adults
Urticaria only	Adults
Large local reaction	None

[a] Assumes positive skin test and/or in vitro test

antibody. Strong positive results are diagnostic, but negative results do not rule out venom allergy. If a false-negative result is suspected from the skin test, then in vitro testing should be performed. Despite a lower sensitivity, in vitro testing may be positive in 5–10% of patients with venom allergy and negative skin tests. It should be viewed as a complementary test in the history-"positive," skin test-negative patient.

The degree of sensitivity on skin tests or in vitro testing does not correlate directly with the severity of a sting reaction. Some patients with the most severe systemic reactions have had minimally positive venom-specific IgE antibodies or mildly positive skin tests (or both). Conversely, patients with large local reactions only are often found to have markedly positive skin tests.

There have been occasional reports of patients with a strong history of allergic reaction to stinging insects in whom the skin tests and in vitro tests have been negative and who have subsequently reacted to later stings, but little guidance has been available for managing these patients. It appears that the chance of another systemic reaction to a sting is smaller for these patients than for those with a positive history and a positive skin test, but it is still significantly higher than for the general population. Therefore, a negative venom skin test or in vitro assay result is not a guarantee of safety in patients with a positive history for a systemic stinging insect reaction. Currently, no formal guidelines are in place for these patients; however, it is recommended that they be counseled about avoidance strategies, use of epinephrine injectors, and emergent care of an acute allergic reaction. Consideration can also be given to repeat testing in 6 months.

For people who have never had a reaction to insect stings, testing is not indicated. Approximately 20% of people who have never had a sting reaction will have a positive skin test to venom. This asymptomatic sensitization is associated with

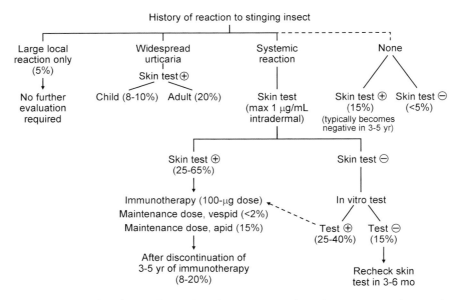

Fig. 12.2 Probability of systemic reaction with subsequent sting. The percentage values are the approximate risk of a systemic reaction with a subsequent sting

approximately a 15% incidence of a systemic reaction with a subsequent sting. Therefore, the presence of venom positivity constitutes some risk for a future systemic reaction, but no variable has been reported that can identify who will have a systemic reaction. Without a clinical history of a systemic reaction, immunotherapy is not indicated. Subsequent risk for a systemic reaction to a stinging insect based on the clinical history is outlined in Fig. 12.2.

12.5 Management

12.5.1 Acute Management

The initial steps in the treatment of anaphylaxis due to insect sting are the same for any cause of anaphylaxis. This includes control of the airway, breathing, and circulation. Epinephrine is the main medication used to counteract anaphylaxis and should be given as soon as possible. It can be given intramuscularly or subcutaneously, but the intramuscular route is preferred. The usual dosage is 0.3–0.5 mL of 1:1,000 epinephrine, which is equivalent to 0.3–0.5 mg. The dosage for children is 0.01 mg kg^{-1}. An oral antihistamine is also usually given. The antihistamine may lessen skin symptoms but is not a substitute for epinephrine, and the use of an antihistamine should not delay the administration of epinephrine. For patients with severe or protracted reactions, multiple doses of epinephrine may be necessary.

In severe anaphylaxis, other supportive measures can be instituted. These include inhaled β-agonists (which may help decrease bronchoconstriction), oxygen, intravenous fluids, and vasopressors. If symptoms persist, systemic corticosteroids should also be administered, but the onset of action is delayed, with a peak effect approximately 4 hours after administration. If the stinging apparatus is identified, it should be gently removed, with care taken not to squeeze the venom sac because this could result in the deposition of more venom.

All patients with a history of anaphylaxis to Hymenoptera should carry self-injectable epinephrine kits. Patient education on the proper use of the injectable epinephrine should be performed in the office. The patient should demonstrate correct use with a sham injectable epinephrine device. It is important that the patient be comfortable with the use of the device before the need for use arises. EpiPen delivers 0.3 mg of epinephrine and EpiPen Jr, 0.15 mg. EpiPen Jr should be used by patients who weigh 20 kg or less. It needs to be emphasized that if a situation arises that requires self-injection of epinephrine, the patient should proceed to the emergency department for further evaluation and management. The patient should not take a "wait and see" approach after self-injecting epinephrine.

12.5.2 Avoidance Measures

The risk for subsequent Hymenoptera stings can be reduced by following simple precautions. The tips for avoidance most often recommended include the following:

- Wear gloves while performing yard work.
- Avoid wearing bright colors or black clothes which attract insects; white or light-colored clothing is preferred.
- Avoid drinking from unattended soda cans.
- Wear shoes and long pants when in fields.
- Keep garbage well wrapped and covered.
- Have professionals remove Hymenoptera nests.

12.5.3   Venom Immunotherapy for Hymenoptera

Patients with a clinical systemic reaction to a stinging insect and a positive skin test or positive in vitro test results are candidates for venom immunotherapy. Those with a negative skin test and negative in vitro test results are not candidates. A positive venom skin test or in vitro test result in the absence of a systemic reaction is not an indication for immunotherapy. This situation can arise when testing is requested because of a family history of Hymenoptera sensitivity or an allergic person is curious about whether he or she is also sensitive to Hymenoptera. Testing in these situations is discouraged because up to 20% of the population can show transient positivity to venom testing. However, in the absence of a history of reaction, this positivity is associated only slightly with an increased risk with a subsequent sting, and the test positivity tends to wane over a few years.

Venom immunotherapy has been shown to be highly effective in reducing the risk of a subsequent sting reaction in patients with sensitivity. Approximately 5–10% of persons allergic to insect sting receive potentially life-saving therapy, because of lack of knowledge of venom immunotherapy. Several studies have indicated that venom immunotherapy prevents systemic symptoms in 97% of patients. However, some studies have shown less efficacy for honeybee than for vespid immunotherapy, with honeybee immunotherapy showing an 80–90% prevention rate. The reason for this is not clear, but it may be related to the amount of venom injected, because the venom inoculum is 2–20 μg for yellow jackets compared with 50 μg for honeybees. For this reason, some experts have favored increasing the maintenance dose to 150–200 μg in those not responding to the traditional 100 μg honeybee immunotherapy.

The immunotherapy mixture is identical to the materials used for skin testing. Because of the difficulty with accurately identifying the stinging insect and the possibility of multiple sensitizations, skin testing should be performed to the five stinging Hymenoptera. In most cases, the immunotherapy should include all venoms that cause a positive skin test, even though some positive results may be due to a vespid cross-reactivity. There have been cases in which immunotherapy was targeted to only one suspected culprit, but the patient subsequently had reactions to the other stinging insects that had produced a positive test. The venoms are available individually and as a "mixed vespid" preparation that contains the full dose (100 μg each) of white-faced hornet, yellow hornet, and yellow jacket. This preparation helps decrease the number of injections required for immunotherapy, but it does not provide wasp coverage. Positive honeybee skin test results are not due to cross-reactivity with the vespids and clearly need to be treated separately. Typically, a patient has skin tests that are positive to honeybee and negative to all the vespids or negative to honeybee and positive to multiple vespids.

There are varying schedules for venom immunotherapy. Most schedules initiate immunotherapy with 0.1 µg mL^{-1} for Hymenoptera venoms and 1:100,000 w/v for fire ant extract and reach a maintenance dose of 100 µg for the Hymenoptera and 0.5 mL of 1:100 w/v for fire ant extract. Some allergists have advocated 50 µg as the maintenance dosage for Hymenoptera, but there is concern about decreased protection. The amount of time to reach maintenance can vary depending on the aggressiveness of the dosing. Ultraquick desensitizations from 1–3 days have been performed; however, these regimens can be associated with a high number of systemic side effects and usually need to be performed in the hospital. The "rush" and "rapid" immunotherapy schedules can attain maintenance dosage in approximately 2–3 weeks. These can be used when the risk of exposure is high, as with patients who work outdoors or those whose locations or schedules do not allow for standard immunotherapy. Standard immunotherapy dosage schedules consist of injections once or twice weekly and reach a maintenance dosage in approximately 3–6 months.

Once the maintenance dosage has been reached, immunotherapy injections are typically given every 4–6 weeks. Studies are under way to determine if the time between maintenance immunotherapy injections can be lengthened. Initial studies have supported giving maintenance injections every 3 months; quarterly maintenance injections have a similar pattern of injection reactions and provide similar protection during immunotherapy and after completion of immunotherapy. Currently, this is not the standard of practice, and additional studies are required to confirm this.

Venom immunotherapy is usually well tolerated. Many patients have slight erythema, itching, or swelling at the injection site. Large local reactions, with swelling more than 2 in. in diameter, occur in approximately 20% of patients and are more common in children. Unless the local reaction is very large, the regular progression in dosage is usually maintained because these reactions are not associated with an increased risk for systemic reactions with subsequent injections. Systemic reactions to venom immunotherapy occur in approximately 10% of patients. These rates are similar to those seen with aeroallergen immunotherapy. The rate underscores the importance of observation for 30 min after an immunotherapy injection. In the setting of a systemic reaction, the next dose should be decreased, often by 50%, with further buildup occurring from this point. A systemic reaction typically occurs early during the "buildup" phase, but it can occur at any point in the program, including at maintenance dosage. Rarely does a patient have repeated systemic reactions to immunotherapy. The only fatalities reported have involved patients with mastocytosis. To decrease allergic side effects from immunotherapy, pretreatment with antihistamines has been shown to decrease both local and systemic side effects when given on days of immunotherapy.

The absolute length of immunotherapy treatment required for prolonged protection from a stinging insect reaction is still being determined. Earlier studies, which observed patients for 1–3 years after discontinuation of 3–5 years of venom

Table 12.3 Risk factors for the development of an allergic reaction
to insect sting after discontinuation of venom immunotherapy

Severe initial anaphylactic reaction
Apid (bee) venom sensitivity
Older age
Allergic reactions to immunotherapy injections
Allergic reactions to stings during immunotherapy
Short duration (<3 years) of immunotherapy

immunotherapy, showed a protection rate of 83–100%. One of the criteria for discontinuing immunotherapy has been the conversion from a previously positive skin test to a negative skin test. However, this occurs in only approximately 20% of patients undergoing 3–5 years of immunotherapy. Despite a conversion to a negative skin test, some patients experience a systemic reaction with a subsequent sting. Because repeat skin testing has not always been helpful in predicting a subsequent reaction, other risk factors have been elucidated. The severity of anaphylaxis before treatment has a role in determining future risk. Subsequent anaphylactic reactions to sting after discontinuation of immunotherapy were seen in approximately 5% of those with initial mild and moderate anaphylaxis and in 15% of those with initial severe anaphylaxis. In addition, significant reactions to stings after immunotherapy appear to be more common with honeybees than with vespids.

Clearly, the risk of a systemic reaction to a sting is higher after the discontinuation of immunotherapy (5–20%) than it is while receiving the maintenance injections for vespids (<2%) and apids (10%). Although earlier studies suggested that venom immunotherapy could be stopped after 3–5 years, the optimum length of therapy should be individualized. Risk factors for a systemic reaction after the discontinuation of immunotherapy include honeybee as opposed to vespid allergy, severity of anaphylaxis before the onset of immunotherapy, older age, and reaction during therapy to either a field sting or the immunotherapy itself (Table 12.3). One approach to counseling patients without risk factors about whether to continue or discontinue immunotherapy after 5 years is to outline their risks as follows: (1) the chance of a systemic reaction with a subsequent sting approaches 10%, even if the sting occurs 10 years later; (2) although most reactions are mild, there is a small chance of a life-threatening reaction; and (3) the only way to maintain the lowest possible risk is to continue venom immunotherapy.

12.6   Conclusion

Stinging insect allergy is a potentially life-threatening situation. The diagnosis and treatment for Hymenoptera allergy has improved considerably over the last 20 years, but it is not perfect. Difficulties arise in the management of the negative skin test reactor and in determining the optimum duration of immunotherapy. Continued improvement in the sensitivity of in vivo and in vitro diagnostic testing, optimization of available treatments, and the consideration of other immunomodulating treatments are challenges for the future.

12.7   Clinical Vignettes

12.7.1   Vignette 1

A 24-year-old woman reports being stung approximately 1 month ago while clearing brush in her backyard. She was not able to identify the insect and did not identify a stinger. She was stung on the left hand and within an hour had continuous swelling from her hand through the forearm to her elbow. Accompanying this was erythema and pruritus in the forearm. She said she did not have any hives or swelling elsewhere, breathing difficulties, or other symptoms. The swelling resolved over 3 days. Further evaluation included positive skin testing to yellow jacket, white-faced hornet, and yellow hornet. Testing was negative to honeybee and wasp.

Comment: The patient had a large local reaction to the sting. There was no evidence for a systemic reaction. Although skin testing was performed, it was not indicated. The positive skin tests are not unexpected because a significant number of patients with large local reactions have positive skin tests. The risk for a systemic reaction with a subsequent sting is approximately 5%. Venom immunotherapy is not recommended in this clinical situation.

12.7.2   Vignette 2

A 10-year-old boy reports getting stung by a "bee" 1 year ago. At the time of the sting, hives developed throughout his body. There was pruritus with the hives. He had neither dyspnea nor hypotension. The reaction was treated in the emergency department. Review of the emergency department visit documented normal vital signs, and the only abnormality on physical examination was the hives. The reaction responded within 2 hours to treatment with diphenhydramine. The boy and his parents were told at that time that "the next sting could be his last" and because of this, his parents have kept him mainly indoors for the past year.

Comment: This is not an uncommon scenario due to popular myths about insect sting allergy. The reaction described is a cutaneous-only reaction without other systemic involvement. His risk of a systemic reaction with a subsequent sting is less than 10%. In children, skin testing would not be indicated in this situation because venom immunotherapy typically is not recommended for this type of reaction in children. In contrast, an adult with this clinical presentation has a higher risk, approximately 20%, for a systemic reaction with a subsequent sting. In adults, skin testing would be indicated and consideration would be given to subsequent venom immunotherapy that targeted the venoms producing positive skin test results.

12.7.3   Vignette 3

A 44-year-old beekeeper reports a honeybee sting that produced widespread hives, wheezing, and feeling of faintness. The emergency department report documents a pulse of 110 beats per min, respiratory rate of 20 breaths per min, and blood pressure of 90/50 m Hg at presentation. Physical examination findings were remarkable for widespread urticaria and scattered expiratory wheezes. He responded to treatment with intramuscular epinephrine, oral diphenhydramine, and albuterol nebulization, and his symptoms resolved. One week later, skin testing to honeybee was negative.

Comment: The reaction described is consistent with a severe systemic reaction (anaphylaxis). The negative test is likely due to the timing of the test. False-negative results to skin testing are common when performed within 4 weeks after the allergic reaction.

Four weeks later, skin testing was repeated, with a positive response to honeybee.

Comment: This result is fitting with his clinical presentation. At this point, his risk for a systemic reaction with a subsequent sting is approximately 60%. With venom immunotherapy, the risk would be approximately 10%.

The patient started venom immunotherapy. A "rush" regimen was used to advance to the maintenance dose over a 3-week period. He tolerated the progression from the initiation of immunotherapy to the maintenance dose without a significant reaction.

Comment: In a patient such as a beekeeper, the risk for a subsequent sting is very high. Because his environment was high risk, the "rush" regimen was used to quickly obtain a maintenance dosage, which provides protection, in a timely manner.

The patient completed 5 years of immunotherapy. During this time, he did not have any significant reactions to the immunotherapy injections. However, he sustained three bee stings that resulted in one large local reaction and two reactions of widespread hives without any other systemic symptoms.

Comment: It has been shown that 3–5 years of venom immunotherapy does not result in life-long protection at the same protective level as continuing immunotherapy. Repeat skin testing at this point is usually not helpful because only 20% will have negative test results, and even in this group, a negative test does not guarantee that a significant reaction will not occur with a subsequent sting. If immunotherapy is stopped at this time, the patient's risk for a reaction with a subsequent sting is approximately 10–15%. If he continued receiving immunotherapy, the risk would be approximately 5%.

On the basis of his high risk for a subsequent sting because of his environment and widespread cutaneous reactions that occurred to stings while receiving immunotherapy, the patient chose to continue venom immunotherapy indefinitely.

Suggested Reading

Freeman, T. M. (2004) Clinical practice: hypersensitivity to Hymenoptera stings. N. Engl. J. Med. 351, 1978–1984.
Goldberg, A. and Confino-Cohen, R. (2001) Maintenance venom immunotherapy administered at 3-month intervals is both safe and efficacious. J. Allergy Clin. Immunol. 107, 902–906.

Golden, D. B. (2005) Insect sting allergy and venom immunotherapy: a model and a mystery. J. Allergy Clin. Immunol. 115, 439–447.

Golden, D. B., Kagey-Sobotka, A., Norman, P. S., Hamilton, R. G., and Lichtenstein, L. M. (2001) Insect sting allergy with negative venom skin test responses. J. Allergy Clin. Immunol. 107, 897–901.

Golden, D. B., Kwiterovich, K. A., Kagey-Sobotka, A., and Lichtenstein, L. M. (1998) Discontinuing venom immunotherapy: extended observations. J. Allergy Clin. Immunol. 101, 298–305.

Lerch, E. and Muller, U. R. (1998) Long-term protection after stopping venom immunotherapy: results of re-stings in 200 patients. J. Allergy Clin. Immunol. 101, 606–612.

Lockey, R. F., Turkeltaub, P. C., Olive, E. S., Hubbard, J. M., Baird-Warren, I. A., and Bukantz, S. C. (1990) The Hymenoptera venom study. III: safety of venom immunotherapy. J. Allergy Clin. Immunol. 86, 775–780.

Mauriello, P. M., Barde, S. H., Georgitis, J. W., and Reisman, R. E. (1984) Natural history of large local reactions from stinging insects. J. Allergy Clin. Immunol. 74, 494–498.

Portnoy, J. M., Moffitt, J. E., Golden, D. B. et al., the Joint Task Force on Practice Parameters, the American Academy of Allergy, Asthma and Immunology, the American College of Allergy, Asthma and Immunology, and the Joint Council of Allergy, Asthma and Immunology. (1999) Stinging insect hypersensitivity: a practice parameter. J. Allergy Clin. Immunol. 103, 963–980.

Reisman, R. E. (1992) Natural history of insect sting allergy: relationship of severity of symptoms of initial sting anaphylaxis to re-sting reactions. J. Allergy Clin. Immunol. 90, 335–339.

Reisman, R. E. (1993) Duration of venom immunotherapy: relationship to the severity of symptoms of initial insect sting anaphylaxis. J. Allergy Clin. Immunol. 92, 831–836.

Stafford, C. T. (1996) Hypersensitivity to fire ant venom. Ann. Allergy Asthma Immunol. 77, 87–95.

Volcheck, G. W. (2002) Hymenoptera (apid and vespid) allergy: update in diagnosis and management. Curr. Allergy Asthma Rep. 2, 46–50.

Index

Printed in the United States of America